D1611801

PHYSIOLOGY OF THE EAR

Physiology
of the Ear

Editors

Anthony F. Jahn, M.D.

*Chief
Section of Otolaryngology–
Head and Neck Surgery
New Jersey Medical School
University of Medicine and
Dentistry of New Jersey
Newark, New Jersey*

Joseph Santos-Sacchi, Ph.D.

*Director
Laboratory of Otolaryngology
New Jersey Medical School
University of Medicine and
Dentistry of New Jersey
Newark, New Jersey*

Raven Press 🦅 New York

Raven Press, 1185 Avenue of the Americas, New York, New York 10036

Made in the United States of America

Library of Congress Cataloging-in-Publication Data

Physiology of the ear / editors, Anthony F. Jahn, Joseph Santos-Sacchi.
    p.   cm.
    Includes bibliographies and index.
    ISBN 0-88167-437-0
    1. Ear—Physiology. I. Jahn, Anthony F. II. Santos-Sacchi,
Joseph.
    [DNLM: 1. Ear—physiology.   WV 201 P578]
QP461.P534 1988
612'.85—dc19
DNLM/DLC
for Library of Congress   88-12198
                                     CIP

9 8 7 6 5 4 3 2 1

To our mentors in auditory physiology,
Professor Juergen Tonndorf (A.F.J.) and the
late Professor Ira Ventry (J.S.S.).

Preface

During the past few years, there has developed a new and broad-based interest in ear physiology. Previously the province of the auditory scientist, ear physiology has suddenly entered the clinical arena, through the dramatic success of the cochlear implant. The expanding interface between clinical otology and biomedical engineering has focused the attention of both physician and engineer on the basics of auditory function. Further refinements in cochlear implantation, implantable and semi-implantable hearing aids, are just some of the exciting applications this area of study holds for the immediate future.

Although auditory function is the chief point of convergence for physicians and engineers, many other aspects of ear physiology hold interest for the clinical practitioner, who deals with problems that range from ear wax to vestibular dysfunction, facial paralysis, and Meniere's disease. A textbook of ear physiology, to be complete, must include these areas.

We have attempted to make *Physiology of the Ear* unique in several ways. First, by dividing contributions between basic scientists and clinicians, we have tried to keep the overall perspective relevant to the clinical practitioner. As such, the book is not a compilation of research contributions but a comprehensive and up-to-date exposition of how the ear as a whole functions. We asked each author to be substantial and didactic but also to include some of the controversies and uncertainties inherent to his or her area of interest. Residents, audiologists-in-training, and new auditory scientists will find that each chapter was written in enough depth to be read alone as an introduction to the underlying scientific aspects of a particular topic.

Second, the design of the book is complete in a chronologic sense. Following an introductory historic chapter, the main text deals with current concepts of ear structure and function, followed by a few brief but intriguing glimpses at techniques that promise to provide new insights in this field.

Finally, to further enhance its usefulness to practicing otologists and residents, the book includes several chapters on nonauditory physiology. Topics such as skin migration in the ear canal, mucosal function in the middle ear, and bone physiology of the otic capsule, although not directly relevant to hearing, are of interest in the management of ear disease.

The challenge to our authors was not an easy one: to be didactic but controversial, comprehensive but detailed, impartial but persuasive. We hope you will enjoy the results of their work as much as we have.

Anthony F. Jahn, M.D.
Joseph Santos-Sacchi, Ph.D.

Contents

ix

Contributors

Jont B. Allen
AT&T Bell Laboratories
Murray Hill, New Jersey 07974

Matti Anniko
Department of Oto-Rhino-Laryngology and
Head and Neck Surgery, and
Otologic Research Laboratories
Umeå University Hospital
S-901 85 Umeå, Sweden

Alf Axelsson
Department of Otolaryngology
Sahlgrenska Hospital
413 45 Göteborg, Sweden

Joel M. Bernstein
Department of Speech–Language
Pathology and Audiology
State College of New York at Buffalo, and
Departments of Otolaryngology and
Pediatrics
State University of New York at Buffalo
Buffalo, New York 14214

Sanford C. Bledsoe, Jr.
Kresge Hearing Research Institute
Department of Otolaryngology
The University of Michigan
Ann Arbor, Michigan 48109-0506

Richard P. Bobbin
Kresge Hearing Research Institute of the
South
Department of Otolaryngology and
Biocommunication
Louisiana State University Medical School
New Orleans, Louisiana 70112-2234

H. A. Dengerink
Department of Psychology
Washington State University
Pullman, Washington 99164-4830

James P. Dilger
Departments of Anesthesiology, and
Physiology and Biophysics
State University of New York
at Stony Brook
Stony Brook, New York 11794-8480

Frank H. Duffy
Department of Neurology
Children's Hospital and Harvard Medical
School
Boston, Massachusetts 02115

Bernt Falk
Department of Otolaryngology
Västerviks Sjukhus
S-593 00 Västervik, Sweden

Robert V. Harrison
Department of Otolaryngology
The Hospital for Sick Children
Toronto, Ontario, Canada M5G 1X8

Michael Hawke
Department of Otolaryngology
Temporal Bone Histopathology Laboratory
University of Toronto
Toronto, Ontario, Canada M5G 1L5

Joseph E. Hawkins, Jr.
Kresge Hearing Research Institute
Department of Otorhinolaryngology
University of Michigan Medical School
Ann Arbor, Michigan 48109-0506

Ivan M. Hunter-Duvar
Department of Otolaryngology
The Hospital for Sick Children
Toronto, Ontario, Canada M5G 1X8

Anthony F. Jahn
Section of Otolaryngology–Head and Neck
Surgery
New Jersey Medical School
University of Medicine and Dentistry
of New Jersey
Newark, New Jersey 07103-2757

Alan Johnson
Department of Otolaryngology
Queen Elizabeth Hospital
Birmingham and Midland Ear and Throat
Hospital
Birmingham, B15 2TH, England

xi

Lloyd Kaufman
Neuromagnetism Laboratory
Departments of Physics and Psychology
New York University
New York, New York 10003

Bengt Magnuson
Department of Otolaryngology
Linköping University Hospital
S-581 85 Linköping, Sweden

D. Marbey
Laboratory of Otolaryngology
New Jersey Medical School
University of Medicine and Dentistry
of New Jersey
Newark, New Jersey 07103-2757

Joseph R. McPhee
Laboratory of Developmental Otobiology
Albert Einstein College of Medicine
Bronx, New York 10461

Steven M. Parnes
Division of Otolaryngology
Albany Medical College
Albany, New York 12208

D. P. Phillips
Department of Psychology
Dalhousie University
Halifax, Nova Scotia, Canada B3H 4J1

Jean-Luc Puel
Kresge Hearing Research Laboratory of
the South
Department of Otolaryngology and
Biocommunication
Louisiana State University Medical School
New Orleans, Louisiana 70112-2234

Evan M. Relkin
Institute for Sensory Research
Department of Bioengineering
Syracuse University
Syracuse, New York 13244-5290

Edwin W Rubel
Department of Otolaryngology
University of Washington
Seattle, Washington 98195

Allen F. Ryan
Department of Otolaryngology
University of California Medical Center
Veterans Administration Medical Center
San Diego, California 92103

Alec N. Salt
Department of Otolaryngology
Washington University School of Medicine
St. Louis, Missouri 63110

Dan H. Sanes
Departments of Otolaryngology and
Physiology and Biophysics
New York University Medical Center
New York, New York 10016

Peter A. Santi
Department of Otolaryngology
University of Minnesota Medical School
Minneapolis, Minnesota 55455

Joseph Santos-Sacchi
Laboratory of Otolaryngology
New Jersey Medical School
University of Medicine and Dentistry
of New Jersey
Newark, New Jersey 07103-2757

Heinrich Spoendlin
ENT Department
University Hospital Innsbruck
A-6020 Innsbruck, Austria

Ruediger Thalmann
Department of Otolaryngology
Washington University School of Medicine
St. Louis, Missouri 63110

Juergen Tonndorf
Bronx, New York 10471

Thomas R. Van De Water
Laboratory of Developmental Otobiology
Albert Einstein College of Medicine
Bronx, New York 10461

Samuel J. Williamson
Neuromagnetism Laboratory
Departments of Physics and Psychology
New York University
New York, New York 10003

J. W. Wright
Department of Psychology
Washington State University
Pullman, Washington 99164-4830

Physiology of the Ear,
edited by A. F. Jahn and J. Santos-Sacchi.
Raven Press, New York © 1988.

Auditory Physiological History: A Surface View[1]

Joseph E. Hawkins, Jr.

Kresge Hearing Research Institute, Department of Otorhinolaryngology, University of Michigan Medical School, Ann Arbor, Michigan 48109

In past ages many men of inquiring and philosophical turn of mind have tried to explain how the ear hears sound. Even now our answer to this fundamental question, our "theory of hearing," remains partial at best. Knowledge of the ear seems always to have lagged behind that of the eye, for reasons both anatomical and technical. Whereas the entire globe, including the retina itself, is relatively accessible for examination, most of the ear is concealed within the head, its essential sensory structures surrounded by the hardest bone of the entire body. Even after the main features of the inner ear had come to be recognized during the 17th and 18th centuries, no one had reason to suppose that much of the labyrinth is concerned not with hearing but with orientation to gravity and control of postural equilibrium. This unsuspected dual function long remained a cause of fanciful misinterpretation and confusion among anatomists and other students of the ear.

An appreciation of the fine structure of the inner ear had to wait until the development of microscopy during the 19th and 20th centuries. In the same way, detailed study of auditory physiology had to wait until the advent of electroacoustic technology. Until physical acoustics became an exact science, sound stimuli could not be adequately controlled or measured, so that only the most primitive evaluation of auditory function was possible. Auditory physiology as we know it is therefore largely a product of the late 19th and the 20th centuries, even though its beginnings extend back to the remote threshold of historic times.

ANCIENT HISTORY

The physicians of Egypt may have been the first medical specialists. The earliest among them was Imhotep, the royal physician of the 30th century B.C., who was later deified. Breasted (10) tells us that it was he who was adopted by the Greeks under the name Asclepios (Aesculapius to the Romans). According to Homer, his

---

[1]Portions of this chapter were presented as a paper entitled "An Historical Background for ORL Research," at the First National Conference on Research Goals and Methods in Otolaryngology, Bethesda, Maryland, April 1982, and as the Fifth Annual James A. Harrill Otolaryngology Lecture, given at the Bowman Gray School of Medicine of Wake Forest University, Winston-Salem, North Carolina, April 1985.

1

two sons served centuries later under Agamemnon as military surgeons in the Trojan War.

For the Egyptian physicians diseases of the eye were especially important, even as in present-day Egypt, but their medical papyri hint that they may have included among their number some whose practice was limited to afflictions of the ear (Politzer[2]). Lines cited by Curto (20) from the Maxims of Ptahhotep (2400 B.C.) indicate that they were well aware of the deafness that comes with age. The Edwin Smith Surgical Papyrus (3000–2500 B.C.), hailed by Breasted (10) as the earliest known scientific document, includes several descriptions of patients with wounds or fractures in the temporal region. In one of them the injury was so close to the ear that hearing sounds was said to be painful. Another patient, with a compound comminuted fracture of the temporal bone, was without speech. Having also a stiff neck and bleeding from the nostrils and ear, he was appropriately diagnosed as having "an ailment not to be treated." The Ebers Papyrus, a sacred Egyptian pharmacopoeia thought to date from about 1500 B.C., contains among its 39 chapters one entitled "Medicines for the ear with weak hearing" (23).

Being a highly practical people—apart from their overriding preoccupation with funeral arrangements and the preservation of the body for the afterlife—the Egyptians seem to have been unconcerned with such abstruse matters as how the ear hears sound. No pertinent hieratic speculations or theories of hearing have come down to us in the few surviving medical papyri.

EARLY GREEK NATURAL PHILOSOPHERS

Among the Greeks there were always thinkers who spent their lives inquiring into the how and why of natural phenomena; fortunately, some of their thoughts, observations, and speculations have been preserved. The first acoustician among them seems to have been the philosopher-mathematician-musician Pythagoras, whose school at Croton in southern Italy (Magna Graecia) flourished in the sixth century B.C., attracting many disciples. His particular contribution to acoustics was to establish by experiment the law relating the pitch of a note produced by the monochord to the length of its vibrating string, thus demonstrating the mathematical basis of the musical scale. Unfortunately, this discovery so enthralled him and his followers that it led them away from physics into fantasies about the sacred character and magical powers of numbers, and into theories about the migrations of the soul (33).

A more solid if less imaginative scientist of the same city and century was the physician Alcmaeon, who made the first anatomical dissections. Sad to say, almost nothing has survived of his writings, but from the accounts left by later Greek authors he deserves to be remembered as the progenitor of both neuroanatomy and physiology. He was the first to take note of the cranial nerves, and the first to recognize

---

[2]Adam Politzer's two-volume *Geschichte der Ohrenheilkunde* (46) is the most complete and authoritative account of the history of otological research and clinical practice, from antiquity to the early years of the 20th century. It is said to have been translated recently into English. Some additional information, especially about British contributions, is included in the smaller *History of Oto-laryngology* by R. S. Stevenson and D. Guthrie (54). Victor Robinson's brief, lively "Chronology of Otology" (49) is also recommended, as well as his challenging "Examination in the History of Otology" (50).

the brain as the seat of the intellect. Blindness and deafness, he said, can be caused by concussion, because the brain is made to shift its position, thus blocking the passages by which visual and auditory impressions reach it. Aristotle attributes to him the curious notion that goats breathe through their ears, which has led some modern readers to infer that Alcmaeon in his dissections may have encountered the Eustachian tube some 20 centuries before Eustachi himself described it. Hearing, he surmised, occurs when movements of the air strike the void within the ear, because every empty space is resonant (45).

The Sicilian philosopher Empedocles, the favorite son of Acragas (modern Agrigento), deserves to be saluted as the founding father of chemistry, since it was he who devised the long-lived theory of the four elements: earth, water, air, and fire. He also had ideas about hearing, and it is even possible that he discovered (or imagined) the *cochlea*. At all events, he was the first to apply that difficult word to the ear, taking it from κοχλοs, the name of the spiral-shelled *murex* or Tyrian mollusc that yielded up the coveted purple dye—written in Greek with the *omicron* or *short o*, which is nowadays mysteriously lengthened in the American tongue. Empedocles is said to have taught that hearing occurs when air strikes that part suspended within the ear which is coiled like the shell of a snail, making it ring like a bell. Later, the fourth-century Athenian philosophers Diogenes and Plato seem to have been entirely unaware of such a structure, but they both regarded the "air in the head" as the resonant space that responds to sound and causes the sensation of hearing (45,55). There is no reason to infer that either of them had performed any anatomical dissections. In fact, at least one author (60) warns us against assuming that the Greeks had even the slightest anatomical knowledge of the inner ear before Galen.

PLATO AND ARISTOTLE

In the *Timaeus* (44), Plato (427–347 B.C.) characterizes sound as a shaking of the air, which is transmitted by way of the ears and the brain to the liver, the seat of the soul. It is Aristotle (384–322 B.C.), however, the younger associate, rival, and interpreter of Plato, who has long received both credit and blame for the doctrine of the "implanted air," which for 2,000 years both dominated and inhibited thought about the anatomy of the ear and the physiology of hearing.

ARISTOTLE AND THE EAR

This extraordinary thinker and observer, who must have been the first to take all knowledge as his province, discusses hearing in at least four of his books dealing with psychology and zoology (1–5). In his *De Sensu* (2) he attributes to hearing a greater share in the development of intelligence than to vision, because speech is instrumental in causing us to learn. "A consequence," he writes, "is that of those who from birth have been without one or other of those two senses, the blind are more intelligent than deaf-mutes" (translated by G. R. T. Ross). In the *De Anima* (1), in which he considers each of the five senses in turn, he adheres to the prevailing view that air confined within a cavity is essential for hearing. The air inside the ear "is lodged fast within walls to make it immoveable, in order that it may perceive exactly all the varieties of auditory movement" (translated by R. D. Hicks). This single sentence seems to have been the origin of the persistent illusion of the *aer implantatus*, purer than other air, with which it never mixes, and placed in the ear, either in the womb or at birth, to remain there for a lifetime. In all likelihood, what Aristotle has in mind is the air contained within the tympanic cavity, but he holds that it in turn is connected by a passage to an air-filled space at the occiput, where he localizes the sense of hearing. Since, as with Plato, all natural phenomena must be explained in terms of the four Empedoclean elements, Aristotle's description is entirely in harmony with his classification of hearing as the air-sense, just as vision is for him the water-sense, smell the fire-sense, and touch, together with taste, the earth-sense.

His Influence

Later anatomists assumed that the *aer ingenitus* must fill the inner ear as well. The encyclopedic Stagyrite can hardly be held responsible for the stultifying burden of *idées fixes* cherished by those who came after him. The massive corpus of Aristotelian writings, once they had been rediscovered through the help of Arab and Jewish scholars and physicians (16), came to enjoy not merely the sanction of the Church, but a status little below that of the Scriptures themselves. Certainly, none of the excellent anatomists of the Italian Renaissance, presumably aware of the rumor [apparently false, according to O'Malley (41)] that Vesalius and his *De Fabrica* (59), because of rude contradictions of the equally revered Galen, had to be protected from the Inquisition by Philip of Spain himself (Barthélemy-Saint Hilaire, 1891), was foolhardy enough to risk excommunication or worse by questioning this well-entrenched doctrine. Admittedly, their studies of the inner ear, based largely on dried temporal bones, gave them little reason to do so. We shall see that it was not until late in the 17th century that the first criticisms appeared, and not until 1760 that Cotugno of Naples showed the implanted air to be a hoary Greek myth.

HIPPOCRATES

The accomplishments of Hippocrates (460–377 A.D.) having to do with the ear, and those of his school on the island of Cos, lie mainly in the realm of ear disease and its treatment. One of his few recorded anatomical observations, however, has to do with the external canal, which leads to a bone of extraordinary hardness, whereas the surrounding bone is full of air spaces. He also recognizes the tympanic membrane as a part of the organ of hearing, describing it as "thin as a cobweb," and especially suited by its dryness for the reception of sounds (46).

THE ALEXANDRIAN ANATOMISTS

The anatomical school of Alexandria, where the dissection of human cadavers was not only permitted but encouraged, flourished more than a century later, after the time of Alexander the Great. Since it included such important investigators as Erasistratus (330–250 B.C.) and Herophilus (335–280 B.C.), it played a significant part in the history of gross and neuroanatomy, but it recorded almost no advances in knowledge of the ear.

THE ROMANS

Occupied with conquest, law, and government, the Romans excelled also in the administration of public health and hygiene, but they tended to leave medical and scientific matters to the Greeks. An anatomist of the first century A.D., Rufus of Ephesus, gave the names *pinna, lobe, helix, concha,* etc., to the various features of the external ear. There was progress in the medical and surgical treatment of ear diseases, as recorded in the writings of Aulus Cornelius Celsus (17), the most important Roman medical writer and the first medical historian. In his sixth book Celsus has a chapter on *Aurium morbi,* in which he recommends remedies for otitis, deafness, tinnitus, and foreign bodies in the ear, and in the seventh and eighth books, brief chapters on *Morbi aurium chirurgici,* including atresia of the external meatus and injuries to the cartilage of the pinna. The exact dates for Celsus are not known, but there is evidence that he lived in the reign of Tiberius, i.e., in the first decades of the present era.

GALEN

Just as the works of Aristotle dominated science and philosophy for centuries, those of Galen (130–200 A.D.) dominated medical thought and practice until the time of the Renaissance. He was born in Pergamon in Asia Minor, studied philosophy, then anatomy, and gained clinical experience by serving as physician and surgeon to the local gladiators. During the reign of Marcus Aurelius he spent two periods in Rome as a highly successful practitioner and physician to the Emperor, before returning to Pergamon for the remainder of his 70 years (51).

Galen was an indefatigable writer and polemicist, whose works covered the known fields of medical science. So far as the anatomy of the ear is concerned, however, his chief contribution seems to have been the introduction of the term *labyrinth.* Probably, as Politzer suggests, it was more an expression of ignorance than of understanding of the complex structures within the petrous bone. He somehow got the idea that the external canal extends inward as far as the dura mater, and thus failed to appreciate the significance of the tympanic membrane. However, he was able to differentiate for the first time between the facial and the auditory nerves, and to follow the course of the former through its canal in the temporal bone to its exit at the styloid process. His dissections were made on dogs and monkeys, and there is apparently no evidence that he ever dissected the human body, even though he had studied anatomy in Alexandria.

Politzer (46) gives an account of Galen's views and contributions concerning the pathology of the ear and the treatment of its diseases. As for its physiology, to illustrate the value of the pinna as a collector of sound, Galen was content to cite the example of the Emperor Hadrian, who was hard of hearing and had the habit of holding his hand behind his ear. Unlike Plato and Aristotle, Galen recognized that the function of the auditory nerve is to convey auditory sensations to the brain.

It was his psychoacoustic judgment that the most suitable and agreeable stimulus for the ear is the human voice.

THE DARK AND THE MIDDLE AGES

Whatever Galen's virtues as a physician or his faults as an anatomist, he was unique, not only for his own time but for more than a thousand years thereafter. The Decline and Fall, the Migration of the Nations (otherwise known as the Barbarian Invasions), and the Dark Ages that ensued, brought little to medicine and nothing to medical science. The Byzantines squandered their classical heritage, and the chief contribution of the Arabs and Jews was to preserve and comment on it rather than to enhance it. Throughout the Middle Ages professional preparation for the practice of medicine seems to have consisted for the most part of learning by rote a Latin poem of almost interminable length (362 to 3,520 lines, depending on the edition), which Castiglioni (16) calls "the backbone of the entire medical literature up until the Renaissance." It was known as the *Flos medicinae* or *Regimen sanitatis salernitanum,* after the renowned school of Salerno, which was at the height of its fame late in the 11th century, when Arab influence was most pronounced. For an account of this interesting but essentially sterile period of medical history, the reader should consult Castiglioni.

THE ITALIAN RENAISSANCE

In the art of painting, the Renaissance began in Florence early in the 14th century, according to Vasari (1511–1574) (58), with Giotto and his revolt against the static Byzantine tradition. In anatomy it may be said to have begun almost simultaneously, but haltingly enough, with the Bolognese Mondino dei Liuzzi and his *Anothomia.* Although he and his successors at Bologna, as at Padua, Montpellier, Paris, and elsewhere, presided over dissections by barber-surgeons for the instruction of their students, they remained faithful followers and expositors of Galen. The illustrations in their books were crude in the extreme, as shown in the reproductions published by Lind (37). Anatomical illustration, as an art form, began appropriately enough with Leonardo da Vinci (1452–1519), but his now-famous notebooks remained incomplete and largely unknown, except by hearsay. The publication that he had planned for the edification of artists and anatomists alike never appeared. Among many other organs, he had studied the eye and the larynx, but not the ear. For him the ear seems to have remained a mystery, even as it had been for Galen. Of it Leonardo wrote only that sound must "resound in the concave porosity of the petrous bone, which is to the inner side of the ear," to be carried from there to the *sensus communis,* i.e., the brain (39).

THE 16TH CENTURY

Although Burckhardt (1901) (12) in his well-known study of the Italian Renaissance devotes scant attention either to *Naturwissenschaft* or to *morbus gallicus,* it was in the 16th century that Anatomy, along with Art, Religion, and the Great Pox, reached unprecedented heights. An irreverent but fortunately anonymous soul has dared to suggest that the last-named Renaissance phenomenon may have been an underlying cause of the first three, just as it has so often been strongly associated with outstanding individual achievement in Politics, War, or Music [cf. (38)]. Be that as it may, a long series of great anatomists appeared in Italy during this century, beginning with Bartolomeo Eustachi (1510–1574), Filippo Ingrassia (1510–1580), and Andreas Vesalius (1514–1564), and continuing with Gabriele Falloppia (1523–1562), Girolamo Fabrizi (1537–1619), Giulio Casseri (1561–1616), and several others. Vesalius, a native of Brussels and a student in Louvain, Montpellier, Paris, and, most important, Padua, was the leader of the anti-Galenic revolt. His historic book, *De humani corporis fabrica,* first published in 1543 when he was 29 years old, is properly regarded as the cornerstone of human gross anatomy. With its superb plates, attributed by Vasari to the Fleming Stefan Calcar, a sometime pupil of Titian, it set an entirely new standard for medical illustration, one that was followed but scarcely equaled in the later publications of Eustachi (24) and of Casseri (15).

Several biographies of Vesalius have been written, one of the best of them by O'Malley (41). His career included service at the courts of the emperor Charles V and of his son, Philip II. The alleged brush with the Holy Office, or the jealousy of his professional rivals, eventually drove Vesalius from Madrid. He died on the return voyage from a supposedly expiatory visit to the Holy Land, while en route to Padua, where he hoped to resume his professorship of anatomy. [For brief sketches of his life, and of the lives of a number of his contemporaries mentioned above, see Politzer (46), Castiglioni (16), and especially Capparoni (14).] So far as the ear is concerned, Vesalius, perhaps unaware of his predecessors, reports his discovery of the malleus and the incus, but he does not mention the stapes, which, as he later admitted, he had failed to notice. The *De Fabrica* has a small, rather crudely drawn marginal sketch of the two ossicles and the inner ear, clearly not from the pencil of Stefan Calcar, but possibly from that of the author himself (Fig. 1).

Ingrassia, a native of Sicily, was also at one time a professor in Padua, but he eventually returned to Palermo, where his lectures attracted large audiences. He himself was greatly admired there and throughout Italy as the "Sicilian Hippocrates," especially because of his service in organizing public health measures during the plague of 1575. He is generally given credit for discovering the stapes, but claim to that tiny bone is also made by Eustachi and by Realdo Colombo (ca. 1515–1577), the prosector, rival, and chief detractor of Vesalius, who was a pre-Harveian exponent of the circulation of the blood, and the first to mention the vessels of the inner ear. There have been other claimants as well. The vexed question of the earliest discovery of the ossicles has been carefully examined by Fioretti and Concato (29,30), and by O'Malley and Clarke (42). For the malleus and incus the latter authors give due credit to Berengario da Carpi (1470–1550). While commenting on the text of Mondino, Berengario in his *Anatomia* (9), published in Bologna in 1521, writes of *duo ossicula parva* in the ear. Eustachi (24), like Vesalius in the *De Fabrica,* points out the resemblance of the middle ossicle to a molar tooth, but his claim to the stapes is dismissed by O'Malley and Clarke in favor of Ingrassia, whose right to it had been admitted by Vesalius and supported by Falloppia among other contemporaries. It seems more than likely, however, that several Renaissance anatomists discovered the ossicles at about the same time and quite independently of one another. As with the long-debated question of the origin of lues, such lingering

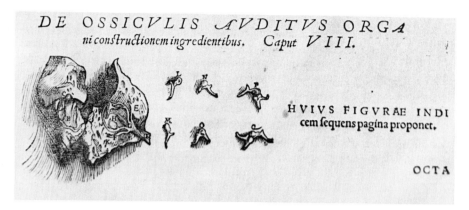

DE OSSICVLIS AVDITVS ORGA
ni conſtructionem ingredientibus. Caput VIII.

HVIVS FIGVRAE INDI
cem ſequens pagina proponet.

OCTA

FIG. 1. Vesalian dissection of the temporal bone and the auditory nerve. The middle ear has been divided so as to show the malleus, C (*ossiculum malleolo assimilatum*), and the inner surface of the tympanic membrane, E (*membrana transversim foramini obducta, quod ab aure in cavitatem fertur*) at the left. At the right are the incus, H (*ossiculum quod incudi & molari denti comparatur*) and the author's impression of the ramifications of the "fifth" (auditory) nerve, D, E, F, G. (*quinti nervorum cerebri paris nervus*). The smaller sketches show various views of the two ossicles. (From ref. 59, marginal sketch, page 33.)

disputes as to priority of discovery become, after four centuries, ever more difficult to resolve.

Eustachi, during his long career at the Sapienzia in Rome, where he had papal dispensation to receive and dissect the bodies of patients who had died in hospital, steadfastly supported the teachings of Galen in opposition to those of Vesalius while making a great many anatomical discoveries of his own, to which the names of others have since become attached as eponyms. Eustachi published his *Opuscula anatomica* in 1564, but entrusted the beautiful copper plates, completed later and intended as illustrations for the text, to an assistant for publication after his death. Instead, they were lost for well over a century, until rediscovered in the Vatican Library by Lancisi. The latter published them in 1714, in a handsome folio volume, *Tabulae anatomicae,* which also lists the numerous but forgotten prior discoveries of Eustachi. As for the ear, Politzer gives him credit for an exact description of the tensor tympani, which is illustrated in the *Tabulae*, as well as for recognizing the chorda tympani as a nerve rather than a blood vessel. His greatest contribution was his precise description of the tube, the only structure that bears his name. In the *Tabulae* he shows a longitudinal section through the temporal bone, with the tympanic cavity, the semicircular canals, and the spiral of the cochlea properly located.

One of the most accomplished and at the same time most beloved figures of this period, according to the testimony of his students and biographers, was Gabriele Falloppia. (As with Shakespeare, the proper spelling of his family name is uncertain. One biographer, Favaro (28), devotes an entire chapter to an examination of the abundant and conflicting evidence before concluding that the question of orthography is unanswerable. The form given here is that used by the *Enciclopedia Italiana*.) As professor of anatomy at Padua, Falloppia established the international renown of that school, and as surgeon he was hailed as the "Aesculapius of his Century." Recounting his discovery and exploration of the Falloppian aqueduct or facial canal in his brief work, *Observationes anatomicae* (27), published in 1561 shortly before his death, he gives also a careful account of the middle ear cavity, likening it to a military drum and naming it for the first time the *tympanum*. He describes the tympanic membrane, the coordinated movement of the ossicles, and the inner ear with the "second and third cavities," i.e., the vestibule and the cochlea, pointing out that there is little change in the size of these structures after birth. He is, of course, entirely unaware of the membranous labyrinth, and sensible enough not to propose a theory of hearing. In his *De morbo gallico* (26) Falloppia gives the first, remarkably graphic account of the almost intolerable tinnitus that can accompany lues. Nevertheless, there is no evidence to suggest that he had actually heard it himself.

THE SUCCESSORS OF FALLOPPIA

Space does not permit more than a brief mention of the other famous members of the Padovan school, who were direct intellectual descendants of Falloppia. His prosector was the Frisian, Volcher Koyter of Groningen (1534–1600), an enthusiast who, understandably enough, considered the complicated structure of the ear as one of the most sublime works of Nature. As a physiologist he argued that the tympanic membrane prevents the mixing of the unclean outside air with the pure *aer implantatus,* and facilitates sound conduction. The tympanic cavity contains most of the implanted air, receiving it from the mastoid air cells, where it is warmed and purified. In any case, he holds that it was not placed there from the beginning by the Creator. In the windings of the cochlea and labyrinth sound is strengthened, as in a musical instrument.

A more familiar name is that of Girolamo Fabrizi (1537–1619), otherwise known as Fabricius ab Aquapendente—to distinguish him from the German Fabricius Hildanus (1560–1634), a prolific writer, but more important as an ear surgeon than as an anatomist. As the protégé and successor to Falloppia in Padua, Fabrizi was honored by the University and the Venetian senate and so richly rewarded by his wealthy patients that he was able to build the well-known *Theatrum anatomicum* at his own expense. Among his works are his *De aure, auditus organo* and *De formato foetu* (25). In the former he expresses a theory of hearing that involves a mixing of the implanted air with "animal spirits" from the auditory nerve. The cavities of the inner ear are there to absorb sound and prevent echo. In the latter he mentions that the middle ear of the fetus is filled with mucus. For ear surgery he insists on the importance of adequate illumination of the external canal and the protection of the tympanic membrane from injury. According to Morgagni (40), he had devised two methods for lighting the canal, one with sunlight passing through a small hole in the window shutter, the other with candlelight passed through a condensing lens formed by water in a flask.

Giulio Casseri (1561–1616) started at Padua as diener and assistant to Fabrizi, who recognized his talents and saw to it that he soon obtained the doctorate and eventually the professorship in succession to his master. He is best remembered for his book, *De vocis auditusque organis historia anatomica* (15), with its excellent plates, which were made, according to his publisher, with the cooperation of painters and an engraver who lived in his house (46). They illustrate, *inter alia,* tracheotomy in a vociferously protesting adult male patient, and the forms of the auditory ossicles and the intra-aural muscles in several species of domestic animals. Thus, Casseri can be regarded as perhaps the earliest comparative anatomist in this field. He also gives the first exact description of the round window membrane, previously seen by the Florentine Guido Guidi (the Vidius of the Vidian nerve), who had been one of the teachers of Vesalius at Paris.

THE 17TH CENTURY

The focus shifts in the next century to other countries than Italy, but before it does at least one more Italian should be mentioned, if only in passing. He is the short-lived but historically important neuroanatomist of Bologna, Constanzo Varoli (1543–1575), whose name is attached to the pons, and who gave the first clear description of the stapedius muscle. From a functional point of view, he was the first to liken the action of the intra-aural muscles to that of the iris.

Let us consider first the French. In Montpellier, and later in Paris, André du Laurent (d. 1609) seems to have been the first to deny that the implanted air could have the significance attributed to it by Aristotle. He regarded it simply as the inner medium; for him the most important part of the ear was the "fifth" (i.e., the eighth) cranial nerve. A more important French scientist, a native Parisian of remarkable gifts, was Claude Perrault (1613–1688), skilled in physics and distinguished for his achievements in architecture as well as in anatomy and physiology. One of his special interests was comparative anatomy, for which he had the resources of the royal menagerie at his disposal. His death at the age of 75 is said to have been the result of an injury received during the autopsy of a camel (46).

One of Perrault's *Essais de Physique* entitled "Du Bruit" ("On Noise") is an extensive exposition of the theories of sound of the day and of his own, often highly original ideas about the anatomy and physiology of the ear. In the cochlea he describes the "spiral membrane" as soft and flexible, attached only to the modiolus and not to the opposite wall. Hence it is the osseous and not the membranous spiral lamina that he has in mind. He believes that the nerve fibers enter the spiral lamina and unite with the substance of the bone to form the true organ of hearing. Unfortunately, he blithely accepts the *aer implantatus*, but places it in the labyrinth rather than in the tympanum. In his scheme of the auditory process, the vibrations of the drum membrane are transferred to the air in the middle ear, and thence to the membrane of the round window. In turn, the implanted air is set in motion, which is attenuated by the "membranous structures" of the labyrinth, transmitted to the spiral membrane, and thence to the true organ of hearing. He also has theories of noise-induced and presbyacusic loss of hearing. Impairment of hearing is caused by sound, he says, because the spiral lamella is shattered like a glass by the strong vibrations. In old age the spiral membrane becomes too dried out to respond properly.

We must also mention Jean Mery (1645–1722), anatomist and surgeon of the Hotel-Dieu, because he rediscovered the membranous spiral lamina, which had been seen by Eustachi to divide the cochlea into two scalae but had since been forgotten. He also discovered at the apex of the cochlea "un petit trou" (a little hole), later to be named by Breschet the *helicotrema*. He was the bitterly jealous rival of the accomplished anatomist to be discussed next.

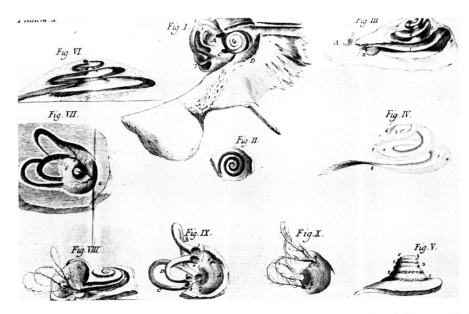

FIG. 2. Duverney's dissections of the inner ear, showing the cochlea with its spiral lamina (III, IV, VI), the modiolus (V), and the vestibule with the semicircular canals, their nerves, and blood vessels (VII–X). In III, B indicates "la fenestre ronde fermée par une membrane mince comme la peau du tambour." The spiral membrane (basilar) shown in IV serves to attach the spiral lamina to the inner wall of the spiral canal. (From ref. 22, plate X.)

Duverney

The life of Joseph Guichard Duverney (1648–1730) covers much the same period as the long reign of Louis XIV. In Paris his demonstrations won him such applause in the highest circles that the position of Court Anatomist was created for him, and he gave Royal tutorials to the Dauphin. He was also the teacher of a majority of the most distinguished French anatomists of his century. Since he was especially attracted to the study of the ear, his extraordinary *chef d'oeuvre, Traité de l'organe de l'ouïe* (22), is an enduring monument to the subject and to its author. For a précis of it, see Politzer (46); better yet, go to the rare book room of your favorite well-endowed medical library and examine its interesting text and its elegantly engraved illustrations for yourself. However, you will not find a portrait of the author himself, for unfortunately none seems to exist.

Duverney's treatise is remarkable not only for its anatomical presentations but for its author's thoughts on the physiology and pathology of the ear. For him, sound is transmitted by the ossicular chain to the oval window, not by air conduction to the round window. There, he believes, it still encounters the implanted air in the vestibule. Nevertheless, Duverney is a true forerunner of Helmholtz, putting forward a resonance theory before its time. He calls attention to the width of the osseous spiral lamina, which gradually narrows from the base to the apex (Fig. 2). He infers, therefore that the tones of low pitch are received at the basal end of the cochlea, those of high pitch at the apical end. In developing this theory he had the aid of the physicist Mariotte. Since they were not in a position to examine the basilar membrane, they can perhaps be forgiven that they got their theory backwards.

Two Englishmen who contributed to auditory physiology should also be recalled. The first is the philosopher Francis Bacon (1561–1626), who was courtier and counsel to Elizabeth I and, as Baron Verulam and Viscount St. Albans, Lord High Chancellor under James I. Some have tried to claim him as the author of Shakespeare's plays. He was, in fact, much too busy with other writing tasks, establishing the inductive method for science and attempting, without success, to thwart his political enemies, who finally managed to discredit him and to have him confined for a period in the Tower. The physics of light and sound, and the nature of sight and hearing were of special interest to him. Unfortunately, he seems never to have got around to writing the work on acoustics and audition that he had promised his readers, but the fragments of thought on these subjects that are included in his other volumes are not without interest. In his *Sylva Sylvarum* (6) he has several accounts of acoustic phenomena, including echoes and whispering galleries, bone conduction of sound via the teeth or the temple, and articulation—labial, dental, guttural, and so forth. He is aware of auditory masking and overexposure, pointing out that "the stronger species drowneth the less, as the light of the sun the light of a glow-worm; the report of an ordnance the voice." Also, "an object of surcharge or excess destroyeth the same; as the light of the sun the eye; a violent sound (near the ear) the hearing." Furthermore, he reminds the reader, "It is an old tradition that those that dwell near the cataracts of Nilus are stricken deaf"; adding, "but we find no such effect in cannoniers, nor millers, nor those that dwell upon bridges." (Obviously, he moved very little in such circles, or else he would have known better.) Finally, he describes the design of an "ear-spectacle," or ear trumpet. There is no indication that he ever constructed one, but he has heard that "there is in Spain an instrument in use to be set to the ear, that helpeth somewhat those that are thick of hearing." More or less the same phraseology might well be used in recommending a hearing aid for a presbyacusic patient.

The second Englishman is the great Oxford physician and member of the Royal Society, Thomas Willis (1622–1675), who flourished there and in London in the troubled times of the Stuarts, the Puritan Rebellion, Cromwell's Commonwealth, and the Restoration. He should be more gratefully remembered for his work as a founder of neurology than for his arterial circle. Throughout his life Willis fought against the Aristotelian and Galenical tradition that he had been taught at Christ Church, in favor of a rational medical approach based on chemical principles. In particular, we should recall that in his *De anima brutorum* (63) he was the first to recognize the cochlea as the true organ of hearing, and to mention the possibility of diplacusis. In his *Cerebri anatome* (63) he demonstrates the origins of the facial, auditory, and accessory nerves. Of course it was he who called attention to the phenomenon of "paracusis Willisii," i.e., the ability of certain hard-of-hearing persons to hear better in noise than in quiet. He also suggested a theory of the distribution of tones in the cochlea that anticipated Duverney's.

In anticipation of the later importance of his fellow countrymen as students of the ear, we should mention at this point Gunther Christoph Schelhammer (1649–1712), a professor at Jena and other German universities. He launched an attack on that everhardy perennial, the implanted air, reminding his contemporaries of its strange hypothetical wanderings over the centuries, being lodged first in the occipital region, then in the cavities of the inner ear, then in the tympanum, and once again in the labyrinth, to the accompaniment of ever more complicated attempts at explanation.

It could not be the receptor organ as postulated. Instead, it is the auditory nerve that is essential, together with the "animal spirits." Of more practical importance was the method he suggested for differentiating between impaired hearing because of injury to the tympanic membrane and that owing to defect of the auditory nerve. Using a musical instrument held between the teeth, he anticipated the 19th-century otologists with their tuning forks. However, as so often in matters of music and science, the Italians had been there first. Politzer points out that a similar test of hearing had been proposed by Hieronimo Capivacci (alias Capo di Vacco) of Padua, who died in 1589. As for deafness, a distinction was drawn between the congenital and the acquired types in a book of 1680 by François de la Boe Sylvius (the Sylvius of the lateral sulcus, not Jacques Dubois Sylvius of the cerebral aqueduct, more than a century earlier).

THE 18TH CENTURY

Once again we must turn our thoughts toward Italy, to pay our respects to a series of men belonging to an unusually robust intellectual family tree, rooted in Bologna, that was scientifically fruitful for well over a century and a half. For our limited purpose, the first of them is the indefatigable Antonio Maria Valsalva (1666–1723), but we must not forget that his teacher was the great Marcello Malpighi (1628–1691), whom he succeeded as professor. Valsalva's *Tractatus de aure humana* (56) is said to have been based on 16 years of work and the dissection of more than a thousand heads. As published in Venice in 1740 by his pupil Morgagni, it consists of two sections of text, one anatomical, the other physiological (Fig. 3). Ten superb plates provide illustrations, among them dissections of the outer, middle, and inner ear. His anatomical and functional studies of the auditory tube, which he named in honor of Eustachi, are classical. His universally known maneuver, however, which he recommended for expelling pus from an infected middle ear, was hardly new, having been mentioned in the writings of Arabian and early European physicians. He recognized the importance of the ossicular chain as a series of levers transmitting sound to the oval window. In one case of deafness he was able to demonstrate disarticulation of the incudo-stapedial joint, in another ankylosis of the stapes. In his theory of hearing, Valsalva went beyond Duverney, pointing to the membranous portions of the labyrinth rather than the spiral osseous lamina as the sites of termination of the branches of the auditory nerve, and regarding them as receptors for sound ("zonae sonorae"). In comparing these areas to musical instruments with strings of different length he was more than a century ahead of Helmholtz.

The gifted and prolific Giovanni Battista Morgagni (1682–1771), having been Valsalva's prosector at the age of 19, was called in 1712 to the professorship of anatomy in Padua, where he remained for 60 years, laying the foundations of pathology. Of his 20 *Epistolae anatomicae*, seven have to do with the ear, presenting important anatomical details supplementary, and sometimes contrary, to the descriptions of Valsalva. In the 13th he reports the effects of experimental perforation of the tympanic membrane in a dog. His pathological studies are presented in his classical work, *De causis et sedibus morborum*, published in Venice in 1761. In one section he considers the relation between otitis media and brain abscess. Unlike many of his contemporaries and successors, he concludes that the ear infection is primary.

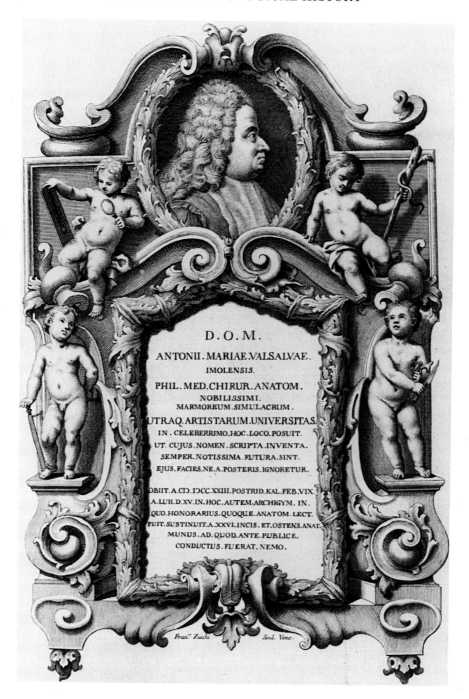

FIG. 3. Tribute to Valsalva in his posthumously published *Tractatus de Aure Humana,* 1740. Note the scalpel and the beautiful dissection of the outer, middle, and inner ear in the hands of the putto at the lower right.

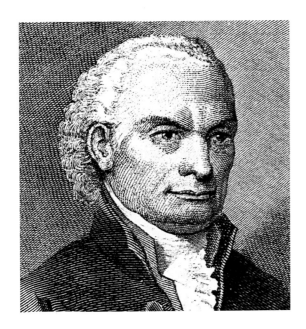

FIG. 4. Domenico Cotugno (1736–1822). (From ref. 46, vol. 1, plate xv.)

For a précis of his monumental work, see Politzer (46); better still, look up a copy of Benjamin Alexander's 1769 translation of the *De causis* in facsimile (40).

We think now of the two men whose work at long last gave the *coup de grace* to Aristotle's implanted air: Domenico Cotugno (1736–1822) of Naples (Fig. 4), and Antonio Scarpa (1747–1832) of Modena and Pavia (Fig. 5). Cotugno's story is one of rags to success, if not to riches. Born into a poverty-stricken family of Apulia in southern Italy, he was enabled, thanks to the generosity of the local nobleman, to study medicine at Naples, where, at the age of 24, he published his epoch-making *De aquaeductibus auris humanae internae anatomica dissertatio* (19). It is based on a departure from tradition, the dissection of the fresh rather than the macerated temporal bone. In it he describes both the cochlear and the vestibular aqueducts, and the clear liquid (later christened *liquor Cotunni,* and still later *perilymph*) that he has seen filling the bony labyrinth. He is not aware of the membranous labyrinth within.

After a period as a student of Morgagni, Cotugno was called back to Naples at the age of 30 to become professor of anatomy and surgery, and there he stayed for the rest of his long and productive life. Although his dissertation had already made him famous, he added to his renown by his discovery of the *liquor cerebrospinalis,* and of the albumin in the urine of patients with nephritis. He introduced helpful prophylactic measures against the spread of tuberculosis, and gave such an excellent description of sciatica that it came to be known as *la malattia di Cotugno.* As a crowning honor, his name was also attached to a form of lead chloride found in the lava of Vesuvius, *cotunnite.*

The *De aquaeductibus* is a small but impressive volume of just over 100 pages; its simple medical Latin is well worth the reader's effort. There is abundant evidence that the young author knows what he is about, and he writes with clarity and authority while bringing the venerable doctrine crashing to earth. As an example, the heading

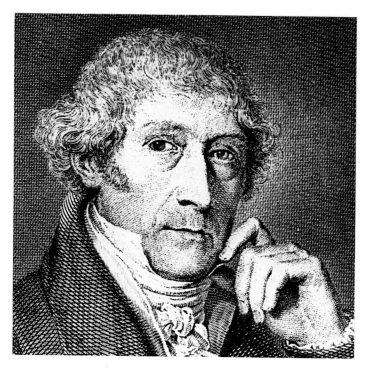

FIG. 5. Antonio Scarpa (1747–1832). (From ref. 46, vol. 1, plate xvi.)

of one of his many short chapters is: *Tota labyrinthi cavitas humore est plena, & aer naturaliter semper abest, nec penetrare in eam potest.* (The entire cavity of the labyrinth is full of liquid, and air is by nature always absent, nor can it enter therein.) In another chapter he gives a magisterial put-down of his predecessors and their numerous errors of observation and interpretation.

Antonio Scarpa's background was much more favorable. His medical studies were divided between Padua, where he became the secretary and favorite pupil of Morgagni, and Bologna, where he acquired his skill in surgery. His first book, *De structura fenestrae rotundae,* was published in 1772, shortly after he had been made professor of anatomy and chief surgeon at Modena. In it his physiological argument is that sound is transmitted to the labyrinth both by way of the ossicular chain to the oval window and by way of the air in the middle ear to the round window and what he called its secondary tympanic membrane. The possibility of a reciprocal relation between the two windows apparently has not occurred to him. His greatest contribution to this field came in the revolutionary year 1789, with the publication of his book, *Disquisitiones anatomicae de auditu et olfactu.* There he presents his discovery of the membranous labyrinth, including the "spiral passage," i.e., the cochlear duct, which he finds to be filled with a watery fluid, later to be called Scarpa's fluid, or the *endolymph.* He also follows the various branches of the auditory nerve to their respective terminations in the labyrinth, making the assumption, not unreasonable for his time, that all parts of the complex structure are concerned with hearing. The same publication deals also with the comparative anatomy of the labyrinth in various animal species beginning with the elasmobranchs, and thus anticipates the studies of Retzius almost 100 years later. There Scarpa devotes considerable attention to the auditory system in birds, an interest that was shared by the discoverer of "animal electricity," Luigi Galvani of Bologna (1737–1798).

THE 19TH CENTURY

On the threshold of the Victorian age, in which anatomy triumphantly became both microscopic and morbid, physiology experimental and not merely speculative, the anatomy of the ear and its nomenclature were clarified by Gilbert Breschet (1784–1845), who was born in the Auvergne and studied medicine in Paris. In 1836 he was appointed to the chair of anatomy of the Faculté de Médecine, as successor to Cruveilhiers. In the same year he published his *Recherches anatomiques et physiologiques sur l'organe de l'ouïe et sur l'audition dans l'homme et les animaux vertébrés* (11), culminating an investigation he had begun in 1815. Taking as his model the taxonomic achievements of Carl von Linné (Linnaeus) in Sweden, he defined vague old terms with precision and coined important new ones, among them *endolymph, perilymph, helicotrema, otolith,* and *otoconia.* His monograph, with its lucid exposition and beautiful engravings, can still be read with pleasure (Fig. 6).

The creator of modern experimental physiology was François Magendie (1783–1855) of the Collège de France, the teacher of Claude Bernard. Active in many fields of physiological research, Magendie was concerned with such auditory problems as directional hearing and the cause of diminished hearing in old age, which he attributed in part to a reduced sensitivity of the auditory nerve and in part to a decrease in the amount of labyrinthine fluid. He held that the function of the Eustachian tube was to renew the air in the tympanic cavity. One of his important findings was that ataxia can be produced in an animal by section of a cerebellar peduncle. That observation helped to motivate Flourens in his experiments on the semicircular canals, which demonstrated the hitherto unsuspected function of the vestibular organs.

An equally influential physiologist was Johannes Müller (1801–1858) of Berlin, the teacher of Helmholtz, whose interest extended to all aspects of sensation, and who formulated the often-cited but not always clearly understood doctrine of specific nerve energies. He was apparently the first physiologist to examine experimentally the passage of sound waves from air to water, and thus became the remote ancestor of impedance audiometry.

Among the anatomical contributors of this period to the study of the ear, we must not overlook Friedrich Christof Rosenthal (1780–1829) of Greifswald, who found, in the course of dissecting a great number of cochleas, the canal in the modiolus that carries his name. We should also mention the Hungarian-born Joseph Hyrtl (1811–1894), professor in Prague and Vienna, who first used the corrosion technique in examining the blood supply of the temporal bone, and who did extensive research on the comparative anatomy of the ear. There is also Emil Huschke (1797–1858) of Jena, who discovered the *zona dentata* of the limbus during his study of the avian inner ear and is thus remembered for "Huschke's teeth." He took them to be the site of termination of the auditory nerve fibers. Perhaps because he was using birds rather than mammals, he failed to discover the true endorgan, an achievement that was reserved to Corti.

Alfonso Corti (1822–1876) was born at Gambarana in Lombardy, the scion of an

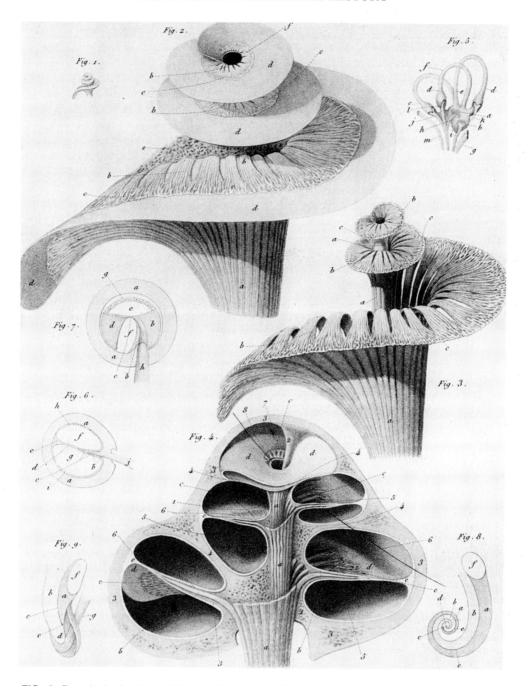

FIG. 6. Breschet's drawings of the cochlea, the spiral lamina, and the cochlear nerve, showing the helicotrema but lacking the vestibular membrane and the spiral ganglion. The smaller sketches show differences between the mammalian and the avian organs of hearing. (From ref. 11.)

ancient family with strong military, scholarly, and medical traditions. Against the wishes of his father, the Marchese di Corti di San Stefano Belbo, young Corti chose to study medicine, enrolling at the University of Pavia. His choice had apparently been inspired by the memory of Scarpa, who had been a family friend. From Pavia he moved on to Vienna, where he became a pupil of Hyrtl. He received his degree in medicine in 1847, and with it an appointment as second prosector. During the troubled year of 1848, Corti left revolutionary Vienna and saw service for some months with the Italian forces. Following that, he resumed his anatomical studies, first in Paris and then in the laboratory of Albert von Kölliker at Würzburg. His interest in the labyrinth had been awakened at Pavia and fostered by Hyrtl, but his efforts to preserve its contents long enough for microscopic examination were successful only after Harting of Delft suggested that he suspend the perishable tissues in fluid while he tried to dissect them. In his single all-important paper, "Recherches sur l'organe de l'ouïe des mammifères" (18), published in 1851 in the *Zeitschrift für wissenschaftliche Zoologie,* he described for the first time the sensory epithelium resting on the basilar membrane, the tectorial membrane, the stria vascularis, the spiral ganglion, and much more (Fig. 7).

In the same year Corti succeeded, upon the death of his father, to the family title. In spite of the disappointment of his learned colleagues throughout Europe, he withdrew completely from scientific activity, to devote himself to his family and the estate, and to the scientific cultivation of his vineyards. It was Kölliker who first used the term *organ of Corti,* and who wrote of "that zealous and intelligent observer," its discoverer: "His work was the starting point of our knowledge of the cochlea."

Corti's success inspired a burst of activity on the part of other anatomists, whose names often became affixed to individual cochlear tissues and epithelial cells. One of these was Ernst Reissner (1824–1875) of Dorpat in Estonia, who confirmed Corti's observations and in 1852 reported his discovery of the vestibular membrane, which closes off the cochlear duct and carries the eponym. Another was Otto Friedrich Deiters (1834–1863) of Bonn, who in his brief lifetime discovered not only the highly specialized cells that sustain the outer hair cells and the reticular lamina of Corti's organ, but also the large multipolar cells of his own lateral vestibular nucleus. Arthur Böttcher (1831–1889), also of Dorpat, was the first to furnish a description of the reticular lamina itself. The darker staining cells resting on the basilar membrane in the basal turn are his. They are covered by the pale cells near the outer sulcus, first pictured by Matthias Claudius (1821–1869) of Copenhagen. Closer to the reticular lamina are the darkish cells (containing lipid droplets in the guinea pig) that are called after Viktor Hensen (1835–1924) of Kiel, to whom we also owe the ductus reuniens, linking the cochlea and the saccule.

Belonging to the next generation of late Victorian anatomists there is the multifaceted Stockholmer of Renaissance stature, Magnus Gustaf Retzius (1842–1919), the son of the anatomist-anthropologist Anders Retzius (Fig. 8). To students of hearing he is best known for his exemplary work on the comparative anatomy of the vertebrate labyrinth, *Das Gehörorgan der Wirbelthiere* (47), for which he himself drew the superb illustrations, and which he published in two folio volumes dated 1881 and 1884. Latter-day students of hearing owe it to their education to become familiar with them both. His later researches on the ear, together with those on neuroanatomy, histology, anthropology, and the comparative morphology of sper-

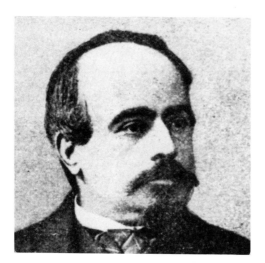

FIG. 7. (Top) Alfonso Corti (1822–1876). **(Bottom)** Two drawings from his famous paper of 1851. The upper figure shows a cross section of the spiral lamina, with apparent autolytic changes that have left the various features of Corti's organ virtually unrecognizable. In the lower figure a surface preparation is shown, in which the inner and outer hair cells, the pillars, the Hensen (?) cells, and the basilar membrane are clearly displayed.

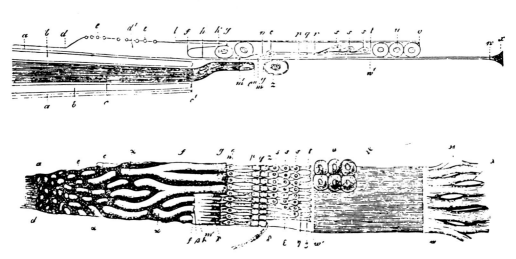

matozoa, *inter alia,* are to be found in his own privately published, folio-sized scientific journal, *Biologische Untersuchungen* (48) (Fig. 9). Retzius employed with great skill the method of microdissection of the labyrinth, making surface preparations of the organ of Corti and other tissues, often fixed and stained with osmic acid (Fig. 10). (That indispensable but highly toxic substance had been added to the histologist's armamentarium by Max Schultze in 1858.)

Thinking once again about physiology, we look back to Hermann Ludwig Ferdinand von Helmholtz (1821–1894), whose life presents a singularly harmonious synthesis of physics and medicine, physiology, psychology, and music. The son of a Prussian schoolmaster, he displayed his many-sided talents even as a pupil at the Potsdam Gymnasium, where he distinguished himself in classical languages, including Hebrew and Arabic, as well as in scientific studies. Lacking the requisite funds for a university career in physics, he accepted a scholarship to study medicine in Berlin, obligating himself to serve for eight years as a military surgeon.

Helmholtz's zeal for the application of physical principles to physiological prob-

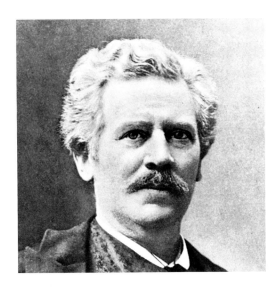

FIG. 8. Gustaf Retzius (1842–1919). (Frontispiece to the final (19th) volume of his *Biologische Untersuchungen*, 1922.)

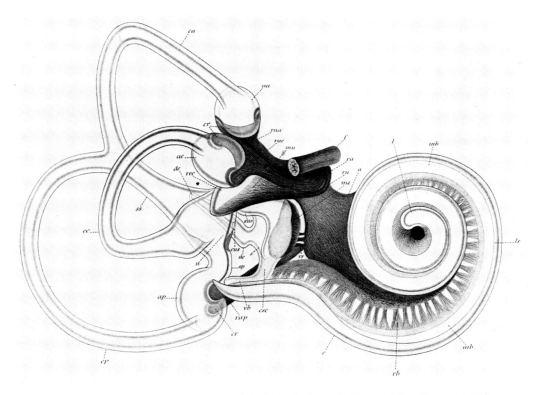

FIG. 9. Dissection of the membranous labyrinth of a 6-month human fetus. (From ref. 48.)

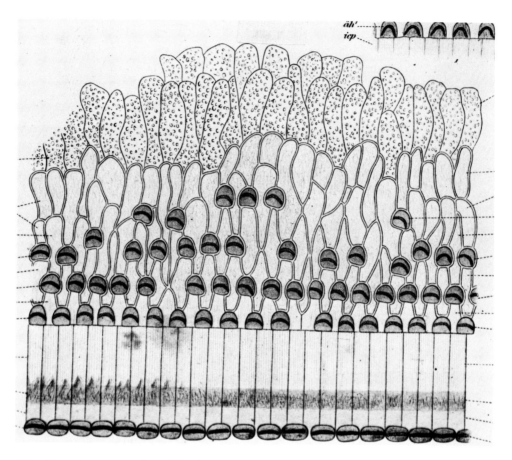

FIG. 10. Surface preparation of the human organ of Corti from the middle of the second turn of an adult male, showing the mosaic pattern of the reticular lamina, with the single row of inner hair cells, the head plates of the inner pillars, and the three rows of outer hair cells, separated by the phalangeal plates of the outer pillars and the Deiters' cells. A fourth row is represented by a few additional outer hair cells, and typical phalangeal scars replace those missing from the first three rows. (From ref. 47, vol. 2, plate xxxvii.)

lems ripened through his close association in Berlin with Johannes Müller and his students, including du Bois-Reymond, Brücke, and Ludwig, and through his long friendship with William Thomson, Lord Kelvin. After completing his peaceful and scientifically productive military duties with a Prussian guard regiment, he became professor of physiology, first at Königsberg and later at Bonn and Heidelberg. Finally he returned to his first love, as professor of physics at the University of Berlin. His contributions to science are numerous and well-known. Among them are the demonstration of the conservation of energy in muscular work, the measurement of the speed of the nerve impulse, the invention of the ophthalmoscope, and fundamental investigations in physiological optics. He is an unforgettable figure in the history of auditory physiology for his studies on the nature of combination tones and on the mechanism of the tympanic membrane and the ossicular chain, as well as for the resonance theory of hearing, developed in the successive editions of his *opus magnum, Die Lehre von den Tonempfindungen als physiologische Grundlage fur die Theorie der Musik* (34), first published in 1862.

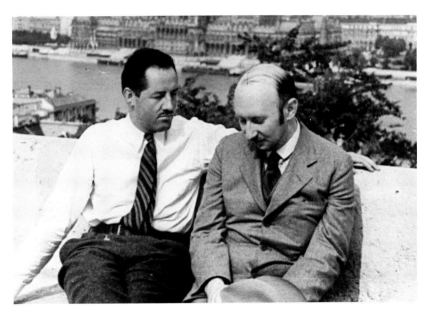

FIG. 11. S. Smith Stevens **(left)** and Georg von Békésy, in Budapest in the summer of 1937. (The photograph was supplied by Mrs. Geraldine Stevens and is reproduced with her kind permission.)

THEORIES OF HEARING

The resonance theory of Helmholtz was not the first, and certainly not the last, of the theories put forward to explain how the ear analyzes complex sounds and noises into their component frequencies. They have been painstakingly reviewed by Theodore Bast and Barry Anson (7) and by E. G. Wever (61), where the interested reader can find them summarized and criticized. Great ingenuity had been invested in their making, but until the studies by the Hungarian telephone engineer and winner of the 1961 Nobel prize for physiology and medicine, Georg von Békésy (1899–1972) (Fig. 11), and the more recent adaptations of the Mössbauer technique by his successors, the experimental foundation had been too flimsy to support such top-heavy theoretical constructions. In general the theories have been of two types: those that located the site of analysis in the cochlea (place theories), and those that assigned it to the auditory nerve and the central auditory neurons (frequency theories). The resonance theory was clearly of the first type, whereas William Rutherford's "telephone theory" (1886), formerly regarded as the major competitor, was of the second. However, the resonators postulated by Helmholtz were nowhere to be found in the cochlea, and it soon became clear that even the fibers of the eighth nerve could not transmit such high frequencies as would be required by the telephone theory. Von Békésy's (8) demonstration of the traveling wave along the basilar membrane seemed to clinch the matter in favor of a cochlear analyzer and a place theory of analysis. It depends on the reciprocal relation between stiffness and mass along the length of the cochlear duct. Wever's volley theory finds a role for the telephone principle in the coding of frequency information for low tones in terms of the frequency of response of the nerve fibers.

AUDITORY PHYSIOLOGY IN THE 20TH CENTURY

Like the rest of neuroscience, the field of auditory physiology has been expanded and transformed in this century by a number of technical and scientific factors: the burgeoning of electroacoustic technology; the rapid development of electrophysiology that followed; the introduction of the computer; the invention of electron microscopy in its several forms; and the adaptation of biochemical, microchemical, and immunochemical techniques to the narrow confines of the inner ear. Since most of these matters are to be dealt with elsewhere in this volume, their recent history will not be recounted here. Furthermore, 20th-century developments in auditory neurophysiology, biophysics, and ultrastructural research have been dealt with admirably in chapters by Hallowell Davis, Josef Zwislocki, and Hans Engström, appearing in Dawson and Enoch's *Foundations of Sensory Science* (21). Nevertheless, a few seminal and direction-giving contributions deserve to be pointed out. One of them is that of von Békésy, as mentioned above, in revealing the nature of wave propagation along the cochlear partition. Others are the discovery of the electrical potentials of the cochlea by Glen Wever and Charles Bray (1930) at Princeton, and their analysis by Hallowell Davis and his colleagues at Harvard into the AC cochlear microphonic potential and the compound action potentials of the cochlear nerve [Stevens and Davis (53)]. The DC endocochlear potential was first reported by von Békésy in 1952. Glen Wever and Merle Lawrence (62) used the cochlear potentials in their analysis of the mechanics of the ossicular chain, which found useful application in middle-ear surgery. We should note also the discovery in 1954 by Catherine Smith, Oliver Lowry, and Mei-Ling Wu at Washington University (St. Louis) of the striking difference in ionic composition between the endolymph and the perilymph.

A more gradual phenomenon has been the development of otopathology from its beginnings in London with Joseph Toynbee (1815–1866), its growth in Imperial Germany, and its flowering in America, with Stacy Guild (1890–1966) at Michigan and Johns Hopkins, John Lindsay (1898–1981) at Chicago, and their respective colleagues and pupils. Experimental otopathology, largely concerned with injuries to the cochlea by noise and ototoxic agents, got its start in Germany with Karl Wittmaack (1876–1972), whose initial publications on these subjects appeared early in this century (1903, 1907). Psychoacoustics was launched in the 1920s at the Bell Telephone Laboratories by Harvey Fletcher (1884–1978) and his collaborators, and notably accelerated in the 1940s and 1950s at the Harvard Psycho-Acoustic Laboratory, under the guidance of S. Smith Stevens (1906–1973) (Fig. 11). The clinical science of audiology, which developed rapidly after World War II, may be said to have had its origin in those two institutions.

VESTIBULAR PHYSIOLOGY

It remains only to give some account of the beginnings of our present understanding of the activity of the vestibular half of the labyrinth. As we have already seen, its gross anatomy had been described with considerable accuracy by Scarpa in the 18th century. Its function, however, had not even been surmised before the investigations of Marie-Jean-Pierre Flourens (1794–1867), an ingenious experimentalist, philosopher of science, and *savant célèbre*. In 1824 he reported that he had cut individual semicircular canals in pigeons and had observed dramatic effects on the motions of the head and on the behavior of the birds. Apparently, each canal responded to and governed movements in its corresponding plane. Although his surgical intervention appeared to have produced vertigo in his subjects, it was only after his later publications in 1842 and 1861 that the significance of his observations gradually came to be appreciated. After the death of Flourens, his eulogy was spoken at the Académie Française by Claude Bernard, who had succeeded to his vacant seat in that august body. Among the well-merited words of praise, however, the revolutionary experiments on the vestibular system seem to have been forgotten.

In the 1870s the independent work of Fr. Goltz (Königsberg, 1870), Ernst Mach (Prague, 1873), J. Breuer (Vienna, 1873), and A. Crum Brown (Edinburgh, 1874) showed conclusively that the vestibular system is concerned with postural equilibrium and not with hearing, as had for so long been assumed. The last three authors independently reached the conclusion that the semicircular canals constitute the sense organ for rotation. E. de Cyon (Paris, 1878) related the direction of nystagmus to the stimulation of the individual canals. J. R. Ewald (Strassburg, 1892) showed that nystagmus in either direction can be evoked by stimulation of either labyrinth. Later he demonstrated the influence of the labyrinth on tone in the limb muscles. Interestingly enough, it was the philosopher-psychologist William James (1842–1910) at Harvard who reported (1882) the absence of vertigo in many deaf-mutes, as well as their resistance to seasickness. Rudolf Bárány, a Hungarian and a Nobel laureate, working first in Politzer's clinic in Vienna and later in Uppsala, systematized clinical vestibular studies, with his introduction of the rotational and caloric tests (1906). One should recall, however, that the first scientific observations of nystagmus and vertigo in response to rotation and to galvanic stimulation had been made long before in Prague by Johannes Evangelista Purkinje (1787–1869), who reported them in the 1820s. [For a more extensive chronicle of pioneer explorations of the vestibular system, see the books of Bast and Anson (7), Camis and Creed (13), or Politzer, all of whom give references to the articles mentioned above.]

THE CENTURY TO COME

Professional historians are not often given to prophecy, but an amateur may be forgiven a clouded and presbyopic glance into the future. It seems reasonable to suppose that important lessons will be gained from studying the effects of electrical stimulation of the auditory system in deaf patients with cochlear implants. Obviously, we still have much to learn about the handling of complex auditory information by the CNS, for most of us have for too long confined ourselves to the periphery, and single unit responses at any level, instructive and essential as they are, can tell us only so much. As in the past, progress in auditory physiology will follow and depend on technical advances in many other fields. Those in neurochemistry should continue to make vital contributions to our understanding of auditory function, and should eventually help us to solve the riddle of the transduction processes of the inner ear. In this connection it may not be amiss to keep a watchful eye on progress in the field of vision. As for cochlear mechanics, it has long seemed passing strange to this observer that the cochlear hair cells should be stimulated by motion of their substratum, whereas the vestibular hair cells are undoubtedly stimulated by motion of their suprastructures. The difference may indeed be real, but one suspects that sooner or later we may become convinced that in the cochlea the *primum mobile* is the *membrana tectoria* and not the *membrana basilaris,* and that our "theory of hearing" may once more be in need of revision.

ACKNOWLEDGMENTS

The author acknowledges with gratitude his indebtedness to the staffs of the various libraries where he has had the privilege of reading relevant portions of the original publications of many of the early anatomists and other contributors to auditory physiology mentioned in the text. In addition to the Taubman Medical Library and the Harlan Hatcher Graduate Library of the University of Michigan, they include the Biblioteca Nazionale Centrale and the Biblioteca Laurenziana, Florence; the Biblioteca Universitaria, Bologna; the Bodleian Library and the Worcester College Library, Oxford.

REFERENCES[3]

1. Aristotle. *De Anima* (Transl., R. D. Hicks). Arno Press, New York, 1976.
2. Aristotle. *De Sensu and De Memoria* (Transl., G. R. T. Ross). University Press, Cambridge, 1906.
3. Aristotle. *Historia Animalium* (Transl., A. L. Peck). Harvard University Press, Cambridge, MA, 1965.
4. Aristotle. *Les Problèmes d'Aristote* (Transl., J. Barthelémy-Saint Hilaire). 2 vols. Hachette, Paris, 1891.
5. Aristotle. *Traités des Parties des Animaux* (Transl., J. Barthelémy Saint-Hilaire). vol. 1, Hachette, Paris, 1885.
6. Bacon, F. Natural History; Sylva sylvarum. In: *The Works of Francis Bacon,* Vols. III and IV. London, 1730.
7. Bast, T. H., and Anson, B. J. *The Temporal Bone and the Ear.* C. C. Thomas, Springfield, IL, 1949.
8. Békésy, G. von. *Experiments in Hearing* (Transl., ed., E. G. Wever). McGraw-Hill, New York, 1960.
9. Berengario da Carpi, J. *Anatomia: Carpi commentaria cum amplissimis additionibus super anatomia mundini.* Bononiae, 1521.
10. Breasted, J. H. *The Edwin Smith Surgical Papyrus.* 2 vols. University of Chicago Press, Chicago, 1930.
11. Breschet, G. Recherches anatomiques et physiologiques sur l'organe de l'ouïe et sur l'audition, dans l'homme et les animaux vertébrés. *Mémoires, Académie de Médecine, Paris,* 5:229–524, 1836.
12. Burckhardt, J. C. *Die Cultur der Renaissance in Italien.* 2 vols. E. A. Seemann, Leipzig, 1901; Phaidon-Verlag, Wien, 1934.
13. Camis, M., and Creed, R. S. *Physiology of the Vestibular Apparatus.* Clarendon Press, Oxford, 1930.
14. Capparoni, P. *Profili Bio-bibliografici di Medici e Naturalisti Celebri Italiani dal Sec. XVo al Sec. XVIIIo.* 2 vols. Instituto Naz. Medico Farmacologico "Serono." Roma, 1928 and 1932.
15. Casseri, G. *De vocis auditusque organis historia anatomica.* V. Baldinus, Ferrariae, 1601.
16. Castiglioni, A. *Histoire de la Médecine* (Trad., J. Bertrand et F. Gidon). Payot, Paris, 1931.
17. Celsus, A. *Medicinae: Libri octo ex recensione Leonardi Targae* (Ed., E. Milligan). Maclachlan et Stewart, Edinburgi, 1831.
18. Corti, A. Recherches sur l'organe de l'ouïe des mammifères. *Ztschr. wiss. Zool.,* 3:109–169, 1851.
19. Cotugno, D. *De aquaeductibus auris humanae internae anatomica dissertatio.* Typographia Sanctae Thomae Aquinatis, Neapoli et Bononiae, 1775.

---

[3]Citations of individual articles published within the past century or so are generally omitted from the References, since they are to be found in the more recent works cited there, including among others those of Bast and Anson, Camis and Creed, Stevens and Davis, Wever, and Wever and Lawrence.

20. Curto, S. *Medicina e Medici nell'Antico Egitto*. Fratelli Pozzo, Torino, 1972.
21. Dawson, W. W., and Enoch, J. M. *Foundations of Sensory Science*. Springer Verlag, Berlin, Heidelberg, 1984.
22. Duverney, J. G. *Traité de l'organe de l'ouïe, contenant la structure, les usages, et les maladies de toutes les parties de l'oreille*. E. Michallet, Paris, 1683.
23. Ebers, G. *Papyros Ebers: Das hermetische Buch über die Arzeneimittel der alten Ägypter, in hieratischer Schrift*. 2 vols. W. Engelmann, Leipzig, 1875.
24. Eustachi, B. Epistola de auditus organis. In: *Opuscula Anatomica*. V. Luchinus, Venetiis, 1564.
25. Fabrizi, G. *Opera omnia anatomica & physiologica. De aure, auditus organo; De formato foetu*. Gleditschius, Lipsiae, 1687.
26. Falloppia, G. De morbo Gallico. In: *Gabrielis Falloppii Mutinensis Opera Omnia*. A. Wechel, Francofurti, 1600.
27. Falloppia, G. *Observationes anatomicae*. M. A. Ulmus, Venetiis, 1562.
28. Favaro, G. *Gabriele Falloppio, Modense*. Modena, 1928.
29. Fioretti, A., and Concato, G. Problemi di storia dell'anatomia dell'orecchio. Nota I: É individuabile lo scopritore dell'incudine e del martello? *Acta medicae historiae Patavina*, 3:47–91, 1956–57.
30. Fioretti, A., and Concato, G. Problemi di storia dell'anatomia dell'orecchio. Nota II: Polemiche cinquecentesche intorno alla scoperta della staffa. *Acta medicae historiae Patavina*, 4:59–120, 1957–58.
31. Flourens, M. J. P. Expériences sur les canaux semi-circulaires de l'oreille dans les oiseaux. *Mém. Acad. Roy. Sci. Paris*, 9:455–466, 1830 (cit., Camis and Creed).
32. Galen. De usu partium corporis humani. In: *Omnia Cl. Galeni Opera*. Froben, Basileae, 1542.
33. Gomperz, T. *Griechische Denker. Eine Geschichte der antiken Philosophie*. 3 vols. Veit, Leipzig, 1896.
34. Helmholtz, H. L. F. *Die Lehre von den Tonempfindungen als physiologische Grundlage für die Theorie der Musik*. F. Vieweg, Braunschweig, 1877.
35. Helmholtz, H. Die Mechanik der Gehörknöchelchen und des Trommelfells. *Pflügers Arch.*, 1:1–60, 1868.
36. Holl, M. Die Anatomie des Leonardo da Vinci. *Arch. Anat. Physiol.*, 1905, 177–262.
37. Lind, L. R. *Studies in Pre-Vesalian Anatomy: Biography, Translations, Documents*. American Philosophical Society, Philadelphia, 1975.
38. Mann, T. *Dr. Faustus. Das Leben des deutschen Tonsetzers Adrian Leverkühn, erzählt von einem Freunde*. Bermann-Fischer, Stockholm, 1948.
39. McMurrich, J. P. *Leonardo da Vinci the Anatomist (1452–1519)*. Carnegie Institution of Washington and Williams & Wilkins, Baltimore, 1930.
40. Morgagni, J. B. *The Seats and Causes of Diseases, Investigated by Anatomy* (Transl., B. Alexander, M.D.). Facsimile of the London, 1769 edition. New York Academy of Medicine, Hafner, New York, 1960.
41. O'Malley, C. D. *Andreas Vesalius of Brussels, 1514–1564*. University of California Press, Berkeley, 1964.
42. O'Malley, C. D., and Clarke, E. The discovery of the auditory ossicles. *Bull. Hist. Med.*, 35:419–441, 1961.
43. Pirsig, W., and Ulrich, R. Karl Wittmaack: His life, temporal bone collection, and publications. On the 100th anniversary of his birth. *Arch. Oto-Rhino-Laryng.*, 217:247–262, 1977.
44. Plato. *Spätdialoge: Philebos, Parmenides, Timaios, Kritias* (Übertr. R. Rufener). Artemis, Zurich, 1965.
45. Plutarch[4]. *Scripta Moralia: De Placitis Philosophorum* (Ed., F. Dübner). Firmin-Didot, Paris, 1890.
46. Politzer, A. *Geschichte der Ohrenheilkunde*. 2 vols. F. Enke, Stuttgart, 1907.
47. Retzius, G. *Das Gehörorgan der Wirbelthiere*. 2 vols. Samson & Wallin, Stockholm, 1881, 1884.
48. Retzius, G. Die Gestalt des membranösen Gehörorgans des Menschen. *Biol. Untersuch.*, 2:1–32, 1882.
49. Robinson, V. Chronology of Otology. *Bull. Hist. Med.*, 10:199–208, 1941.
50. Robinson, V. Examination in the history of otology. *Laryngoscope*, 51:315–329, 1941.
51. Sarton, G. *Galen of Pergamon*. University of Kansas Press, Lawrence, 1954.
52. Scarpa, A. Delle parti molli del laberinto umano. In: *Opere del Cav. Antonio Scarpa* (Ed., D. P. Vannoni). Tip. della Speranza, Firenze, 1836.

---

[4]The author of the De Placitis Philosophorum, sometimes referred to as "Pseudoplutarch" (Werner), is now thought to have been the less known Aetius of Armida (Mesopotamia), who studied at Alexandria and served as court physician to the Byzantine Emperor Justinian in the 6th century A.D., rather than the philosopher-biographer Plutarch, who flourished in the earlier years of the Roman Empire (ca. 46–120 A.D.).

53. Stevens, S. S., and Davis, H. *Hearing: Its Psychology and Physiology*. John Wiley & Sons, New York, 1938.
54. Stevenson, R. S., and Guthrie, D. *History of Oto-laryngology*. E. and S. Livingstone, Edinburgh, 1949.
55. Theophrastus. Deperditorum scriptorum excerpta et fragmenta: De sensu et sensibilibus. In: *Theophrasti Eresii Opera, Quae Supersunt, Omnia* (Ed., F. Wimmer, pp. 321–340). Firmin-Didot, Paris, 1931.
56. Valsalva, A. M. *Tractatus de aure humana*. F. Pitteri, Venetiis, 1740.
57. Vasari, G. *Le Vite de'piú eccellenti pittori, scultori et architettori*. 3 vols. Giunti, Fiorenza, 1568; repr., Batelli, Firenze, 1948.
58. Vasari, G. *Lives of the Artists* (Transl., G. Bull). Penguin Books, Harmondsworth, Middx., 1965.
59. Vesalius, A. *De humani corporis fabrica*. I. Oporinus, Basileae, 1543.
60. Werner, H. Antike Ohranatomie und Gehörsphysiologie. *Arch. Gesch. Med.,* 18:151–171, 1926.
61. Wever, E. G. *Theory of Hearing*. Constable, London, 1949; Dover, New York, 1970.
62. Wever, E. G., and Lawrence, M. *Physiological Acoustics*. Princeton University Press, Princeton, 1954.
63. Willis, T. Cerebri anatome; De anima brutorum. In: *Opera omnia*. S. de Tournes, Genevae, 1680.

Physiology of the Ear,
edited by A. F. Jahn and J. Santos-Sacchi.
Raven Press, New York © 1988.

The External Ear

Juergen Tonndorf

Bronx, New York 10471

Interest in the auditory function of the ear was initially focused mainly on middle and inner ears. The role of pinna and external canal was treated rather briefly, mostly with reference to problems of binaural, directional hearing. Information was derived chiefly from theoretical concepts (7). The function of the ear canal from the psychoacoustic and physiological standpoints was first studied by von Békésy (2) when he calculated the difference between sound pressure in a free field (i.e., in a situation in which there are no obstacles or walls present) and that acting on the tympanic membrane. The first experimental study dealing with this problem was that of Wiener and Ross (14). Later more detailed studies were carried out by Shaw and his group (8). Zwislocki (16) determined the impedance of the ear canal before designing his ear-like coupler for earphone calibration. This chapter relies largely on these sources. A more extensive bibliography is available for interested readers in the paper by Shaw (8).

ANATOMY OF PINNA AND EAR CANAL

The external ears, or pinnae, protrude from each side of the head, around the entrances of the external ear canals. In humans, the two pinnae are nearly symmetrical in size and shape. (In one species of owls the right pinna is much larger than the left.) The shape of the pinna is determined by its cartilaginous frame, which gives it some rigidity. The skin and underlying tissues are quite firmly attached to the cartilage. Only the earlobe is free of it. Figure 1 gives a lateral view of the left pinna showing and naming its various parts, mainly the helix, the fossa of the helix, the antihelix, the earlobe; the crus of the helix; the tragus and antitragus demarcate the concha, which leads directly into the ear canal. The border between concha and ear canal is not sharply delineated; one reason why, as Shaw (8) remarked, the measured length of the canal varies slightly from author to author. (There are of course also some small individual variations in the same way as there are large and small pinnae.) The ear canal is approximately 2.5 cm long and its lumen has an average diameter of approximately 0.7 cm (Fig. 2). In the lateral one-third, the walls consist of several quasi-independent pieces of cartilage, separated by the fissures of Santorini, which lend it some flexibility. The medial two-thirds are formed by the tympanic portion of the temporal bone, which is a tube, open at the top, but firmly fused to the squamous portion that closes it off, thus completing the tube. Hence, the osseous ear canal lies at the base of the skull.

Medially, the ear canal terminates at the tympanic membrane. The membrane is

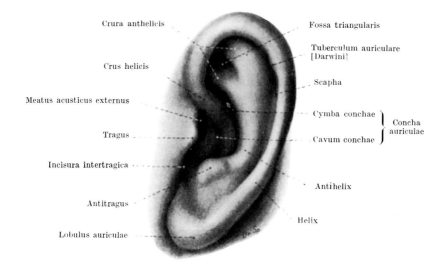

FIG. 1. Left pinna with its various parts labeled. (From ref. 3.)

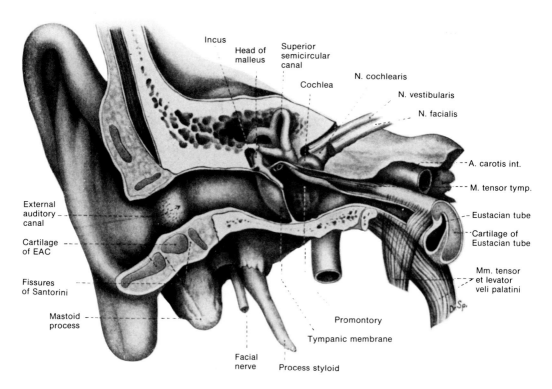

FIG. 2. Frontal view of a cross section through the right ear. Pinna and ear canal are shown in some detail. Note the elevation of the canal floor where the capitulum of the lower jaw protrudes (although the latter is not shown). (From ref. 3.)

inclined from superior-lateral to inferior-medial, more in small children, where it lies almost horizontal, and less in adults. Moreover, its flared cone shape makes its position rather complex.

Although there is ample, mobile layer of subdermal tissue in the outer portion of the ear canal, the skin of the medial portion adheres directly to the periosteum subdermal tissue intervening; this makes it immobile but quite sensitive to the touch. A branch of the vagus nerve supplying this area is responsible for the cough reflex elicited when the osseous wall is touched.

TRANSFORMATION OF SOUNDS FROM A FREE-FIELD SITUATION TO A POSITION IN FRONT OF THE TYMPANIC MEMBRANE

Sound pressure existing in a free field is transformed in several steps on its way to the ear drum. The listener's torso, head, and external ear represent a series of acoustic baffles, barriers, and resonators that significantly modify the sound prior to its impact on the tympanic membrane. Without analyzing these in a qualitative and quantitative manner, one cannot predict the sound pressure acting on the tympanic membrane from free-field measurements.

Effects of Torso and Head

It is not only the ear canal that affects the transformation of sound pressure impinging on the head. The torso, i.e., mainly shoulders and neck, tends to absorb some sound energy, more so when heavy clothing is worn and less so when clothing is light or absent. Even in the latter case there is some interference between the direct wave incident on the ear and that reflected from the shoulder (15). The effect also varies with the angle of impact and frequency.

For frequencies the head can, in first approximation (below approximately 1 kHz), be considered a somewhat hard-walled sphere, a notion that goes back to Lord Rayleigh (7). Based on this concept, Stewart (11) derived interaural phase differences and interaural pressure differences that were valid and quite accurate below 1 kHz. Figure 3 shows that, in order to reach the ear that lies on the offside of the head (on the right in Fig. 3), the sound has to travel farther than to the nearer ear. The difference in distance of travel (d) depends on the diameter of the head (a) and the azimuthal angle (θ), the angle between the midplane of the head, a midplane of the head (A *to* A'), and the direction of the incident wave: $d = a\sin\theta + a\theta$. The associated interaural time difference t is given as $t = d/c = (a/c)(\sin\theta + \theta)$ (c being the velocity of sound in air, i.e., approximately 340 m/sec). The actual shape of the head and signal frequency have virtually no effect. Based on this information, Feddersen et al. calculated the interaural time differences for various azimuthal angles (Fig. 4). Shaw (8) gave a composite figure (Fig. 5) for calculated interaural phase differences, using data from several authors.

Binaural, Directional Hearing

When sounds arrive at the two ears, they are fused into a single image. However, when there is an interaural time difference, low-frequency sounds appear to be lo-

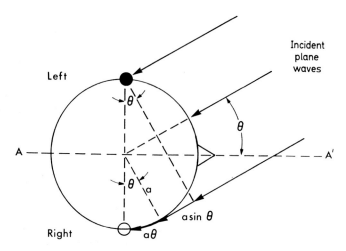

FIG. 3. Top view of the head (schematic) with sound impinging from the left. The sound clearly has to travel farther to the right ear than to the left one. (From ref. 8.)

cated on the side of the earlier arrival, the more so the larger the difference. The common image then appears localized to that side. Whereas low frequencies are bent around the head, high frequencies are attenuated at the offside ear, because the head provides a shadow for that ear, shielding it from sound waves originating on the contralateral side. The resulting interaural intensity difference provides an important clue for localization of high frequencies. This is known as the duplex theory that was first formulated by Lord Rayleigh (6). The closer the sound source is to the head, the more pronounced the head-shadow effect becomes. The separation of the effects of time and intensity differences is given by the ratio of wavelength/diameter of the head. It lies in the frequency region between 1.5 and 3.0 kHz. When

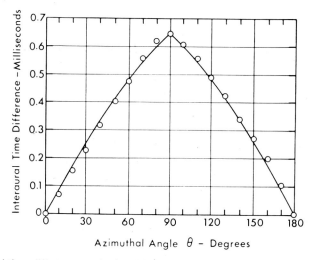

FIG. 4. Interaural time differences calculated for a spherical head with a diameter of 17.5 cm as a function of the azimuthal angle of the incident (plane) sound wave (After ref. 8.)

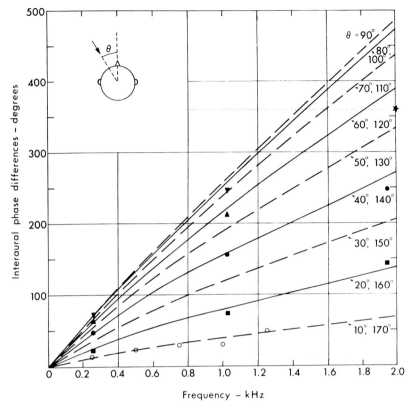

FIG. 5. Interaural phase differences calculated for a spherical head with a diameter of 17.5 cm. Actual data from various authors. Phases are ambiguous when differences are larger than 360°. (From ref. 8.)

one listens under earphones, time or intensity differences may determine the outcome, now called lateralization, because the source is reported close to the head or even within it. The reader who wishes more detailed information on directional hearing is referred to appropriate texts, e.g., Green (4).

Effects of Pinna, Concha, and Ear Canal

The ear canal itself can be considered a small sound-pressure detector located on the surface of a hard sphere (11). This situation affects the gain (or loss) of sound pressure at the ear from that in the free field, depending mainly on the angle of incidence but also on the diameter of the head (Fig. 6).

Figure 7 shows the average gain (or loss) produced by the various structures of the ear as well as the effects of torso and neck already mentioned, for an angle of incidence of 45° in the horizontal plane. At this angle the total pressure gain happens to be largest between 2 kHz and 5 kHz.

The gain produced by the pinna is not very large, approximately 3 dB at 4 kHz. Because of its shape, the effect of the pinna varies considerably with the angle of

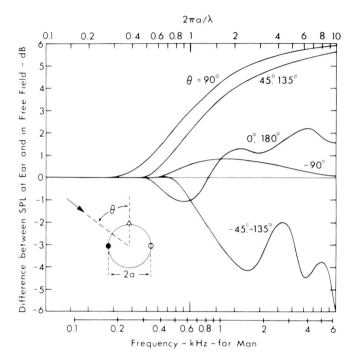

FIG. 6. Transformation of sound-pressure levels (calculated) from free field to an ear assumed to be a point receiver on the surface of a hard spherical head of radius *a* for various azimuthal angles of the incident wave. The frequency scale at the bottom is for a sphere of radius *a* = 8.75 cm. (From ref. 8.)

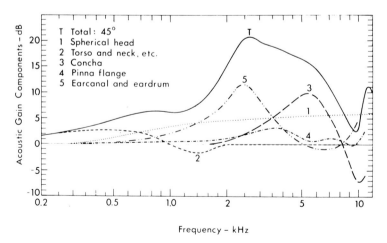

FIG. 7. Sound-pressure gain (or loss) induced by various components of the human ear (averages) for an azimuthal angle of 45°. (From ref. 8.)

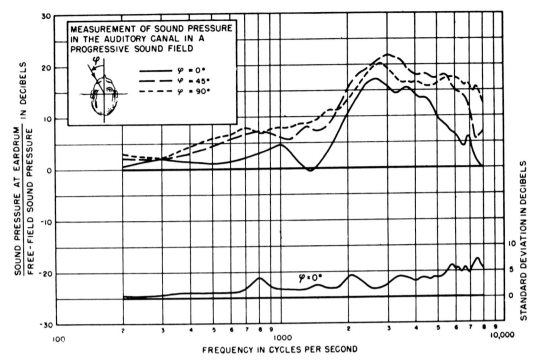

FIG. 8. Sound-pressure gain in front of the tympanic membrane in a progressive sound field for three azimuthal angles as shown. Results of actual measurements. (From ref. 14.)

incidence of the sound. The concha produces a gain of approximately 10 dB at 4 kHz to 5 kHz, but a loss of approximately 5 dB at 10 kHz (10,15).

The ear canal represents a tube open at one end and closed at the other. Therefore, when its length is 2.5 cm, it has a first resonance of approximately 2.6 kHz. However, its acoustic behavior at higher frequencies is not that easily accounted for. At these short wavelengths, transversal resonance modes come into play. Consequently, for frequencies greater than approximately 16 kHz, there is no longer a uniform wavefront at the tympanic membrane, but the sound pressure varies by as much as 10 dB to 15 dB for small lateral distances, i.e., sometimes fractions of a millimeter. For this reason, precalibrated earphones cannot be used at these high frequencies. Even measurements at one spot taken by a probe microphone located in front of the tympanic membrane, which are quite helpful at frequencies between approximately 6 kHz to 15 kHz to compensate for uncertainties in earphone calibration, have little if any use. One would have to take readings at at least six different places and integrate them, a virtual impossibility at present (12).

Figure 7 shows that the effects of concha and ear canal plus tympanic membrane complement each other in that they broaden the gain between 2 kHz and 5 kHz, a region important for speech perception. The total gain from combining all components is approximately 20 dB at 2.5 kHz. There is a rather broad maximum between 2 kHz and 5 kHz, as previously mentioned.

Figure 8 presents some older data of Wiener and Ross (4), since they show the effect of three different angles of incidence, the gain for a 45° angle being once more the largest.

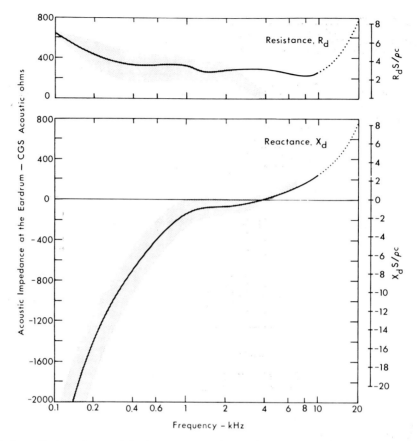

FIG. 9. Acoustic impedance of the human tympanic membrane, separated as its resistance and reactance components, based on data of various authors. (From ref. 8.)

The pronounced gain for the high frequencies shown in Figs. 6 and 7 has a consequence for the hearing loss occurring after noise exposure. Tonndorf and Cajazzo (*unpublished data*) argued as follows: Postexposure losses are always maximal, approximately $\frac{1}{2}$ octave above the exposure frequency. Therefore, when the frequency of 2.6 kHz is elevated because of the canal resonance and exposure is sufficiently strong, the maximal induced loss must be expected to occur at about 4 kHz, corresponding the well-known 4-kHz notch. The authors were able to prove their contention by doubling the length of the ear canal. The resonance point shifted downward to half its value and with it the point of maximal loss.

Impedance of the Tympanic Membrane

The impedance of the tympanic membrane was first determined by Tröger (13) and later on by several others, among them Zwislocki and Møller (5). Figure 9, originally published by Shaw (8), combines data from six different authors. The impedance is given separately in terms of its resistance and reactance components.

Definition of the Acoustic Input

It would be desirable to define the acoustic input, e.g., that at the auditory threshold, in terms of the sound power acting on the tympanic membrane. Although the sound pressure at this point can be easily and accurately measured with the aid of probe microphones, to determine the power one would also need the exact values of the tympanic membrane impedance, i.e., the reactance and resistance; but these values vary somewhat from the average given in Fig. 9, and their measurement in individual cases is time-consuming to say the least. [Consult textbooks on audition, e.g., Green (4), for currently accepted audiometric reference values, their determinations in free-field situations or under earphones, and the pitfalls of such measurements, some of which have to do with the position of the tympanic membrane at the end of the ear canal.]

Noise in Enclosed Ears

Everyone who has ever held a large sea shell or other such cavity close to his/her ear heard a noise. The same phenomenon is observed when an ear is covered by an earphone. These noises have been repeatedly measured [e.g., Shaw and Piercy (9)]. Their spectrum decreases with frequency and their magnitude becomes higher the larger the air volume enclosed under the cushion. The masking produced by this noise on low-level signals at or near the auditory threshold has been determined (8).

The origin of this noise is not quite clear. A vascular origin, as assumed by several authors, e.g., Shaw (8), is not very likely, because the noise does not pulsate. The needed clue may be provided by the previously mentioned fact, i.e., the noise becomes more intense the larger the air volume enclosed under the cushion. Furthermore, the 200-cc chamber, recommended by von Békésy (1) to minimize the occlusion effect in bone-conduction testing, produces, in the experience of this writer, an even higher noise level than that existing under earphone cushions. This author therefore suggests that the noise represents the Brownian movement of the enclosed air molecules.

Earphone Calibration Couplers

Earphones employed in audiometry are usually precalibrated. Probe microphones inserted into the ear canal, with their tips located in front of the tympanic membrane, provide of course more accurate calibration at all audiometric test frequencies. This would take care of individual variations and also give more precise results at frequencies from 6 kHz to 15 kHz, where precalibration is not too reliable. However, most audiologists probably do not have the necessary skill to insert the probes safely, and the cost is at present still too high, although widespread use would probably lower it. Therefore, the use of precalibrated earphones is currently the method of choice. The calibrator consists of a microphone that is coupled to the earphone in question by means of a specially designed device.

The simplest case, although not representing the oldest attempt of its kind, is that of a coupler for insert earphones. In that instance, the impedance the earphone faces is essentially that of the tympanic membrane (see Fig. 9), plus that of an air volume

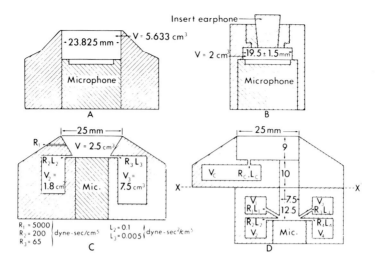

FIG. 10. Schematic cross sections through various couplers used for earphone calibration. Dimensions as shown. The resistances (R) and masses (L) are specified. The Zwislocki coupler (D) may either be used in its entirety for supra-aural earphones or its lower portion only for insert earphones. (After ref. 8.)

of about 2 cc, thought to represent the space between the insert and the membrane and its effective impedance. Recent measurements have shown that this cavity is actually approximately 0.8 cc too large, since the earphone occupies a considerable portion of the ear canal. Figure 10B shows the coupler currently in use, the HA 1 coupler, approved by the American Standards Institute (ANSI).

Couplers to be employed with supra-aural earphones, equipped, for instance, with an MX-41 cushion, are less reliable because the cushion compresses the pinna in an unpredictable manner, thus altering the enclosed air volume by an unknown amount. A coupler for that purpose, the National Bureau of Standards type 9(A), has already been in use for a fairly long time. The cavity volume of the current version is approximately 5.7 cc, again to match the effective volume of the ear canal and of the cavities formed by the pinna. It is once more approved by ANSI and is shown in Fig. 10A.

The least reliable coupler by definition is that designed for use with circumaural earphones, since one cannot, at present, determine how much of the enclosed volume is occupied by the pinna. The currently used version, approved by the IEC, the appropriate international standards organization, is presented in Fig. 10C.

Many years of use showed that the 9(A) coupler gives results that do not conform well to the performance of real ears, Zwislocki undertook a series of measurements (16–18) to determine once more the acoustic properties of real ears and then proceeded to design his ear-like coupler (Fig. 10D). Its performance is much superior to that of previous designs, although it represents the impedance of an *average* ear; real ears may still deviate from its performance, which is a slight but unavoidable shortcoming. For scientific purposes, the use of probe microphones is much preferred. Figure 10 gives schematic presentations of the various couplers. Readers who wish more detailed technical information, e.g., the numerical values of the various resistances (R) or masses (L) are referred to the appropriate technical literature cited in Shaw (8).

REFERENCES

1. Békésy, G. von (1932a): Zur Theorie des Hörens bei der Schallaufnahme durch Knochenleitung. *Ann. Phys.*, 13:111–136.
2. Békésy, G. von (1932b): Ueber den Einfluss der durch den Kopf und den Gehörgang bedingten Schallfeldverzerrungen auf die Hörschwelle. *Ann. Phys.*, 14:51–58.
3. Falk, P. (1943): *Einführung in die Hals-Nasen-Ohren-Heilkunde*. Thieme, Leipzig.
4. Green, D. M. (1976): *An Introduction to Hearing*. Lawrence Erlbaum Associates, Hillsdale, NJ.
5. Møller, A. R. (1960): Improved technique for detailed measurements of middle ear impedance. *J. Acoust. Soc. Am.*, 32:250 (abstract).
6. Rayleigh, Lord (J. W. Strutt) (1888): *The Theory of Sound*, vol. 2, pp. 440–443. (reprint) Dover, New York, 1945.
7. Rayleigh, Lord (J. W. Strutt) (1876): Our perception of the direction of a sound source. *Nature*, 14:32–33.
8. Shaw, E. A. G. (1974): The external ear. In: *Handbook of Sensory Physiology*, vol. V/1, edited by W. D. Keidel and W. D. Neff. Springer, Berlin.
9. Shaw, E. A. G., and Piercy, J. E. (1962): Physiological noise in relation to audiometry. *J. Acoust. Soc. Am.*, 34:745 (abstract).
10. Shaw, E. A. G., and Teranishi, R. (1968): Sound pressure generated in an external ear replica and real human ears by a nearby point-source. *J. Acoust. Soc. Am.*, 44:240–249.
11. Stewart, G. W. (1914): Phase relations in the acoustic shadow of a rigid sphere; phase difference at the ears. *Physiol. Rev.*, 4:252–258.
12. Tonndorf, J., and Kurman, B. (1984): High-frequency Audiometry. *Ann. Otolaryngol.*, 93:576–582.
13. Tröger, J. (1930): Die Schallaufnahme durch das äussere Ohr. *Phys. Z.*, 31:26–47.
14. Wiener, F. M., and Ross, D. A. (1946): The pressure distribution in the auditory canal in a progressive sound field. *J. Acoust. Soc. Am.*, 18:401–408.
15. Yamagushi, Z., and Sushi, N. (1956): Real ear response of receivers. *J. Acoust. Soc. Am. (Japan)*, 12:8–13.
16. Zwislocki, J. J. (1970): An acoustic coupler for earphone calibration. Special Report LCS-S-7, Syracuse University, Syracuse, New York.
17. Zwislocki, J. J. (1971): Ear-like coupler for earphone calibration. *J. Acoust. Soc. Am.*, 50:110 (abstract).
18. Zwislocki, J. J. (1971): An ear-like coupler for earphone calibration. Special Report LSC-S-9, Syracuse University, Syracuse, New York.

Physiology of the Ear,
edited by A. F. Jahn and J. Santos-Sacchi.
Raven Press, New York © 1988.

The Nonauditory Physiology of the External Ear Canal

*Alan Johnson and **Michael Hawke

*Department of Otolaryngology, Queen Elizabeth Hospital, and Birmingham and Midland Ear and Throat Hospital, and University of Birmingham, Birmingham, B15 2TH, England; and **Department of Otolaryngology, and Temporal Bone Histopathology Laboratory, University of Toronto, Toronto, Ontario, Canada M5G 1L5*

FUNCTIONS OF THE EXTERNAL EAR CANAL

The external ear canal carries out two different physiological functions: these are referred to as auditory and nonauditory functions. The auditory function of the external ear canal allows efficient sound transmission from the environment to the tympanic membrane. The acoustic or auditory functions of the canal are considered elsewhere in this volume. The nonauditory functions of the canal are the protection of the tympanic membrane and deeper structures from injury and the maintenance of a clear passage through which sound can be conducted to the tympanic membrane.

The protective function of the external ear canal is related to its anatomical structure. The shape and depth of the external canal and the rigidity of its walls provide some protection to the tympanic membrane from direct injury. The deeper, narrower, and more tortuous the canal, the less chance there will be for direct injury to the tympanic membrane and underlying middle ear structures.

The self-cleansing function of the canal prevents the accumulation of debris within the lumen (which would prevent the transmission of sound down the air column of the external canal). This function of keeping the canal free of debris may appear relatively simple at first glance; however, when considered more closely there are significant technical problems that must be solved in the self-cleansing of a blind-ended, skin-lined canal that opens onto the side of the head. The tympanic membrane, which is situated at the "blind" or medial end of the canal, must remain thin in order to vibrate efficiently when stimulated by sound waves, and at the same time the lateral surface of the tympanic membrane must be covered with a thin layer of epidermis (skin) to remain exposed to the external atmosphere.

This epidermal covering provides a barrier that protects the underlying tissues from the potentially harmful effects of the surrounding environment, i.e., drying, wetting, abrasion, chemical damage, or bacterial invasion. This protective function is provided by the most superficial epidermal layer, the stratum corneum. The stratum corneum consists of layers of dead keratinocytes that constitute a relatively impervious but flexible surface layer. Because the cells of the stratum corneum have terminally differentiated, they are incapable of either self-regeneration or repair. The integrity of the stratum corneum must therefore be maintained by the continuous production of keratinocytes from those cells in the deeper layers of the epidermis that have not yet terminally differentiated, i.e., the cells of the stratum basale and stratum spinosum. These replacement cells that arise in the stratum basale undergo differentiation as they rise through stratum granulosum. At the upper layer of the stratum granulosum, these rising cells undergo terminal differentiation into keratinocytes joining the deepest layer of the stratum corneum. When the keratinocytes reach the upper surface of the stratum corneum they are continuously shed from the surface of the body. This process is known as desquamation.

The thickness of the epidermis is relatively constant over most of the body, measuring 75 to 150 μm; however, the relatively thicker epidermis (thick skin) covering the soles of the feet or the palms of the hands must withstand much pressure and friction and measures between 400 and 600 μm. Mechanisms exist within the epidermis that produce an increase in the mitotic rate of the deeper layers if the stratum corneum is removed at an increased rate, so that the production of keratinocytes is regulated to maintain an adequately thick outer protective barrier (the stratum corneum). Mechanisms also exist within the skin that allow for the rapid regeneration or repair of wounded stratum corneum.

The epidermis lining the external ear canal is in a unique situation; because of its location, the epidermis is not subject to the usual surface contact (friction) that normally removes those keratinocytes that have desquamated from the surface of the stratum corneum elsewhere in the body, i.e., the keratinocyte debris that results from the continuous movement of epidermal cells from the stratum basale upwards. This means that an alternative mechanism for the removal of the superficial layer of stratum corneum of the tympanic membrane and the protected (deep) portion of the ear canal must exist. If such a mechanism did not exist, the lumen of the canal would gradually become occluded by keratin debris, and the transmission of sound would be impaired.

If viewed in teleologic terms, as land animals evolved deeper external ear canals for the protection of the tympanic membrane, they simultaneously had to develop a self-cleansing mechanism to keep the canal free of debris (a deaf animal would not be able to compete successfully for food and self-protection). The mechanism that developed was that of epithelial migration. Epithelial migration is a unique physiological response to the problems produced by a unique anatomical situation.

The external ear canal is also protected by the arrangement of hairs and the production of wax within the outer (cartilaginous) portion. The hairs and ceruminous glands assist in preventing foreign bodies, alive or dead, from entering the ear canal, and they also play an important role in assisting the process of desquamation and skin migration out of the ear canal.

ANATOMY OF THE EXTERNAL EAR CANAL (4,35,41,47,53)

The adult human external ear canal consists of an outer cartilaginous third and an inner osseous or bony two-thirds. As with all anatomical features, there is a considerable variation between individuals in the actual dimensions of the external ear canal. The distance from the annulus of the tympanic membrane to the anterior lip of the concha is about 25 mm. The canal runs mainly medially, but the cartilaginous part is inclined slightly posterosuperiorly and the bony part is inclined anteroinferiorly; as a result the axis follows a lazy S-shaped course. The narrowest portion of the canal is the isthmus, which is located about 6 mm lateral to the tympanic annulus. When viewed in cross section, the canal displays an elliptical shape. These variations in both the direction of the axis and the caliber of the canal serve to increase the protection afforded to the tympanic membrane.

The outer or cartilaginous portion of the canal can be straightened if the examiner retracts the pinna gently in a posterosuperior direction (posteriorly in children). This maneuver pulls the anterior rim of the concha backwards to reveal the deep or bony canal. A posterior bulging of the anterior medial wall of the bony canal is frequently encountered. This prominent bulge may obscure the anterior portion of the tympanic membrane and the anterior recess of the canal, making access difficult during cleansing or reconstructive surgery.

The outer cartilaginous canal is surrounded by an incomplete cylinder of elastic cartilage, which is continuous at its lateral end with the conchal cartilage. This surrounding cylinder of cartilage is deficient superiorly and posteriorly, where the gap is bridged by dense fibrous tissue that is also attached to the squamous temporal bone.

There are two fissures in the cartilage of the canal; the incisures of the cartilaginous meatus or the fissures of Santorini, which are located anteroinferiorly. These fissures provide a path for infection or neoplasm to spread between the parotid gland and the external ear canal. The medial end of the cartilage is firmly attached to the lateral lip of the bony part of the canal. Both the epidermis and dermis of the skin covering this part of the canal are thick (providing a significant degree of protection from trauma), and within the dermis there are numerous hair follicles and sebaceous and ceruminous glands. The arrangement of these structures is important to their function and is described in detail below.

The inner or bony portion of the external canal is composed of a complete cylinder of bone extending from the junction with cartilage to the tympanic annulus. The tympanic bone forms the anterior and inferior walls and the lower part of the posterior wall. There is sometimes a foramen in its anteroinferior surface (the foramen of Huschke). The remainder is formed by the squamous and mastoid parts of the temporal bone. The medial end of the canal is sealed by the tympanic membrane, a disk of fibrous tissue approximately 9 mm in diameter, which is set obliquely, facing slightly anteriorly and inferiorly. It has two parts, the pars tensa and pars flaccida. Most of the membrane consists of the pars tensa, which is between 30 and 230 μm thick and is tented medially from the annulus to its center by the handle of the malleus. The pars tensa has an inner layer of circumferential fibers and an outer layer of radial fibers, which are not collagen (27,28). At the superior limit of the handle of the malleus is its lateral process, and from this the anterior and posterior mallear folds run to the bony margin of the drum. Above these folds lies the pars flaccida, which, as its name indicates, is not held taut like the rest of the drum, and the fibrous tissue within it does not have the same organized pattern as that of the pars tensa. The medial aspect of the drum is covered by the respiratory mucosa of the middle ear.

The lateral aspect of the tympanic membrane and the bony canal are covered by an extremely thin epidermis, which measures between 15 and 30 μm in depth on conventional histological sections. Over the pars tensa it has three to five layers of cells and over the pars flaccida, five to ten (28). The thickness of the epidermis is not uniform over the pars tensa. The epidermis is thicker over the handle of the malleus and at the annulus, and thinner midway between the umbo (the inferior end of the malleus handle) and the tympanic annulus (37). The dermis is indistinct from the rest of the lamina propria in the pars flaccida, but in the pars tensa its depth is similar to that of the epidermis.

During surgical procedures that involve raising flaps of skin and soft tissue including periosteum off the canal wall, it is apparent that the connective tissue layer is thicker over the pars flaccida and the posterosuperior part of the bony canal than it is along the floor and anterior wall of the canal. This facilitates dissection posterosuperiorly, whereas on the floor and anterior wall of the canal it is very easy to tear the skin when raising it off the bone.

The blood supply of the superficial portion of the external ear canal is derived from the posterior auricular artery and the auriculotemporal branch of the superficial temporal artery, whereas the deep canal is supplied by the deep auricular branch of the maxillary artery that enters the canal through the squamotympanic fissure. The tympanic membrane also receives blood from its medial aspect, and there is a circular anastomosis at its periphery.

The lymphatic drainage is to the pre-auricular and occipital nodes and then to the upper deep cervical nodes. The sensory innervation of the canal and membrane is derived from the Vth, VIIth, IXth, and Xth cranial nerves. The auricular branch of the vagus (Arnold's nerve), which comes off the superior vagal ganglion, picks up a contribution from the inferior ganglion of the glossopharyngeal nerve, and may also receive a contribution from the facial nerve at or just above the stylomastoid foramen. A branch of Arnold's nerve supplies the posterior part of the canal and the corresponding segment of the tympanic membrane. This nerve enters the external ear canal through the tympanomastoid suture. Arnold's nerve can be identified during dissection or surgery as it exits from the tympanomastoid suture line, and it can be blocked with local anesthetic injected in this area. The auriculotemporal nerve (which is derived from the mandibular division of the Vth cranial nerve) supplies the anterior and superior walls of the external ear canal and the corresponding segments of the tympanic membrane, usually by two branches.

Both unmyelinated and myelinated nerve fibers are found and these are particularly numerous in the pars flaccida. No specialized nerve endings have been identified in the deep canal skin, but the canal is obviously well innervated, as can be seen when it is traumatized. Of current interest in relation to the innervation of the external ear canal is the discovery by Alm et al. (3) that if the skin of the external ear canal in rats is stimulated by friction or cold, an effusion develops in the middle ear not only on the stimulated side but on the contralateral side as well. Nerve fibers have also been identified in association with the ceruminous glands, and these may have a secretomotor function.

The anatomical relations of the external ear canal are the temporomandibular joint (anterior) and the parotid gland (anteriorly and inferiorly), the middle cranial fossa (superiorly), the mastoid air cells (posteriorly), and the tympanic bone (inferior).

Embryology

The external ear canal is derived from the ectoderm of the first branchial groove between the first (mandibular) and second (hyoid) arches. In early fetal life the canal becomes obstructed by a plug of ectodermal cells that resorbs during development, and by birth the epidermis has thinned to adult thickness. In the neonate the tympanic bone and mastoid are not fully developed, so that although the canal is only slightly shorter (20 mm) (41) than in the adult, a larger proportion of the canal is cartilaginous. As a result, the shape of the canal differs from the adult, being more oval, and the tympanic membrane lies in a more horizontal plane, although it is of adult size. As the skull bones grow, the canal gradually assumes the adult shape and dimension.

DETAILED PHYSIOLOGY OF THE EXTERNAL EAR CANAL

Protective Function

The protective function of the canal is achieved in part by its anatomy, and the relevant features of this have already been described. The other features that contribute to the protective function are the arrangement of the hairs in the canal and the secretion of wax. Both of these also have an important role in desquamation of stratum corneum from the deep part of the canal, part of the self-cleansing mechanism.

The Hairs

Hairs are found in the outer cartilaginous part of the external ear canal where they surround the meatus and in the posterosuperior part of the osseous canal as described by Politzer in 1902 (47). If studied closely under an operating microscope or with an otoscope it can be seen that all the hairs point outward so that the ends provide an obstruction to any object small enough to fit down the canal, whether it be animate (such as an insect) or inanimate. The hairs are short, and the most medial hairs lie at a very oblique angle, almost flat, against the canal wall (Figs. 1 and 2), whereas laterally they become more upright and therefore more obstructive to anything entering the canal (22). In males the hairs at the outer end of the canal and over the tragus become thicker and longer as a secondary sexual characteristic. The most lateral hairs guarding the entrance to the ear canal may provide a complete lattice, which is counterproductive since the hairs then prevent the emigrating skin debris from exiting the canal, leaving a mass of keratin squames and cerumen to accumulate within the canal and creating an acoustic barrier.

In addition to the trap-like arrangement of the hairs in the canal, the nature of the surface of individual hairs may contribute to the one-way system in the canal. If the hair surface is viewed under a light or preferably a scanning electron microscope, the overlapping arrangement of the cuticular plates resembles tiles on a roof; this arrangement may facilitate movement from the root toward the tip of the hair but not in the opposite direction (Fig. 3). Although this feature can be seen on the surface of any hair, in the external ear canal it may actually contribute to the one-way (lateral movement) system.

Wax

Wax or cerumen is a combination of desquamated keratinocytes and the secretions from the glands of the superficial part of the external ear canal. Two types of se-

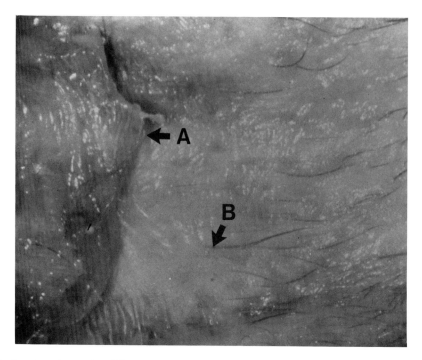

FIG. 1. A cadaveric canal wall illustrating the detaching edge of the stratum corneum (A), and how the most medial canal hairs have been pushed down (B) as the advancing sheet of outwardly migrating stratum corneum is "levered" upwards.

cretory glands are found in the external canal: sebaceous glands, which are closely associated with the hair follicles, and ceruminous glands, which are a type of apocrine gland. There are no conventional eccrine sweat glands in the canal (41). The sebaceous glands are simple or branched alveolar glands, which produce a holocrine (whole cell) fatty secretion of triglycerides and wax esters that empties into the canal at the base of the hair follicles. Sebaceous glands are not capable of active secretion and form their secretion by a passive breakdown of cells. Sebum has slight antibacterial and antifungal properties, as well as a waterproofing effect on the surface of the epithelium (60).

Genetics

The existence of two distinct types of ear wax, wet and dry, was first investigated in Japan (34). The majority of Japanese ($\geq$80%) have dry wax, which is a light gray or brownish gray color and has a dry and flaky consistency. This type of wax has been called "rice bran" ear wax. By contrast, the other type of wax is golden brown, moist, and sticky and is called "honey wax" or wet wax. Investigation of families revealed that wax type is a hereditary dimorphic trait carried by one pair of genes. The wet wax gene is dominant, and wet wax homozygotes and heterozygotes are phenotypically identical. The findings among American Indians were the same (45). Another interesting feature of the wet wax phenotype is the strong association of

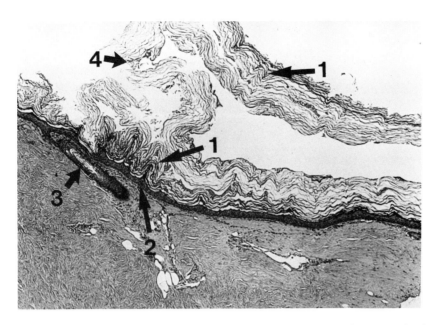

FIG. 2. Longitudinal section showing the wrinkles in the stratum corneum (1) that can also be seen persisting in the sloughed keratin within the canal. The cellular ridges (2) can be seen directly under the wrinkles. Note how the most medial hair (3) has been pushed downwards by the stratum corneum, and how the stratum corneum is detaching at the deep-superficial junction (4).

axillary odor, which is absent in the dry wax phenotype. This is presumably related to some type of genetic difference in apocrine gland function, and geneticists have pondered over the evolutionary significance of this difference. There is some evidence that the wax types were present before Homo sapiens evolved, because wet and dry wax types have been identified in chimpanzees.

Wet wax is the predominant form in Caucasians and Negroes, whereas dry wax is dominant in Mongoloid peoples. There is considerable geographic variation in the

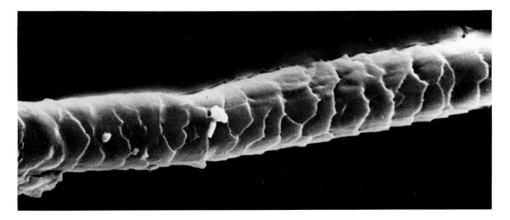

FIG. 3. Scanning electron micrograph picture illustrates the "roof tile" pattern of the scales on the surface of this external canal hair.

wax types (46). An interesting relationship between the ceruminous glands and the milk glands of the breast has been noted. Several studies have shown that there is a very low incidence of carcinoma of the breast among Oriental women who have dry wax when compared with those Oriental women who have the "Western" type of wet wax. The incidence of carcinoma of the breast among Oriental women with wet wax approaches the incidence in Caucasian women.

Biochemistry and Bacteriology

Wax was first analyzed by Nakashima (38); he and subsequent authors (1,6,17,66) have looked in detail at its constituents. It contains a mixture of lipids, protein, free amino acids, and mineral ions. The protein content of dry wax is greater than that of wet wax (34), and the lipid content is higher in freshly secreted wax than it is in stale wax (17).

The antibacterial effect of wax is debatable. A bacterial flora normally exists in the external ear canal (14). Baumann et al. (7) found no significant difference in the lipid content of wax in subjects susceptible to otitis externa when compared with normal individuals. Perry and Nichols (43) tried to colonize normal ears with a pathogenic strain of *P. aeruginosa* and found that this inoculum rapidly died out, with none of the subjects developing otitis externa. They concluded that other factors beside pathogenic bacteria must be present to facilitate the development of otitis externa.

Creed and Negus (18) and Perry and Nichols (43) looked for an antibacterial effect in cerumen and concluded that it did not have any. However Chai and Chai (16) made a 3% solution of dry wax and found this to be highly bactericidal (99%) against *S. marcescens, H. influenzae,* and one strain of *E. coli* but less so against another *E. coli, streptococci, S. aureus,* and notably *P. aeruginosa* (30%–80%). Another study using wet wax (60) demonstrated similar findings. It is interesting to note that even in those studies in which an antibactericidal effect was shown, *Pseudomonas,* the most common pathogen in the external ear canal, showed considerable resistance to the antibacterial properties of ear wax.

Lysozyme and immunoglobulin G have also been identified in cerumen (44). Both substances were found more frequently in dry wax than in wet, which is of interest in view of the similar antibacterial effects of the two types. It is not clear what the significance of this difference is, but there is no epidemiological evidence that one wax type has any specific advantage over the other.

CERUMINOUS GLANDS

The ceruminous glands number between 1,000 and 2,000 in a normal ear canal and have a distribution similar to the hairs in the external ear canal (41). Ceruminous glands are tubular glands whose ducts may open either directly into the base of the hair shafts superficial to the sebaceous gland duct or separately onto the skin surface. The glandular epithelium is cuboidal, and the cells have a distinct intracellular

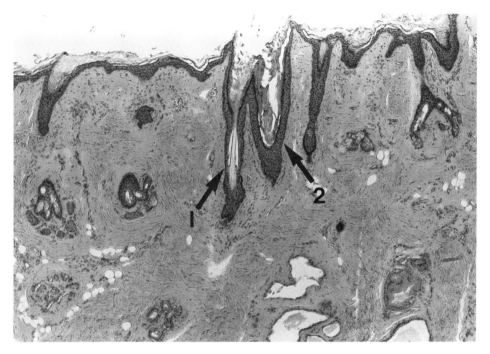

FIG. 4. Longitudinal section shows how the hairs in the more lateral part of the canal are more upright (1). A ceruminous gland (2) can be seen opening into the upper part of a hair follicle.

pigment in some areas. They also have cytoplasmic extrusions into the lumen of the gland, and their secretion is extruded at the luminal surface of the cell. Deep to the glandular epithelium there is a layer of myoepithelial cells.

Cerumen Secretion

Contraction of the myoepithelial cells causes the contents of the ceruminous glands to be secreted. Perry et al. (42) identified sympathetic nerve fibers closely associated with these cells, although a more recent study was not able to confirm their findings (8). Both studies, however, found that the ceruminous glands were stimulated to secrete by adrenergic stimuli, such as locally or systemically injected adrenaline, or pain and anxiety. Local pressure on the skin and movement such as clenching the teeth also stimulated secretion. Cholinergic stimuli and heat did not cause secretion.

Shelly and Perry (54) described in detail the manner in which cerumen is secreted. The secretion is milky at first but changes into a brown waxy material soon after exposure to the air. The close association of the duct openings to the base of the hair shafts allows the hairs to be coated with both sebum and the secretion from the ceruminous glands (Fig. 4). These secretions also coat the skin of the superficial part of the canal. The physical stickiness of these secretions may have some protective function in that objects coming into contact with it are more likely to stick to the skin and hairs of the superficial canal.

In clinical practice wax is often found in the canal deep to the area in which it is secreted, which poses the question as to how it got there. Undoubtedly in many cases it is pushed there by cotton-tipped buds (5). The obsession that many people have that wax is dirty leads them to attempt to remove it from both their own and their children's ears. Unfortunately, the standard cotton swab is just the right size in many ear canals to act as a ram rod, and so rather than extract the wax, it impacts it deeper into the external ear canal.

The telltale sign on examination is a smooth concave impression in the lateral surface of the lump of wax, sometimes with a wisp of cotton wool stuck to it, where the head of the bud has made its impression. Once the deep canal has become filled with wax in this way, the normal physiological cleansing mechanism fails, and skilled help is usually required to remove the wax.

This is, however, probably not the only way in which wax gets into the deep part of the canal. On some occasions a thin layer of wax can be seen coating part of the deep canal. This may sometimes be seen in canals that are too narrow to admit a cotton bud. One likely explanation is that the wax trickles medially when in its liquid state, before solidifying. Finally, as has already been mentioned, thick hairs may totally obstruct the lateral end of the canal in some males, and thus over a long period of time a plug of hairs, wax, and desquamated skin accumulates medial to this barrier, with progressive accumulation eventually extending into the deep canal.

Wax in the external ear canal can cause difficulties when attempting to diagnose acute otitis media. Some clinicians have stated that in the presence of the "hot" inflamed middle ear of patients with acute otitis media, wax in the canal will liquify and run out of the canal. The implication is that if there is wax obstructing the canal, the patient does not have the condition. This is, however, not true (52), and if a patient is suspected of having any middle ear pathology, the external ear canal needs to be cleaned sufficiently to enable the entire surface of the drum to be properly visualized.

THE SELF-CLEANSING FUNCTION

Epithelial Migration

History

The finding that markers that were stuck to the surface of the skin over the tympanic membrane moved was probably first documented by Blake in 1882 (11). He made this observation when the paper disks he was using to repair perforations in the membrane migrated off the drum and out along the canal. Blake went on to use the same markers to plot the rate and direction of migration in normal individuals. He also observed that the stratum corneum of the deep canal became detached from the underlying skin in the region of the junction of the deep, osseous, and superficial cartilaginous parts of the canal.

Since this original description was made, the experiment has been repeated by many investigators, mainly in humans and guinea pigs (2,13,29–31,33,39,59). Alberti's study (2), published in 1964, gave a detailed description of the patterns and rates of migration in 40 young adults. He used dots of India ink as surface markers and identified two main patterns of migration. The most common was radial, away from the umbo (found in 80%); the other pattern was horizontal, away from the handle of the malleus but otherwise radial in the inferior half of the drum and over the pars flaccida. He also calculated that the mean rate of migration was 0.07 mm/ day. His findings were similar to but more detailed than those of Blake (11); not all authors, however, agreed with his findings. Notably Stinson (59) felt that the center from which migration occurred was in the anterior recess of the canal over the tympanic annulus. All authors have agreed that in the normal ear canal the surface of the skin moves laterally from the medial end of the canal.

The Mechanism of Migration

The purpose of this migratory phenomenon is clearly to keep the canal free of debris, but the actual mechanism of the process has puzzled otologists since it was first recognized. Skin at other sites in the body does not normally migrate, and so the phenomenon is often overlooked (21).

Although many of the authors describing migration have pondered over the details of this phenomenon, the most serious attempts to identify it precisely were those of Litton (31) and Boedts (13). Litton (31) labeled mitoses in the epithelium of guinea pig external ear canals using tritiated thymidine and then followed the progress of the label over periods as long as 14 days.

The rapid migration rate of skin of the external ear canal of guinea pigs is between 0.5 and 1 mm/day (31,39), and the thinness of the tympanic membrane makes the guinea pig a useful experimental animal for this work in spite of the awkward shape of its external canal, which makes access to the inferior half of the membrane difficult.

The pattern of migration over the surface of the tympanic membrane in guinea pigs is quite different from that in humans. In the guinea pig migration occurs in a superior direction over the whole tympanic membrane, and Litton (31) identified a generation center of epidermal mitoses around the inferior part of the tympanic annulus. During a period of days the labeled cells moved in all directions away from this generation center. Litton considered that the two possible mechanisms for migration were displacement of the skin away from the generation center by the production of new cells and active migration of skin cells off the drum and along the canal wall. He concluded from his study that a displacement mechanism was the most probable, and his reasoning was based on the finding of a generation center. He drew an analogy with nail growth. The rate of nail growth is similar to the rate of migration in the external ear canal in humans. There are, however, several defects in this argument.

First, the nail is a thick structure, measuring 0.3 to 0.65 mm in depth. The epidermis in the deep part of the human ear canal is the thinnest in the body, measuring as little as 15 μm (37), one-twentieth the thickness of the thinnest nail. In the guinea pig it measures as little as 0.3 μm (23) and migrates about 10 times faster than in the human. The nail also consists of hard keratin and this rigidity, along with its thickness means, provides it with the mechanical strength to be physically displaced. The extremely thin migratory epidermis of the external ear canal is soft, and when its migration is obstructed it accumulates. This is clearly seen in both human and guinea pig ear canals, where the deep layers of the skin heap up into cell ridges (Fig.

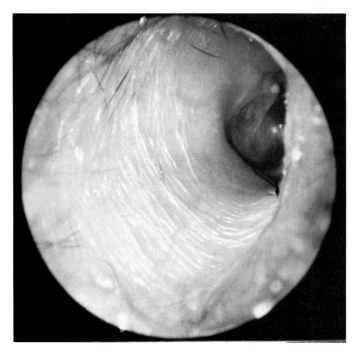

FIG. 5. A series of transverse wrinkles can be seen along the floor of the bony canal of this patient.

2), and the stratum corneum forms a series of wrinkles when the fixed structures, the hairs, are encountered in the lateral part of the external ear canal (Fig. 5) (22,23). If migration were a passive displacement phenomenon, this thin layer of skin would accumulate close to the generation center; however, it migrates 15 to 20 mm in the human ear canal before accumulating.

Either a generation center or an area of increased skin production has to exist, whatever the mechanism of cell movement is. When skin is migrating off the tympanic membrane and along the external ear canal, cells have to be generated to replace those leaving. The existence of a generation center provides no evidence in favor of either mechanism. Litton (31) stated that by analogy the generation center in humans would be expected in the region of the umbo, because this is the point away from which surface markers move. Such a generation center has never been identified in humans, and indeed mitotic figures can be found elsewhere on the tympanic membrane (24). Smelt and Hawke (55) demonstrated in a model that migration could occur from the center of the drum even if mitoses occur over the whole drumhead as random events.

Another feature of Litton's experiment that is not explained is the discrepancy between the rate of movement of the labeled cells and surface markers away from the generation center. Even after 13 days there were labeled cells within 3 mm of the generation center, whereas from his own measurements surface markers moved at an average rate of 0.67 mm/day. This discrepancy is difficult to explain if we postulate that cell generation is the sole mechanism for movement, since one would expect all the cells to be indiscriminately pushed along at the same rate.

Apart from the reasons already stated against a displacement mechanism, there are other factors to support the possibility of an active migration. It is known that if cells are migrating under their own power, they adopt an asymmetrical shape, and the long axis of a migrating cell is aligned in the direction of movement (56). In sections of migratory epidermis there is marked asymmetry of the epidermal cells, and this is most striking in the deeper layers, the stratum basale and spinosum. Furthermore, such alignment of skin cells is not found in skin from other sites on the body, including the skin in the cartilaginous part of the external ear canal. The long axis of the spindle-shaped cells in migratory epidermis of the external ear canal coincides to a remarkable extent with the recognized pattern of migration (24). Obviously a static observation on fixed tissue does not tell us what is happening in the living organism, but cell alignment in the direction of migration was found in all specimens studied and requires an explanation. If a cell was being passively displaced away from a generation center, one expects that it would adopt an axis at right angles to the direction in which it was being displaced.

It is now recognized that many cells have the cytoskeletal elements that would permit them to move (19), and epidermal cells are no exception (10,36,57). Filamentous actin (F-actin) has been identified in the migratory epidermis of the guinea pig drum, and its distribution documented (12). Thus epidermal cells have the mechanism to migrate, and it is well recognized that they do so in wounds and cell culture (48,64).

Another question to be answered is which cells in the skin are responsible for migration, and therefore where is the plane of cleavage. If the ultrastructure of the canal wall skin is studied, it is reasonable to exclude the possibility of migration within the dermis, because in this layer cells are relatively sparse and collagen is prominent (23,28). Boedts (13) considered that the stratum corneum was the probable plane of migration, but this is a layer of dead cells, and electron microscope evidence indicates that movement within this layer is highly improbable (49). For these reasons it seems that the plane of cleavage is between the basement membrane and the stratum granulosum, and thus would involve the stratum basale, the stratum spinosum, or both (23). Further evidence that this is the level of migration comes from a labeling experiment in guinea pigs (25). This experiment demonstrated that ink particles inserted into the skin at one point on the drum moved laterally in the deep layers of the epidermis, indicating that these cells are involved in migration.

Corroborative evidence exists in that the greatest concentrations of contractile proteins within the epidermis are found in the stratum basale and spinosum (36,58). Also, accumulations of nucleated epidermal cells (stratum basale, spinosum, and granulosum) are found where migration stops (Fig. 2), and these cells represent an accumulation of cells that have migrated and are undergoing differentiation before desquamating into the lumen of the external ear canal (22).

Desquamation

The emigrating epidermis has to come to a halt at some point in the external ear canal. The ultimate fate of all the emigrating cells must be the same as that of keratinocytes at all other sites. This is differentiation into the dead cells of the stratum corneum followed by detachment (desquamation) from the skin surface. If normal human canals are examined, wave or wrinkle patterns can be seen building up as the most medial hairs are approached, like waves on a shore (Fig. 5). If this region is sectioned and studied by light microscopy, it can be seen that the waves are made up of two elements. Superficially there are convolutions of stratum corneum, and deep to these there are heaps or ridges of nucleated epidermal cells (stratum basale and stratum spinosum cells), and these ridges are capped by accumulations of stratum granulosum cells (Fig. 2).

In the sectioned tissue the relationship between the most medial fixed epidermal structures, the hairs and gland ducts, and the emigrating skin can be clearly seen (Fig. 2). The hairs at this site are very much flattened onto the canal wall (Fig. 1), and they act as ramps to detach the advancing edge of the epidermis from the underlying tissue. The ducts of the glands are also deep to the advancing edge here, so that their secretions help to lubricate and detach the epidermis at this point. Several authors (2,11,20) noted that this is the point at which their surface labels become detached, and Bezold and Siebenmann (9) noticed that the desquamated skin could be stretched to a considerable length. This is possible because as the superficial layer of the stratum corneum moves laterally and desquamates, it wrinkles up in an accordian-like fashion. Stretching the layer amounts actually to straightening out the wrinkles.

Wrinkles and Ridges

The term wrinkles was first used by Johnson (22) to describe the surface corrugations seen in the external canals of both living patients and cadaveric specimens. This term was also used by Johnson to describe the corrugation that was seen in the stratum corneum on histologic sections of canal skin specimens (and which were responsible for the surface wrinkles seen on gross examination). Johnson also introduced the term ridges of the external canal skin to describe the localized thickenings of the nucleated layer of the epithelium of the external canal that was seen in the histologic sections of the canal skin. These localized thickenings of the nucleated cell layer of the deep external canal epithelium were present directly underneath the wrinkles of the stratum corneum. Johnson identified two different types of wrinkles in the skin of the deep external canal: transverse wrinkles, which ran at right angles to the long axis of the canal and longitudinal wrinkles, which ran parallel to the long axis of the canal. These wrinkles develop because the stratum corneum is a flexible sheet migrating laterally along the deep canal wall.

The transverse wrinkles were most obvious on the posterior bony canal wall and least visible on the inferior bony canal wall. They always became larger and more frequent as the junction between the deep (bony) and superficial (cartilaginous) canal (deep-superficial junction) was approached from the deep canal. Transverse wrinkles are produced as the flexible sheet of laterally migrating stratum corneum is blocked by the stationary adnexal structures (hairs) at the deep-superficial junction. This arrangement of the hairs at the deep-superficial junction is invariable and provides a mechanism for the elevation and desquamation of the stratum corneum of the deep canal at this point.

The longitudinal wrinkles were most commonly seen on the floor of the canal in the bony isthmus and just lateral to it. They were also seen on the anterior and posterior walls of the same area. Longitudinal wrinkles are less obvious than transverse wrinkles and do not become larger as the deep-superficial junction is approached. The outwardly migrating flexible sheet of stratum corneum of the deep canal produces longitudinal wrinkles (in the axis of the canal) as it is compressed circumferentially as it passes through the narrowing of the isthmus.

CONCLUSION

The hypothesis put forward here for the self-cleansing mechanism of the deep part of the external ear canal is that migration proceeds as an active process in the deeper layers of the epidermis. There is a requirement for an area of increased epidermal production at the medial end of the canal to replace the emigrating cells, but no such requirement along the canal wall because the surface area is not increasing here. The stratum corneum is carried out by the underlying cells as a passive flexible sheet covering the canal wall, and its surface is thrown into patterns of wrinkles because of the shape of the canal and the obstruction and elevating action of the hairs at the lateral end, where it becomes detached by the action of the hairs and secretions. The cells in the deeper layers of the epidermis are responsible for the active migratory process, and when they are arrested by the static structures laterally, they have no alternative but to differentiate into stratum corneum, and desquamate along with the cells they carried out (22,23).

How the desquamated material is shed from the lumen of the canal is uncertain. It has been suggested that the action of chewing may move the material laterally particularly since movements of the mandibular condyle alternately compress and expand the cartilaginous canal (15), but there is no evidence to substantiate this theory. It may fall out, be extracted by the finger nail, or accumulate, as has been discussed.

There remain many unanswered questions regarding the physiology of the external ear canal. The argument about whether the process is one of active migration or displacement remains unsettled. Beyond this lie the questions regarding which factors influence the skin to move laterally. Could it be light, a temperature gradient, or the electric fields (32) within the canals? Much research is yet to be done.

PATHOLOGICAL CONSIDERATIONS

Disturbance of migration is related to a number of pathological conditions in the middle ear and external ear canal. The development of cholesteatoma of the middle ear represents a failure of skin to emigrate successfully. Cholesteatoma remains a major cause of middle ear disease. The successful surgical management of cholesteatoma depends on the provision of a smooth surface over which the epidermis can travel laterally. The reason the debris accumulates in an attic retraction is almost certainly related to the mechanical barrier caused by the acute angle of the lateral bony lip (51). If the skin cannot migrate, it differentiates and desquamates. If it then becomes infected, the rate of epidermal production increases, leading to a more rapid accumulation of debris, with its erosive consequences. However, it seems unlikely that the development of the retraction pocket itself is attributable to a defect in the migratory process.

Very little has been published about the migratory process in pathological conditions of the external ear canal. Saad (50) carried out ink dot studies on patients with various otological conditions and found that in otitis externa, desquamation occurred in the deep canal and migration was retarded. Similarly, desquamation *in situ* or delayed migration occurred in a number of other conditions, but the number of patients in each group was small. The migratory process is undoubtedly disturbed in inflammatory conditions of the middle and external ear. This may represent an increase in the production and differentiation of cells, a decrease in migration, or a combination of these factors.

The migratory process is the key factor in the healing of small perforations in the guinea pig (26), and it undoubtedly has great importance in myringoplasty in humans. This became apparent when nonmigratory skin was used to repair defects in the early days of middle ear reconstructive surgery (62,65). If such skin was used, keratin debris accumulated in the canal and required constant removal. Current techniques rely on stimulating the healing process at the edges of the perforation and providing a scaffold over which local epidermal cells can migrate. Obviously normal wound-healing factors are involved in the healing process initially, but when the defect has been closed, the epidermis covering it is able to participate in the self-cleansing process.

The role of the migrating sheet of epidermis in the extrusion of grommets placed in the drum has been debated, and O'Donoghue (40) carried out a study on this topic and concluded that migration was unlikely to be the only factor responsible for grommet extrusion. Once extruded, however, the tube is often transported laterally by the normal process of migration.

REFERENCES

1. Akobjanoff, L., Carruthers, C., and Senturia, B. H. (1954): The chemistry of cerumen: A preliminary report. *J. Invest. Dermatol.,* 23:43–50.
2. Alberti, P. W. R. (1964): Epithelial migration on the tympanic membrane. *J. Laryngol. Otol.,* 78:808–830.
3. Alm, P. E., Bloom, G. D., Hellström, S., Stenfors, L.-E., and Widemar, L. (1983): Middle ear effusion caused by mechanical stimulation of the external auditory canal. *Acta Otolaryngol. (Stockh.),* 96(1–2):91–98.
4. Anson, B. J., and Donaldson, J. A. (1973): *Surgical Anatomy of the Temporal Bone and Ear.* W. B. Saunders, Philadelphia.
5. Baxter, P. (1983): Association between the use of cotton tipped swabs and cerumen plugs. *Br. Med. J. [Clin. Res.],* 287(6401):1260.
6. Bauer, W. C., Carruthers, C., and Senturia, B. H. (1953): Free amino acid content of cerumen. *J. Invest. Dermatol.,* 21:105–110.
7. Baumann, E. S., Carr, C. D., and Senturia, B. H. (1961): Studies of factors responsible for diseases of the external auditory canal. III. A comparison of lipids in normal and infestation susceptible ears. *Ann. Otol. Rhinol. Laryngol.,* 70:1055–1061.
8. Bende, M. (1981): Human ceruminous gland innervation. *J. Laryngol. Otol.,* 95(1):11–15.
9. Bezold, F., and Siebenmann, F. (1908): *Textbook of Otology* (translated by J. Holinger), p. 109. E. H. Colgrove, Chicago.
10. Bhatnager, G. M., and Santana, H. (1980): Immunofluorescent staining of myosin, actin and α-actinin in normal epidermis and cultured human epidermal cells. *J. Invest. Dermatol.,* 74:258.
11. Blake, C. J. (1882): The progressive growth of the dermoid coat of the membrana tympani. *Am. J. Otol.,* 4:266–268.
12. Boden, P., Johnson, A., Weinberger, J. M., Hawke, M., and Gotlieb, A. I. (1986): In situ localization of F-actin in the normal and injured guinea-pig tympanic membrane. *Acta Otolaryngol. (Stockh.),* 101:278–285.

13. Boedts, D. (1978): The tympanic epithelium in normal and pathological conditions. *Acta Otorhinollaryngol Belg.*, 32:293–420.
14. Brook, I. (1981): Microbiological studies of the bacterial flora of the external ear canal of children. *Acta Otolaryngol. (Stockh.)*, 91(3–4):285–287.
15. Carne, S. (1980): Ear syringing. *Br. Med. J.*, 280:374–376.
16. Chai, T. J., and Chai, T. C. (1980): Bactericidal activity of cerumen. *Antimicrob. Agents Chemother.*, 18(4):638–641.
17. Chiang, S. P., Lowry, D. H., and Senturia, B. H. (1957): Microchemical studies on normal cerumen. *J. Invest. Dermatol.*, 28:63–68.
18. Creed, E., and Negus, V. E. (1926): Investigations regarding the function of aural cerumen. *J. Laryngol. Otol.*, 41:223–230.
19. Goldman, R. D., Milsted, A., Schloss, J. A., Starger, J., and Yerna, M.-J. (1979): Cytoplasmic fibres in mammalian cells: Cytoskeletal and contractile elements. *Ann. Rev. Physiol.*, 41:703–722.
20. Gülzow, J. (1973): Beobactungen am Selbstreinigungsmechanismus des Ohres. *Z. Laryngol. Rhinol.*, 52:781–788.
21. Ham, A. W., and Cormack, D. H. (1979): *Histology*, 8th ed., pp. 929–930. J. B. Lippincott Company, Philadelphia.
22. Johnson, A., Hawke, M., and Berger, G. (1984): Surface wrinkles, cell ridges, and desquamation in the external auditory canal. *J. Otolaryngol.*, 13:345–354.
23. Johnson, A., and Hawke, M. (1985): An ultrastructural study of the skin of the tympanic membrane and external ear canal of the guinea-pig. *J. Otolaryngol.*, 14:357–364.
24. Johnson, A., and Hawke, M. (1985): Cell shape in the migratory epidermis of the external auditory canal. *J. Otolaryngol.*, 14:273–281.
25. Johnson, A., and Hawke, M. (1986): An ink impregnation study of the migratory skin in the external auditory canal of the guinea-pig. *Acta Otolaryngol. (Stockh.)*, 101:269–277.
26. Johnson, A. and Hawke, M. (1987): The function of migratory epidermis in the healing of tympanic membrane perforations in guinea-pig. *Acta Otolaryngol. (Stockh.)*, 103:81–86.
27. Johnson, F. R., McMinn, R. M. H., and Atfield, G. N. (1968): Ultrastructural and biochemical observations on the tympanic membrane. *J. Anat.*, 103:297–310.
28. Lim, D. J. (1970): Human tympanic membrane. *Acta Otolaryngol.*, 70:176–186.
29. Link, R. (1952): Uber die Gefassversorgung des trommelfelles und des ausseren Gehorganges. *Arch. Ohr Nas Kehlkofh.*, 160:561–572.
30. Litton, W. B. (1963): Epithelial migration over tympanic membrane and external canal. *Arch. Otolaryngol.*, 77:254–257.
31. Litton, W. B. (1968): Epidermal migration in the ear: The location and characteristics of the generation center revealed by utilizing a radioactive desoxyribose nucleic acid precursor. *Acta Otolaryngol. [Suppl.] (Stockh.)*, 240.
32. Luther, P. W., Peng, H. B., and Lin, JJ-C. (1983): Changes in cell shape and actin distribution induced by constant electric fields. *Nature*, 303:61–64.
33. Magnoni, A. (1938): Osservazioni sulla migrazione dell epitelio della membrani timpanica. *Valsalva*, 5:234–240.
34. Matsunaga, E. (1962): Dimorphism in human normal cerumen. *Ann. Hum. Genet.*, 26:273–286.
35. Mawson, S. R., and Ludman, H. (1979): *Diseases of the Ear*, 4th ed. Edward Arnold Ltd.
36. McGuire, J., Lazarides, E., and DiPasquale, A. (1977): Actin is present in mammalian keratinocytes. In: *Biochemistry of Cutaneous Epidermal Differentiation*, edited by M. Seiji and I. A. Bernstein. University Park Press.
37. Naiberg, J. B., Proops D. W., and Hawke, M. (1984): Thickness of the migratory epithelium of the external auditory canal. *Arch. Otolaryngol.*, 110:253–257.
38. Nakashima, S. (1933): Uber die chemische zussammensetzung des cerumens. *Z. Physiol. Chem.*, 216:105–109.
39. O'Donoghue, G. M. (1983): Epithelial migration on the guinea-pig tympanic membrane: The influence of perforation and ventilating tube insertion. *Clin. Otolaryngol.*, 8:297–303.
40. O'Donoghue, G. M. (1984): The kinetics of epithelial cells in relation to ventilating tubes. *Acta Otolaryngol. (Stockh.)*, 98:105–109.
41. Perry, E. T. (1957): *The Human Ear Canal*. Charles C. Thomas, Springfield, IL.
42. Perry, E. T., Hurley, H. J., Gray, M. B., and Shelly, W. B. (1955): Adrenergic innervation of the apocrine gland of the human ear canal. *J. Invest. Dermatol.*, 25:219–221.
43. Perry, E. T., and Nichols, A. C. (1956): Studies on the growth of bacteria in the human ear canal. *J. Invest. Dermatol.*, 27:165–170.
44. Petrakis, N. L., Doherty, M., Lee, R. E., Smith, S. C., and Page, N. L. (1971): Demonstration and implications of lysozyme and immunoglobulins in human ear wax. *Nature*, 229:119–120.
45. Petrakis, N. L., Molohon, K. T. and Tepper, D. J. (1967): Cerumen in American Indians: Genetic implications of sticky and dry types. *Science*, 158:1192–1193.

46. Petrakis, N. L., Pingle, U., Petrakis, S. J., and Petrakis, S. L. (1971): Evidence for a genetic cline in the earwax types in the Middle East and South East Asia. *Am. J. Phys. Anthropol.,* 35:141–144.
47. Politzer, A. (1902): *Diseases of the Ear* (Translated by M. J. Ballin and C. L. Hellier), 4th Ed., Bailliere Tindall and Cox, London.
48. Proops, D. W., Hawke, M., and Parkinson, E. K. (1984): Tissue culture of migratory skin of the external ear and cholesteatoma: A new research tool. *J. Otolaryngol.,* 13:63–69.
49. Raknerud, N. (1975): The ultrastructure of the interfollicular epidermis of the hairless (hr/hr) mouse. III. Desmosomal transformation during keratinization. *J. Ultrastruct. Res.,* 52:32–51.
50. Saad, E. F. (1977): The epidermis of the drumhead in some otologic conditions. *Arch. Otolaryngol.,* 103:386–388.
51. Sadé, J., Avraham, S., and Brown, M. (1981): Atelectasis, retraction pockets and cholesteatoma. *Acta Otolaryngol.,* 92:501–512.
52. Schwartz, R. H., Rodriguez, W. J., McEveny, W., and Grundfast, K. M. (1983): Cerumen removal: How necessary is it to diagnose acute otitis media? *Am. J. Dis. Child.,* 137(11):1064–1065.
53. Senturia, B. H., Morris, M. D., and Lucente, F. E. (1980): *Diseases of the External Ear Canal.* 2nd Ed. Grune and Stratton, New York.
54. Shelly, W. B., and Perry, E. T. (1956): *J. Invest. Dermatol.,* 26:13–20.
55. Smelt, G., and Hawke, M. (1986): A paradigm for tympanic epithelial dispersion. *J. Otolaryngol.,* 15:336–343.
56. Solomon, F. (1981): Organizing the cytoplasm for motility. *Cold Spring Harbor Symp. Quant. Biol.,* 46(1):17–22.
57. Steinert, P., Peck, G., Yuspa, S., McGuire, J., and DiPasquale, A. (1976): Isolation of an actin-like protein from epidermal tumors and cultured epidermal cells. *J. Invest. Dermatol.,* 66:276.
58. Steinert, P., and Yuspa, S. H. (1978): Biochemical evidence for keratinization by mouse epidermal cells in culture. *Science,* 200:1491–1493.
59. Stinson, W. D. (1936): Reparative processes in the membrana tympani. *Arch. Otolaryngol.,* 24:600–605.
60. Stone, M., and Fulghum, R. S. (1984): Bactericidal activity in wet cerumen. *Ann. Otol. Rhinol. Laryngol.,* 93(2pt1):183–186.
61. Strauss, J. S., Downing, D. T., and Ebling, F. J. (1983): Sebaceous glands. In: *Biochemistry and Physiology of the Skin,* edited by L. A. Goldsmith, pp. 569–595. Oxford University Press.
62. Thorburn, I. B. (1960): A critical review of tympanoplastic surgery. *J. Laryngol. Otol.,* 74:453–474.
63. Tos, M., and Poulsen, G. (1980): Attic retractions following secretory otitis. *Acta Otolaryngol.,* 89:479–486.
64. Vizian, C. B., Matoltsy, A. G., and Mescon, H. (1964): Epithelialization of small wounds. *J. Invest. Dermatol.,* 43:499–507.
65. Wright, W. K. (1960): Myringoplasty. *Arch. Otolaryngol.,* 71:369–375.
66. Yassin, A., Mostafa, M. A. and Moawad, M. K. (1966): Cerumen and its microchemical analysis. *J. Laryngol. Otol.,* 80:933–938.

Physiology of the Ear,
edited by A. F. Jahn and J. Santos-Sacchi.
Raven Press, New York © 1988.

Middle Ear Mucosa: Histological, Histochemical, Immunochemical, and Immunological Aspects

Joel M. Bernstein

Department of Speech–Language Pathology and Audiology, State College of New York at Buffalo, and Departments of Otolaryngology and Pediatrics, State University of New York at Buffalo, Buffalo, New York 14214

Otitis media with effusion (OME) is an inflammation of the mucoperiosteal lining of the eustachian tube, middle ear, and mastoid cavity. The disease is associated with an accumulation of fluid that may be purulent, serous, seromucinous, or mucoid.

Almost 100 years ago, Politzer (22) gave a thorough and still valid description of the clinical features and treatment of OME. In his *hydrops ex vacuo* theory, he postulated that the pathogenetic mechanism of OME involved the development of negative pressure in the middle ear cleft secondary to mechanical obstruction of the eustachian tube. In 1950, Hoople (13) presented a classical treatise on OME in which he considered the disease a major challenge to otolaryngology. The increased use of antibiotics in the 1940s to treat purulent otitis media and the aviation-related study of barotrauma stimulated much interest in OME.

Today, OME represents the most common inflammatory disease in young children after the common cold. It is the most common cause of acquired hearing loss in children today and also represents the most common precursor of chronic irreversible otitis in older children and young adults. Because this disease represents an enormous epidemiological and socioeconomic problem and because a fair number of children with this disease develop progressive damage to the hearing mechanism despite all modalities of medical and surgical treatment, it is necessary to study carefully the pathogenesis of this inflammatory disease.

The purpose of this chapter is to present the histological, histopathological, and histochemical aspects of the middle ear mucosa in OME in humans and the immunological reactivity in middle ear effusions (MEE) and middle ear tissues in this disorder. It is hoped that an understanding of the immunological reactivity will allow one to interpret the histopathology and immunopathology of OME in humans and lead to rational approaches to diagnosis and treatment.

NORMAL HISTOLOGY

The middle ear, or cavum tympanicum, lies between the outer ear canal and the labyrinth (11). Its boundaries are largely formed by the tympanic membrane laterally and the bony labyrinth medially. The cavity contains the auditory ossicles, the ten-

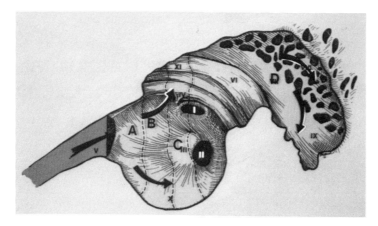

FIG. 1. Schematic representation of the medial wall of the middle ear cleft showing the potential routes by which the mucociliary system transports mucus from the anterior/superior portion of the middle ear and the anterior/inferior portion of the middle ear toward the eustachian tube.

dons of the tensor tympani and stapedial muscles, the semicanal for the tensor tympani, and connective tissue trabeculae. The cavity continues anteriorly into the auditory or eustachian tube, which opens into the nasopharynx. The posterior part of the tympanic cavity is connected through the tympanic antrum to air-filled cavities or cells in the mastoid process of the temporal bone. The middle ear cleft can be defined as the eustachian tube, middle ear cavity, entrance to the mastoid antrum (aditus ad antrum), and mastoid cavity proper.

The mucous membrane lining of the lumen of the eustachian tube has a low columnar ciliated epithelium whereas near the pharynx, a taller pseudostratified ciliated epithelium is found (19). At the pharyngeal opening, numerous goblet cells appear. Furthermore, there are many mixed glands in the lamina propria of the cartilaginous portion of the eustachian tube. Thus, the eustachian tube has a mucociliary system characterized by true cilia and abundant goblet cells and submucosal mucous glands. The epithelium of the middle ear cavity is of the simple squamous type, although near the opening of the auditory tube, it is ciliated, cuboidal, or columnar in type.

Using temporal bone specimens and biopsies from children with otitis media, Sade (23) described a progressive loss of ciliated epithelium as one proceeds from the eustachian tube anteriorly to the tip of the mastoid posteriorly. This information is summarized in Figs. 1 and 2. Sade has suggested that the normal middle ear cleft was lined with both mucus-producing elements and cilia. Further evidence that the normal middle ear epithelium possesses secretory cells was provided by the investigation of Lim and Hussl (17) and Kawabata and Paparella (15) who demonstrated at least four different types of secretory cells by electron microscopy. These include goblet cells, light and dark granulated cells, and lamellar granulated cells. The mucus-secreting cells converge in large numbers near the ciliated cells. However, other electron microscopic studies of human middle ear mucosa have revealed that the normal middle ear mucosa contains five types of cells: nonciliated cells with secretory granules, ciliated cells with secretory granules, ciliated cells without secretory granules, intermediate cells, and basal cells (12).

Goblet cell densities have been extensively studied in normal middle ear and eu-

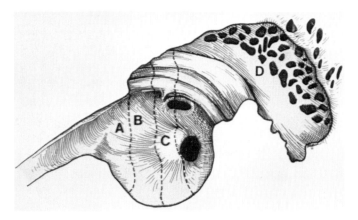

FIG. 2. Schematic representation of the medial wall of the middle ear cleft showing the following anatomic landmarks: **(A)** ciliated epithelium and goblet cells always present; **(B)** ciliated epithelium and goblet cells usually present; **(C)** ciliated epithelium and goblet cells rarely present; **(D)** ciliated epithelium and goblet cells never present.

stachian tube mucosa (29). In normal middle ears, there is a low density of goblet cells and no mucous glands. Production of mucus from the goblet cells occurs to some extent. Few inflammatory cells are found in the lamina propria of the normal middle ear; however, a few lymphocytes and plasma cells may be seen in the middle ear mucosa of the normal squirrel monkey (18). In addition, lysozyme is found in the middle ear mucosal cells (31). The source of this enzyme is thought to be from mucosal secretory granules (18). Acid phosphatase has also been demonstrated in the secretory granules in the surface epithelium of the normal middle ear mucosa (14). Thus, like the eustachian tube, the mucosa of the anterior third of the normal middle ear cavity appears to be supplied with a mucociliary system (24).

The normal mastoid cavity is lined by a single layer of low cuboidal epithelium with a minimal amount of subepithelial connective tissue. For the most part, these cells lack cilia, and there are no goblet cells or glands in the normal mastoid mucous membrane (19).

The work of Mirko Tos (27) in Copenhagen has contributed enormously to our understanding of the normal morphology of the middle ear mucosa and has greatly increased our knowledge about the histopathological process that takes place in the middle ear mucosa during the development of otitis media. He considers the normal middle ear mucosa to be devoid of glands, but the epidemiological studies of otitis media in both clinical patients as well as a study of temporal bones demonstrated that 90% of children will develop otitis media within the first 3 years of life (28). Therefore, it is difficult to establish whether the glands that are found in biopsies and temporal bones of older children and young adults can be accepted as part of the normal middle ear mucosa. Tos considers that it is much more likely that these changes are the result of pathological processes that have occurred at some time early in life. Nevertheless, most studies of the middle ear mucosa seem to agree that the anterior/inferior portion of the middle ear does contain a mucociliary system that is capable of handling a normal production of mucus from the goblet cells that are present in the anterior third of the middle ear mucosa.

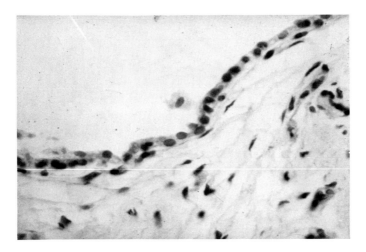

FIG. 3. Simple squamous-cuboidal epithelium of the promontory from a patient with Meniere's disease. The submucosa has an occasional capillary and scattered inflammatory cells. (Hematoxylin-eosin × 100)

More recent work by Albiin et al. (1) has noted the codistribution of ciliated and secretory cells in the human middle ear and has been extensively reviewed in the literature. In their study of rat mucosa, the findings demonstrated striking similarities to that in the human middle ear.

In conclusion, the normal histology of the middle ear would include at least two tracts of ciliated cells and goblet cells that connect the epitympanum with the eustachian tube and the anterior/inferior portion of the middle ear mucosa with the eustachian tube (Fig. 1). The remaining parts of the tympanic cavity and mastoid cavity appear to be lined by a simple squamous-cuboidal nonciliated epithelium (Fig. 2). Finally, the presence of glands in the middle ear mucosa most likely represents the result of previous inflammation rather than a part of the normal middle ear mucosa. Normal middle ear mucosa, as seen from a biopsy of the promontory of a patient with Meniere's disease, is shown in Fig. 3. This demonstrates simple squamous-cuboidal epithelium with no glands, an occasional capillary, and a few inflammatory cells.

PATHOGENESIS OF OTITIS MEDIA WITH EFFUSION

There is general agreement that eustachian tubal dysfunction is the primary etiology of OME. If normal eustachian tube function is defined as the ability to equalize both a negative and positive pressure, all patients who develop OME have poor tubal function at the time that they develop otitis media (8).

The act of opening the eustachian tube is accomplished primarily by the tensor veli palatini muscle (9). In normal tubal function, intermittent opening of the tube maintains near-ambient pressure in the middle ear cavity. Bluestone et al. (10) have suggested that there are two types of eustachian tube obstruction that could result in MEEs: mechanical and functional. Mechanical obstruction may result from inflammation from bacteria, virus, allergy, or hypertrophic adenoids or tumors of the

TABLE 1. *Types of mucosal epithelium found in 107 biopsy specimens from patients with otitis media with effusion*

Epithelium	No. of specimens	%
Squamo-cuboidal	54	52
Columnar	9	8
Pseudostratified columnar	39	36
Stratified squamous (no keratin)	2	2
Stratified squamous (with keratin)	3	2

nasopharynx. Functional obstruction can result from persistent collapse of the cartilaginous tube attributable to increased tubal compliance or inadequate opening mechanisms, or both. Functional obstruction of the eustachian tube appears to be the single most common type found in children with recurrent OME. This simplistic account of the eustachian tube dysfunction leading to a negative pressure in the middle ear cleft and the subsequent transudation of fluid into the middle ear probably accounts for the early stage of OME. The chronicity of MEE appears to depend not only on the maintenance of eustachian tube dysfunction but on the metaplastic and inflammatory changes, which will be discussed later in this chapter. Furthermore, several experimental models suggest that even after the patency of eustachian tube has been restored, inflammatory changes in the middle ear cleft may continue (25). However, experimental long-term occlusion in cats demonstrates that the only way in which middle ear mucosa can become normalized is if the eustachian tube can become functional. The investigations of Tos et al. (26,30) in both short- and long-term eustachian tube obstruction experiments demonstrate the great importance of tubal patency in the prognosis of otitis media. In ears with anatomically occluded tubes, no recovery occurs, whereas in ears with normalized tubal function, the middle ear mucosa and goblet cell density return to normal. Thus, following eustachian tube dysfunction or obstruction, the middle ear mucosa undergoes a significant metaplastic change, and the normal simple squamous-cuboidal epithelium often changes into a pseudostratified columnar ciliated or respiratory epithelium. A summary of the mucosal epithelial changes that occur in chronic OME following eustachian tube obstruction in humans is summarized in Table 1. Pseudostratified columnar epithelium appeared to be the most common change from squamous-cuboidal epithelium, although in 52% of the patients, the squamous-cuboidal epithelium was maintained at least at the level of the promontory biopsy. Stratified squamous epithelium with keratin is an extremely rare event but did occur in three patients in this study. The findings in the lamina propria in OME in which chronic eustachian tube obstruction in humans is present are shown in Table 2. Gland formation was evident in 60% of the biopsy specimens. In most instances the epithelium lining the glands was identical to that lining the lumen of the middle ear space, suggesting invagination of surface epithelium to form glands. An example of this is shown in Fig. 4, in which a gland invaginating from the epithelial surface is observed. The invaginated portion had cells with material that reacted positively to staining with PAS-Alcian Blue. The epithelium in OME often demonstrates a secretory sheet as seen in Fig. 5. These

TABLE 2. *Submucosal changes in 35 biopsy specimens obtained from promontory area of middle ear in otitis media with effusion*

Findings	No. of specimens	%
Presence of glands	21	62
Presence of inflammatory cells	21	62
Presence of capillaries	18	52
Presence of increased fibrous tissues	27	74

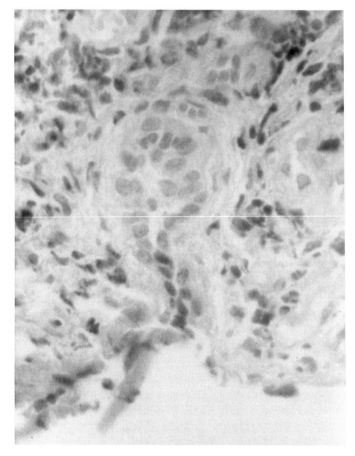

FIG. 4. Surface epithelium of the middle ear mucosa invaginating to form a submucosal cyst or gland. (Hematoxylin-eosin ×100)

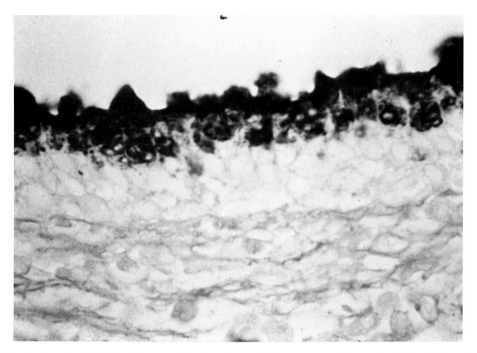

FIG. 5. Pseudostratified columnar epithelium from middle ear mucosa in a patient with otitis media with effusion. Alcian blue positive material is prominent in the apical portions of the cells. Most of these cells are goblet cells. (Alcian blue-PAS reaction ×500)

cells are primarily all goblet cells, which demonstrates the extremely significant increase in the number of goblet cells in the middle ear mucosa in patients with OME. In regard to these changes, it should be emphasized that Tos (26) has demonstrated that the most likely source of the increased glands in the middle ear mucosa is the result of hyperplasia of the basal cells of the normal epithelium, which forms subepithelial glands. These glands are often branched and complex and secrete mucosubstances. The presence of increased mucous secretions, which are mainly glycoproteins in the middle ear fluid, is the result of mucosubstances secreted from the increased number of mucous glands and goblet cells that occur in the middle ear mucosa following chronic eustachian tube obstruction. Sometimes a glue-like nature of the fluid is present, and it is likely that this may be attributed to some extent to resorption of water. However, this has not yet been determined, and it is just as likely that the viscous nature of the mucoid effusion is the result of increased carbohydrate synthesis in the goblet cells and mucous glands, giving rise to glycoproteins.

The submucosal glands in middle ear mucosa in OME demonstrate mucosubstances both in the cell and in the lumen of the gland (Fig. 6). The lamina propria in the normal middle ear mucosa from the promontory normally does not possess any glands or any significant number of inflammatory cells.

Unfortunately, the nature of the mucus in OME has not been carefully studied. There have been very few studies to date on the exact biochemical nature of the mucus, although it is believed that the mucus in the middle ear is most likely similar

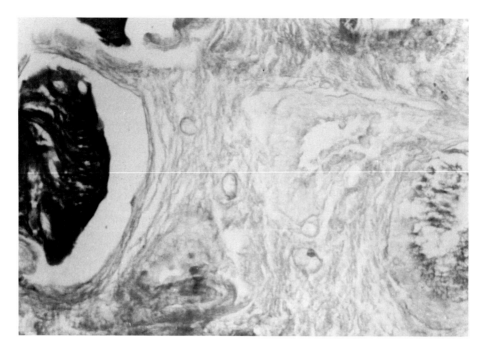

FIG. 6. Lamina propria of middle ear mucosa of a patient with otitis media with mucoid effusion. PAS positive material is present in the lumen of the gland on the left and in the apices of the glandular cells on the right. (PAS reaction ×500)

to that of mucus in other areas of the respiratory tract and probably consists of a long core of amino acids with side branches of carbohydrates in which neuraminic acid and fucose very often occur as terminal sugars (2). In addition, blood group substances are most likely present in the MEE, although this has not yet been specifically demonstrated. This is one area where further research is absolutely necessary in order to determine the nature of the mucus, which may play a role not only in the mucociliary system but also in the immunopathology of the middle ear mucosa. It seems likely, however, that bacteria play an important role in the metaplasia of the middle ear production of mucus because eustachian tube obstruction in germ-free animals never gives rise to glandular development of mucus production. (16).

Several years ago, our laboratory demonstrated that neuraminidase changes the staining properties with Alcian blue-PAS stain from the dark blue characteristic of acid mucins to the purple stain characteristic of neutral mucins, suggesting that neuraminic acid may be a terminal sugar in the mucus secreted by the glands of the middle ear mucosa (2).

Inflammatory cells in the lamina propria appear to be mainly mononuclear, including plasma cells, lymphocytes, and macrophages (Fig. 7). Polymorphonuclear cells were uncommon and eosinophils were rarely seen. In several biopsies perivascular accumulation of mononuclear cells (Fig. 8) were present occasionally, and the development of mononuclear follicles was evident in a few biopsy specimens.

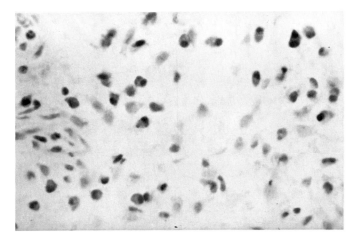

FIG. 7. High-power photomicrograph of the lamina propria of the mucous membrane of the middle ear in a patient with otitis media with a mucoid effusion. There is an abundance of plasma cells and small lymphocytes. (Hematoxylin-eosin ×500)

In summary, eustachian tube obstruction produces a metaplasia of the middle ear mucosa with the development of increased numbers of glands and goblet cells and a significant inflammatory infiltrate that consists mainly of chronic inflammatory cells, such as lymphocytes and macrophages. Plasma cells are very often seen. It is likely that they play an important role in the immune defense against both bacterial and viral pathogens; however, if eustachian tube obstruction becomes long-standing, these inflammatory cells may release enzymes as well as immunological mediators of inflammation, which subsequently causes tissue injury and chronic irreversible damage to the middle ear mucosa. This concept will be explored later in this chapter.

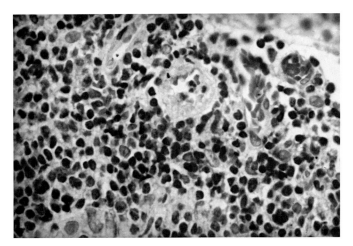

FIG. 8. Lamina propria of mucous membrane of the middle ear in a patient with otitis media with a mucoid effusion. There is a dense accumulation of predominantly mononuclear cells around the small capillary. (Hematoxylin-eosin ×100)

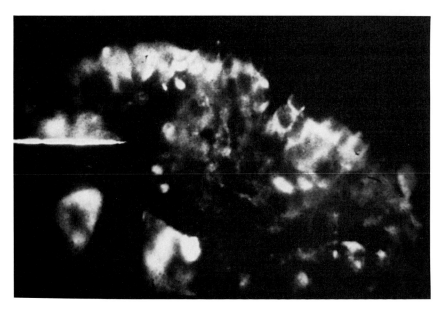

FIG. 9. Immunohistological localization of IgA in the epithelium and lamina propria of the mucous membrane from a child with otitis media with a mucoid effusion, stained with specific antisera for IgA. IgA is found in the apical region of the epithelial cells as well as the interepithelial area of these epithelial cells. In the lower insert on the left, a plasma cell synthesizing IgA is seen.

IMMUNOHISTOLOGICAL STUDIES

Direct fluorescent antibody staining demonstrates tissue localization of IgA and IgG classes of immunoglobulin and secretory component in the middle ear mucosa obtained from patients with OME. Minimal staining is observed rarely for IgM. IgE staining is notably absent in most middle ear mucosal biopsies. As shown in Figs. 9 and 10, pronounced staining was observed for IgA in the surface epithelial basement membrane and plasma cells in the lamina propria in the middle ear mucosa in OME.

The distribution and immunohistological localization of secretory component were similar to that observed in other external surfaces. Specific staining was found in the apical cells in the glandular areas of the mucosal epithelium (Fig. 11). No immunocompetent lymphoid tissue or specific cellular staining for immunoglobulin was present in the mucosa obtained from three patients with otosclerosis and two patients with Meniere's disease. The lumens of many glands were filled with fluid containing IgA and IgG. The presence of the third component of complement (C_3) in tissue sections was not often found but did appear occasionally in the polymorphonuclear cells and rarely in the endothelium of capillaries (Figs. 12 and 13). Six middle ear mucosal specimens have been studied for the synthesis of various proteins. Synthesis of lactoferrin and lysozyme was observed in all cultures. Secretory component was synthesized by all cultures, as shown in Fig. 14. Both IgA and IgG were synthesized by all cultures. The levels of serum immunoglobulins were within the normal age-adjusted range in all the patients studied. The distribution of immunoglobulins and the secretory component in 20 MEEs is presented in Table 3. Because of the varying degrees of dilution that occurs during the collection of MEEs, no attempt has been

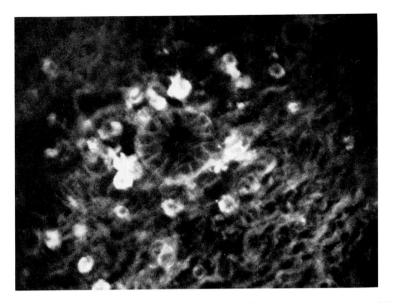

FIG. 10. Immunohistological localization of IgA plasma cells in the lamina propria of the middle ear mucosa from a child with otitis media with mucoid effusion, stained with specific antisera for IgA. There are abundant plasma cells surrounding a small gland in the lamina propria. Most of these plasma cells are synthesizing IgA.

made to quantitate precisely the concentration of various immunoglobulins in the middle ear. However, detectable amounts of IgG and IgA were found in all middle ears tested. IgM was found in 50% of the specimens and IgE was detected in low amounts in five specimens. Secretory component was detected in all but two specimens. Although both IgG and IgA were readily detectable in MEEs, the individual

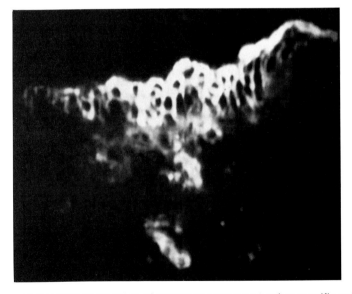

FIG. 11. Immunohistological localization of secretory component using specific antisera for secretory component. There is demonstration of secretory component in the apical region of the epithelial cells of the middle ear mucosa.

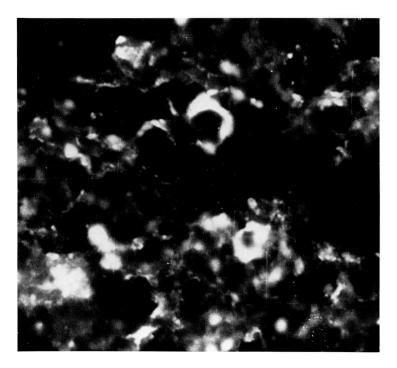

FIG. 12. Immunohistological localization of C3 in inflammatory cells found in the middle ear mucosa. In adjacent sections, these cells are primarily neutrophils. The deposition of C3 in the neutrophils may be nonspecific, although they may represent the incorporation of immune complexes.

and mean ratios of IgG to IgA in the ear fluids were about twofold lower than the ratios observed in the prepared specimens of serum. The mean IgG to IgA ratio in serum was 11 and in the ear fluids was about 5.6. Sucrose density gradients were performed on three MEEs in which secretory component was present. This was performed to determine whether secretory component was attached to IgA or whether it was present in the free form. Analysis of the various fractions from the gradient is demonstrated in Fig. 15. Secretory component was found with IgA, and furthermore, IgA was present in a heavier fraction than IgG. Thus, it is apparent that secretory IgA is present in MEEs.

TABLE 3. *Distribution of immunoglobulins and secretory component in 20 middle ear effusions from patients with otitis media with effusion*

Immunoglobulin	No. of middle ear washings with detectable levels
IgG	20
IgA	20
IgM	10
IgE	5
Secretory component	18

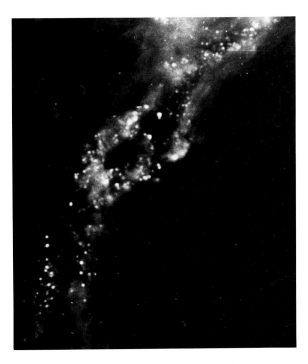

FIG. 13. Immunohistological localization of C3 found in a granular pattern in a small capillary in the middle ear mucosa of a patient with otitis media with mucoid effusion. It is apparent that the receptor for C3 is present in the capillary wall. It is unlikely that this represents an immune complex deposition because neither immunoglobulin nor antigen could be identified in these sections.

Available information on the mucosa of the normal middle ear reviewed earlier in this chapter has suggested that ciliated epithelium with secretory glands is a distinct feature of the eustachian tube and the contiguous areas of the middle ear cavity. However, the remainder of the normal middle ear cavity consists largely of nonciliated cells with secretory granules, basal cells, and less frequently ciliated cells with or without secretory granules. Thus, the normal middle ear cavity contains a paucity of mucous glands, a low density of goblet cells, a characteristic absence of lymphoid follicles, and a very sparse presence of plasma cells and lymphocytes. However, following eustachian tube obstruction, the middle ear mucosa bears a striking resemblance to the immunological features observed in the peripheral mucosal site of the common mucosal immune system (7). These features are summarized in Table 4. The results of immunological studies performed on middle ear secretions and tissues strongly indicate that the effusion in OME is attributable to a local reaction. Secretory component is a protein unique to external secretions and is found in serum in only small amounts, usually below the level detectable by the routine techniques in immunochemistry. In the studies performed in our laboratory and mentioned earlier, secretory component has been identified in more than 80% of the MEEs and appears to be combined with dimeric IgA.

An observation of particular importance is viral-specific IgA antibody activity in MEEs (21). These observations provide evidence for the distinct system of local immunity functioning in the middle ear of patients with OME. The mechanism un-

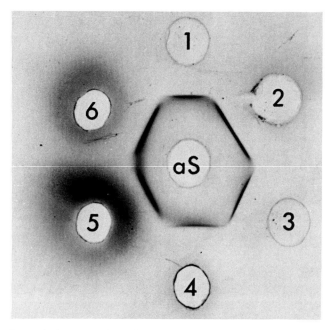

FIG. 14. Autoradiograph demonstration of *in vitro* synthesis of secretory component in the tissue cultures of middle ear mucosa. Supernatant fluid from six radioactive-labeled mucosal tissue cultures was placed in the peripheral wells and diffused against antiserum to human secretory component (aS). Specific labeled precipitant bands for secretory component were observed in all cultures. Cultures frozen immediately after the addition of labeled culture failed to demonstrate any labeled precipitant.

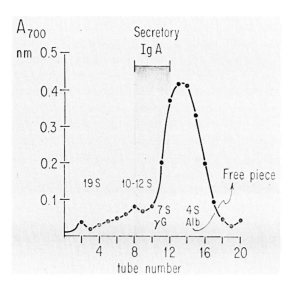

FIG. 15. Sucrose density gradient of a middle ear effusion. Analysis of the fractions with specific antisera demonstrated the presence of secretory component in tubes 10 to 12. IgA was also present in these fractions. Free piece was not found in the albumin fraction. This density gradient study strongly suggests that most of the secretory component present in the middle ear fluid was incorporated into dimeric 10S IgA.

TABLE 4. *Comparison of common mucosal immune system and middle ear mucosa in OME*

Characteristic	Mucosal system in intestinal and respiratory tracts[a]	Mucosal system in middle ear in OME[b]
Ciliated epithelium	+	+
Mucus production	+ + +	+ +
Predominance of 11S IgA	+ + + +	+
IgG/IgA ratio	0.5–1.0	3–4
In vitro synthesis of		
IgA	+ + +	+ +
IgG	+	+
SC	+ +	+ +

[a] Strong minimal evidence.
[b] Otitis media with effusion.

derlying the production of secretory IgA in MEE appears to be the local availability of immunologically active antigen to immunocompetent cells in the middle ear mucosa or to immunocompetent tissue in the nasopharynx. In our studies, although both IgG and IgA classes of viral specific antibody were detected in the middle ear, the proportion of viral specific antibody of the IgA class was two to six times higher than those of the IgG antibody (Table 5). In view of these observations and the findings mentioned previously, it is suggested that the middle ear mucosa is capable of mounting a specific local antibody response after appropriate antigen stimulus. Recent evidence also suggests a local antibody response in MEE against a variety of bacterial agents, including the M protein of *Streptococcus pyogenes* (20) and the outer membrane proteins of *Hemophilus influenzae*. The specific antibody directed

TABLE 5. *Summary of the ratio of IgG to IgA antibody mean titers in the serum of middle ear against polio, mumps, measles, and rubella*

Virus	No. of paired specimens tested	Ratio of γG:γA antibody titer (mean)	
		Serum	Middle ear
Polio-I	13	10:2	1:4
Mumps	10	10:1	1:2
Measles	10	10:1	1:1
Rubella	9	10:3	1:6

The serum ratio of antibody suggests that IgG is the major immunoglobulin. However, the middle ear ratio suggests that IgA is found in significantly higher concentrations in the middle ear fluid than in the corresponding sera. These viral specific antibody titers of the IgA class strongly suggest the concept of a local IgA antibody response after appropriate antigen stimulation. However, it is most likely that the IgA plasma cells are resident in the middle ear only after arriving from areas of antigen stimulation such as the nasopharynx, tonsils, or GALT or BALT.

against the M protein may prevent adherence of the bacteria to the middle ear mucosa and suppurative otitis media, and the specific antibodies of all isotypes directed against all five outer membrane proteins of *Hemophilus influenzae* may play a role in the eradication of this organism, which is becoming more important in otitis media because of its increasing frequency and resistance to most antibiotics used in the treatment of otitis media today (5).

CELL-MEDIATED IMMUNITY IN THE MIDDLE EAR

Little information is available regarding the role of the cellular immune mechanism in the protection from or the pathogenesis of otitis media. In an earlier report using cell surface receptors on T and B lymphocytes and macrophages, our laboratory suggested that T cells predominate in the serous effusions and B cells were more common in the mucoid effusions (6). Macrophages represent the most common mononuclear cell in the sediment of all effusions, except for the purulent form of otitis media in which the neutrophil was the most common.

Using monoclonal antibodies directed against specific determinants on the surface of T cells and T-helper and -inducer cells and T-suppressor cytotoxic cells, new data regarding T-cell subsets and B cells in different MEEs have been described. The data are presented in Table 6 and reflect the number of T and B cells in different types of MEEs. The data suggest that the total number of T cells and B cells in greatest in mucoid effusions. The lowest number of B cells is seen in serous effusions. These results are not surprising inasmuch as the total number of lymphocytes appears to be higher, in general, in mucoid effusions than in serous effusions. It is apparent the T cells predominate in all effusions. There was no MEE in which B cells were present in larger numbers. Nevertheless, B cells appear to be present in significantly greater numbers in mucoid effusions than in serous effusions as suggested in our previous report.

The ratio of T-helper to T-suppressor cells in MEEs is also shown. In general, T-helper cells are more predominant; however, there are significantly more T-suppressor cells in mucoid effusions than serous effusions and the T helper-T suppressor ratio is significantly less in mucoid effusions. The number of specimens is small at

TABLE 6. *Summary of T-cell subpopulations and B cells in different middle ear effusions*

	Serous (n = 14)	Mucoid (n = 13)	Purulent (n = 4)
T	485 ± 204[a]	705 ± 344	441 ± 119
B	188 ± 69	423 ± 196	416 ± 277
	$P < 0.01$		
T_h	450 ± 202	481 ± 197	353 ± 16
T_s	170 ± 48	309 ± 204	156 ± 23
	$P < 0.01$		
T_h/T_s	264	1.5	2.26
	$P < 0.01$		

[a] Cells/μl of middle ear effusion.

this time, and there is some question as to the validity of the unpaired *t* test. However, several conclusions can be stated cautiously at this time. T cells predominate in all effusions; B cells appear to be less frequent than T cells but are significantly greater in mucoid effusions than in serous effusions. T-suppressor cells are also greater in mucoid effusions, although T-helper cells predominate in all effusions. The importance of this T- and B-cell distribution in different MEEs remains to be determined. The source of T and B cells in middle ear mucosa is unknown, although the tonsils, adenoids, or GALT, BALT, or both are distinct possibilities.

LYMPHOCYTE-MACROPHAGE INTERACTION IN MEEs

Recent studies (7) from our laboratory have suggested that macrophages may play a critical role in the modulation of T- and B-cell activity in the middle ear. The characteristics of cellular elements in the MEEs, peripheral blood, and adenoid tissue, as well as the effect of middle ear macrophages on the functional activity of lymphocytes, have been examined in 50 patients with chronic OME. The proliferative responses induced by phytohemagglutinin or pokeweed mitogen in middle ear lymphocytes were generally low compared with the responses observed in peripheral blood and adenoidal lymphocytes. Cocultures of middle ear macrophages and adenoidal lymphocytes resulted in a significant depression of the proliferative response in both immunoglobulin synthesis and lymphocyte transformation. These observations have suggested that macrophages in the middle ear may have a profound influence on the regulation of the immune response in OME.

Additional experiments from our laboratory (J. M. Bernstein and S. Cohen, *unpublished data*) have shown that MEEs may also inhibit the incorporation of tritiated thymidine into mouse thymocytes. Thus, the suppressive effect of middle ear fluid on the incorporation of radioactive-labeled DNA into peripheral blood lymphocytes or adenoidal lymphocytes and mouse thymocytes suggests that middle ear fluid may down regulate immune responses. Whether this down regulation is a result of monokines released by macrophages or lymphokines released by lymphocytes cannot be stated at this time.

However, taken together, these observations suggest that the adherent cell population of MEEs, which are most likely macrophages, are functionally distinct from the peripheral blood monocytes and exert a suppressive effect on the proliferative response of peripheral blood lymphocytes to pokeweed mitogen as well as on the *in vitro* synthesis of the major immunoglobulins. On the basis of these observations, we have proposed that in certain chronic forms of OME there is a relative preponderance of macrophages that are actively immunosuppressive for the proliferative response to mitogen and specific antigens as well as suppressive to the synthesis of specific immunoglobulins. Finally, such immunological hyporesponsiveness may be related to the pathogenesis of chronic OME.

The secretory immune system is a composite of T cells and T-cell subsets, antibody, macrophage, and other cellular effectors that function in a unique and somewhat compartmentalized manner. Available evidence to date suggests that B cells and antibody production and function, and T-cell-mediated reactivity in the mucosal surfaces of the gastrointestinal tract, respiratory tract, genital tract, mammary glands, nasopharynx and salivary glands, and upper respiratory mucosa exhibit a commonality. The bulk of the secretory IgA reactivity observed in these mucosal sites appears to be a reflection of initial antigenic exposure and lymphoid activation in the GALT and BALT. The mucosa of the middle ear during inflammatory states, following eustachian tube obstruction and bacterial invasion, has now been shown to function in a similar manner to other secretory sites listed earlier and appears to respond to antigenic stimuli in a similar manner.

The role of immunological reactivity in middle ear pathology, however, remains to be exactly defined. The source of immunocompetent cells in the middle ear particularly needs to be elucidated to aid further development of efficient vaccines against middle ear infection.

Another area that is being actively investigated in our laboratory is the possible role of food immune complexes in OME, as well as the role of delayed hypersensitivity in chronic OME.

IMMUNOLOGICAL FACTORS

IgE-mediated hypersensitivity is present in approximately 35% to 40% of children with recurrent OME who are unselected in a clinical population (4). The middle ear mucosa may be a target organ, but in probably less than 10% of patients seeking an otolaryngologist for treatment. However, the eustachian tube mucosa, or the orifice of the eustachian tube in the nasopharynx, is probably the most likely site for the effect of mediators of inflammation following antigen-antibody complexing on the surface of either mucosal mast cells or connective tissue mast cells. There also appears to be evidence (32) now that certain viral infections such as respiratory syncytial virus or parainfluenza virus, may induce IgE-mediated responses in the nasopharynx. This would, in turn, give rise to IgE-mediated responses in this area with the release of both histamine and membrane-associated mediators such as prostaglandins, thromboxanes, and leukotrienes. These mediators could lead to eustachian tube edema and suppurative otitis media. Thus, IgE-mediated hypersensitivity may occur at the level of the middle ear mucosa, the eustachian tube, and the nasal mucosa. Mediators released from an allergic rhinitis may, by mucociliary activity of the nasal mucosa, reach the eustachian tube and produce dysfunction and eventual obstruction of the tube. Nasal blockage alone does not appear to produce eustachian tube dysfunction.

A high percentage of MEEs may possess heterophile antibodies of high titers, and in some cases, these heterophile antibody titers in the MEEs may actually be higher than those of the corresponding sera (3). Absorption studies on selected middle ear fluids have shown that high sheep red blood cell (SRBC) antibody titers and low bovine red blood cell (BRBC) titers suggest that Forssman antibodies are present in the MEE. On the basis of other results, we have also concluded that some of the heterophile antibodies in the middle ear fluid may be mixtures of both Forssman and Hanganutziu-Deicher antibodies. The latter antibody is a serum sickness antibody. The antigenic stimulants responsible for formation of Forssman or Hanganutziu-Deicher antibodies in patients with otitis media remain to be determined, but certainly some strains of bacteria such as *Streptococcus pneumoniae* and *Beta hemolytic streptococci* are known to possess Forssman or Forssman-like antigen. It is possible that the Forssman antibodies demonstrated in MEEs of patients might have been produced by bacterial infection. Alternatively, it might be suggested that the Hanganutziu-Deicher antigen may appear as a neo-antigen or an altered antigen as a result of a pathological process on the surface of the middle ear mucosa cell. The presence of higher lytic titers against SRBC and BRBC in some MEEs lends support again to the concept of a local immune system operating in the middle ear. It is also tempting to speculate that the source of some of the B cells producing these heterophile antibodies could be the palatine tonsils.

Immune complexes have frequently been demonstrated in the middle ear fluid, but they may only represent the normal immunoregulatory process by which antibodies and complement opsonize bacteria for phagocytosis or for lysis. Immune-complex deposition in the blood vessels of the middle ear mucosa or the basement membrane of the middle ear epithelium has never been demonstrated. Therefore, at the present time, there is no evidence to support the concept of immune complex disease as a pathological mechanism in the production of OME.

Moreover, not only are microbial antigens found in the middle ear but in nutritional antigens as well. Immune complexes consisting of food and the corresponding antibody have been demonstrated in the middle ear fluid. Again, whether these nutritional immune complexes play any role in otitis media has not been resolved.

Finally, delayed hypersensitivity in OME is a reasonable mechanism because the putative mediators of delayed hypersensitivity are present in MEE. Macrophage-inhibition factor, macrophage-activating factor, interferons, activated T cells, lymphocyte transformation, and chemotactic factors have all been found in middle ear fluids. Thus, mediators of delayed hypersensitivity are present and can certainly add to the maintenance of the inflammatory response in the middle ear mucosa.

MEDIATORS OF INFLAMMATION IN MIDDLE EAR EFFUSIONS

The resolution of otitis media requires the eradication of bacteria or virus from the middle ear space and a return of normal ventilation to the tympanum as a result of normalization of eustachian tube function. However, when eustachian tube dysfunction continues and MEE persists, the immunological reactivity in these effusions is maintained by the persistence of antibody or mediators of cell-mediated immune mechanisms. The persistence of these mediators of inflammation may then lead to tissue injury to both the soft tissue and the bony structure in the middle ear cleft. Inflammatory mediators may arise from at least three different sources: (a) Serum protein may enter the middle ear as a result of transudation and be broken down nonspecifically by enzymes released from either epithelial cells of the middle ear cleft or by inflammatory cells in the middle ear space. Such proteins as fibrinogen, the complement cascade, the clotting factor, and plasminogen may all be broken down into active inflammatory products. (b) The release of mediators from inflammatory cells may infiltrate the middle ear space and tissue following an inflammatory response. Neutrophils, eosinophils, and mast cells may all be involved. These cells can release lysosomal enzymes that are capable of breaking down tissue protein thus leading to tissue necrosis in the middle ear space. (c) The breakdown and necrosis of tissue in the middle ear itself may lead to collagen lysis, and the products of collagenolysis may be chemotactic even in nanogram amounts and capable of attracting neutrophils, aggregating platelets, and clumping of erythrocytes. These inflammatory reactions in the middle ear space can be looked on in terms of two key elements that characterize the inflammatory reaction: vasopermeability changes and the arrival of leukocytes from the circulation.

Mediators of inflammation that have been identified in the middle ear fluid are histamine, chemotactic factors (C3A, C5A bacterial factors), bradykinin, plasminogen-plasmin system, prostaglandins, leukotrienes, platelet-activating factor, lysosomal enzymes, and other nonspecific biochemical agents.

A unifying concept for inflammation in the middle ear mucosa could propose that the earliest changes in the inflammatory response in otitis media is the production of modified tissue proteins in the middle ear mucosa as a result of viral and/or bacterial infection associated with eustachian tube dysfunction. These proteins can alter the complement system and lead to the release of histamine, kinins, and prostaglandins. In addition the coagulation system may become activated, which in turn could activate certain complement components and lead to release of vasoactive amines. The complement system also contains characteristic factors that may play a role in a nonimmune inflammatory response. Other mediators such as the leukotrienes and platelet-activating factor are also present in MEEs and may play a role in both increased vascular permeability and the migration of inflammatory cells into the middle ear space. Whether this acute inflammation will lead to healing or chronic inflammation depends on the persistence of chronic inflammatory cells such as macrophages, lymphocytes, and neutrophils and the mediators that can be released from these cells. Perhaps the most important message to leave with the reader is that these inflammatory mediators can cause tissue injury and may lead to permanent damage to the mucous membrane of the middle ear, the tympanic membrane, and the ossicular chain. Furthermore, there is some evidence that these inflammatory mediators may penetrate the round window and cause permanent sensorineural hearing loss. For all these reasons, it should be strongly emphasized that these effusions should be evacuated if they persist for more than 90 days and do not respond to medical management.

CONCLUSIONS

In this chapter the histological, histopathological, and histochemical nature of mucous membrane in otitis media has been partially characterized. The mucous membrane of the mucoid effusion appears to retain the blue stain of Alcian blue at pH 1. This would strongly suggest the presence of sulfated glycoproteins as part of the biochemical makeup of mucus in mucoid MEEs. This type of mucous substance does not appear to be present in the mucous membrane of the serous effusion. This difference in mucosubstances could result in a heightened difficulty of the mucociliary system to handle this type of mucus in OME with a mucoid effusion. Furthermore, the change in the nature of the mucus could give rise to new antigenic determinants on the surface of epithelial cells and in turn could result in an altered immune response to the epithelial cell. It is imperative that further work be done on the biochemistry of mucins in the middle ear fluid.

Examination of the histopathology discloses a consistent pattern of perivascular mononuclear infiltration. Abundant plasma cells appear throughout the lamina propria and give rise to predominantly IgA, although IgG is often produced as well.

The presence of IgA-producing plasma cells, the *in vitro* synthesis of immunoglobulins and secretory component, and the specific IgA antiviral and antibacterial antibody activity in MEEs all indicate the presence of a local secretory immune system in the middle ear mucosa. The cytologic examination of the middle ear fluid demonstrates a significant difference in the lymphocyte subpopulations in the serous and mucoid categories of OME. Whether these kinds of effusions result from different immune mechanisms or different forms of the same inflammatory process cannot be resolved at the present time.

It is possible that the predominance of macrophages in the long-standing middle ear fluid may produce an immunosuppressive effect on lymphocyte function and humoral immunological mechanisms in OME.

Finally, the chemical mediators of inflammation that may result from immunological processes or the release of enzymes from inflammatory cells may cause in permanent tissue damage to the middle ear and sensorineural hearing loss, if the fluid is not evacuated in a reasonable period of time.

REFERENCES

1. Albiin, N., Hellstrom, S., Stenfors, L. E., and Cerne, A. (1986): Middle ear mucosa in rats and humans. *Ann. Otol. Rhinol. Laryngol.* 95(suppl. 126):2–15.
2. Bernstein, J. M., Boerst, M., and Hayes, E. R. (1979): Mucosubstances in otitis media with effusion. *Ann. Otol. Rhinol. Laryngol.,* 88:334–338.
3. Bernstein, J. M., and Kano, K. (1982): Heterophile antibodies in middle ear effusions. *Arch. Otolaryngol.,* 108:267–269.
4. Bernstein, J. M., Lee, J., Conboy, K., et al. (1985): Further observations on the role of IgE mediated hypersensitivity in recurrent otitis media with effusion. *Otolaryngol. Head Neck Surg.,* 95(5):611–615.
5. Bernstein, J. M., Wilson, M., Murphy, T. F., Dryja, D. M., and Ogra, P. L. (1988): The presence of specific antibodies against outer membrane proteins of nontypable hemophilus influenzae in middle ear effusions: Functional and isotypic characteristics. In: *Fourth International Symposium on Middle Ear Effusions,* edited by D. J. Lim, C. D. Bluestone, J. Klein, and J. D. Nelson. B. C. Decker, Inc., Philadelphia/Toronto (*in press*).
6. Bernstein, J. M., Szymanski, C., Albini, B., et al. (1978): Lymphocyte subpopulations in otitis media with effusion. *Pediatr. Res.,* 12:786–788.
7. Bernstein, J. M., Tsutsumi, H., and Ogra, P. L. (1985): The middle ear mucosal immune system in otitis media with effusion. *Am. J. Otolaryngol.,* 6:162–168.
8. Bluestone, C. D., Beery, Q. C., and Andrus, W. S. (1974): Mechanics of eustachian tube as it influences susceptibility to and persistence of middle ear effusions in children. *Ann. Otol. Rhinol. Laryngol.* 83(suppl. 11):27–34.
9. Bluestone, C. D., Wittel, R., Paradise, J. L., and Felder, H. (1972): Eustachian tube function as related to adenoidectomy for otitis media. *Trans. Amer. Acad. Ophthalmol. Otol.,* 76:1325–1339.
10. Bluestone, C. D., Paradise, J. L., and Beery, Q. (1972): Physiology of the eustachian tube in the pathogenesis and management of middle ear effusions. *Laryngoscope,* 82:1654–1670.
11. Grant, J. C. B. (1952): *A Method of Anatomy,* pp. 782–790. Williams and Wilkins, Baltimore.
12. Hentzer, E. (1970): Ultrastructure of the normal mucosa in the human middle ear, mastoid cavities and eustachian tube. *Ann. Otol. Rhinol. Laryngol.,* 79:1143–1157.
13. Hoople, G. D. (1950): Otitis media with effusion: A challenge to otolaryngology. *Trans. Amer. Acad. Ophth. Otol.,* 54:531–541.
14. Juhn, S., Huff, J., and Paparella, M. M. (1971): Biochemical analyses of middle ear effusions. *Ann. Otol. Rhinol. Laryngol.,* 80:347–353.
15. Kawabata, I., and Paparella, M. M. (1969): Ultrastructure of the normal human middle ear mucosa. *Ann. Otol. Rhinol. Laryngol.,* 78:125–132.
16. Kuijpers, W., and van der Beek, J. (1987): The effect of eustachian tube obstruction on middle ear mucosal transformation. In: *Immunology of the Ear,* edited by J. M. Bernstein and P. L. Ogra, pp. 205–230. Raven Press, New York.
17. Lim, D. J., and Hussl, B. (1969): Human middle ear epithelium. An ultrastructural and cystochemical study. *Arch. Otolaryngol.,* 89:57–67.

18. Lim, D. J., and Shimoda, D. L. (1971): Secretory activity of normal middle ear epithelium. *Ann. Otol. Rhinol. Laryngol.,* 80:319–330.
19. Maximow, A. A., and Bloom, W. (1957): *A Textbook of Histology.* W. B. Saunders, Philadelphia.
20. Mogi, G., Maeda, S., Umehara, T., et al. (1983): Secretory IgA, serum IgA and free secretory component in middle ear effusion. In: *Recent Advances in Otitis Media with Effusion,* edited by D. J. Lim, C. D. Bluestone, J. O. Klein, and J. D. Nelson, pp. 147–149. B. C. Decker, Philadelphia-Toronto.
21. Ogra, P. L., Bernstein, J. M., Tomasi, T., and Coppola, P. R. (1974): Characteristics of secretory immune system in human middle ear: Implications in otitis media. *J. Immunol.,* 112:448–495.
22. Politzer, A. (1984): *A Textbook of Diseases of the Ear and Adjacent Organs: For Students and Practitioners,* p. 739. Lea Brothers, Philadelphia.
23. Sade, J. (1966): Middle ear mucosa. *Arch. Otolaryngol.,* 84:137–143.
24. Sade, J. (1970): The mucociliary system in relation to middle ear pathology and sensorineural hearing loss. In: *Sensorineural Hearing Loss, Ciba Symposium,* edited by G. E. W. Solstenholm and J. Knight, pp. 79–99. J. and A. Churchil, London.
25. Sade, J., Carr, C. D., and Senturia, B. H. (1959): Middle ear effusions produced experimentally in dogs. I. Microscopic and bacteriologic findings. *Ann. Otol. Rhinol. Laryngol.,* 68:1017–1028.
26. Tos, M. (1981): Experimental tubal obstruction: Changes in middle ear mucosa elucidated by quantitative histology. *Acta Otolaryngol.,* 92:51–61.
27. Tos, M. (1984): Anatomy and histology of the middle ear. *Clin. Rev. Allergy,* 2:267–284.
28. Tos, M. (1985): Normalization of the middle ear mucosa. *Auris Nasus Larynx,* 12(suppl. I):S30–S32.
29. Tos, M., and Bak-Pedersen, P. (1972): The pathogenesis of chronic secretory otitis media. *Arch. Otolaryngol.,* 95:511–521.
30. Tos, M., Wiederhold, M., and Larsen, P. (1984): Experimental long-term tubal occlusion in cats. *Acta Otolaryngol. (Stockh.),* 97:580–592.
31. Veltri, R. W., and Sprinkle, P. M. (1973): Serous otitis media immunoglobulin and lysozyme levels in middle ear fluids and serum. *Ann. Otol. Rhinol. Laryngol.,* 82:297–301.
32. Welliver, R. C. (1987): Allergy and middle ear effusions—fact or fiction? In: *Immunology of the Ear,* edited by J. M. Bernstein and P. L. Ogra, pp. 381–390. Raven Press, New York.

Physiology of the Ear,
edited by A. F. Jahn and J. Santos-Sacchi.
Raven Press, New York © 1988.

Physiology of the Eustachian Tube and Middle Ear Pressure Regulation

*Bengt Magnuson and **Bernt Falk

*Department of Otolaryngology, Linköping University Hospital,
S-581 85 Linköping, Sweden, and **Department of Otolaryngology, Västerviks Sjukhus,
S-593 00 Västervik, Sweden*

Like many other physiologic functions, pressure regulation in the middle ear is hardly noticeable under normal conditions, making itself felt only when disturbed. When one is exposed to rapid changes in ambient pressure, most vivid sensations may be experienced, signaling that the ears are in trouble. When flying in an aircraft making a fast descent before landing, for example, a person with healthy ears may experience pain indicating that something is wrong. Of what relevance is this observation in the context of normal physiology? Is this pain in the ear caused by a malfunctioning eustachian tube or is it caused by the specific pressure environment? The answers to these questions are essential when considering our current views on eustachian tube physiology.

In this chapter we will not give a single definitive description of the physiology of the eustachian tube. At the moment we are in a transition period in which two different theories of tubal function exist side by side. One emerged during the early years of otology, more than 100 years ago, and is now enjoying general acceptance, being supported by an extensive literature and the force of tradition. The other theory is relatively new, having evolved during the past decade, and still under development. The two theories are different in several respects; on some points they are antipodal. After reviewing the anatomy and mechanics of the eustachian tube we describe and discuss both theories. Recent studies have revealed new information concerning the function of the eustachian tube in diseased ears, and a special section is devoted to pathophysiology. The next section outlines possible future developments. Finally, a number of tubal function tests that are in current use are described.

REVIEW OF ANATOMY AND MECHANICS

The anatomy of the eustachian tube forms the basis of its function, even though the details of its physiology may be interpreted differently depending on the point of view. The eustachian tube is of entodermal origin and formed from a dorsal pouch in the upper part of the primitive gut, the first branchial pouch. During fetal development the pocket divides into different sacs that form the middle ear cavity, the epitympanum, and the mastoid air cell system (2). The cell system continues to expand during childhood and early adult life. Detailed accounts of the embryology

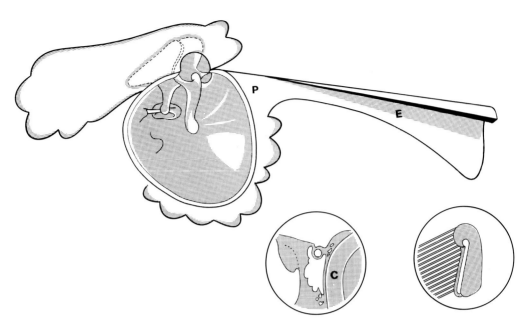

FIG. 1. Rendering of the right middle ear and eustachian tube. **Top,** lateral aspect: The protympanum (P) constitutes an open cavity in direct continuation with the middle ear cavity. The eustachian tube proper (E) is closed in the resting position. **Bottom,** transverse sections: The protympanum (left) is located medial to the mandibular joint and separated from it by a plate of bone. Part of the medial wall is constituted by an extremely thin bone lamella covering the internal carotid artery (C). The eustachian tube (right) is opened by contraction of the tensor veli palatini muscle; striped area indicates direction of pull.

and the macroscopic and microscopic anatomy of the eustachian tube are found in otolaryngological textbooks (2).

The Protympanum

The protympanum, often called the bony tube, is an open cavity forming a direct anterior continuation of the mesotympanum (the middle ear cavity) (Fig. 1). The protympanum is about 10 mm long in the adult human. The lateral wall of the protympanal cavity is separated from the mandibular fossa by a plate of bone (Fig. 1, bottom left). An extremely thin bone plate covering the carotid artery constitutes the medial wall. The bottom of the protympanum is raised above the level of the hypotympanum. The threshold is made up of cellular bone, the protympanal cells, an extension of the hypotympanal cell tracts. The superior boundary of the protympanum is formed by the semicanal of the tensor tympani muscle. The protympanal cavity becomes narrower in the anterior direction and ends at the tubal isthmus. Here the lumen is oval shaped, being approximately 2 to 3 mm high and 1 to 1.5 mm wide. At the isthmus the protympanum connects to the mobile cartilaginous tube or the eustachian tube proper.

The Cartilaginous Tube

The cartilaginous tube points in a medial and inferior direction from the isthmus to the nasopharyngeal ostium; the length is approximately 25 mm in the adult. In children the tube is shorter and takes a more horizontal position than in adults (24). The tube is lined by respiratory columnar epithelium with ciliated cells and goblet cells. In the cartilaginous tube there is also an abundance of submucosal glands (48). A thin film of mucus is propelled by ciliary activity from the middle ear through the eustachian tube to the nasopharynx; this mucociliary activity protects the ear from ascending infection. The tubal cartilage is located on the medial side, and the lateral side is formed by a thick fibrous sheet. The opening muscle is found on the lateral side, attached to the superior edge of the crook-shaped cartilage and to the fibrous sheet that forms the lateral wall of the tube (Fig. 1, bottom right).

In contrast to the protympanum, there is no open lumen in the cartilaginous tube (although it may appear to be so in histological sections). The cartilaginous tube forms a closed slit and, in the true meaning of the word, does not resemble a tube since there is no open communication. The structure resembles more a valve that closes off the middle ear from the respiratory passages, thereby protecting the ear from strong sounds and pressure variations evoked by phonation and respiration. A person with a wide-open auditory valve avoids speaking in a loud voice since a person's voice can be one of the most powerful natural sound sources.

Tubal Closure and Pressure Opening

In the resting position the mucosal membranes of the lateral and medial walls of the tube are closely approximated and adherent to each other. The force of closure is passive, being derived from the adhesive force of the mucous blanket covering the mucosal surfaces, the elastic forces of adjacent supportive tissues, and the hydrostatic pressure of venous blood. Under physiologic circumstances, the lumen of the cartilaginous tube is normally opened in two ways: passively by positive middle ear pressure and actively by muscular contraction. In the closed, resting position the tube offers limited resistance to passage in the down direction (from the middle ear to the nasopharynx), while effectively preventing passage in the updirection. Pressure opening occurs when the middle ear pressure exceeds the nasopharyngeal pressure by a certain amount. The pressure difference forces the tube open, and the pressure is reduced as gas passes out of the ear through the tube. Negative pressure is not released in the same manner.

Active Dilation of the Tube

Active opening of the tube is mainly accomplished by the medial portion of the tensor veli palatini muscle (10,44,45). This muscle division has appropriately been named the dilator tubae muscle. The levator veli palatini muscle may help to dilate the most anterior part of the tube, but contraction of the levator muscle alone does not open the tube all the way to the isthmus (26). The dilator tubae muscle is activated by swallowing and yawning, and sometimes by mandibular movements. The tensor and levator veli palatini muscles, as well as the tensor tympani muscle, are all innervated by the trigeminal nerve and activated on swallowing (28). On swallowing, the tube opens only a fraction of a second (0.3 to 0.5 sec); on yawning, the opening time is considerably longer.

The Tensor Tympani Muscle

The tensor tympani muscle is located in close proximity to the eustachian tube and the middle ear, but the function of this muscle is not fully understood. It is attached to the neck of the tympanic membrane medially. The tensor tympani muscle, together with the tympanic membrane, makes up a diaphragm pump, and one of the functions of this muscle may be to facilitate elimination of positive pressure in the middle ear. Since the muscle shares its innervation, line of pull, and insertion with the tensor veli palatini it has been hypothesized that the tensor tympani may assist in opening the eustachian tube at its tympanic end by forcing intratympanic air into the tube, in coordination with the tensor veli palatini. Like the stapedial muscle, the tensor tympanic muscle can be also activated by strong sound. However, the tensor tympanic muscle seems to play only a minor role in sound protection (37).

THE EUSTACHIAN TUBE IN AVIATION AND DIVING

During the last few decades the limits of our ability to equalize pressure across the tympanic membrane have been increasingly tested as we expose ourselves to rapid pressure changes in connection with air travel and diving. It is important to realize that the rate of pressure changes experienced in a small unpressurized airplane or the elevator of a skyscraper is "unphysiologic" in the sense that it is not part of a human's natural environment. The pressure changes that occur in diving are even greater than those experienced during flight owing to the difference of density of water compared to air. Underwater pressure increases linearly with depth: 101 kPa (1 atm) for every 10 m of depth. Atmospheric pressure decreases exponentially with altitude. Pressure changes are fully experienced in small taxi planes and rotary wing aircraft that are not equipped with a pressurized cabin. A passenger plane with a pressurized cabin may be cruising at an altitude of 10,000 to 12,000 m where the ambient pressure is reduced by more than three quarters. Without the pressurized cabin the passengers would experience severe anoxia. The pressurized cabin, however, prevents the pressure from falling below the 2,000-m level. Even though the cabin mitigates pressure changes, a substantial difference of pressure is still experienced; the pressure difference from ground level to cruising level amounts to about 22 kPa, or nearly one-quarter of the normal atmospheric pressure.

Elimination of Positive Pressure

Positive pressure in the ear relative to the environment occurs during ascent in an airplane or when rising to the surface after diving. This positive pressure is perceived as a feeling of fullness in the ear that is interrupted by a popping sound when the eustachian tube is forced open and the pressure released. A positive intratympanic pressure is thus reduced by "pressure opening" but, in order to open the tube, the pressure difference must be large enough. The magnitude of pressure needed to open the tube (the so-called opening pressure) varies from individual to individual, between right and left ears, and also shows variations with time (17). In healthy ears the opening pressure is about 4 kPa (400 mm water pressure) (14,21). A positive intratympanic pressure is not always eliminated totally on pressure opening. When the tube closes again a small residual pressure usually remains in the middle ear (the closing pressure). If the middle ear pressure is less than the opening pressure, active dilation of the tube by contraction of the tensor veli palatini muscle certainly helps release the pressure. It is possible that the tensor tympani muscle may also be involved in releasing positive pressure as mentioned earlier. During flight and diving a large difference in pressure between the right and left ears may develop because opening pressures are unequal. This can give rise to disturbed vestibular function and nystagmus, so-called alternobaric vertigo (47).

Elimination of Negative Pressure

Negative pressure in the ear relative to the environment occurs on descent from altitude in an airplane and in diving. Negative pressure is not eliminated spontaneously and can give rise to barotrauma. In order to eliminate negative pressure in the middle ear the tube must be dilated actively by muscular contraction. The closed tube, however, is made to close even more firmly in the presence of negative pressure and the tube may thus become locked (3,20). As a result, muscular contraction no longer suffices to open the tube. If the negative pressure is allowed to increase still further, sharp pain is felt in the ear. Effusion of fluid in the middle ear and submucosal or intraluminal bleeding may occur. Finally the tympanic membrane may rupture. In order to avoid tubal locking and barotrauma the negative pressure must be eliminated early by inflation. The Valsalva maneuver or the Frenzel maneuver can be used (see section on functional tests at end of chapter).

The ability to eliminate negative pressure in the ear by swallowing varies considerably between individuals; this ability, for example, is more developed in adults than in children (9). If the pressure equalization ability is investigated in healthy ears, the result will depend on the criteria used for selection of test subjects and the specific experimental method. However, some subjects are always found who, despite having healthy ears, are seemingly unable to equalize pressure through swallowing (14,21). A person who cannot equalize negative pressure may thus have perfectly healthy ears but may make a poor candidate for a fighter pilot.

EUSTACHIAN TUBE FUNCTION: CLASSICAL VIEW

In the previous section the basic anatomy and mechanics of the eustachian tube and related structures were described. In this section we outline the cognitive structure or the "conceptual anatomy" associated with eustachian tube function, beginning with the classical theory. In the classical theory much attention is paid to pressure equalization. Sound protection and drainage functions are naturally recognized as being of importance, but pressure equalization is seen as the most important physiologic function of the eustachian tube.

This view originated in the middle of the 19th century. It was postulated that the air in the middle ear and the mastoid air cell system is continually absorbed, with the result that the pressure decreased. The principal role of the eustachian tube was to ventilate the ear; the tube must open intermittently for releasing the negative pressure by supplying new air. Should the tube not open, the absorption of air and the decrease in pressure would continue until subsequently transudation of fluid would fill the middle ear cavity. This is called the *hydrops ex vacuo theory*, as stated by Politzer (40) and Bezold (4). The classical theory of eustachian tube function is thus based on three fundamental principles: *gas absorption, ventilation, and obstruction*. We will now define and discuss these principles, trying to obtain an overview without going into the finer details.

Gas Absorption

It is assumed, *a priori*, that gas is absorbed from the closed middle ear cavity. This assumption is justified by analogous reasoning, theoretical calculations, and experiment. Gas is absorbed from other cavities in the body, e.g., when air is introduced into the pleural or peritoneal cavities this is absorbed, and bronchial occlusion is followed by pulmonary atelectasis. Absorption of air has been studied in experimentally applied subcutaneous gas pockets in the rat (39,43). It was found that a difference in partial pressures developed between the gas mixture in the air-filled pocket and gases dissolved in the blood—a total difference amounting to 6.7 kPa. Absorption of gas is therefore inevitable. In a hypothetical closed and non-ventilated cavity with rigid walls a negative pressure of 6.7 kPa would ultimately be reached (39). The same would apply to the middle ear. Of course, the middle ear cavity is not rigid. Furthermore, negative pressure, when reaching a certain level, promotes transudation of fluid that prevents further pressure decrease. Owing to the process of transudation, the maximum negative pressure caused by absorption of gas would therefore be limited to approximately −1 kPa.

Absorption of gas has also been studied after experimental occlusion of the eustachian tube in various test animals such as monkeys, dogs, and cats (11,25,42). Effusion of fluid ensues when the experimental procedure is successful, and the pressures measured usually have not exceeded −1 kPa. The effects of gas absorption have also been studied in human ears by serial tympanometry or using the microflow technique (see section on functional tests). The initial middle ear pressure is first assessed and, after the subject has refrained from swallowing for 10 minutes, a second measurement usually shows a lower pressure (13,36). The result has then been extrapolated to 1 hour, or to 24 hours. The pressure decrease during 1 hour with a closed tube has been estimated to be 0.5 kPa, and the amount of gas absorbed during 24 hours would be approximately 1 ml (13).

Ventilation of the Middle Ear

The normal function of the eustachian tube is described in terms of ventilation or pressure equalization. Ventilation, according to the classical theory, is equivalent to the ability of the eustachian tube to equalize negative pressure. Experimental confirmation of the fact that negative pressure can be harmful was first presented by Magnus (29), who studied the effects of pressure on the ear. In 1864 a railway bridge was being constructed over the Rhine river and the ground work under water was made possible with the aid of a pressurized caisson. When entering the caisson through the pressure lock, some workers experienced pain in the ears and Magnus found that the tympanic membrane appeared severely retracted. He concluded that the tube is normally closed and the pressure could be released only by tubal opening.

In the years following, this view gained general acceptance. Ability to equalize pressure has become synonymous with good function, and inability to equalize pressure is supposed to be characteristic of poor tubal function.

Pressure equalization studies performed with modern equipment confirm earlier findings: positive intratympanic pressure is usually equalized without much effort, either passively by pressure opening or actively by muscular opening. Negative pressure is more difficult to equalize; impaired ability to equalize pressure is not uncommon in healthy ears. The ability to equalize negative pressure is thus not the decisive criterion of normality.

Tubal Obstruction

The development of ear disease, such as middle ear effusion and atelectasis with retraction of the tympanic membrane, is explained by assuming that the eustachian tube is obstructed. It is still widely accepted that obstruction of the tube is of prime importance in the development of acute and chronic middle ear disease and is one of the main themes in the classical theory. Tubal obstruction prevents pressure equalization, and therefore gas absorption leads to the development of high negative pressure and ear disease. Obstruction of the tube can be intraluminal, caused by inflammatory edema or polyps, or extraluminal in the presence of a tumor. The latter cause of obstruction is unusual. In middle ear surgery one can sometimes find a polyp or a cholesteatoma occluding the protympanum and blocking passage, but it is questionable whether such changes are involved in the etiology of ear disease or are secondary changes in a diseased ear.

In temporal bone preparations and investigations using X-ray contrast media in diseased ears, it has been found that obstruction is usually absent; in fact anatomical obstruction of the tube is very unusual (6). The same has been found in studies of tubal function employing manometry (12,31,34). In the light of these findings an amendment of the original obstruction hypothesis was necessary. In exchange for the concept of anatomical obstruction, a new concept was introduced—functional obstruction. This qualification means that inability to equalize negative pressure with swallowing, not anatomical obstruction, is the characteristic finding in a diseased ear.

OBJECTIONS TO CLASSICAL THEORY

Some of the experimental results that are in keeping with absorption hypothesis are based on surgical ligation or electrocautery of the eustachian tube in animals. The procedure involves surgical trauma with resulting inflammatory edema. The blocking of the tube occludes the natural pathway of egress for any secretions formed in the middle ear, and accumulation of fluid is inevitable. Here one may ask if the result of the surgical procedure in a test animal is a good analogy of physiologic processes in the human ear—healthy or diseased. These experiments have not succeeded in demonstrating the development of high negative pressure in the middle ear. On the other hand, high negative pressure is frequently found in diseased ears. One must ask, therefore, if negative pressure in the middle ear can be explained in a different manner.

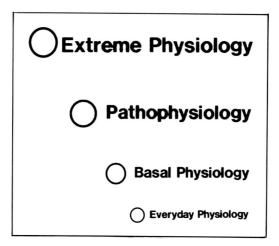

FIG. 2. Scheme to emphasize how our traditional knowledge has been dominated to a large extent by observations made in extreme physiologic situations. The physiologic pressure-regulating system looks different when studied under other experimental conditions.

Measurements of middle ear pressure in humans during 10-minute periods of refraining from swallowing have been extrapolated to 1 hour or to 24 hours as mentioned previously, but such extrapolated results have proved to be erroneous (11). It has also been shown that it is necessary to maintain the physiologic gas mixture in the middle ear when studying the effects of gas exchange (11). In experiments of this type no attention has usually been paid to the pulmonary ventilation that can influence the result (23).

In the classical theory, tubal function is synonymous with pressure equalization. This assumption has led to previous research designed around the equalization principle with the result that this view has been perpetuated. In daily life people have not always been exposed to rapid changes in ambient pressure. This occurs during fast movements in the vertical direction as in flying and deep-sea diving or when rapidly driving a car up or down a hill. These man-made situations are of fairly recent origin and certainly not characteristic of the environmental circumstances that influenced the evolution of the eustachian tube. It is difficult to conclude that pressure equalization is the most important physiologic function of the tube. This is illustrated in preoperative evaluation of cases of chronic ear disease; it is not possible to predict the outcome of surgery with conventional tubal function tests (1,15).

The traditional view has largely been built around physiologic features displayed under extreme experimental conditions, but the physiology of the eustachian tube has several facets or levels, as illustrated in Fig. 2. Physiologic functions under basal conditions, during everyday activities, and under pathologic conditions may all have their specific characteristics, and it may be incorrect to apply the conclusions drawn from one of these levels to another. Of course the old view is still useful in connection with rapid fluctuations of ambient pressure, such as with flying and diving activities. Thus the response to artificial test pressures, as studied with tubal function tests, is significant within its own domain but cannot be directly applied to tubal behavior under normal physiologic circumstances. Likewise, experimental results obtained with conventional tubal function tests may not be relevant when evaluating the tube in pathologic conditions.

MIDDLE EAR PRESSURE REGULATION: A NEW APPROACH

The classical theory consists of a series of tested hypotheses: the absorption, ventilation, and obstruction principles. Throughout the years these ideas have become deeply ingrained in our ways of thinking to the extent that they may appear axiomatic, which in itself constitutes a good enough reason to reconsider the issue. Maybe another approach can be of advantage.

Like the classical theory, the new approach builds on inferential reasoning. In the first place, the appearance of the healthy tympanic membrane does not suggest that it is normally exposed to negative pressure. The slight outward curvature of the membrane could indicate the presence of positive pressure in the middle ear cavity. The rock bottom hypothesis of classical theory is challenged: Does continual gas absorption in the middle ear really exist? According to the classical theory, gas is mainly transported in the up direction through the eustachian tube, from the nasopharynx to the middle ear. It may be recalled that this direction of passage is more difficult than the down direction. If this is the order of nature, the choice seems counterintuitive or, at least, the general design of the system appears impractical.

The Pressure-Regulating System

In the new approach the eustachian tube is not seen as the only pressure regulator; rather it is one of three different components, all serving to control the middle ear pressure (Fig. 3). A bidirectional diffusion of gases is postulated: The process of diffusion involves liberation of gas as well as absorption. The pressure-regulating system is constituted by the cooperation and continual interplay between these components.

1. Bidirectional diffusion of gas (liberation and absorption).
2. Tubal passage (up and down).
3. Bidirectional exchange of fluid (production and elimination).

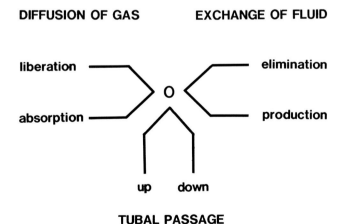

FIG. 3. Representation of the present view on the pressure-regulating system featuring a dynamic balance between three components as the basis for pressure regulation.

In physiologic situations the intratympanic pressure will fluctuate close to the ambient pressure, but not necessarily remaining exactly equal to the ambient pressure; a dynamic equilibrium is maintained (35). If a disturbance occurs, all three components work together in restoring the pressure; if one of the components is incapacitated, the remaining two can take over. It can be seen that an increase in the middle ear pressure will occur if (a) more gas is liberated than absorbed, (b) more gas passes up than down the tube, and (c) if more fluid is produced than eliminated. In the opposite situations the middle ear pressure will decrease (when absorption dominates over liberation of gas, when tubal passage of gas in the down direction dominates over the up direction, and when elimination dominates over production of fluid).

Experimental Findings

Buckingham and Ferrer (7) have reported results showing that gas can be liberated in the middle ear. They sealed small tympanic membrane perforations in noninflamed ears with a thin film of oil-based eardrops in a series of patients. In 54% (38 of 70) the oil film formed a bubble that frequently burst outward, thus indicating liberation of gas with development of positive pressure in the middle ear at rest. Buckingham et al. (8) also performed experiments in dogs with controlled ventilation. The eustachian tube was cannulated with a catheter, and the far end of the catheter was placed under water. As long as the animal was ventilated to maintain the blood gases within normal ranges, bubbles of gas formed at the catheter tip. An increased number of bubbles formed during hypoventilation or when the animal was ventilated with a gas mixture containing carbon dioxide. Bubbles no longer formed when the animal was hyperventilated, instead water started to rise in the catheter, thus indicating the development of negative middle ear pressure. The same pressure changes were seen when the eustachian tube catheter was connected to a water manometer. It can be hypothesized that middle ear pressure is a function of carbon dioxide concentration in the blood, and that CO_2 diffuses into the middle ear cavity.

These findings have been verified in human subjects, using serial tympanometry for measuring pressure changes in response to different breathing patterns (22). Negative pressure developed during hyperventilation; the pressure peaked at -0.3 to -0.4 kPa after 20 min of moderately forced voluntary hyperventilation (this type of breathing cannot be maintained indefinitely). During hypoventilation a positive middle ear pressure developed and increased slowly as long as the subject did not swallow.

The effect of physiologic hypoventilation was studied further by simply measuring the middle ear pressure in the early morning (22). During sleep, breathing is slower and more shallow than during the active hours. The rate of swallowing is reduced and the ability to equalize pressure is reduced as well in the horizontal body position (46). Hence, according to the classical theory, the morning pressure in the middle ear should have been negative. In the majority of ears, however, the pressure was positive with a mean value of 0.48 kPa (range, -0.25 to $+1.95$ kPa). After breakfast, when the subjects had yawned, chewed, and swallowed repeatedly, the middle ear pressure was very close to the ambient pressure in all ears.

In another study middle ear pressure was monitored during rest in a number of subjects by taking tympanograms every second minute (23). Results showed that in the majority of ears, the pressure remained at a level slightly above atmospheric or increased. In some ears a pronounced pressure increase was seen during periods of drowsiness or sleep when the rate of swallowing declined and the carbon dioxide concentration in expiratory air increased. In some ears the pressure showed a slow continuous increase over a 2-hour observation period.

NORMAL PHYSIOLOGY: SUMMARY

The experimental results reviewed above cast doubt on the conventional opinion that the middle ear gas is subject to continuous absorption, and evidence is present to indicate that diffusion is a bidirectional procedure. The 24-hour net result of gas turnover might even show a positive balance. The classical theory offers no explanation for the findings reviewed above. To overcome this difficulty, the new approach considers tubal function in a wider context, thereby creating more room for encompassing situations other than those special situations in which the ear is exposed to rapid changes in ambient pressure.

It is emphasized that rapid changes in ambient pressure encountered during flying and diving do not constitute physiologic stimuli for the eustachian tube. In the new approach less attention is paid to the equalization of artificially applied pressures in experimental situations, and more attention is paid to the protective closing action of the eustachian tube. A reliable tubal closure ensures protection of the ear from the nasopharyngeal environment, including its loud sounds, extensive respiratory pressure variations, and potentially harmful bacterial flora. The opening and closing actions of the eustachian tube are subordinated as part of the pressure-regulating system.

In the healthy ear, pressure regulation is usually smooth and imperceptible, provided the environment is physiologic. In a normal situation fairly stable middle ear pressure is maintained by virtue of the pressure-regulating system with its three components as outlined earlier. During rest and sleep the pressure may increase to positive values. Usually, however, this positive pressure is eliminated easily.

PATHOPHYSIOLOGY

Passage through the eustachian tube is easier in the down direction than in the up direction; this is true for both healthy and diseased ears. In fact, this constitutes a crucial weakness within the system. If tubal passage in the down direction is too easy, pressure opening of the tube might occur in response to sniffing. At the moment of a sharp sniff a negative pressure peak occurs in the nasopharynx. The pressure suddenly becomes much lower than that in the middle ear cavity. The tube cannot withstand the large pressure difference; the pressure gradient forces the tube open, and the ear is evacuated. This is the central issue in development of high negative pressure in the middle ear. Negative pressure is induced by the act of sniffing. Evacuation of the ear is active, not passive, as assumed in the classical theory; for a review see Magnuson (33).

Tubal closing failure with sniff-induced high negative pressure constitutes an important pathogenetic factor. Of course several different factors may be at work in

PHYSICAL FACTORS　　　　**BACTERIAL FACTORS**

high negative pressure ⇥———➤ ascending infection

constant traumatization ⇥———➤ external infection

FIG. 4. Scheme to illustrate the major pathogenic factors. Physical factors include high negative pressure in the middle ear caused by evacuation on sniffing, and traumatization caused by continual scratching and abrasion of the external ear canal so commonly present in patients with chronic otitis media. Infection may invade the ear by two different routes: ascending infection through the eustachian tube and external infection through the external ear canal. *Arrows* indicate that the physical factors may provoke infection.

the development of ear disease; four major factors are given in Fig. 4. When gas is evacuated from the middle ear, the resulting negative pressure locks the tube, and the negative pressure remains for some time. The tympanic membrane is forced to retract, and the middle ear mucosa is also affected by the pressure trauma. Production of fluid comes to dominate over elimination, and effusion of fluid in the middle ear may develop, serous otitis media (SOM). As a secondary effect on the mucosa, the mucociliary function may be influenced. Impairment of the protective mucociliary clearance may lead to increased susceptibility to ascending infection with development of recurrent attacks of acute purulent otitis media. Negative pressure in combination with infection, if induced on a repetitive basis, may lead to chronic changes involving the tympanic membrane, the mucosa, and the mastoid air cell system. In the long run, deep retraction of the eardrum may lead to thinning and atrophy of the membrane. The mucosa may undergo metaplasia with development of an increased amount of goblet cells and mucous glands (the effusion becomes mucoid). The development of the air cell system may be arrested or involution of the air spaces may take place. This leads to the small and sclerotic cell system that is characteristic of chronic ear disease.

Induction of Negative Pressure

Two different factors take part in the induction of negative pressure: failure of the eustachian tube to close firmly enough in the resting position (tubal closing failure) and the sniffing behavior of the subject. Evacuation of the ears on sniffing has been investigated using three-channel manometry in different study populations such as children with persistent middle ear effusion, patients with a cleft palate, and patients with chronic ear disease (cases of adhesive otitis and cholesteatoma) (18,19,31). In such cases the eustachian tube has traditionally been thought of as being obstructed. The consistent finding throughout these studies, however, was that the majority of ears had tubal closing failure. The eustachian tube tended to snap open too easily on sniffing and the ears were evacuated. A three-channel pressure recording (nasopharynx, right ear, left ear) is reproduced in Fig. 5 to illustrate the induction of negative middle ear pressure. The subject was a woman displaying habitual sniffing behavior; eardrums were severely retracted and effusion of fluid was present in both middle ears. Transmyringeal ventilation tubes were inserted

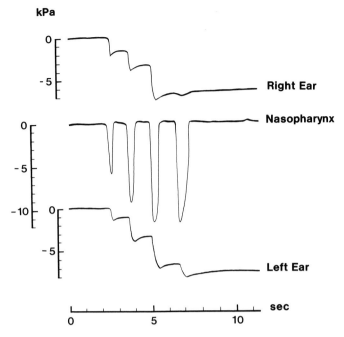

FIG. 5. Simultaneous three-channel manometric recording showing a series of high negative pressure peaks in the nasopharynx evoked by sniffing. A stepwise evacuation of both ears took place.

before the recording to enable measurement of middle ear pressures. Another characteristic finding in our studies was an aggravated one-way valve action; tubal passage in the down direction was favored, but passage in the up direction was often difficult or impossible. In some cases the tube showed an extreme one-way valve action, meaning that the ear could not be inflated by the Valsalva maneuver no matter how hard the patient tried, but the same ear could often be evacuated by sniffing without effort (18,31).

Habitual Sniffing Behavior

It may seem strange to consider harmful effects connected with sniffing since this is such a common behavior for clearing the nose. In a healthy ear, casual sniffing may sometimes give rise to a temporary reduction of the middle ear pressure (16,31). This is soon eliminated and no harm is done. In a case of ear disease, however, a combination of tubal closing failure and habitual sniffing behavior is often present. Sniffing leads to evacuation of the ears especially during periods when the subject is suffering from a common cold, but subjects often continue to evacuate the ears on a habitual basis even when no respiratory infection is present. Some persons seem to develop the habitual sniffing behavior very early in life; the process is seemingly that of a conditioned reflex (30). This demands some consideration.

Autophonia and Hyperacusis

Two different auditory stimuli seem to be involved in maintaining the sniffing habit: autophonia and hyperacusis (30,34). Autophonia is experienced when the eustachian tube is wide open. This highly disturbing symptom occurs when the sound of one's own voice is transmitted through the open tube to the middle ear, striking the tympanic membrane from the inside. The sound is much too loud and the natural feedback between speech and hearing is distorted. Certain individuals find that the disturbance can be suppressed temporarily by vigorous sniffing. Negative pressure is induced in the middle ear, and the eustachian tube is forced to close. Pressure equalization ability is often excellent in these cases, however, and after a while the person must swallow. The tube reopens and the sound immediately becomes too loud; this initiates more sniffing. These events are repeated in a cyclical manner.

Hyperacusis is related to autophonia but refers to a disturbed perception of environmental sound (30,34). Negative pressure induced by sniffing forces the tympanic membrane to retract. The transmission of sound is changed by the increased stiffness of the membrane and the ossicular chain. Low-frequency sound is attenuated and high-frequency sound is emphasized, permitting the hyperacusic patient to reduce and modify the perceived intensity of the disturbing environmental sound. If middle ear effusion develops as a consequence of habitual sniffing, hearing may also be impaired regarding the higher frequencies. Adaptation is still possible, however, and as time passes the person becomes used to the attenuated sound and comes to prefer this specific sound quality. The sound experienced with retracted eardrums, with or without effusion of fluid in the middle ear, is often preferred over the much stronger sound experienced after the ear has been inflated. Evacuation is no longer carried out in order to suppress the autophonia associated with an open tube but to reduce the intensity of environmental sound and maintain a desirable sound quality.

Clinical Presentation

It must be recognized that tubal closing failure is expressed differently in different individuals. In some cases the eustachian tube may show all signs of being wide open. The middle ear pressure varies continuously with respiration, but no stable negative pressure is induced by sniffing. If the same ear is examined on another occasion the tube may no longer be wide open, and the ear is easily evacuated by sniffing. The tube locks and negative pressure is maintained in the middle ear. In other cases the first impression is that the tube is very firmly closed but later examination shows that negative pressure is induced by sniffing without much effort. The following classification into four different types may be helpful in understanding the various clinical expressions of the disorder (30).

A. The Constantly Wide-Open Tube

In this condition the tube is obviously wide open during examination. On otoscopy the tympanic membrane is seen to be moving in and out in response to the pressure variations with breathing. Despite this fact the subject may not be the least disturbed; he/she may not even be aware of the respiratory movements of the tympanic membrane and does not complain of autophonia. It is probable that the condition has been present for such a long time that the subject has accepted it as natural. Perhaps the tube has remained wide open since birth, in which case the subject has never known anything different, and no habitual sniffing behavior has developed. The appearance of the tympanic membrane may be normal apart from movements with respiration, or the membrane might show some sclerotic or atrophic areas. The constantly wide-open tube is the least common of the four types described here.

B. *The Intermittently Wide-Open Tube*

This condition is seen quite often in young adults with normal tympanic membranes. The tube is closed most of the time but on occasion it opens widely. The difference is experienced very acutely by the subject and no adaptation is possible. When the tube opens, the voice suddenly becomes too loud and echoing, as when one is speaking into an empty barrel. Seemingly, the tube tends to stay open in stressful situations of various kinds, both mental and physical (30). In women the disturbance is sometimes provoked by pregnancy or often by the use of contraceptive pills (38); a history of significant weight loss, such as seen in anorexia, is elicited. In elderly persons the disturbance often begins after a period of debilitating disease or after major surgery whereby the stress and loss of body weight are provoking factors. Intermittent autophonia is experienced as a profound disturbance, but the diagnosis is not always obvious. The tube may not be open at the time of examination, and the patient often cannot describe the symptoms clearly enough. The patient mostly complains of a closed-up sensation, which may lead to the false conclusion that the eustachian tube is obstructed. As a consequence the patient may visit one doctor after another, until finally the real cause of the complaint is revealed.

Closure of the eustachian tube depends, in part, on the hydrostatic pressure of venous blood with the result that autophonia related to a wide open tube occurs almost exclusively in the upright body position. When the person is recumbent the autophonia disappears; this is a characteristic diagnostic criterion. These patients may also report that the sensation of blockage paradoxically lessens during an upper respiratory infection.

C. *The Suppressed Wide-Open Tube*

This condition is frequently found in both children and adults with retracted eardrums, persistent middle ear effusion, or retraction cholesteatoma. Habitual sniffing behavior is firmly established. The behavior may not be too obvious and the subject is often so used to it that he/she may not be aware of the sniffing habit (and still less aware of the cause of the reactive behavior). This can make diagnosis difficult. Furthermore, the primary complaint is frequently not related to the state of the eustachian tubes but rather to some kind of chronic ear disease. The ear disease attracts attention in the first place, and conventional thinking easily leads to the implicit conclusion that the eustachian tube is obstructed. The real disturbance may never be revealed unless the evaluation is specifically designed for finding it. The patient may be suffering from severe middle ear disease requiring surgery, and it is essential that the real disturbance be detected, otherwise the habitual sniffing behavior will continue after surgery, and the result of the surgical procedure may be destroyed (32).

D. Relative Closing Failure

This is the most common of the four conditions described here. It is very frequently found in young children suffering from recurrent episodes of middle ear effusion (18). In this condition the eustachian tube never appears wide open. There is no sharp borderline, however, between this state and the previous one (type C). Many children seem to experience hyperacusis after inflation or nose-blowing and try to avoid this as much as possible. The children suffer from frequent common colds, which is the reason for their constant sniffing. The state of persistent middle ear effusion (serous or mucoid) is apparently induced by casual sniffing during common colds and is then maintained by continued habitual sniffing. The ability to equalize negative pressure by swallowing is mostly absent, and the one-way characteristic of the tubal passage is pronounced. This means that tubal passage in the up direction is difficult, but passage in the down direction takes place readily and is provoked by the sniffing.

Diagnostic Clues

The majority of patients belonging to types C and D have previously been given an incorrect diagnosis. Even so, the right diagnosis can be made clear using simple clinical methods that do not require sophisticated equipment. The patient is asked to inflate the ears by the Valsalva maneuver. The patient may remark that he/she does not like to do that. This is a first clue. When asked why, the patient may express fear that it may hurt or explain that the sound is so strange after inflation. If the patient makes only a half-hearted attempt and does not succeed in inflating the ears, a Politzer inflation may be performed, taking care not to blow too hard. Many patients have experienced extreme discomfort in connection with careless Politzerization (it feels like the ears explode). After successful inflation the patient is observed a short while to see if the positive pressure introduced is immediately eliminated by sniffing. The patient is asked a few questions regarding hearing. Sound may admittedly be heard more clearly than before the inflation, but it may appear too strong and sharp; the sound feels strange and there is some unpleasant quality to it.

The patient may recall previous episodes when hearing was experienced the same way (e.g., after yawning or nose-blowing) and may be able to show how the unpleasant sensation can be relieved by sniffing or by performing a reverse Valsalva maneuver. To obtain objective evidence, the position of the eardrums after inflation and sniffing can be assessed with the otomicroscope or the magnifying otoscope, and the change in middle ear pressure can be measured by tympanometry.

Frequently, the patient finds it very hard to verbalize how the disturbance is experienced. The expression, "My ears feel all closed up," may give a false lead. The closed-up sensation indicates an altered state of hearing and often refers to autophonia or hyperacusis (34). Much can be learned by communicating with the patients, taking a detailed case history, devoting time to listening and learning individual expressions used by patients, and learning to use certain key words that apply to the patients' own experiences.

FUTURE DEVELOPMENTS

A great deal of knowledge is available regarding the responses of the eustachian tube in artificial pressure environments, but understanding normal physiology has

The Toynbee test: In this test the nose is pinched while the subject swallows. A biphasic pressure change occurs in the nasopharynx as the soft palate moves up and then down again. Since the eustachian tube opens during swallowing the same pressure changes are often transmitted to the middle ear. A small positive pressure peak first appears; this is followed by negative pressure. The negative pressure may then remain for a while. In some ears only the negative pressure phase occurs in the middle ear.

Tests of Muscular Opening

Aspiration–deflation test: In this test a positive or negative test pressure of a certain magnitude is induced in the middle ear cavity, and the ability to reduce or eliminate the pressure by swallowing is studied. (In recent years the test has been called the inhalation–exhalation test.) The magnitude of the test pressure used has varied among investigators, but usually 1 to 2 kPa has been used (100 to 200 mm water pressure). In cases of perforated eardrums the test pressure is applied directly to the external ear canal, and the subject is asked to swallow several times. In cases of intact eardrums the test pressures are applied with the aid of a pressure chamber, and pressure changes are measured by serial tympanometry (9,16,19) or the microflow technique (14). The latter procedure is based on measuring the minute airflow caused by movement of the tympanic membrane in response to pressure changes. The result is then integrated with time to assess volume changes.

Forced response test: This test can only be performed when the tympanic membrane is perforated. Positive pressure is applied to the external ear canal, and air is forced through the eustachian tube with a pump until a constant flow is obtained. Swallowing is followed by an increased airflow as the eustachian tube is dilated by muscular contraction. The tubal resistance to airflow is calculated during resting conditions (passive resistance) and at the moment of swallowing when the resistance is expected to be lower (active resistance). In some patients an increased resistance during swallowing has been found, indicating that the tube is constricted rather than dilated by the act of swallowing (12).

Sonotubometry: In this procedure the transmission of sound through the open eustachian tube is studied (49). A loudspeaker presenting a constant tone is connected to the nose, and the sound is recorded by a microphone placed in the external ear canal. The recorded sound level increases as the tube opens on swallowing. This test has the obvious advantage that no pressure is applied to the ear, and the function of the eustachian tube is thus not disturbed by the test procedure. There are, however, technical difficulties in isolating the test tone from noise and therefore the test is not in general use.

REFERENCES

1. Andreasson, L., and Harris, S. (1979): Middle ear mechanics and eustachian tube function in tympanoplasty. *Acta Otolaryngol. [Suppl.] (Stockh.)*, 360:141–147.
2. Anson, B. J. (1973): Embryology and anatomy of the ear. In: *Otolaryngology*, vol. 1, edited by M. A. Paparella and D. A. Shumrick, pp. 3–110. Saunders, Philadelphia, London, Toronto.
3. Armstrong, H. G., and Heim, J. W. (1937): The effect of flight on the middle ear. *J. Am. Med. Assoc.*, 109:417–421.

4. Bezold, F. (1883): Die Verschliessung der Tuba Eustachii, ihre physikalische Diagnose und Einwirkung auf die Funktion des Ohres. *Berl. Klin. Wochenschr.*, 6:551–572.
5. Bluestone, C. D., Cantekin, E. J., and Berry, Q. C. (1976): Effect of inflammation on the ventilatory function of the eustachian tube. *Laryngoscope*, 87:493–507.
6. Bluestone, C. D., Wittel, R. A., and Paradise, J. L. (1972): Roentgenographic evaluation of the eustachian tube function in infants with cleft and normal palates. *Cleft Palate J.*, 9:93–100.
7. Buckingham, R. A., and Ferrer, J. (1980): Observations of middle ear pressures. *Ann. Otol. Rhinol. Laryngol.* (suppl. 68), 89:56–61.
8. Buckingham, R. A., Stuart, D. R., Gieck, H. A., Girgis, S. J., and McGee, T. J. (1984): Experimental evidence against middle ear oxygen absorption. *Laryngoscope*, 95:437–442.
9. Bylander, A., Ivarson, A., and Tjernstrom, O. (1981): Eustachian tube function in normal children and adults. *Acta Otolaryngol. (Stockh.)*, 92:481–491.
10. Cantekin, E. I., Doyle, W. J., and Bluestone, C. D. (1983): Effect of levator veli palatini muscle excision on eustachian tube function. *Arch. Otolaryngol.*, 109:281–284.
11. Cantekin, E. I., Doyle, W. J., Phillips, D., and Bluestone, C. D. (1980): Gas absorption in the middle ear. *Ann. Otol. Rhinol. Laryngol.* (suppl. 68), 89:71–75.
12. Cantekin, E. I., Sez, C. A., Bluestone, C. D., and Bern, S. A. (1979): Airflow through the eustachian tube. *Ann. Otol. Rhinol. Laryngol.*, 88:603–612.
13. Elner, A. (1977): Quantitative studies of gas absorption from the normal middle ear. *Acta Otolaryngol. (Stockh.)*, 83:25–28.
14. Elner, A., Ingelstedt, S., and Ivarsson, A. (1971): The normal function of the eustachian tube. A study of 102 cases. *Acta Otolaryngol. (Stockh.)*, 72:320–328.
15. Ekvall, L. (1970): Eustachian tube function in tympanoplasty. *Acta Otolaryngol. [Suppl.] (Stockh.)*, 263:33–42.
16. Falk, B. (1981): Negative middle ear pressure induced by sniffing, a tympanometric study in healthy ears. *J. Otolaryngol.*, 10(4):299–305.
17. Falk, B., and Magnuson, B. (1984): Test-rest variability of eustachian tube responses in children with persistent middle ear effusion. *Arch. Otorhinolaryngol.*, 240:145–152.
18. Falk, B., and Magnuson, B. (1984): Eustachian tube closing failure in children with persistent middle ear effusion. *Int. J. Pediatr. Otorhinolaryngol.*, 7:97–106.
19. Falk, B., and Magnuson, B. (1984): Eustachian tube closing failure: Occurrence in patients with cleft palate and middle ear disease. *Arch. Otolaryngol.*, 110:10–14.
20. Flisberg, K., Ingelstedt, S., and Ortegren, U. (1963): The valve and "locking" mechanism of the eustachian tube. *Acta Otolaryngol. [Suppl.] (Stockh.)*, 182:57–68.
21. Groth, P., Ivarsson, A., Tjernstrom, O., and White, P. (1985): The effect of pressure change rate on the Eustachian tube function in pressure chamber tests. *Acta Otolaryngol. (Stockh.)*, 99: 67–73.
22. Hergils, L., and Magnuson, B. (1985): Morning pressure in the middle ear. *Arch. Otolaryngol.*, 111:86–89.
23. Hergils, L., and Magnuson, B. (1987): Middle ear pressure under basal conditions. *Arch. Otolaryngol. Head Neck Surg.*, 113:829–832.
24. Holborow, C. (1970): Eustachian tubal function, changes in anatomy and function with age and the relationship of these changes to aural pathology. *Arch. Otolaryngol.*, 92:624–626.
25. Holmgren, L. (1940): Experimental tubal occlusion. *Acta Otolaryngol. (Stockh.)*, 28:587–592.
26. Honjo, I., Okazaki, N., and Kumazawa, T. (1979): Experimental study of the eustachian tube function with regard to its related muscles. *Acta Otolaryngol. (Stockh.)*, 87:84–89.
27. Ingelstedt, S., Ivarsson, A., and Jonson, B. (1967): Mechanics of human middle ear. Pressure regulation in aviation and diving. A non-traumatic method. *Acta Otolaryngol. [Suppl.] (Stockh.)*, 228:1–57.
28. Kamerer, D. B. (1978): Electromyographic correlation of tensor tympani and tensor veli palatini muscles in man. *Laryngoscope*, 88:651–662.
29. Magnus, A. (1864): Verhalten des Gehor-organs in komprimierter Luft. *Arch. Ohrenheilk.*, 1:269–283.
30. Magnuson, B. (1978): Tubal closing failure in retraction type cholesteatoma and adhesive middle ear lesions. *Acta Otolaryngol. (Stockh.)*, 86:408–417.
31. Magnuson, B. (1981): On the origin of the high negative pressure in the middle ear space. *Am. J. Otolaryngol.*, 2:1–12.
32. Magnuson, B. (1981): Tympanoplasty and recurrent disease: Sniff induced high negative pressure in the middle ear space. *Am. J. Otolaryngol.*, 2:277–283.
33. Magnuson, B. (1983): Eustachian tube pathophysiology. *Am. J. Otolaryngol.*, 4:123–130.
34. Magnuson, B., and Falk, B. (1983): Eustachian tube malfunction and middle ear disease in new perspective. *J. Otolaryngol.*, 12(3):187–193.
35. Magnuson, B., and Falk, B. (1984): Diagnosis and management of eustachian tube malfunction. *Otolaryngol. Clin. North Am.*, 17:659–671.

36. Melville Jones, G. (1961): Pressure changes in the middle ear after altering the composition of the contained gas. *Acta Otolaryngol. (Stockh.),* 53:1–11.

37. Moller, A. R. (1974): The acoustic middle ear reflex. In: *Handbook of Sensory Physiology,* edited by H. Autrum, R. Jung, W. R. Loewenstein, D. M. McKay, and H. L. Teuber, pp. 519–548. Springer Verlag, Berlin, Heidelberg, New York.

38. Münker, G. (1980): The patulous eustachian tube. In: *Physiology and Pathophysiology of Eustachian Tube and Middle Ear,* edited by G. Munker and W. Arnold, pp. 113–117. Georg Thieme, Stuttgart.

39. Piiper, J. (1965): Physiological equilibria of gas pockets in the body. In: *Handbook of Physiology,* edited by W. O. Fenn and H. Rahn, pp. 1205–1218. American Physiological Society, Washington, DC.

40. Politzer, A. (1867): Diagnose und Therapie der Anammlung seroser Flussigkeit in der Trommelhohle. *Wien. Med. Wochenschr.,* 17:244–247.

41. Proctor, B. (1967): Embryology and anatomy of the eustachian tube. *Arch. Otolaryngol.,* 86:51–62.

42. Proud, G., Odoi, H., and Toledo, P. (1971): Bulbar pressure changes in eustachian tube dysfunction. *Ann. Otol. Rhinol. Laryngol.,* 80:835–837.

43. Rahn, H., and Canfield, R. E. (1955): Volume changes and steady state behavior of gas pockets within body cavities. In: *Studies in Respiratory Physiology,* edited by H. Rahn and W. O. Fenn. Technical Report 55-357, pp. 395–408. Wright Air Development Center, Dayton, OH.

44. Rich, A. R. (1920): A physiological study of the eustachian tube and its related muscles. *Bull. Johns Hopkins Hosp.,* 352:206–214.

45. Rood, S. R., and Doyle, W. J. (1978): Morphology of tensor veli palatini, tensor tympani and dilator tubae muscles. *Ann. Otol. Rhinol. Laryngol.,* 87:202–210.

46. Rundcrantz, H. (1969): Posture and eustachian tube function. *Acta Otolaryngol. (Stockh.),* 68:279–292.

47. Tjernstrom, O. (1974): Middle ear mechanics and alternobaric vertigo. *Acta Otolaryngol. (Stockh.),* 78:376–384.

48. Tos, M. (1970): Development of mucous glands in the human eustachian tube. *Acta Otolaryngol. (Stockh.),* 70:340–350.

49. Virtanen, H. (1978): Patulous eustachian tube, diagnostic evaluation by sono-tubometry. *Acta Otolaryngol. (Stockh.),* 86:401–407.

50. Zollner, F. (1936): Wiederstandsmessungen an der Ohrtrompete zur Prufung ihrer Wegsamkeit. *Arch. Ohren. Nasen u. Kehlkopfheilk.,* 140:137–154.

Physiology of the Ear,
edited by A. F. Jahn and J. Santos-Sacchi.
Raven Press, New York © 1988.

Introduction to the Analysis of Middle-Ear Function

Evan M. Relkin

*Institute for Sensory Research and Department of Bioengineering, Syracuse University,
Syracuse, New York 13244-5290*

The role of the middle ear is to couple airborne sound waves to the fluid-filled scala vestibuli of the cochlea. Understanding the function of the middle ear, under normal or pathological conditions, requires at least some appreciation of the basics of acoustics and mechanics. Generally, these disciplines are not part of the background of those with a clinical interest in hearing. Yet, measurements of the input admittance (or input impedance or input compliance) are routine steps in an audiological examination. The goal of this chapter is to provide an understanding of the necessary basics of acoustics and mechanics with the aid of graphical interpretations and with little reliance on mathematics beyond simple algebra. There is minimal derivation of results, but rather results are given as mathematical expressions whose interpretation and significance are explored. Questions that are considered are of this nature: How does the additional mass of pathological bone growth on the ossicles affect the middle-ear admittance? I hope that the reader will develop the means to respond to such questions without having to resort to memorization of multiple cause and effect relationships. At times I have attempted to clarify issues that are sometimes confused in the clinical interpretation of measurements of middle-ear function.

The chosen goal of this chapter is an ambitious one. It would be equally or more ambitious to attempt to review all that is known about middle-ear function. By necessity some topics simply cannot be covered. For example, a topic that would require a chapter of its own is the middle-ear reflex (11). The concepts developed in this chapter derive from many years of physiological and theoretical research, beginning with the pioneering work of Helmholtz (4) and the early work of Wever and Lawrence (18) and Békésy (1). Within the context of this chapter it is not possible to cite all the subsequent literature. For more scholarly reviews of the scientific literature the reader is referred to the reviews of Dallos (2), Møller (12), and Zwislocki (21). The results presented in this chapter derive from experiments on several mammalian species, including guinea pigs, cats, and humans. In some cases the human data are from experiments on cadavers. Rather than confuse the discussion with constant reference to the appropriate species, I have presented the material as if it applied to a single generic species. There are many similarities among the middle-ear mechanisms of these species. In general the similarities are much greater than the differences. However, the reader is warned that differences do exist, and generalizations can sometimes be erroneous. The reader is referred to the cited literature for details.

THE MIDDLE EAR AS AN ACOUSTIC TRANSFORMER

When sound waves encounter a boundary between two different materials, as exists at the surface of a body of water, some of the sound energy will enter the second material and some of the energy will be reflected. The fraction of energy that enters the second material is determined by the *acoustic impedances* (Z) of the two materials as shown in Eq. 1 where

$$\frac{E_2}{E_1} = \frac{4Z_2Z_1}{(Z_2 + Z_1)^2} \qquad [1]$$

E_1 is the incoming sound energy in the first material, E_2 is the sound energy transmitted into the second material, Z_2 is the acoustic impedance of the second material, and Z_1 is the acoustic impedance of the first material. Acoustic impedance is a property of any object, be it gas, solid, or liquid, that depends on the density and geometry of the object. The concept of the acoustic impedance will be developed further in subsequent sections. When the impedances of the two materials are equal, this ratio reaches a maximum value of 1.0, meaning that all the energy enters the second material. When the impedances of the two materials are different, the ratio will always be less than 1.0. This condition is known as an *impedance mismatch*. For example, the acoustic impedance of water is 3,470 times the acoustic impedance of air. At the boundary between a large expanse of air and water, it can be calculated using Eq. 1 that only 0.1% of the sound energy enters the water.

For hearing to occur, airborne sound energy must enter the fluid-filled cochlea. Without the middle ear, sound would impinge directly on the oval window of the cochlea and there would be an air–water boundary. The example given above was for such an interface with a large surface area. The surface area of the oval window of the cochlea is small and thus those calculations do not apply exactly. However, through more detailed analysis it can be calculated that about 3.0% of the incoming sound energy would enter the cochlea. This is equivalent to a hearing loss of 15 dB. The role of the middle ear is to change or *transform* the impedance of the cochlea so that when sound impinges on the tympanic membrane, the impedance mismatch is not as severe as it would be if the sound had impinged directly on the oval window. How the middle ear achieves this transformation is our next topic.

The simplest model of the mechanical action of the middle ear is the folded "seesaw" diagramed in Fig. 1. The tympanic membrane and the footplate of the stapes are represented as two circular "seats" with different surface areas. A solid circular surface that moves back and forth is often referred to as a *piston*. The length of the seesaw from the tympanic membrane to the fulcrum, or axis of rotation, represents the manubrium of the malleus. Likewise, the length of the seesaw from the footplate of the stapes to the axis of rotation represents the long arm of the incus. These lengths are often referred to as *lever arms*. Sound pressure applies a force on the piston representing the tympanic membrane and is transferred to the cochlea at the footplate of the stapes through the rotation of the lever mechanism. The difference in the areas of the two pistons and the lengths of the lever arms results in an amplification of the pressure at the footplate of the stapes relative to the pressure at the tympanic membrane. As we will develop, this pressure amplification also results in an impedance transformation so that the impedance at the tympanic membrane is closer to that of air than the impedance at the footplate of the stapes.

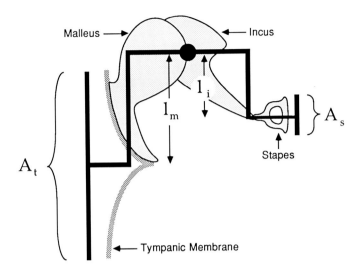

FIG. 1. The seesaw model of the middle ear is superimposed on a diagram of the tympanic membrane and the ossicular chain. A_t and A_s are the areas of the tympanic membrane and the stapes footplate, respectively. l_m and l_i are the lever arms associated with the manubrium of the malleus and the long arm of the incus, respectively.

Pressure P is equal to force F divided by surface area A (Eq. 2). A basic law of

$$P = \frac{F}{A} \qquad [2]$$

mechanics states that at the axis of rotation, the product of the force applied at one piston and the length of the lever arm must equal the same product for the other lever arm. Using this law and Eq. 2, we obtain:

$$P_t A_t l_m = P_s A_s l_i \qquad [3]$$

where P_t is the pressure at the tympanic membrane; A_t, the area of the tympanic membrane; l_m, the lever arm associated with the manubrium of the malleus; P_s, the pressure at the stapes footplate, A_s, the area of the stapes footplate; l_i, the lever arm associated with the long arm of the incus. The subscripts i, m, s, and t will refer to the incus, malleus, stapes, and tympanic membrane, respectively, when used with all variables introduced subsequently. Rearranging Eq. 3 gives the ratio of the sound pressure at the stapes to the sound pressure at the tympanic membrane:

$$\frac{P_s}{P_t} = \frac{A_t}{A_s} \times \frac{l_m}{l_i} \qquad [4]$$

The first fraction on the right-hand side of Eq. 4 is referred to as the *area ratio* and the second fraction is referred to as the *lever ratio*. Since the area of the tympanic membrane is greater than the area of the stapes footplate and the manubrium of the malleus is longer than the long arm of the incus, both of these ratios will be greater than one and the pressure at the stapes will be greater than the pressure at the tympanic membrane.

To continue the development of the impedance transformer it is necessary to

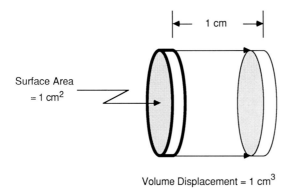

← 1 cm →

Surface Area
= 1 cm²

Volume Displacement = 1 cm³

FIG. 2. Diagrammatic interpretation of the variable *volume displacement*. If a piston with a surface area of 1.0 cm² is moved left to right 1.0 cm, the piston sweeps out a cylinder with a volume equal to the surface area multiplied by the displacement, in this case 1.0 cm³. This is the *volume displacement*. If this motion were to take place in 1.0 sec, then the *volume velocity* would be 1.0 cm³/sec.

introduce the variable known as *volume velocity*. Referring to Fig. 2, if a piston with a surface area of 1.0 cm² moves a distance of 1.0 cm, then the volume swept out by the piston is 1.0 cm³. This product of the surface area and the length of motion is known as the *volume displacement*. If the motion took place in 1.0 sec, then the velocity of the piston was 1.0 cm/sec and the *volume velocity* was 1.0 cm³/sec. Thus for the simple motion of a piston, volume velocity U is the surface area of the piston multiplied by the velocity u of the piston:

$$U = A \times u \qquad [5]$$

A definition that we will need later is that of acoustic impedance Z which is equal to the ratio of sound pressure to volume velocity:

$$Z = \frac{P}{U} \qquad [6]$$

Returning to the model of the middle ear, from simple geometrical considerations it can be shown that the velocity of the piston representing the tympanic membrane divided by the velocity of the piston representing the footplate of the stapes is equal to the lever ratio (Eq. 7).

$$\frac{u_t}{u_s} = \frac{l_m}{l_i} \qquad [7]$$

This makes intuitive sense if you consider the seesaw. Both sides of the seesaw must move back and forth in the same amount of time. The end of the seesaw with the longer lever arm will move a greater distance. Velocity is distance divided by time, so the end of the seesaw with the longer lever arm, the manubrium, will have a greater velocity. Equation 4 can be modified by substituting the ratio of velocities for the lever ratio:

$$\frac{P_s}{P_t} = \frac{A_t}{A_s} \times \frac{u_t}{u_s} \qquad [8]$$

If we substitute volume velocity divided by area (U/A) for the velocities u in Eq.

8 the area terms will cancel and we see that the ratio of the pressures is equal to the ratio of the volume velocities:

$$\frac{P_s}{P_t} = \frac{U_t}{U_s}$$ [9a]

or

$$P_s \times U_s = P_t \times U_t$$ [9b]

Equation 9b describes one of the basic principles of a transformer. The product of pressure and volume velocity, which is equal to energy, is constant. If pressure is increased then volume velocity must be decreased for the product to remain constant. A transformer works by trading the size of one variable against the size of the other. At the stapes, sound pressure is increased while volume velocity is decreased relative to values at the tympanic membrane. Thus the pressure at the stapes is amplified, but because the product of pressure and volume velocity remains constant, no energy has been added.

A few more algebraic manipulations will allow us to derive the impedance transformation. Combining Eqs. 5 and 6 gives the following expression for sound pressure:

$$P = ZuA$$ [10]

If we substitute this expression for the sound pressures in Eq. 8, rearrange terms, and substitute the lever ratio for the ratio of velocities (Eq. 7), we obtain Eq. 11, which gives the ratio of the impedance at the tympanic membrane to the impedance at the footplate of the stapes:

$$\frac{Z_t}{Z_s} = \left(\frac{A_s}{A_t}\right)^2 \left(\frac{l_i}{l_m}\right)^2$$ [11]

Since the area of the stapes footplate is less than the area of the tympanic membrane and the long arm of the incus is shorter than the manubrium of the malleus, the right-hand side of Eq. 11 will be less than 1.0, and the impedance at the tympanic membrane will be reduced relative to the impedance at the stapes footplate. This is the *impedance transformer* action of the middle ear. The acoustic impedance of the fluid in the cochlea at the oval window is decreased at the tympanic membrane to a value that is closer to the acoustic impedance of air. Referring back to Eq. 1 you can see that this will increase the amount of the incoming sound energy that will be transmitted by the middle ear to the cochlea. Calculations show that the expected loss of sound pressure owing to reflection at the tympanic membrane is reduced to 1 to 2 dB compared with the 15 dB mentioned earlier (2).

The model of the middle ear we have been discussing is a highly idealized model. Several qualifications of the model should be discussed. First, although the footplate of the stapes may be well represented by a piston, this is not true of the tympanic membrane. The tympanic membrane is a complex, flexible structure and all its parts do not vibrate with the same displacement. Our understanding of the pattern of motion of the tympanic membrane has been changed drastically in the last two decades. In Fig. 3 the motion of the tympanic membrane is represented by lines of equal displacement that are analogous to the lines of equal elevation on a geograph-

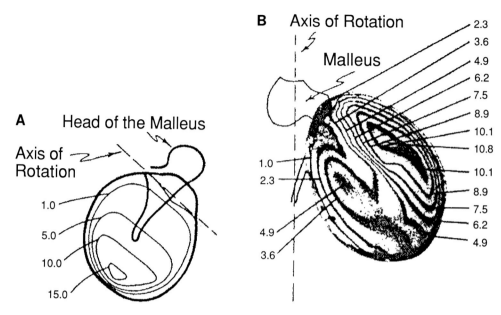

FIG. 3. Displacement contours for motion of the tympanic membrane as described by Békésy **(A)** and Khanna and Tonndorf **(B)**. A: the numbers represent relative displacements for frequencies below 2,000 Hz, and B: the numbers are the displacement in units of 10^{-5} cm at 600 Hz, 111 dB SPL. Note that in A there is a single displacement peak just below the tip of the malleus whereas in B there are two displacement peaks, one on each side of the malleus near the level of the umbo. (Modified from ref. 5.)

ical contour map. Békésy's (1) description of the pattern of motion is shown in Fig. 3A. The point of maximal displacement (the peak of a hill) was at a point below the umbo of the malleus in the center of a region referred to as the *lower fold*. This point was surrounded by irregular rings representing decreasing displacement at points increasingly distant from the point of maximal displacement. Holographic images of the motion of the tympanic membrane show a different pattern of motion (Fig. 3B) (5,16,17). In the latter image, there are two points of maximal displacement on either side of the manubrium roughly at the level of the umbo. Each maximum is surrounded by contours of decreasing displacement. In effect, there are two hills, one on either side of the manubrium.

In either case, it is clear that the motion of the tympanic membrane is not like that of a piston, which has constant displacement across its entire surface. It is possible to calculate the net volume displacement for complex patterns of motion such as those shown in Fig. 3. We can then represent this motion with a piston of appropriate surface area chosen so that the volume displacement is the same as that for the complex motion. The surface area of this equivalent piston is referred to as the *effective area* of the motion of the tympanic membrane. Typically, the effective area is between 60% and 80% of the actual area of the tympanic membrane. The piston in our model of the middle ear whose surface area equals the surface area of the entire tympanic membrane must be replaced with a piston with the correct effective area. The calculation of the effective area is further complicated by the fact that the pattern of motion of the tympanic membrane is not the same at all sound frequencies. Above 2,500 Hz, the pattern of vibration of the membrane becomes increasingly complex relative to the patterns shown in Fig. 3, which only apply for lower frequencies. To be precise, we would need to calculate an effective area for each frequency. Therefore, it is not possible to give a single precise value for the area ratio, a value that is needed to calculate the pressure amplification and the impedance transformation.

A second simplification assumed in the seesaw model involves the lever arm associated with the manubrium. This lever arm has been treated as if all the forces are applied at the end, i.e., at the umbo. This is not the case since the manubrium is attached to the tympanic membrane along much of its length. Forces acting anywhere other than at the umbo act through a lever arm that is less than the length of the manubrium. Again, an equivalent *effective lever* can be calculated (5), but the value of the lever ratio that should be used in the preceding equations is also uncertain.

A final consideration involves the pattern of displacement shown in the holographic images. The displacement, and thus the velocity, to the right and left of the manubrium is greater than that of the manubrium itself. This results in a transformer-type action. At the manubrium, velocity is decreased but is necessarily accompanied by an increase in pressure. As shown before (Eq. 9B), the product of velocity and pressure must remain constant. Therefore there is a pressure amplification and an impedance transformation that occurs within the tympanic membrane. This effect is thought to be attributed to the curvature of the tympanic membrane. This *catenary* effect is the same one that is applied in the design of suspension bridges. You will note the similarity of the curvature of the tympanic membrane to the curvature of the cables used to support a suspension bridge. Khanna and Tonndorf (5) suggested that this *membrane transformer* is the most important determinant of the impedance matching function of the middle ear, having a greater effect than either the *effective* lever ratio or the *effective* area ratio, or the product of both.

From the discussion of the last few paragraphs it should be clear that the simple seesaw model of the middle ear is at best an approximation. The model introduces the concepts that explain the transformer action of the middle ear, but it is difficult, if not impossible, to relate with precise numbers physical structures within the middle ear to the parts of the model.

THE FREQUENCY DEPENDENCE OF THE MIDDLE-EAR INPUT IMPEDANCE

Until now we have been treating the impedance of the middle ear as if it could be represented by a single number that was not a function of frequency. Careful readers may have realized that if the effective area changes with frequency, then the area ratio changes with frequency and the impedance transformation provided by the middle ear must also change with frequency. Even if the impedance at the footplate of the stapes, i.e., the input impedance of the cochlea, were constant with frequency [it is not, see (6)], the impedance at the tympanic membrane would vary with frequency as a result of the concomitant changes with frequency in the area ratio. There are other factors that make the impedance at the tympanic membrane change with frequency. We will now consider those factors and how they contribute to the impedance that is measured at the tympanic membrane.

In the seesaw model of the middle ear, many physical aspects of that system were ignored. The masses of the ossicles and tympanic membrane were not considered. The tympanic membrane, the joints between the ossicles, and the muscles and ligaments attached to the ossicles all have elastic properties; they behave like springs. Throughout the middle-ear system there are sources of friction that dissipate, or waste, vibrational energy. Last, the physical properties at the oval window of the cochlea that determine the impedance of the cochlea are complex, as already indicated. All these factors combine to determine the actual impedance that is measured at the tympanic membrane, referred to as the *input impedance* of the middle ear. As we will see, this impedance is a function that is strongly dependent on frequency.

Before discussing input impedance, we must develop a few mathematical concepts. To describe an impedance that varies with frequency actually requires two functions. There are two alternative, but mathematically equivalent, ways of doing this. The first is to describe the impedance as a complex number as shown in Eq. 12. (Henceforth, complex numbers will be indicated by uppercase, boldface type, e.g., the symbol for complex impedance will be $\mathbf{Z}$.)

$$\mathbf{Z} = R + iX \qquad\qquad [12]$$

The imaginary number i is the square root of negative one. A complex number such as $\mathbf{Z}$ is the sum of a real part R and an imaginary part iX. The real part R is known as *resistance*. The coefficient of the imaginary part X is known as *reactance*. In general, both R and X vary with frequency and together they are one of two possible sets of functions required to describe the complex impedance.

The alternative sets of functions required to specify $\mathbf{Z}$ are the magnitude and phase functions. This description of $\mathbf{Z}$ is best understood by referring to Fig. 4. Here $\mathbf{Z}$ is

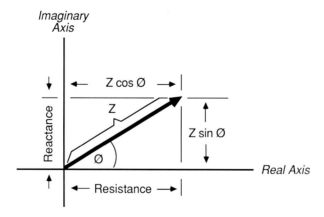

FIG. 4. Graphical interpretation of two mathematical descriptions of complex impedance, $\mathbf{Z} = R + iX$. $\mathbf{Z}$ is represented as a vector, the thick-lined arrow. The angle between the abscissa and the arrow, measured in a counterclockwise direction, is the phase angle $\emptyset$. Resistance (R) is the projection of the vector onto the abscissa or real axis. Reactance (X) is the projection of the vector onto the ordinate or imaginary axis. See text for further explanation.

plotted on a special set of axes known as the complex plane. The real part of **Z** (i.e., *R*) is plotted on the abscissa and the coefficient of the imaginary part of **Z** (i.e., *X*) is plotted on the ordinate. The complex impedance **Z** is represented by a vector, an arrow that extends from the origin of the axes to the corner of the rectangle determined by the real and imaginary parts. The length of the arrow is the vector's *magnitude* (indicated by uppercase, lightface type, e.g., *Z*) and the angle between the abscissa and the arrow, measured in a counterclockwise direction, is the *phase angle* (∅). Negative angles indicate a clockwise rotation from the abscissa. The resistance and the reactance of **Z** are the projections of the arrow onto the abscissa and ordinate, respectively, as indicated in the figure. The mathematical expressions for these projections are also indicated on the figure. The magnitude and phase angle, like the resistance and reactance, depend on frequency. Equations 13a and b give the relationships between the two alternative pairs of functions that can be used to describe the complex impedance **Z**.

$$\text{Magnitude: } Z = \sqrt{R^2 + X^2} \qquad [13a]$$

$$\text{Phase angle: } \emptyset = \arctan \frac{X}{R} \qquad [13b]$$

The customary way of describing a complex number graphically is to plot either resistance and reactance as functions of frequency or magnitude and phase as functions of frequency. We will see several examples of the latter in later discussions.

At this point it is convenient to introduce a variable called admittance (*Y*). We will concentrate on admittance henceforth, because admittance is what is most often measured by clinical devices such as tympanometers and otoadmittance meters. As indicated by the boldface type, admittance is also a complex number that is the reciprocal of **Z**. Referring to Eq. 6, admittance is equal to volume velocity divided by sound pressure. Therefore, for a fixed sound pressure, a greater admittance implies a greater volume velocity, or equivalently a greater response to sound. The magnitude of *Y* is the reciprocal of the magnitude of **Z**, and the phase angle of *Y* is the negative of the phase angle of **Z**. These relationships are summarized below:

$$Y = \frac{1}{Z} \qquad [14a]$$

$$Y = \frac{1}{Z} \qquad [14b]$$

$$\emptyset_{\text{admittance}} = -1 \times \emptyset_{\text{impedance}} \qquad [14c]$$

Admittance is the sum of a real part, conductance *G*, and an imaginary part *i* multiplied by susceptance *B*:

$$Y = G + iB \qquad [15a]$$

$$Y = \sqrt{G^2 + B^2} \qquad [15b]$$

$$\emptyset = \arctan \frac{B}{G} \qquad [15c]$$

It is very important to realize that *G* is not the reciprocal of *R* and *B* is not the reciprocal of *X*. This can be proven easily using the algebra of complex numbers but the proof is not necessary within the context of this chapter. The actual relationships are given below:

$$G = \frac{R}{R^2 + X^2}; \quad B = \frac{X}{R^2 + X^2} \qquad [16]$$

The physical properties of the middle-ear mechanism that contribute to the input admittance are friction, mass, and compliance. Friction is a resistance to motion that results in the conversion of mechanical energy to heat. Thus, the symbol for friction is often taken as R for resistance. We will use lowercase r to avoid confusion with the resistance part of the complex impedance. Energy converted to heat through friction is wasted because it is not transmitted through the middle ear into the cochlea. The mass of an object (M) results in inertia, which is the tendency of an object to resist changes in speed or the direction of motion. The greater the change of speed or direction, the greater the force that is needed to overcome the inertia. Objects vibrating in response to sound are changing speed constantly and must change direction twice every cycle. The higher the frequency of the sound, the greater the speed and the more frequent the changes of directions. Therefore, the effects of mass are more important as frequency increases. Compliance (C) is the reciprocal of stiffness. The less stiff a spring is, the more compliant it is. Membranes, such as the skin of a drum or the tympanic membrane, also are compliant. For a given applied pressure, the more compliant the membrane, the greater will be the indentation of the membrane. In contrast to mass, compliance is more important at low frequencies.

Complex mechanical systems, such as the suspension system of an automobile or the middle-ear mechanism, can be represented by many interconnected mechanical parts that are either resistance elements, masses, or springs. The admittance of the whole device can be derived from the combined admittances of each part of the entire system. How this is done is beyond our scope. However, the admittances of each type of part are given below (the symbol f is for frequency):

$$\text{Resistance: } \mathbf{Y} = \frac{1}{r} \qquad [17a]$$

$$\text{Mass: } \mathbf{Y} = \frac{-i}{2\pi fM} \qquad [17b]$$

$$\text{Compliance: } \mathbf{Y} = (2\pi fC)i \qquad [17c]$$

The admittance of a resistance element does not depend on frequency and has a magnitude of $1/r$ and a phase angle of zero. The admittance of a mass element is purely imaginary with a magnitude of $1/2\pi fM$. Since the admittance of a mass only has a negative imaginary part, its vector will lie along the imaginary axis and point in a negative direction. This vector has a phase angle of $-90°$. Notice that the magnitude of the admittance of a mass element, which is a measure of how much it will vibrate for a fixed applied sound pressure, *decreases* as frequency *increases*; the higher the frequency the lesser the amount of vibration. Also note that the phase angle does not depend on frequency. The admittance of a compliance element is also purely imaginary with a magnitude of $2\pi fC$ and a constant phase angle of $+90°$. Notice that the magnitude of the admittance of a compliance *decreases* as frequency decreases; the lower the frequency the lesser the amount of vibration.

Several complex models of the middle ear have been described in the scientific literature (8,14,19,20). These models can be analyzed mathematically to calculate such things as the input admittance at the tympanic membrane. The results of such calculations agree with experimental data. Appreciating these complex models is difficult for those not well versed in mechanics and mathematics. Fortunately, a simple model can do a reasonable job of reproducing the general trends seen in the more complex models. This model consists of one of each of the mechanical elements: a resistance, a compliance, and a mass (9,13). We will consider this model in detail to gain an understanding of which anatomical features contribute to each of the mechanical elements of the model. The model will also be used to predict changes in the input admittance produced by changes in the size of one of the elements as might occur in pathological conditions. Through this exercise the reader should develop a greater appreciation for the physiological and clinical significance of the admittance measured at the tympanic membrane.

Resistance in the middle ear system exists wherever there is friction between the moving parts, as can occur at the joints between the ossicles. Friction also occurs within the tympanic membrane as a result of the motion of the fibers that make up the membrane. However, the major contributor to resistance in the middle-ear system is the input to the cochlea (19). Since resistance represents expenditure of energy, most of the energy transmitted through the middle ear is used to stimulate the cochlea and is not lost as heat in the middle-ear mechanism.

Mass is often the most confusing element in a mechanical system. Mass is proportional to the weight of an object or equal to weight divided by the acceleration owing to gravity. Any object that has mass has inertia—the greater the mass, the greater the inertia. If an object is moving in a straight line, the mass and inertia are equivalent. However, in a rotating system, such as the seesaw model of the middle ear, the geometry of the moving object is critically important in determining its motion. For an example, a figure skater in a spin rotates very rapidly when his/her arms are tucked close to his/her body, but slows dramatically if his/her arms are extended. The skater has not changed his/her mass, but has changed his/her *moment of inertia* by changing the geometry. The moment of inertia is calculated by multiplying the mass by the square of the distance from the axis of rotation. Therefore, with arms extended more of the skater's mass is far away from the axis of rotation and the skater's moment of inertia is increased, making it more difficult to spin. The axis of rotation of the middle-ear system passes through the head of the malleus and the head of the incus where most of the mass of the ossicles is concentrated. The bulk of the mass is very close to the axis of rotation, thereby keeping the moment of inertia as small as possible. Therefore the energy required to overcome the effects of inertia are minimized. In subsequent discussion, for the sake of simplicity, we will continue to refer to the mass of the middle-ear system and will not make explicit calculations of the moment of inertia. When we increase mass in our model of the middle ear we are really increasing the inertia without specifying whether the change is because of changes in mass, in geometry, or both.

Any object that can expand and contract has compliance. Compliance in the middle-ear system is contributed by the joints of the ossicles, the annular ligament, and the muscles and other ligaments that connect to the ossicles. However, the most important contributors to compliance are the tympanic membrane and the middle-ear space. The net compliance that results from these two elements is often a source

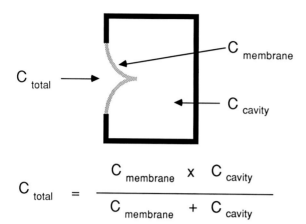

$$C_{total}$$

$C_{membrane}$

C_{cavity}

$$C_{total} = \frac{C_{membrane} \times C_{cavity}}{C_{membrane} + C_{cavity}}$$

FIG. 5. Diagram showing the derivation of the total compliance measured at the tympanic membrane when there is an enclosed cavity, the middle-ear space, behind the membrane. The total compliance depends on the compliance of the membrane itself and the compliance of the enclosed space as given in the equation.

of confusion and some clarification is necessary. The tympanic membrane has a compliance of its own. This is the compliance that would be measured if the tympanic membrane, supported by the tympanic ring, were suspended in free space. The volume of air enclosed by the middle-ear cavity also has a compliance of its own. If a volume of air is squeezed it will, like a spring, exert a force opposite to the applied pressure. If the applied pressure is released the air will expand, like a spring, back to its original volume. The compliance of the cavity depends on the volume V of air as given in Eq. 18:

$$C = \frac{V}{\rho c^2} \qquad [18]$$

where ρ is the density of air and c is the speed of sound. The smaller the volume of air is, the smaller the associated compliance, and the smaller the compliance, the smaller will be the volume change for a fixed applied pressure. As diagramed in Fig. 5, the compliance of the tympanic membrane itself and the middle-ear volume combine to determine the compliance measured at the tympanic membrane when the space behind it is enclosed by the walls of the middle-ear cavity. The mathematical expression for the combined compliance is also given in the figure. A common error is to confuse the compliance of the membrane itself with the total compliance.

By examining the equation given in Fig. 5, we can learn something about the relative contributions of the two compliances to the total compliance. Consider the case in which the middle-ear cavity is so large that the compliance of the cavity is much greater than the compliance of the tympanic membrane. The denominator in the equation for the total compliance is then approximately equal to the compliance of the cavity alone. (The sum of a relatively large number and a relatively small number is approximately equal to the large number, e.g., 1.000 + 0.001 is equal to 1.000 within one-tenth of 1% error.) We can then cancel the denominator and the compliance of the cavity in the numerator. The result is that for a large middle-ear space, the total compliance is approximately equal to the compliance of the tympanic membrane alone. If instead the cavity were very small, its compliance would be very small and the denominator would be approximately equal to the compliance of the tympanic membrane. In this case the total compliance would approximately equal the compliance of the cavity. In summary, if either compliance is much smaller than the other, the total compliance will be approximately equal to the smaller of the two compliances. In humans, under normal conditions, the compliance of the tympanic membrane is smaller than the compliance of the middle-ear space and therefore, the compliance of the tympanic membrane tends to dominate the total compliance (19). The situation can be reversed when fluid partially fills the middle-ear cavity and the air volume is reduced. In this case, the total compliance at the tympanic membrane can be dominated by the reduced compliance of the middle-ear space.

We will now combine each of the three elements, resistance, mass, and compliance, to form a simple model of the middle ear. The complex input admittance at the tympanic membrane for this model will be described by the admittance magnitude and phase angle as functions of frequency. The equations for these functions are:

$$Y = \sqrt{\dfrac{1}{r^2 + \left(2\pi f M - \dfrac{1}{2\pi f C}\right)^2}} \qquad [19]$$

$$\emptyset = \arctan\left(\dfrac{\dfrac{1}{2\pi f C} - 2\pi f M}{r^2}\right) \qquad [20]$$

These expressions have been evaluated and plotted in Fig. 6 for values of r, M, and C chosen such that the results are similar in appearance to actual measurements of

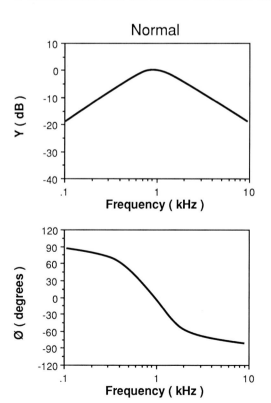

FIG. 6. Admittance magnitude and phase plotted as functions of frequency for the simplified middle-ear model consisting of one resistance element, one compliance element, and one mass element. Frequency is plotted on a logarithmic scale. Admittance magnitude is plotted on a relative decibel scale chosen so that the maximum at 1.0 kHz is at 0 dB. Phase is plotted in degrees. Note that the phase angle equals 0° at the frequency for which the magnitude is maximum and is equal to +90° at the lowest frequency and −90° at the highest frequency.

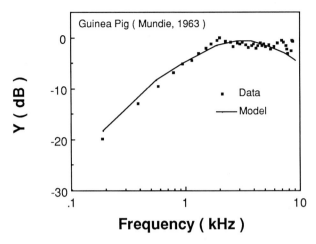

FIG. 7. Relative admittance magnitude for the guinea pig (ref. 13) plotted as a function of frequency. Actual data (*solid squares*) averaged for 10 ears are compared with calculations based on a three-element model of the guinea pig middle ear. Notice the good agreement between the data and the model at all but the highest frequencies.

the input admittance of the human middle ear. Sound frequency is represented on a logarithmic scale from 0.1 to 10.0 kHz. The magnitude function is plotted as relative values, on a decibel scale, such that the peak of the function at 1.0 kHz has a value of 0 dB.

Figure 7 shows actual admittance magnitude data for the guinea pig middle ear (13). In the guinea pig, the peak of the magnitude function is between 3.0 and 4.0 kHz. In humans, the peak is closer to 1.0 kHz as in Fig. 6. The solid line in Fig. 7 is the admittance magnitude calculated for a three-element model of the guinea pig middle ear. You can see that the agreement between the data and the model is very good except at the highest frequencies. To achieve a better agreement, a far more complicated model of the guinea pig middle ear with four resistances, four compliances, and three masses is required (20).

The frequency where the admittance magnitude is a maximum is known as the *resonant frequency*. For a fixed sound pressure, the volume velocity of the tympanic membrane will be greatest at the resonant frequency and the sound energy transmitted by the middle ear to the cochlea will also be maximum. Because of this, hearing thresholds are lowest near the resonant frequency. The resonant frequency (f_{res}) depends on the mass and compliance elements:

$$f_{res} = \frac{1}{2\pi} \sqrt{\frac{1}{MC}} \qquad [21]$$

Any changes in the value of mass or compliance will shift the resonant frequency. We will soon see examples of this. At the resonant frequency, referring to Eq. 19, the term within the parentheses in the denominator of the fraction under the square root sign is equal to zero. Therefore the admittance magnitude is simply equal to $1/r$, which is the same as the admittance of a resistance element (Eq. 17a). *At the resonant frequency*, it can be said that the model behaves as a "pure" resistance.

Notice that the phase angle at the resonant frequency is 0°, the same as that for a resistance element.

An important characteristic of resonant functions is their *bandwidth*. The bandwidth is a measure of the width of the peak of the function. To measure the bandwidth, points on the magnitude function are found that are 3 dB less than the value at the peak, at frequencies less than and greater than the resonant frequency. The bandwidth is the difference between the upper frequency point and the lower frequency point. The bandwidth is a measure of the range of frequencies for which the magnitude function is close to its maximum value. In the middle ear, the bandwidth of the admittance magnitude is a measure of the range of frequencies transmitted by the middle ear with minimal attenuation. As shown in Eq. 22, the bandwidth BW depends on resistance and mass:

$$BW = \frac{1}{2\pi} \frac{r}{M} \qquad [22]$$

Admittance functions are also characterized by their behavior at the low and high frequency extremes. For the magnitude function this can be done by evaluating Eq. 19 as the frequency approaches zero and as the frequency grows to infinity. At high frequencies, the term $2\pi fM$ in the denominator of the fraction under the square root will be the largest term. The term $1/2\pi fC$ gets increasingly smaller as frequency gets increasingly larger. If we go to sufficiently high frequencies, the $2\pi fM$ term will also be much larger than the r^2 term. At these high frequencies, the admittance magnitude function simplifies to be approximately equal to $1/2\pi fM$, which is the same as the admittance magnitude for a single-mass element. Therefore at sufficiently high frequencies, the model can be said to behave like a "pure" mass. Note that the high frequency phase angle is close to $-90°$, which is the phase angle expected for a pure mass. At high frequencies the admittance magnitude is proportional to the inverse of frequency, $1/f$. Functions that are inversely proportional to frequency have a characteristic shape when plotted on log–log axes such as decibels versus log–frequency as in Fig. 6. On these axes the function is a straight line with a slope of -6 dB/octave or -20 dB/decade. A slope of -6 dB/octave implies that the function is halved every time frequency is doubled. Equivalently, -20 dB/decade implies that the function decreases by a factor of one-tenth every time frequency increases by 10. For the magnitude function of our model to behave as a pure mass or for it to be said that the function is dominated or controlled by mass, the slope of the magnitude function should be -6 dB/octave and the phase angle should approach $-90°$ at high frequencies. These conditions occur for frequencies well above the resonant frequency.

Similarly, we can evaluate the characteristics of the model at low frequencies. Here the term $1/2\pi fC$ in Eq. 19 dominates at sufficiently low frequencies. As frequency gets very small this term gets very large. The admittance magnitude is approximately equal to $2\pi fC$ and the phase angle is equal to $+90°$, the same as for a pure compliance element. Thus, at sufficiently low frequencies the model is compliance dominated. This is the condition that is often said to occur in normal adult human ears at 220 Hz, a frequency often used by tympanometers and otoadmittance meters. The slope of the admittance magnitude will be *positive* 6 dB/octave or equivalently, *positive* 20 dB/decade. These slopes correspond to a doubling of magnitude for each doubling of frequency and a 10-fold increase in magnitude for every 10-fold

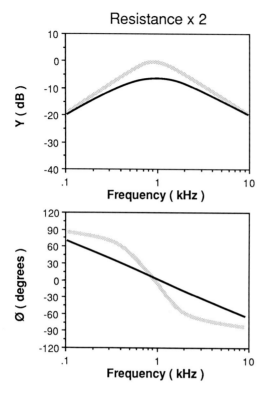

FIG. 8. The normal functions from Fig. 6 (*stippled lines*) are compared with similar functions calculated with resistance, or friction, increased by a factor of 2 (*solid lines*). Note that the magnitude function is decreased in the area of the maximum but that the maximum is still at 1.0 kHz. Also note that the low- and high-frequency phase angles are not equal to +90° and −90°, respectively.

increase in frequency, respectively. To establish that the middle ear is in fact compliance dominated requires that the slope of the magnitude function be 6 dB/octave and that the phase angle be +90° at low frequencies. This can be difficult to prove if measurements are only taken at one or two frequencies as should be evident in the following examples.

One of the real values of models, such as the one we have been discussing, is that it is possible to alter them mathematically to simulate pathological changes. The pathological model can then be compared with measurements made on real pathological ears. From this exercise we can gain a better understanding of the relationship between clinical measurements and the underlying pathologies. We will now consider three examples, in which the values of the elements that make up the model have been altered. We will also consider the effects of increased resistance, decreased compliance, and increased mass.

First, we will investigate the effects of increased friction by increasing r by a factor of 2. Friction might increase because of bone growth at the annular ligament, changes in the joints of the ossicles, changes in the tympanic membrane, or even changes within the cochlea. Figure 8 compares the new admittance magnitude and phase functions with the functions for the normal model. For the magnitude function, the greatest changes occur near the resonant frequency where the magnitude is reduced. That the changes should occur near the resonant frequency makes sense since the height of the magnitude function is controlled by resistance near the resonant peak. As predicted by Eq. 21 the resonant frequency has not changed because it does not depend on the value of r. Thus, the phase angle equals zero at the same frequency.

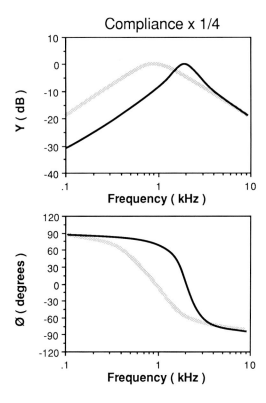

FIG. 9. The normal functions from Fig. 6 (*stippled lines*) are compared with similar functions calculated with compliance decreased by a factor of 4 (*solid lines*) as might happen if the middle-ear space were partially filled with fluid. The size of the change in compliance is exaggerated to make changes in the functions more clear. Note that the maximum of the magnitude function is shifted to higher frequencies. Also notice that the decrease in the magnitude function occurs primarily at low frequencies because the low-frequency admittance is controlled by compliance. The frequency at which the phase angle is zero has shifted and coincides with the new peak in the magnitude function. Finally, see that the phase angle is approximately $+90°$ for a greater range of frequencies.

Note that, as predicted by Eq. 22, the bandwidth has increased, the peak is less sharp. An important change is the change in the shape of the phase function. At the lowest and highest frequencies plotted, the phase angle no longer approaches $+90°$ and $-90°$, respectively. Therefore, it is no longer correct to say that the admittance is dominated by compliance at these low frequencies or by mass at these high frequencies. We would have to go further from the resonant frequency before these statements would be accurate.

In Fig. 9 we see the effects of decreasing compliance by a factor of 4. This might occur if the volume of the middle-ear cavity space were decreased by being partially filled with fluid or if the tympanic membrane were to become stiffer. The size of the change in compliance is exaggerated so that the changes in the functions are easier to see. Note first that, as predicted by Eq. 21, the resonant frequency has shifted to a higher frequency but that the height of the peak is not changed. The zero point on the phase function has shifted with the resonant frequency. It may appear that the bandwidth has decreased, but referring to Eq. 22, we see that bandwidth should not depend on compliance. The apparent change in bandwidth is the result of plotting the data on logarithmic axes. On a linear frequency axis the apparent bandwidth would have remained constant. As expected the greatest decrease in the admittance magnitude function occurs at low frequencies. This reflects the fact that the low-frequency part of the function is determined mostly by compliance. The low frequency phase angle is now approximately equal to $+90°$ up to a higher frequency compared with the original model. Therefore, the new model can be correctly said to be compliance dominated over a larger range of frequencies.

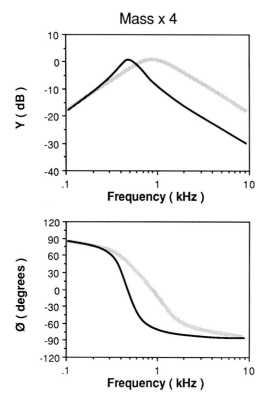

FIG. 10. The normal functions from Fig. 6 (*stippled lines*) are compared with similar functions calculated with mass increased by a factor of 4 (*solid lines*) as might occur with pathological bone growth on the ossicles. The size of the change in mass is exaggerated to make changes in the functions more clear. Note that the maximum of the magnitude function is shifted to lower frequencies along with the zero point in the phase function. The bandwidth of the magnitude function is decreased. Also notice that the decrease in the magnitude function occurs primarily at high frequencies because the high-frequency admittance is controlled by mass. Finally, see that the phase angle approximately equals +90° for a smaller range of frequencies.

In the last of the examples shown in Fig. 10, the mass has been increased by a factor of 4. This might result from pathological bone growth on the ossicles. Again the size of the change has been exaggerated. As predicted by Eq. 21 the resonant frequency has shifted to a lower frequency along with the zero point on the phase function. However, the height of the peak is not affected. Equation 22 tells us that the bandwidth is decreased as it appears in the figure. Note that the decrease in the magnitude function is greatest at high frequencies reflecting the fact that the high frequency part of the function is largely controlled by mass. Importantly, since the phase function has shifted to the left, the range of frequencies for which the model can be said to be compliance dominated has decreased.

The direction of the changes in any of these examples can be reversed simply by changing which of the functions is taken as the reference or starting point. For example, in Fig. 9 the effects of decreasing mass can be seen simply by interchanging the roles of new and normal plots. Decreasing mass shifts the resonant frequency to a higher value. This can be predicted as well by referring to Eq. 21.

An important point can be made from these examples. Often the input admittance of the human ear is described as compliance dominated. It should be clear now that this statement is accurate only if the frequency range and condition of the ear are specified. It may be true that the *normal, adult* input admittance is compliance dominated at 220 Hz, but this may not be true for higher frequencies, for nonadults, or under pathological conditions.

TRANSMISSION OF SOUND BY THE MIDDLE EAR TO THE COCHLEA

In the second section of this chapter we considered the relationship between impedance at the tympanic membrane and the percentage of the sound energy that enters the middle ear. For perfect transmission of sound into the middle-ear system, the impedance of the middle ear must match the impedance of the medium that is carrying the sound, in this case the air in the ear canal. An equivalent statement is that the admittance of the middle ear must be equal to that of the air in the ear canal. Since the admittance of the middle ear is less than that of air, the greater the admittance of the middle ear, the closer it will be to the admittance of air. In the third section of this chapter we established that the admittance varies with frequency. Because admittance is maximum at the resonant frequency, the matching is closest to optimal at that frequency.

Once the sound is accepted by the middle ear, it must be transmitted from the tympanic membrane through the ossicular chain to the cochlea. Any loss of energy in the tympanic membrane or the ossicular chain further reduces the efficiency of the overall transmission of sound from air to the cochlea. The relationship between the response to sound of the tympanic membrane and the response at the stapes is referred to as the *transfer function* of the middle ear. For our simple three-element model, the transfer function is given by the ratio of the sound pressure at the stapes footplate to the pressure at the tympanic membrane. In this case, the transfer function is simply proportional to the input admittance. At the resonant frequency the two pressures are equal and the transfer function is equal to one. At all other frequencies the ratio is less than one.

The actual situation is more complicated. There are additional losses of energy in the middle-ear system that are not included in the model. Evidence for losses within the middle-ear mechanism comes from comparisons of the displacement of the tip of the malleus to the displacement of the footplate of the stapes (3,7,9). The ratio of these two displacements should equal the physical lever ratio for the ossicular chain. However, researchers have found that at high frequencies, above 2,500 Hz, this ratio decreases with increasing frequency. Thus, not all the energy in the motion of the tympanic membrane is transmitted to the cochlea but some is lost in the ossicles, most likely attributable to slippage in the joints. Thus, the performance of the middle ear degrades at higher frequencies and is worse than that predicted by the input admittance. The simple model of the middle ear is closer to reality at low frequencies than it is at frequencies above the resonant peak.

Calculating the overall performance, or efficiency, of the middle ear is very complicated. In the end, what matters is the ratio of the sound power that is delivered to the cochlea to the sound power just outside the tympanic membrane. To make such a calculation requires actual numbers for the properties of a realistic, detailed model for the external and middle ears (15). The results, as far as general trends, are not that different from the admittance magnitude curves for our model. There is a peak in the efficiency curve near 1.0 kHz, where the efficiency is about 40%. Above and below 1.0 kHz, the efficiency decreases to approximately 10% at 100 Hz and to 0.6% at 4.0 kHz.

RELATIONSHIP OF MIDDLE-EAR PERFORMANCE TO THRESHOLDS

We have seen that the properties of the middle ear determine how much sound energy reaches the cochlea and how that energy varies with frequency. If at threshold, the energy required to stimulate the cochlea were constant with frequency, then the shape of a threshold versus frequency curve would be determined by the middle ear. For our simple model, the threshold curve would look like the admittance magnitude curve flipped upside-down. The properties of the cochlea are not quite so simple (6) such that at low frequencies the amount of energy required at threshold is increased (2). In addition, the sound reaching the tympanic membrane depends on the properties of the external ear and ear canal. Nevertheless, it has been established in several mammalian species (2,9,10,15) that the properties of the middle ear, combined with those of the ear canal and external ear, can for the most part account for the frequency dependence of the threshold of audibility for pure tones. Any changes in the admittance of the middle ear produced by pathology, as considered for our three-element model, will be reflected by similar changes in the audibility curve.

REFERENCES

1. Békésy, G. von (1960): *Experiments in Hearing* (Transl. E. G. Wever). McGraw-Hill, New York.
2. Dallos, P. (1973): *The Auditory Periphery, Biophysics, and Physiology*, pp. 83–126, Academic Press, New York.
3. Guinan, J. J., and Peake, W. T. (1967): Middle-ear characteristics of anesthetized cats. *J. Acoust. Soc. Am.*, 41:1237–1261.
4. Helmholtz, H. L. F. (1885): *On the Sensation of Tone*, (Transl. A. J. Ellis). Dover Publications, New York.
5. Khanna, S. M., and Tonndorf, J. (1972): Tympanic membrane vibrations in cats studied by time-averaged holography. *J. Acoust. Soc. Am.*, 51:1904–1920.
6. Lynch, T. J. III, Nedzelnitsky, V., and Peake, W. T. (1982): Input impedance of the cochlea in cat. *J. Acoust. Soc. Am.*, 72:108–130.
7. Manley, G. A., and Johnstone, B. M. (1974): Middle-ear function in the guinea pig. *J. Acoust. Soc. Am.*, 56:571–576.
8. Møller, A. R. (1961): Network model of the middle ear. *J. Acoust. Soc. Am.*, 33:168–176.
9. Møller, A. R. (1963): Transfer function of the middle ear. *J. Acoust. Soc. Am.*, 35:1526–1534.
10. Møller, A. R. (1965): Experimental study of the acoustic impedance of the middle ear and its transmission properties. *Acta Otolaryngol.*, 60:129–149.
11. Møller, A. R. (1974): The acoustic middle ear muscle reflex. In: *Handbook of Sensory Physiology, Volume V/1: Auditory System*, edited by W. D. Keidel and W. D. Neff, pp. 519–548. Springer-Verlag, Berlin.
12. Møller, A. R. (1974): Function of the middle ear. In: *Handbook of Sensory Physiology, Volume V/1: Auditory System*, edited by W. D. Keidel and W. D. Neff, pp. 491–517. Springer-Verlag, Berlin.
13. Mundie, J. R. (1963): The impedance of the ear—a variable quantity. In: *Middle Ear Function Seminar*, edited by J. L. Fletcher, pp. 63–85. U.S. Army Medical Research Laboratory Report, Dept. 576, Wright Patterson A.F.B., Ohio.
14. Onchi, Y. (1961): Mechanism of the middle ear. *J. Acoust. Soc. Am.*, 33:794–805.
15. Rosowski, J. J., Carney, L. H., Lynch, T. J., and Peake, W. T. (1986): The effectiveness of external and middle ears in coupling acoustic power into the cochlea. In: *Peripheral Auditory Mechanisms*, edited by J. B. Allen, J. L. Hall, A. Hubbard, S. T. Neely, and A. Tubis. Springer-Verlag, Berlin.
16. Tonndorf, J., and Khanna, S. M. (1970): The role of the tympanic membrane in middle ear transmission. *Ann. Otol. Rhinol. Laryngol.*, 79:743–753.
17. Tonndorf, J., and Khanna, S. M. (1972): Tympanic-membrane vibrations in human cadaver ears studied by time-averaged holography. *J. Acoust. Soc. Am.*, 52:1221–1233.
18. Wever, E. G., and Lawrence, M. (1954): *Physiological Acoustics*. Princeton University Press, Princeton.

19. Zwislocki, J. (1962): Analysis of middle-ear function. Part I: Input impedance. *J. Acoust. Soc. Am.*, 34:1514–1523.
20. Zwislocki, J. (1963): Analysis of the middle-ear function. Part II. Guinea-pig ear. *J. Acoust. Soc. Am.*, 35:1034–1040.
21. Zwislocki, J. J. (1975): The role of the external and middle ear in sound transmission. In: *The Nervous System, Vol. 3: Human Communications and Its Disorders*, edited by D. B. Tower, pp. 45–55. Raven Press, New York.

Physiology of the Ear,
edited by A. F. Jahn and J. Santos-Sacchi.
Raven Press, New York © 1988.

The Facial Nerve

Steven M. Parnes

Division of Otolaryngology, Albany Medical College, Albany, New York 12208

The facial nerve is an extremely complex cranial nerve from both a basic science and a clinical perspective. Fallopius discovered the canal bearing his name that houses the larger portion of the nerve; but it was Charles Bell who first recognized the clinical importance of this structure. Its lengthy serpentine course through the temporal bone intrigues yet sometimes frustrates the modern otologic surgeon. The many varied functions provide ample opportunity to examine the nerve physiologically with direct application to the clinical evaluation. This chapter explores the known facts and controversial areas concerning the clinically relevant anatomy, structure, and function of this seventh cranial nerve. Pathophysiology, with a brief discussion of idiopathic facial paralysis, is also included.

COURSE AND RELATIONSHIPS

The facial nerve is unique in that it is the longest cranial nerve confined within a bony conduit. Its origin is within the pons, where the facial nucleus forms a column of multipolar neurons in the ventral lateral tegmentum, dorsal to the superior olivary nucleus and ventromedial to the spinal trigeminal nucleus (Fig. 1) (40). The intra-axial fibers loop around the nucleus of the abducens nerve, describing what is referred to as the internal genu.

Once the nerve emerges from the inferior border of the pons in the recess between the olive and inferior cerebellar peduncle, it divides into four segments. The first is the intracranial portion, 12 to 14 mm within the cerebellopontine angle to the internal meatus. The motor segment is medial to the eighth cranial nerve and separated from that structure by the nervus intermedius (15).

The nerve enters the internal auditory meatus, accompanied by the nervus intermedius, cochlear-vestibular nerves, and internal auditory artery and vein. It occupies an anterior rostral position, remaining primarily anterior to the superior vestibular nerve and superior to the cochlear nerve. In 8 to 10 mm it reaches the lateral end of the meatus superior to the crista transversalis and anterior to the vertical crista (Bill's Bar). Exiting the internal auditory canal, the nerve curves gradually anteriorly around the basal turn of the cochlea entering the intratemporal portion for 2 to 4 mm. This is the narrowest portion of the fallopian canal. At the geniculate ganglion there is an expansion, with the greater superficial petrosal nerve leaving at the anterior edge and proceeding through the facial hiatus. The nerve itself makes a 40° to 80° turn (the external or first genu) and courses posteriorly and slightly inferiorly 11 mm across the tympanic cavity. This forms its horizontal position overlapped by

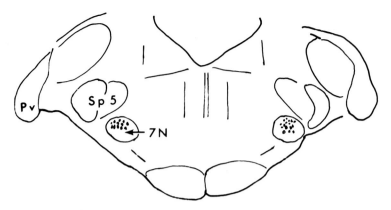

FIG. 1. Facial nerve nucleus (labeled cells) within the pons in the ventral lateral tegmentum. Sp, spinal trigeminal nucleus; Pv, posterior, ventral cochlear nucleus.

the cochleariform process and through most of the horizontal course the facial nerve forms a superior boundary to the fossula at the vestibular fenestra or oval window niche. After leaving the oval window niche, the facial nerve curves more gently to its vertical position (second genu) where it passes anterior and caudal to the lateral semicircular canal. It then passes lateral to the sinus tympani and stapedius muscle to form the vertical (mastoid) portion within the temporal bone. Another important landmark is the short process of the incus just lateral to the facial nerve as it enters its vertical position. The vertical position of the nerve is approximately 13 mm long to the exit at the stylomastoid foramen. During its vertical course, the chorda tympani nerve leaves the facial nerve in an anterosuperior direction, entering the middle ear at the iter chordae posterior, and crossing the middle ear lateral to the long process of the incus and medial to the angle of the malleus exiting at the anterior iter. Here it enters the petrotympanic (Glaserian) fissure. At the stylomastoid foramen the facial nerve widens considerably, becoming the extracranial segment (Fig. 2) (2,12,15,21). At the stylomastoid foramen, it innervates the posterior belly of the digastric muscle. At 15 to 20 mm it enters the parotid gland where it divides at the pes anserinus into two main branches, the temporal-facial and cervical-facial. Terminal ramifications of these branches to the temporal, zygomatic, buccal, mandibular, and cervical regions are variable (Fig. 3) (12,14).

VASCULAR SUPPLY

The facial nerve obtains its blood supply from both the carotid and vertebral systems. The stylomastoid artery, a branch of the posterior auricular artery, anastomoses with the descending branch of the petrosal artery at the junction of the upper and middle thirds of the mastoid segments of the fallopian canal. These two arteries provide most of the supply to the mastoid and tympanic segments of the nerve up to the geniculate ganglion. The vertebrobasilar system gives rise to the anterior inferior cerebellar artery, which supplies the nerve in the cerebellopontine angle. The labyrinthine branches of the artery vascularize the meatal segment of the nerve. The large arteries and veins of the extrinsic circulation form the vascular

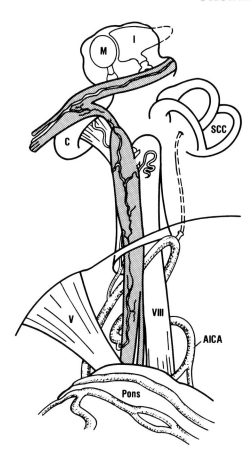

FIG. 2. Intracranial, meatal, labyrinthine, and tympanic segments of facial nerve with their blood supply, superior view. Facial nerve (*shaded*); M, malleus; I, incus; C, cochlea; SCC, semicircular canals; V, trigeminal nerve; VIII, cochlear nerve; AICA, anterior, inferior cerebellar artery. (From ref. 12.)

bundle along the anterior surface of the mastoid segment and then form arcs with penetrating branches into the nerve. The venous draining plexus lies mostly within the epineurium. The circulation in general appears to be oriented longitudinally, although it is very irregular without any specific pattern. The labyrinthine segment, the narrowest portion of the bony canal, has the fewest vessels and may thus represent a potentially weak area in the blood supply (7,21,24).

STRUCTURE OF THE FACIAL NERVE

Sunderland and Cossar (46) had determined that the structure of the facial nerve was not constant along its course. The nerve fibers travel in groups of fascicles and then vary according to the level surrounded by three types of connective tissue. The endoneurium forms the framework of the interior of the fascicle. It separates and surrounds each nerve fiber to form a definitive external sheath. The perineurium is a thin but dense laminated mesothelial layer that covers each fascicle. It imparts considerable tensile strength to the nerve trunk and constitutes a diffusion barrier. The third layer, the epineurium, is loose connective tissue that encloses and forms a protective packing for the fascicles, condensing to a compact structure that anatomists often refer to as the sheath. This sheath may also represent a trilaminate

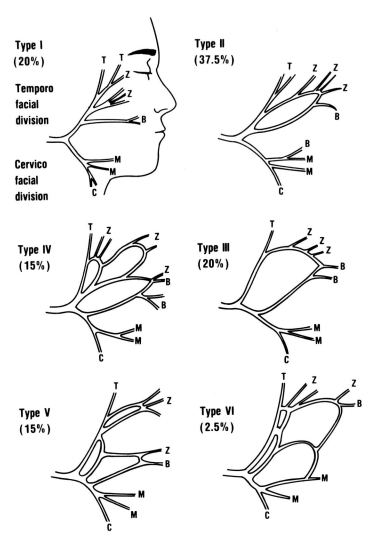

FIG. 3. Peripheral branching of the extratemporal facial nerve. T, ramus temporalis; Z, ramus zygomaticus; B, ramus buccalis; M, ramus marginalis mandibulae; C, ramus colli. (From ref. 12.)

coat consisting of periosteum, vascular connective tissue, along with the epineurium. The nerve fibers at the cerebellopontine angle cross the space loosely arranged in parallel bundles without any epi- or perineurium. The motor fibers and nervus intermedius are in separate but adjacent systems. When the nerve reaches the internal auditory meatus, although the fiber arrangement is retained, the nerve fibers are collected into a single compact structure with a small amount of supportive epineural tissue and a very thin sheath. Distal to the geniculate ganglion, however, the nerve is composed of several bundles, the first beginning as a single fasciculated section but very quickly is replaced by multiple fascicles with a rapid change in its pattern. Each fascicle at the stylomastoid foramen contains fibers for each of the terminal branches given off distal to this level. The final sorting takes place peripherally at the pes anserinus (Fig. 4) (45,46).

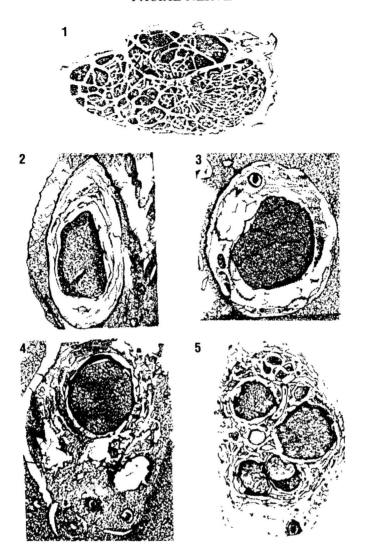

FIG. 4. Diagrammatic representation (transverse sections) of the fascicular patterns in the structure of the facial nerve along its course. **(1)** Section in the internal auditory canal. Facial nerve is superiorly located, demonstrating fine, intraneural framework. **(2)** Preganglionic portion, fibers collected in a single bundle. **(3,4)** Sections between origins of the stapedius and chorda tympani branches demonstrating major fascicular bundles with small satellites. **(5)** Section distal to chorda tympani showing multifasciculated pattern. (From ref. 46.)

Orientation of the individual fibers within the nucleus and nerve trunk has been under considerable investigation. Using horseradish peroxidase studies in cats, Radpour and Gacek (39,40) were able to demonstrate that the facial nerve nucleus demonstrates a specific spatial representation in relationship to the individual branches. The orbicularis oculi muscles are represented in the rostral pole of the lateral division of the facial nucleus dorsally (Fig. 5), whereas the orbicularis oris muscles are represented in the caudal pole of the lateral division of the facial nerves nucleus ventrally (Fig. 6). The platysma muscle is represented in the medial division of the center cell

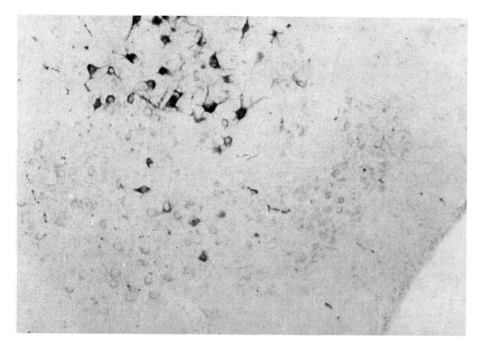

FIG. 5. Facial nerve nucleus of the monkey with labeled cells in the dorsal, rostral pole after injecting orbicularis oculi muscles with HRP (×150).

groups located ventrally. Frontalis representation is also in the medial division but in the dorsal pole. An area of greater dispute is whether this orientation is maintained throughout the facial nerve proper. Although May (27) and Crumley (13) have presented data to indicate this orientation, recent evidence by Thomander et al. (50), Gacek (19), Radpour (41), and Parnes et al. (35) refute this. It appears that no orientation exists until near the stylomastoid foramen. Instead, there is random distribution of the fibers (Fig. 7). Murakami et al. (33) noted similar findings in regards to the stapedial nerve fibers in the facial nerve trunk. Thus, from a practical perspective, an attempt to realign the severed facial nerve within the temporal bone would be without merit.

FUNCTIONS OF THE FACIAL NERVE

The facial nerve is a complex structure containing mixed motor and sensory components. The efferent motor component that originates in the main facial nucleus innervates the muscles of facial expression as well as the posterior belly of the digastric, stylohyoid, postauricular, and stapedius muscles. The anatomical investigation of the corticonuclear projections of the facial nerve nucleus demonstrates the origin at the precentral gyrus. As the fibers pass downward, the majority cross to the contralateral nucleus at the level of the pons, although some fibers continue ipsilaterally. The superior part of the nucleus receives bilateral innervation; the inferior portion receives unilateral uncrossed fibers. A lesion distal to the nucleus

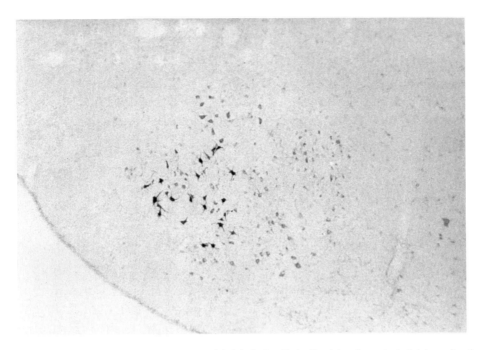

FIG. 6. Facial nerve nucleus of the cat with labeled cells in the lateral, ventral division after injecting orbicularis oris with HRP (×150).

would therefore result in a complete upper and lower facial paralysis, but a lesion proximal to the nucleus, as in the motor complex, would result in maximal involvement in the musculature of the middle and lower face, sparing the frontal and upper zygomatic regions (43). Evidence also suggests that there are other projections from the facial nucleus to the trigeminal complex—in particular the mesencephalic system—that may accompany the motor fibers to provide proprioception to the facial musculature (Fig. 8) (36). Trigeminal facial nerve communications may also occur peripherally (8).

The superior salivary nucleus projects efferent (parasympathetic preganglionic) fibers for tearing along the nervus intermedius to the geniculate ganglion where the fibers leave the main trunk at the anterior part of the geniculate ganglion to exit the facial hiatus along the greater petrosal nerve. These fibers are joined by sympathetic fibers of the deep petrosal nerve and synapse at the sphenopalatine ganglion. The postganglionic fibers then innervate the lacrimal glands and mucous glands of the nose. The nervus intermedius also contains afferent fibers that provide the sensory innervation of Ramsay Hunt's cutaneous zone (posterior wall of the auditory canal, zone near the tympanum, the auditory meatus, external ear, the tragus, helix, antihelix fossa, and part of the lobe) and the gustatory innervation of the anterior two-thirds of the tongue. These latter fibers follow pathways of the lingual nerve and chorda tympani to the geniculate ganglion and then pass to the nucleus tractus solitarius (11,12).

From the superior salivary nucleus another set of parasympathetic preganglion fibers leaves via the facial nerve trunk to the level of the mastoid segment where

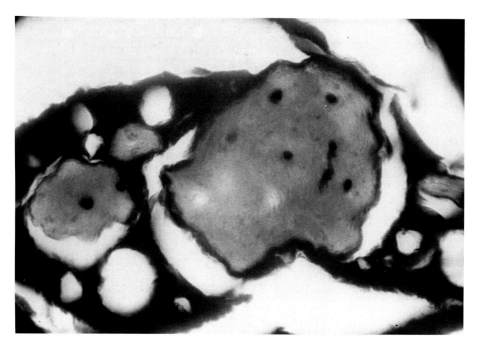

FIG. 7. Cross section of the intratemporal (mastoid) segment of the facial nerve in the cat demonstrating multiple fascicles with random distribution of labeled axons after injecting the orbicularis oris muscle with HRP ($\times$150).

the fibers then follow the chorda tympani to the submandibular ganglion. Postganglionic fibers for secretion of saliva pass to the submandibular and sublingual glands (11).

Control of ocular blood flow may be mediated via the facial nerve. Bill and Nilsson (9) have shown that electrical stimulation of the facial nerve at both the posterior cranial fossa and deep petrosal nerve level leads to marked increase in choroidal blood flow and vasodilatation in the uvea (Fig. 9).

The facial nucleus receives other projections that modulate other systems, such as the vestibular, sympathetic, and vagal systems. Synaptic actions of vagal afferents on the facial motor neurons in the cat indicate possible coordination between mastication and facial activity (47). Similar connections demonstrated through horseradish peroxidase (HRP) techniques probably involve the coordination of facial movements with eye and head movements (44). Sympathetic innervation is also likely via the facial nerve in some capacity, as evidenced by Thomander et al. (49) who indicate the presence of postganglionic sympathetic axons within the facial nerve.

DIAGNOSTIC TESTS OF FACIAL NERVE FUNCTION

Because of the many different functions of the facial nerve, it provides a unique opportunity to evaluate nerve function in many capacities, providing both prognostic and topographical information (5,12,25).

Facial motion: Initially, the affected individual should be carefully examined to

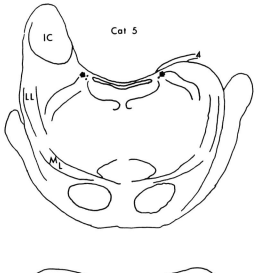

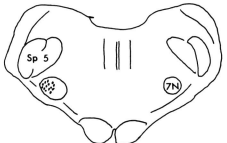

FIG. 8. Projection drawing of pons **(bottom)** and midbrain **(top)** of cat demonstrating labeled cells of lateral portion of left seventh cranial nerve nucleus and bilateral labeling of mesencephalic cells in midbrain (*arrows*) after injecting orbicularis oris with HRP. 7th, seventh nerve; Sp 5, spinal trigeminal nucleus; ML, medial lemniscus; LL, lateral lemniscus; and IC, inferior colliculus. (From ref. 21.)

detect even the slightest facial movement to determine if the facial nerve is intact. One must be cautious not to misinterpret upper eyelid movement owing to levator palpebral activity (occulomotor nerve) for a functioning facial nerve. Forehead sparing indicates a lesion of central origin, although there may be exceptions (27,32). Intact frontal innervation and paralysis of the remainder of mimetic muscles on that side indicate a contralateral central lesion. In the opercular syndrome, the cortical type of pseudobulbar paralysis, normal facial movements exist only during involuntary emotional expressive movements like laughing and yawning.

Test for lacrimation: The Schirmer test is performed by comparing tearing from the eye on the paralyzed side with that of the eye on the normal side. The amount of tearing is measured on small tapes, and a reduction of 30% or more on the involved side is considered a positive test. This specifically looks at injury at the petrosal nerve level indicating a lesion proximal to the geniculate ganglion. Unfortunately, the test is not 100% accurate since unilateral lesions can produce bilateral reduction for unexplained reasons and conversely compression by extensive lesions can still allow parasympathetic fibers to remain intact and insure normal lacrimation. It is also possible that the unmyelinated parasympathetic fibers react differently to injury than the myelinated motor fibers, again resulting in variable results (5,17).

Stapedial reflex test: The stapedius muscle contracts reflexively in response to loud sound, usually at 85 dB above threshold. When the stapedius muscle contracts, it stiffens the ossicular chain, causing an increase in the acoustic impedance of the

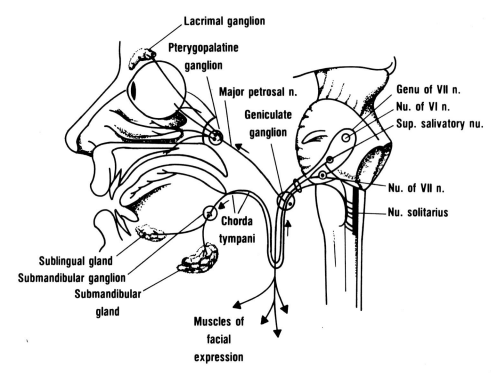

FIG. 9. Distribution of the facial nerve—four nuclei. 1. Motor fibers (from facial nerve nucleus) to muscles of expression and mastication. 2. Sensory fibers (from superior salivary nucleus or spinal nucleus of N.V.) to Ramsay Hunt's cutaneous zone (via nervus intermedius). 3. Parasympathetic fibers (from superior salivary nucleus) to submandibular and sublingual glands (via chorda tympani) and lacrimal gland and orbital vasculature (via greater petrosal nerve). 4. Taste fibers (from nucleus solitarius) to the anterior two thirds of tongue (via chorda tympani nerve). (Based on Noback, C. and Demarest, R., *The Human Nervous System*, McGraw-Hill, New York, 1981.)

sound transmission of the mechanism of the middle ear. An acoustic impedance probe may detect this change objectively. An absence of the reflex in a normal ear may indicate a lesion proximal to the take-off of the stapedius nerve, but, like the Schirmer test, it has not been completely reliable because degeneration may affect myelinated fibers differently according to their size and position (5,12).

Chorda tympani nerve: Afferent fibers for taste arise distal to the stapedial branch and pass upward to the facial ridge and exit at the petrotympanic fissure to join the lingual nerve. Galvanic current applied to the tongue is "tasted" and the threshold for current needed to evoke this taste may be measured through electrogustometry. An elevation of threshold would indicate the dysfunction of the chorda tympani nerve and again imply the presence of a lesion proximal to the origin (12,25).

Measurement of submandibular flow: This is another attempt to evaluate chorda tympani function. May et al. (28) have noted that a 25% reduction from the abnormal to normal side would indicate a positive test and imply a poor prognosis for recovery in patients with idiopathic facial paralysis.

Electrodiagnostic Tests

Nerve excitability: A current-stabilized electrical stimulator with a maximum output of 20 mA can be used for prognostic information. The facial nerve is stimulated at the site of branching with square pulses of 0.3-msec duration, and the intensity is increased until minimal muscle contraction is noted. A difference of 3.5 mA between the normal and paralyzed side is considered positive, suggesting degeneration, and carries with it an unfavorable prognosis. A variation of this is the maximal stimulation test in which the comparison is made of the currents required to produce maximum rather than minimum muscle contraction (12,29).

Electroneuronography (evoked electromyography) (ENOG): The ENOG provides a quantitative analysis of both nerve excitability and maximal stimulation tests. Bipolar electrodes with a diameter of 7 mm are placed 18 mm apart for stimulation and recording. Square wave impulses of 0.2 msec duration and 50- to 100-V amplitudes with a frequency of 1/sec are delivered percutaneously in front of the tragus. The second bipolar electrode placed securely in the nasolabial fold with the superior electrode beside the alar rim captures the summation potentials of the underlying facial muscles. The oscilloscope will display the summating potentials, which can be recorded. The amplitude of the evoked summating potentials of the intact and involved side of the face are measured peak to peak. The difference in amplitude corresponds to the percentage of degenerated nerve fibers tested. Maximum responses are used for calculation. Unfortunately, information provided by ENOG represents a delay of 24 to 48 hours in regards to the events that occur, because of the time required by wallerian degeneration to progress from the site of injury to the site of testing. ENOG assesses only the percentage of motor fibers that have undergone degeneration. Facial nerve subjected to traumatic injuries of the magnitude requiring surgical intervention undergo more than 90% degeneration within 6 days of the injury. Patients whose injury demonstrates 95% or more degeneration within 14 days have a poor prognosis (Fig. 10) (12,35).

Electromyography (EMG): By itself, EMG is of limited clinical value in early facial paralysis. Denervation potentials are sought but do not occur until 14 to 21 days after onset of complete paralysis. Thus, if denervation is discovered at this time, certainly it would indicate severe injury to the facial nerve. The other role of EMG is to indicate incipient recovery, when polyphasic potentials are noted prior to actual clinical visualization of facial movement (5,16).

Antidromically evoked facial nerve response: To overcome the difficulties in delay of evaluation due to the 48-hour response to wallerian degeneration, a new technique has been devised to preclude this problem. Antidromic conduction testing is an alternative that provides direct and immediate assessment of proximal nerve function (opposite to normal direction). The technique uses opposite direction electrical activity and computerized averaging of evoked potentials (34). Because of the newness of the test, prognostic implications have not been totally determined; however, the test has been used for electrophysiologic monitoring during facial nerve surgery within the temporal bone, particularly during the removal of cerebellopontine angle tumors. This facilitates identification of the facial nerve in large cerebellar pontine angle tumors while minimizing the mechanical trauma (42).

Roentgenograms: Computerized tomography (CT) can assist in delineating lesions adjacent to the nerve in the IAC, cerebellopontine angle, and deep lobe of the parotid. This has proved to be very effective with the high resolution CT. The entire fallopian canal can be visualized in two planes (axial and coronal) so that one can concentrate on the labyrinthine segments, geniculate ganglion fossa, and proximal portion of the tympanic segment. Magnetic resonance imaging may also be complementary to this

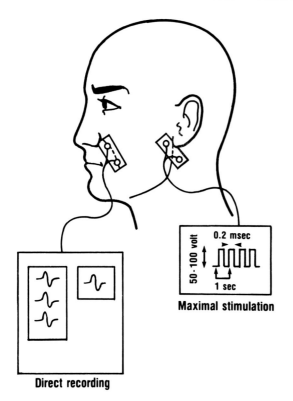

FIG. 10. Electroneurography: two bipolar electrodes for stimulation and recording of evoked summation potential of facial muscles directly recorded on oscilloscope. (From ref. 12.)

radiologic evaluation. However, lack of bony detail may limit the usefulness of this test.

Other diagnostic studies include auditory and vestibular function tests such as pure tone audiometry, tympanometry, auditory-evoked potentials, electronystagmography, and sinusoidal harmonic acceleration, since the auditory and vestibular nerves share common anatomical boundaries.

FACIAL NERVE INJURY

General Comments

Nerve fibers transmit information encoded as a sequence of uniform impulses, the action potentials, that consist of brief changes in membrane polarization. This is effected via a transient flow of sodium ions into the fiber followed by outflow of potassium ions. The movements take place at discrete membrane sites, called ionic channels, which are pore-like structures within the axonal membrane. There are at least three types of ionic channels in the axon membrane: sodium, potassium, and leakage channels.

Myelinated axons are covered by a myelin sheath but left uncovered at the nodes of Ranvier. In myelinated axons there are physical differences between the nodal axolemma and the internodal axonal membrane. Ionic channel densities are much higher in the nodal axolemma, rendering them more excitable. Thus, currents flowing

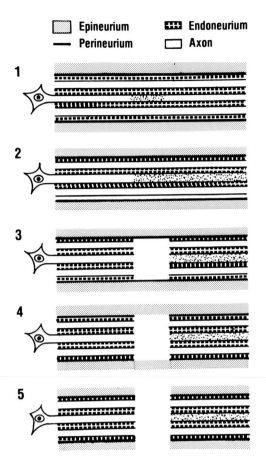

Epineurium **Endoneurium**
Perineurium **Axon**

FIG. 11. Five types of nerve injury. **(1)** neu-ropraxia, impulse conductive block; **(2)** axon-otmesis, loss of structural continuity of the axon with intact endoneural sheath; **(3)** en-doneurotmesis, loss of structural continuity of the axons and endoneural sheaths within a fas-cicle; **(4)** perineurotmesis, loss of structural continuity of the perineurium with intact epi-neurium; **(5)** neurotmesis, loss of continuity of the nerve trunk. (From ref. 45.)

along the internode are always in an outward direction without excitation. The ma-jority of the inward currents generated during a nodal action potential passes down the axon and exits across the next nodal region since a more distal node represents a lower resistance pathway and thus completes the local circuit. The propagation along the internode region is passive and serves only to excite the next nodal region, a phenomenon known as a saltatory conduction. By contrast, nonmyelinated neu-rofibers with the same diameter conduct in a continuous fashion to achieve maximal velocities of only 10 to 15 m/sec. Optimally constructed myelinated fibers can prop-agate an impulse at speeds in excess of 50 m/sec (20).

Injuries will interrupt the conduction process. Sunderland (45) classified these injuries based on the histology of the nerve trunk (Fig. 11).

In first-degree injury (neuropraxia) there is an interruption of conduction without loss of axonal or myelin continuity at the site of injury. Although clinically, voluntary motor function is either decreased or absent, electrical stimulation distal to the lesion is still possible. This type of injury is believed to be attributable to ischemia or direct mechanical deformity—perhaps owing to direct pressure on the axoplasm or sec-ondary ischemia obstructing the venous outflow, which is most sensitive to compres-sion (22,45).

Second-degree injury is owing to axonal degeneration without loss of endoneurial continuity (axonotmesis). Degenerative changes become evident on both sides of the lesion and the distal axon then demonstrates wallerian degeneration involving axon and myelin degeneration with removal by Schwann cell and macrophage phagocytosis. Schwann cells apparently play a key role in this process in which activity first increases to remove the debris followed by a decline of activity by the third week. A central core is formed in the endoneurial tubule setting the stage for reinnervation. The columns of Schwann cells are then thought to provide a biochemical attraction for regenerating axons. The interruption of retrograde transport is a signal to the cell body that an injury has occurred and thus for a variable distance of approximately a few millimeters proximal, fiber degeneration also occurs. Within the cell body Nissl granules of the parent neuron begin to disintegrate and disperse through the cytoplasm. The cell nucleus is displaced to the periphery and neurofilaments are lost. The cell remains in this state for approximately 2 to 3 weeks. The first 3 weeks are concerned with cell survival. Following this, there is an increase in axoplasmic transport in which axonal regeneration begins. The tip of the regenerating axon exhibits intense activity with reinnervation following the original pattern since the endoneurial tubules are intact (23,52). Clinically, there is usually full recovery in these types of injuries (22,45).

In the third-degree injury (endoneurotmesis) not only does wallerian degeneration of the axon and myelin sheath occur, but endoneurial tubule and fascicular organization is disrupted. The perineurium remains intact. This degree of injury also produces trauma to the intrafascicular vascular network, with hemorrhage, edema, and ischemia. These lesions are caused by traction crush injuries or compression through either direct or indirect means. The implication of the extensive architectural disorganization seen with this injury is that aberrant regeneration of axonal sprouts may occur due to misalignment in the fascicles. Clinically, this may result in some synkinesis and mass motion. Thomander (48) and Aldskogius et al. (4) have demonstrated a reorganization of the facial motor nucleus after peripheral nerve regeneration, confirming misdirected axonal sprouts. Comparing natal to adult rats, Aldskogius noted that the degree of disorganization after injury is much less in the neonate, implying that surviving neurons in the less mature animal effect a more appropriate pathway. It is not clear whether this is because of peripheral mechanisms or because the less mature central nervous system has more flexibility to compensate for the injury.

Fourth-degree injury (perineurotmesis) results in trauma extending to the perineurium permitting regenerating axons not only to enter the incorrect tubule in its own fascicle but adjacent fascicles as well. This carries a worse prognosis clinically in which more synkinesis and mass movement is likely. Neuroma formation is also common.

Fifth-degree injury (neurotmesis) is the most severe in that the entire nerve trunk is severed, providing little hope for spontaneous recovery. Neuroma formation, neuronal loss, and misdirection of axonal sprouts are usually maximal and thus microsurgical repair of this lesion is necessary if one hopes to gain any significant recovery. It is controversial whether the repair should be epineurial or perineurial. Recent evidence suggests that spatial orientation is not maintained; therefore, it is more likely that epineurial suturing is more appropriate. Repairs should be done free of tension, thus a nerve graft is preferable over mobilization with tension despite two anastomic sites that must be traversed. Timing is another controversial subject, but most agree that if possible, injuries should be repaired within 24 hours. In complex wounds, however, when the condition of the nerve is not always certain, a delay of 3 to 5 weeks is advisable because intraneural changes are more precisely delineated, the epineurium may be thicker and stronger, and there is maximum axoplasmic flow where the neuron is in an optimal state to undergo the additional trauma of surgery (22).

Sunderland (45) has pointed out that degrees of facial nerve injury can also be affected by location. At the cerebellopointine angle, the nerves are loosely arranged and not confined within a strong perineurial sheath. They are more readily displaced, thus able to accept much more stretching, spreading, and compression in contrast to the area distal to the geniculate ganglion where the nerve is confined within the fallopian canal. The same may be said for the nerve beyond the stylomastoid foramen where benign lesions in the parotid gland can stretch the nerve without causing significant clinical dysfunction.

IDIOPATHIC FACIAL PARALYSIS

The aforementioned discussion logically addresses the issue of idiopathic facial paralysis or Bell's palsy, which is generally attributed to edematous swelling of the facial nerve within the rigid confines of the facial nerve and a secondarily induced compression ischemia. Although a viral etiology such as herpes zoster or Coxsackie (37,51), as well as a prevalence of concurrent diabetes mellitus (3) is suspected, the cause of this disorder is unknown. The various pressure systems in the facial canal, the (a) arteries in the epineurium, (b) capillary pressure inside the fascicle, (c) intrafascicular pressure, (d) venous pressure in the epineurium, and (e) pressure within the facial canal are in a delicate balance, which offer little margin for compensation in the event of an increase in pressure within the canal. Neural edema initially causes an obstruction in venous outflow. This leads to an increase in intrafascicular capillary pressure that then further compromises the circulation. Further progression to the capillary circulation leads to damage to the endothelium. This will then leak protein to the tissues rendering them edematous. The edema further increases intrafascicular pressures resulting in anoxia that threatens the survival of nerve fibers by interfering with their nutrition and metabolism, deforming them, and promoting proliferation and increased activity of fibroblasts with the formation of constrictive endoneurial connective tissue (45).

As the pathologic process is hidden, the pathogenesis is still speculative. Clinically, the natural history of idiopathic facial paralysis has been well described by Peterson (38). His investigation included 10,011 patients seen over a 15-year period. Other than supportive treatment, none of these patients received any definitive treatment such as steroids or surgery. Seventy-one percent attained full recovery of their mimetic motion. Taste, stapedial reflex, and lacrimal function recovered 80%, 86%, and 97%, respectively. Thirteen percent had only slight disfigurement and another 16% resulted in moderate to severe deformities with often associated mass movement or synkinesis.

Some important observations were made: There was no patient who did not show at least some movement. Several prognostic factors were identified: early return of movement, younger patients, and incomplete paralysis were favorable signs, whereas decreased tearing, postauricular pain, absence of stapedial reflex, association of diabetes, and positive maximum stimulation tests were considered poor prognostic indicators (2,38).

Studies evaluating effective management of facial paralysis must therefore measure against this standard. Clinical studies advocating steroids, surgical decompression, immunotherapy, and other treatment modalities often fail to demonstrate any improvement over the natural history.

When presented with a patient with a facial paralysis, one must first rule out an identifiable underlying cause. This may be infectious (acute suppurative otitis media, chronic otitis media, herpes zoster, malignant external otitis), congenital (Moebius syndrome, osteopetrosis), tumors (acoustic and facial neuromas, adenois cystic carcinoma), or autoimmune disorders (sarcoidosis). It is then imperative to identify the patients in the poor prognostic group based on the aforementioned findings as well as abnormalities on electrical and topognostic testing, recognizing their limitations. Since a possible pathologic mechanism is edema of the nerve confined within the bony canal leading then to ischemia, steroids have become the mainstay in treatment for their known effect on moderating the inflammatory responses (1).

Does surgical decompression play a role? Yamamoto and Fisch (53) have demonstrated in animals that an artificially created compression injury will have a better prognosis if surgical decompression follows the injury. This does not necessarily translate to the clinical entity, however, and it is yet to be proven that surgical decompression actually influences the natural course of the disease in patients with a poor prognosis (10,18,30). It is possible that a total decompression applied early in the course of the disease may have a positive effect, but unfortunately a prospective, randomized study will probably never be possible.

REFERENCES

1. Adour, K. (1982): Current concepts in neurology. Diagnosis and management of facial paralysis. *N. Engl. J. Med.*, 307:348–351.
2. Adour, K., Hilsinger, R., and Callan, E. (1985): Facial paralysis and Bell's palsy: A protocol for differential diagnosis. *Am. J. Otol.*, (Nov.):68–73.
3. Adour, K., Wingerd, J., and Doty, H. (1975): Prevalence of concurrent diabetes mellitus and idiopathic facial paralysis (Bell's palsy). *Diabetes*, 24:449–451.
4. Aldskogius, H., and Thomander, L. (1986): Selective reinnervation of somatotopically appropriate muscles after facial nerve transection and regeneration in the neonatal rat. *Brain Res.*, 375:126–133.
5. Alford, B., Jerger, D., Coats, A., Peterson, L., and Weber, J. (1974): Diagnostic tests of facial nerve function. *Otolaryngol. Clin. North Am.*, 7:331–342.
6. Anson, B., Donaldson, J., Warpeha, R., Rensink, M., and Shilling, B. (1973): Surgical anatomy of the facial nerve. *Arch. Otolaryngol.*, 97:201–213.
7. Balkany, T. (1986): The intrinsic vasculature of the cat facial nerve. *Laryngoscope*, 96:70–77.
8. Baumel, J. (1974): Trigeminal-facial nerve communications. *Arch. Otolaryngol.*, 99:34–44.
9. Bill, A., and Nilsson, S. (1985): Control of ocular blood flow. *J. Cardiovasc. Pharmacol.*, 7(suppl.):596–602.
10. Brown, J. (1982): Bell's palsy: A 5 year review of 174 consecutive cases: An attempted double blind study. *Laryngoscope*, 92:1369–1373.
11. Chouard, C. (1977): Wrisberg intermediary nerve. In: *Facial Nerve Injury*, edited by U. Fisch, pp. 24–39. Aesculapius, Birmingham.
12. Coker, N., and Fisch, U. (1984): Disorders of the facial nerve. In: *Otolaryngology*, vol. 1, edited by G. English, pp. 1–43. Harper and Row, Philadelphia.
13. Crumley, R. (1980): Spatial anatomy of the facial nerve fibers—a preliminary report. *Laryngoscope*, 90:274–280.
14. Davis, R., Anson, B., Budinger, J., and Kurth, R. (1956): Surgical anatomy of the facial nerve and parotid gland based upon a study of 350 cervicofacial halves. *Surg. Gynecol. Obstet.*, 102:385–412.

15. Donaldson, J., and Anson, B. (1974): Surgical anatomy of the facial nerve. *Otolaryngol. Clin. North Am.*, 7:289–308.
16. Esslen, E. (1977): Electromyography and electroneuragraphy. In: *Facial Nerve Surgery*, edited by U. Fisch, pp. 93–100. Aesculapius, Birmingham.
17. Fisch, U. (1977): Lacrimation. In: *Facial Nerve Surgery*, edited by U. Fisch, pp. 147–153. Aesculapius, Birmingham.
18. Fisch, U. (1981): Surgery for Bell's palsy. *Arch. Otolaryngol.*, 107:1–11.
19. Gacek, R., and Radpour, S. (1982): Fiber orientation of the facial nerve: An experimental study in the cat. *Laryngoscope*, 92:547–556.
20. Ge, X., Spector, G., and Carr, C. (1982): The pathophysiology of compression injuries of the peripheral facial nerve. *Laryngoscope*, 92(suppl. 31):1–15.
21. Guerrier, Y. (1977): Surgical anatomy, particularly vascular supply of the facial nerve. In: *Facial Nerve Surgery*, edited by U. Fisch, pp. 13–23. Aesculapius, Birmingham.
22. Horn, K., and Crumley, R. (1984): The physiology of nerve injury and repair. *Otolaryngol. Clin. North Am.*, 17:321–333.
23. Kreutzberg, G. (1977): Neurobiology of the regenerating facial motor unit. In: *Facial Nerve Surgery*, edited by U. Fisch, pp. 44–46. Aesculapius, Birmingham.
24. Kukwa, A., Czarnecka, E., and Oudghiri, J. (1984): Topography of the facial nerve in the stylomastoid foramen. *Folia Morphol.*, 43:311–314.
25. Manni, J., and Stennert, E. (1984): Diagnostic methods in facial nerve pathology. *Adv. Otorhinolaryngol.*, 34:202–213.
26. Matsumoto, Y., Yanaghara, N., Murakumi, S., and Fujita, H. (1984): Effects of facial nerve compression on the stapedial nerve. *Laryngoscope*, 111(suppl.):7–11.
27. May, M. (1973): Anatomy of the facial nerve (spatial orientation of fibers in the temporal bone). *Laryngoscope*, 88:1311–1329.
28. May, M., Blumenthal, F., and Taylor, F. (1981): Surgery based on prognostic indicators and results. *Laryngoscope*, 91:2092–2103.
29. May, M., Harvey, J., Marovitz, W., and Stroud, M. (1971): The prognostic accuracy of the maximal stimulation compared with that of nerve excitability in Bell's palsy. *Laryngoscope*, 81:931–938.
30. May, M., Klein, S., and Taylor, F. (1984): Indications for surgery for Bell's palsy. *Am. J. Otolaryngol.*, 5:503–512.
31. Miehlke, A. (1964): Normal and anomalous anatomy of the facial nerve. *Trans. Am. Acad. Ophthalmol. Otolaryngol.*, 68:1030–1044.
32. Miehlke, A. (1973): *Surgery of the Facial Nerve*, W. B. Saunders, Philadelphia.
33. Murakami, S., Yanagihara, N., Matsumoto, Y., and Okamura, H. (1984): Orientation of stapedial nerve fibers in the facial nerve trunk. *Ann. Otol. Rhinol. Laryngol.*, 111(suppl.):3–6.
34. Niparko, J., Kartush, J., Bledsoe, J., and Graham, M. (1985): Antidromically evoked facial nerve response. *Am. J. Otolaryngol.*, 6:353–357.
35. Parnes, S., Strominger, N., and Gummer, E. (1982): Spatial anatomy of the facial nerve in the cat. *Surg. Forum*, 33:557–559.
36. Parnes, S., Strominger, N., Silver, S., and Goldstein, J. (1982): Alternate innervations of facial musculature. *Arch. Otolaryngol.*, 108:418–421.
37. Paun, L., Parvv, C., and Ceausu, E. (1985): Detection by immunofluorescence of possible viral implications in ''idiopathic'' peripheral facial paralysis. *Rev. Roum. Med.*, 36:285–288.
38. Peitersen, E. (1982): The natural history of Bell's palsy. *Am. J. Otol.*, 4:107–111.
39. Radpour, S. (1977): Organization of the facial nerve nucleus in the cat. *Laryngoscope*, 87:557–574.
40. Radpour, S., and Gacek, R. (1980): Facial nerve nucleus in the cat. Further study. *Laryngoscope*, 90:685–692.
41. Radpour, S., and Gacek, R. (1985): Anatomic organization of the cat facial nerve. *Otolaryngol. Head Neck Surg.*, 93:591–596.
42. Richmond, I., and Mahla, M. (1985): Use of antidromic recording to monitor facial nerve function intraoperatively. *Neurosurgery*, 16:458–462.
43. Schmitt, J., and Gacek, R. (1986): Anatomical investigation of the corticonuclear projections to the facial nerve in the cat. *Laryngoscope*, 96:129–134.
44. Shaw, M., and Baker, R. (1983): Direct projections from vestibular nuclei to facial nucleus in cats. *J. Neurophysiol.*, 50:1265–1280.
45. Sunderland, S. (1977): Some anatomical and pathophysiological data relevant to the facial nerve injury and repair. In: *Facial Nerve Surgery*, edited by U. Fisch, pp. 47–61. Aesculapius, Birmingham.
46. Sunderland, S., and Cossar, D. (1953): The structure of the facial nerve. *Anat. Rec.*, 116:147–162.
47. Tanaka, T., and Asahara, T. (1981): Synaptic actions of vagal afferents on facial motor neurons in the cat. *Brain Res.*, 212:188–193.
48. Thomander, L. (1984): Reorganization of the facial motor nucleus after peripheral nerve regeneration. *Acta Otolaryngol.*, 97:619–626.
49. Thomander, L., Aldskogius, H., and Arvidsson, J. (1984): Evidence for a sympathetic component

in motor branches of the facial nerve: A horseradish peroxidase study in the cat. *Brain Res.*, 301:380–383.

50. Thomander, L., Aldskogius, H., and Grant, G. (1981): Motor fiber organization in the intratemporal portion of the cat and the rat facial nerve studied with the horseradish peroxidase technique. In: *The Facial Nerve Complex*, vol. 3, edited by L. Thomander, pp. 1–19. Acta Universitatis Upsaliensis, Upsala; and *Acta Otolaryngol.*, 93:397–405, 1982.

51. Tomita, H. (1977): Viral etiology of Bell's palsy. In: *Facial Nerve Surgery*, edited by U. Fisch, pp. 356–363. Aesculapius, Birmingham.

52. Williams, P., and Hall, S. (1971): Prolonged in vitro observations of normal peripheral nerve fibers and their acute reactions to crush and deliberate trauma. *J. Anat.*, 108:397–408.

53. Yamamoto, E., and Fisch, U. (1977): Experimental decompression of the facial nerve. In: *Facial Nerve Surgery*, edited by U. Fisch, pp. 350–355. Aesculapius, Birmingham.

Physiology of the Ear,
edited by A. F. Jahn and J. Santos-Sacchi.
Raven Press, New York © 1988.

Bone Physiology of the Temporal Bone, Otic Capsule, and Ossicles

Anthony F. Jahn

Section of Otolaryngology–Head and Neck Surgery, New Jersey Medical School,
University of Medicine and Dentistry of New Jersey, Newark, New Jersey 07103-2757

Bone is connective tissue that has specialized to gain strength. Its strength stems from its resilience and hardness. The primary applications of bone are for weight bearing, attachment of muscles, and protection of delicate contents. Secondary but equally important are bone's function as a calcium reservoir and marrow stores for the manufacture of blood.

In the temporal bone, all of these functions of skeletal bone may be found. The petrous pyramids are weight-bearing struts that form the main cross beams of the skull base; the otic capsule isolates and protects the delicate membranous labyrinth; the external surface of the mastoid process and the undersurfaces of the petrous and tympanic bones afford attachment for major muscles that balance and turn the head on the neck; the petrous apex represents the largest marrow stores in the skull, and, like the rest of the skeleton, the temporal bone is involved to a minor degree in calcium homeostasis. Additionally, the auditory ossicles represent a unique application of bone to transmit and modify acoustic/mechanical vibrations.

Bone consists of a collagen matrix, minerals, and a minute amount of intercellular ground substance. It owes its hardness or rigidity to its minerals, its resilience to its collagen bundles, and its strength to the combination of the two. Mature bone is analogous to reinforced concrete: whereas the concrete (i.e., mineral salts) provides hardness and weight, the embedded steel rods (represented by collagen) provide its ultimate strength.

GENERAL OVERVIEW OF BONE FORMATION

In the developing embryo, the cranial and axial skeleton is first modeled in mesenchyme and cartilage. This permits more rapid growth, and given the protective environment of the amniotic fluid, provides adequate structural support. Ossification takes place in two ways: either by progressive breakdown of the cartilage matrix and its replacement with bone (endochondral ossification) or direct ossification of the pre-existing mesenchymal matrix without breakdown (intramembranous ossification). According to the mode of initial ossification, bones are classified as cartilage bone or membrane bone. The two modes of ossification do not differ significantly in the kind of bone ultimately formed, but merely describe the environment in which initial bone formation occurs. In general, long bones are formed by endochondral ossification, whereas the bones of the skull are formed by intramembranous ossification.

143

The time of onset of ossification of the cartilage matrix varies greatly, depending on the location and also among species: as extreme examples, in the human embryo, endochondral bone development begins in the 7th to 8th week after conception (23), whereas in the rat and hamster the otic capsule is still completely cartilaginous at birth and does not begin to ossify until the neonatal period (35).

Ossification is a twofold process consisting of the deposition of osteoid and its subsequent calcification. Osteoid is manufactured by osteoblasts, cells that are most likely derived from the perivascular mesenchyme. Osteoid consists of collagen fibers and intercellular ground substance. The arrangement of the collagen is determined by numerous factors and in turn defines the kind of bone (woven, lamellar, or skein) that is formed.

Although the manufacture of osteoid is essentially similar in most locations, the density of the bone produced differs: bone may be compact, with orderly tight layers as seen in cortical bone, or it may be cancellous, with sponge-like spaces to accommodate marrow, as seen in medullary bone. The trabeculae criss-crossing medullary bone are formed in accordance with lines of stress (Wolff's law).

Mature cortical bone consists of layers or lamellae that are disposed either along the surface (periosteal bone) or in concentric layers around a vascular channel (Haversian bone). Bone laid down along the walls of the marrow cavity lacunae is called endosteal bone and resembles periosteal bone. The cellular and chemical composition of periosteal and Haversian bone is identical; the only differences are its contours (flat versus concentric) and its location (superficial versus deep). Other forms of bone are also found in the mature temporal bone, which will be discussed later.

Mature bone has three components: cells, a noncellular organic matrix, and an inorganic mineral component. The osteocytes of mature bone are derived from the osteoblasts, which in the process of osteoid formation and calcification become immured within the developing bone. The osteocytes obtain their nutrition via their long cytoplasmic processes that extend through minute bony channels to maintain contact with one another and ultimately with the arteries supplying the bone. These arteries may course through the substance of the bone or run on its surface. In Haversian bone, the lamellae and osteocytes surround the central nutrient artery in concentric rings; the physiologic unit of central nutrient vessel and related osteocytes form an osteon. Periosteal osteocytes derive their blood supply from the overlying periosteum. A unique variant of this is the blood supply to the ossicles, which is derived in great part from the overlying mucosa (2).

Osteocytes continue to live for decades and in more subtle ways continue to control bone formation, mineralization, and even resorption (32). As the osteocyte ages, well-described progressive cytoplasmic and nuclear changes mark its senescence (46). Physiologic bone turnover is effected by bone breakdown and new bone formation and may be a feature of growth, remodeling, or repair. Bone is broken down by osteoclasts, giant multinucleated cells that probably originate in the lymphoid organs and travel via the bloodstream to the site of bone remodeling (47). Osteoblasts, osteocytes, osteoclasts, and their precursors form the physiologic cell population of bone.

The noncellular organic matrix of bone, or osteoid, is made of intercellular ground substance and collagen. The intercellular ground substance contains glycoproteins and acid proteoglycans, as well as gamma-carboxyglutamic acid, phosphorylated polypeptides, and lipids (4). Both ground substance and collagen are synthesized by the active osteoblast and, to a much lesser extent, the mature osteocyte (29).

Collagen, which forms at least 96% of unmineralized bony matrix, is a fibrous protein formed of long (300 nm) rod-like molecules. There are three types of interstitial collagen, each characterized by distinct polypeptide chains.

Type I is found in bone, dentine, and fibrous cartilage. Type II is seen in hyaline and elastic cartilages and also found in the bony otic capsule as cartilage islands in the endochondral layer. Type III is found in smooth muscles, arteries, endoneurium, and viscera (28). Collagen molecules aggregate to form fibrils, and the fibrils are arranged in specific patterns, depending on the kind of bone formed. Primary, or woven, bone has its collagen bundles in a woven, quasirandom arrangement. Woven bone is typically seen only at initial ossification or during the first phase of bony repair. It is usually replaced by secondary, or lamellar, bone, whose collagen bundles are packed into tight parallel bundles; this is the collagen pattern seen with mature periosteal or Haversian bone. Exceptions to this rule regarding primary and secondary bone (i.e., collagen patterns) are found in the temporal bone and will be discussed later.

The inorganic mineral component of bone is mostly calcium phosphate, which forms 35% to 65% of the dry weight of bone (24). About 45% of the total mineral content is amorphous calcium phosphate and the rest, calcium hydroxylapatite. Calcium deposition follows osteoid formation and completes the process of ossification. The mineral is derived from the circulation, and its rate of deposition is governed by a number of factors, including the type of bone (i.e., primary or secondary) (4), hormonal influences (36), and the tissue pH (38). The calcium salts form needle- and tablet-shaped crystals that infiltrate the collagen fibrils to add rigidity to the strength and resilience of the collagen (4). The calcium salts of the skeleton represent a large reservoir of this mineral, which can be used to maintain appropriate serum calcium levels in concert with the actions of the gastrointestinal tract and parathyroid glands. The osteocytes are thought to play some role in the release of calcium into the circulation without concomitant resorption of bone matrix, a process termed halisteresis (32).

With this brief outline as general background, we are now in a position to consider the specific features of bony physiology that distinguish the temporal bone. For the sake of convenience, the discussion to follow is divided into three areas: the temporal bone encasing the ossicles and inner ear, the bony otic capsule, and the auditory ossicles. For each area we will discuss the physiologic features of embryologic development, maturity in the adult, and degenerative changes of aging. We will refer to any clinical implications in the course of the discussion.

THE TEMPORAL BONE

The temporal bone is a fused complex of four parts: the petrous (or petromastoid) bone, the squamous bone, the tympanic bone, and the styloid bone. Since each component forms independently, from the developmental point of view they are best considered as separate bones that are secondarily joined once their basic development is complete. Of the four bones, the petrous and squamous are well formed at birth, whereas the styloid and tympanic bones continue to develop well into infancy.

The four components of the temporal bone are formed in cartilage and mesen-chyme as part of the embryonic chondrocranium. The pars squamosa and pars tym-panica are membrane bones with direct intramembranous ossification, whereas the pars petromastoidea and the styloid process are endochondral bones with breakdown of the cartilage anlage and replacement by bone (31). The squamous bone begins to ossify from a single center, in the 8th week. This ossification extends also into the root of the zygomatic process (18) and continues during most of intrauterine de-velopment. At birth, the peripheral extremes of the pars squamosa are not yet com-pletely ossified and the temporoparietal junction is soft.

The pars tympanica in the embryo is a flat ring, dehiscent at the top. It begins to ossify in the 10th week, from a single center located medially and ventrally (18). After birth, the tympanic ring continues to grow laterally and inferiorly. By 6 months, it extends anteroinferiorly to partially adhere to the petromastoid portion. Between 1 and 2 years, the bone extends laterally to enclose an anteroinferior dehiscence along the floor of the developing bony external canal, and by $2\frac{1}{2}$ years the dehiscence is surrounded to form the foramen of Huschke. The bone continues its posteroinferior growth to define the vaginal process, ensheathing the styloid, and completes its development by obliterating the foramen of Huschke to form the definite bony ex-ternal canal (48). The pars tympanica is unusual in that its development into the external bony canal takes place postnatally, during the early infant years; at birth, there is no bony external canal, and on the neonate skull the tympanic ring and tympanic membrane lie flat, directly on the surface. Even after it has fully formed, the tympanic ring seems to maintain a greater potential for growth, since the reactive new bone formation seen with exostoses is confined exclusively to the tympanic ring and is not seen on the squamous plate bridging the notch of Rivinus superiorly.

Intramembranous ossification in the squamous and tympanic bones proceeds from a single central center and its rate is rather rapid. This permits continued peripheral growth and flexibility. By contrast, the petromastoid and styloid bones undergo endochondral ossification from multiple centers, a more laborious process with less potential for continued peripheral growth.

The petromastoid bone begins to ossify during weeks 20 to 24 of gestation. Os-sification proceeds from multiple separate centers and is essentially complete by the 28th to 30th weeks (18,31). The styloid bone, the proximal portion of Reichert's cartilage, ossifies from two centers, the proximal one beginning before birth and the lateral one soon after.

The process of endochondral ossification involves several stages. Robles-Marin and co-workers (38) in a study of ossifying embryonic vertebral bodies found that the degenerating chondrocyte itself initiates osteogenesis by producing a proto-plasmic secretion that forms a ground substance for calcium precipitation. The initial calcium precipitation, which may be the result of local pH changes, induces vascular invasion and the beginning of osteogenesis. Internal development of the marrow-containing petrous apex occurs secondarily, during the bone-remodeling phase, as sinusoids within the bone enlarge by confluence (36).

Since much of this work has been carried out in other experimental systems, the exact timing for these phenomena in the temporal bone cannot be given. By birth, however, the petrous apex contains major stores of red marrow, which over time becomes inactive (yellow).

Postnatal growth of the temporal bone is significant, and relates partly to the growth of the brain (40). In part, however, its growth is independent of the environment. The remarkable changes of the tympanic bone have already been described. The squamous bone also continues to grow, initially more in height, then more in length (41). The pars petrosa undergoes rapid development during the second year of life (40). This initial growth period is followed by a second growth spurt at puberty (8). During the postnatal period, there is also a realignment of the long axis of the petrous bone, a phenomenon believed to compensate for the change from quadripedal to bipedal posture (42).

Variations in the dimensions of the temporal bone relate to the side studied (41), the race of the individual (40), and the degree of pneumatization (3).

The adult temporal bone is for the most part lamellar (secondary) bone, mostly periosteal rather than Haversian. Its thickness varies from the filigree-like septa of the mastoid to the thick compact bone of the tympanic bone and skull base. An exception to this generalization is the unique area of hypermetabolic bone that is consistently found in the anterior epitympanic recess (15). This rim of nonlamellar (woven) bone is consistently seen and its significance is unclear.

With regards to aging, there are no specific distinguishing features in this part of the temporal bone as compared with lamellar bone elsewhere.

THE OTIC CAPSULE

The otic capsule, or bony labyrinth, is unique in morphology and physiology and has posed a challenge for temporal bone histologists for more than a century. Anson (1) summarized the key distinguishing features of the otic capsule: (a) Despite its small size, it originates from 14 ossification centers, appearing within a period of 6 weeks. (b) There is fusion of the centers peripherally, without intermediate zones of epiphyseal growth. (c) Each center has a trilaminar structure that is maintained throughout the entire capsule. (d) There is an independent timetable of growth for each layer of every center. (e) There is a self-governing schema in attaining mature histologic architecture, a fetal architecture that is maintained throughout adult life, with a total absence of those processes that elsewhere convert fetal bone into Haversian.

Although the above features are the most immediately striking, the apparent arrest in maturation obscures the fact that there are subtle but documented changes representing continuing metabolic turnover, injury, and healing as well as maturity and aging in the otic capsule. These will be described below.

The otic capsule is trilaminar, consisting of three distinct bony layers. The outer covering layer is lamellar compact bone that blends peripherally with the rest of the petrous bone (Fig. 1). This outer periosteal layer grows by external deposition of lamellae. The inner lining layer forms the walls of the perilymphatic spaces of the labyrinth and provides attachment to the membranous structures of the labyrinth (Fig. 2). This thin, compact lamellar bone is inaccurately called endosteal bone, although its proper designation is internal periosteal bone, since the term endosteal in bone morphology refers specifically to the bone lining the marrow cavities. Anson (1), who calls this the internal periosteal layer, uses endosteal to designate bone deposited on the cartilage islands of the endochondral layer.

It is the middle, or endochondral, layer that is histologically unique. Modeled in

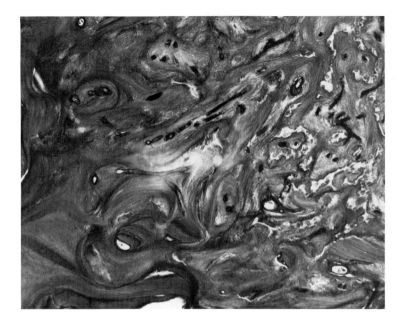

FIG. 1. Otic capsule low-power view. Note the gradual blending between the endochondral bone (right) and the lamellar compact periosteal bone (left) that represents the outermost layer of the otic capsule.

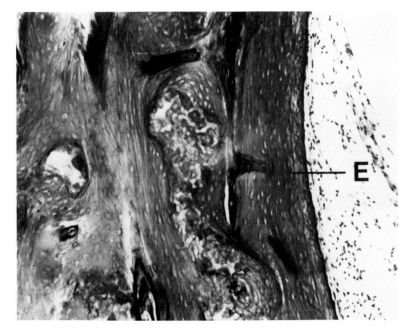

FIG. 2. Endosteal layer of otic capsule (E). In this high-power view note the compact thin endosteal bone layer lining the cavity of the membranous labyrinth.

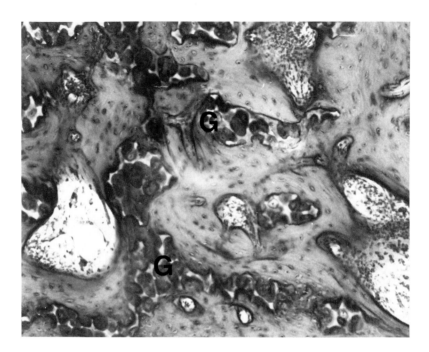

FIG. 3. Globuli interossei (G). In this high-power view the cartilage islands characteristic of the endochondral (middle) layer of the otic capsule are clearly seen. Note also the numerous capillary spaces lined by fibrous connective tissue.

cartilage like the rest of the skeleton, the endochondral layer never completely ossifies but maintains islands of cartilage cells that are surrounded by finger-like processes of bone (Fig. 3). The histologic appearance of the bone suggests loosely coiled yarn and has been termed *embryonic skein bone* (*Strähnenknochen*) (27). This unique arrangement of bone is probably a structural adaptation to the physical constraints imposed by the persistent islands of cartilage. Why these islands of cartilage persist (and they persist throughout life) is unknown; we will discuss some hypotheses later.

The terminology applied to the islands of cartilage and surrounding bone has become confused. The original investigators found that the finger-like extensions of bone sectioned perpendicularly looked like small balls. The term *globuli ossei* was used by Manasse (25) to refer to these bony masses, which were interspersed amid the islands of cartilage that he called "cartilage containing interglobular spaces." Subsequent investigators unfortunately designated the cartilage rests as *globuli interossei*. Since the term no longer refers to the globuli of intrachondral bone, it is strictly speaking meaningless; nonetheless, globuli interossei referring to the cartilage rests has become enshrined in the literature (9,11,39).

Embryology of the Otic Capsule

The otic capsule initially appears as a mesenchymal and cartilaginous condensation around the developing otocyst. Ossification is initiated at 14 separate centers, beginning in the 15th to 16th weeks. At 17 weeks, some of the ossification centers fuse.

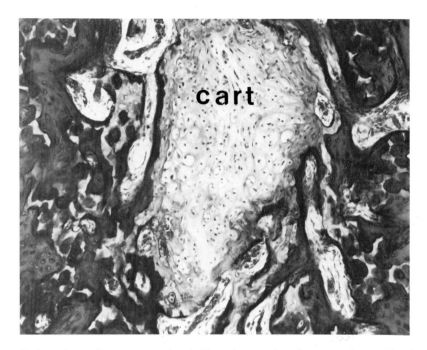

FIG. 4. Embryonic cartilage remnant (cart). The otic capsule adjacent to the cochlea in this 6-hour-old neonate displays a remnant of embryonic cartilage. It is large, cellular, and undergoing active resorption at its edges. Note the numerous capillaries surrounding the cartilage and the more familiar globuli interossei at the periphery of the photograph.

By 18 weeks, much of the otic capsule is ossified. The cochlea, which begins to ossify at the base, is still cartilaginous at the apex this time. At 19 weeks, ossification is mostly complete, except over the posterior and horizontal canals. At 20 and 21 weeks the final (14th) ossification center appears, overlying the posterolateral portion of the posterior canal. The area of the fissula ante fenestram is the last to ossify, beginning in the 22nd to 23rd weeks (9,46). A detailed and illustrated description of the process is given by Schuknecht and Gulya (40) (Fig. 4).

The source of the bone in the endochondral layer has been a topic of controversy. Manasse (25) originally suggested that ossification was an *in situ* process, and the osteocytes were "metaplastic" embryonic cartilage cells. More recent investigators have shown that the osteocytes of intrachondral bone originate extrinsically, the process involving the removal of chondrocytes and intercellular substance by mononuclear cells, followed by the invasion of osteogenic vascular buds (12,35). Cells that originate from the perivascular elements of these capillary buds enter the empty lacunae of cartilage remnants to become osteoblasts (35). The mature osteocytes of the fine-fibered alamellar "skein bone" are similar to osteocytes found in long bones (35). Fueling the controversy regarding the origins of intrachondral bone has been the suggestion that some effete chondrocytes in the cartilage rests calcify directly (5) and further that chondrocytes occasionally transform directly into chondroid bone (12).

Although there was some doubt regarding metabolic turnover in the mature otic capsule, it is now clear that there is a continuous, albeit slow, process of bone

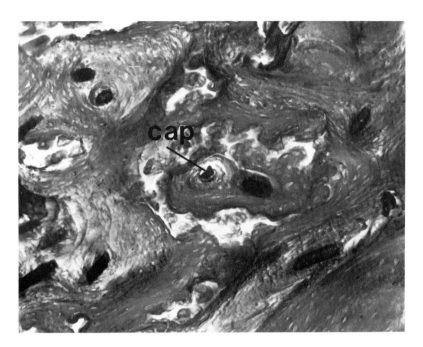

FIG. 5. Bony turnover, endochondral layer. The capillary (cap) runs through a cartilage island. It is surrounded by concentric layers of compact bone. This is the mechanism by which new bone is formed. The appearance of this island of bone, surrounded by cartilage, gave origin to the term *globuli ossei* (see text).

formation and destruction in adult endochondral bone (Fig. 5). Gussen (12) has described continuing partial replacement of cartilage rests by new endochondral bone and has further suggested that new cartilage is formed by mesenchymal cells lining the labyrinth. In the noncellular ground substance component of the endochondral layer, Zechner and Altmann (52) demonstrated a constant low-level metabolic activity, evidenced by changes in staining characteristics of the mucopolysaccharides. In 1975, in a study of adult temporal bones from premortem tetracycline-treated patients, we described an active uptake of this label by newly synthesized bone in the perivascular areas of the endochondral layer (16).

In examining the physiology of endochondral bone, a fundamental question remains: what is the purpose (if any) of the cartilage rests in the otic capsule? Their distribution is irregular and has been the subject of numerous studies (5,12,20,26). Rauchfuss (35) has suggested that the persistence of cartilage rests is a function of the distance between neighboring ossification centers. A higher concentration of cartilage remnants was noted at the anterior border of the oval window, medial margin of the round window, and superior margin of the internal auditory canal by Costa and Covell (5), who examined a possible relationship with predilective sites of otosclerosis. Persistent chondrocytes were demonstrated in the stapes footplate by Marovitz and Shapiro (26) and Gussen (12), supporting the labyrinthine origin of the footplate.

The reason for the persistence of cartilage rests may be a negative one: lack of mechanical stress, phylo- and ontogenic factors that have persisted. As to positive reasons, Sercer (42,43) has pointed out that the otic capsule rotates rostrally during embryonic and postnatal development, a reorientation that may represent a recapitulation of the phylogenic ascent from the quadriped to the upright posture. This rotation may be more easily accommodated in a cartilage shell. This reorientation was demonstrated in monkeys by Daniel et al. (6). Zechner and Altman (51,52) have speculated that the cartilage remnants, which are rich in mucopolysaccharides, could be regarded as metabolic energy stores for the cochlea. Equally speculative are suggestions that the cartilage rests serve to cushion the cochlea (44) or in some fashion permit it to vibrate as a form of bone conduction (30).

Injury and Repair

Bony fractures normally heal by the formation of a fibrous scar that subsequently ossifies and remodels. The initial reparative bone is woven, with disorganized collagen fibrils. It is replaced by lamellar bone with orderly collagen deposition and a commensurate gain in tensile strength. Irritative or inflammatory foci are also capable of evoking the reparative response. This is exemplified elsewhere by the involucrum seen in osteomyelitis.

Both of these healing responses may be seen in the outer and inner periosteal layers of the otic capsule but are notably missing the endochondral layer. Although this layer is clearly not metabolically inert (see above), it seems to lack the osteogenic reserves to heal any disruptions in a substance. This is readily demonstrated by the microfractures seen in adult temporal bones.

Microfractures are microscopic fissures seen crossing the otic capsule in certain predictable patterns. These fractures are most commonly seen between the round window niche and posterior canal ampullae, around the oval window, and between the utricle and fallopian canal (17). They are more common with increasing age, suggesting that they may be the result of chronic mechanical stress. It has been suggested that they are caused by the vector forces of mastication acting on the otic capsule. Examination of these microfractures reveals that the diastasis is often filled by cellular fibrous tissue, but never by new bone (Fig. 6). If the fracture extends into the periosteal lining bone, there may be evidence of exuberant bony healing, but only localized to that site. This lack of bony healing is seen more dramatically in labyrinthine fractures following temporal bone trauma. Schuknecht (39) has utilized this lack of endochondral healing in the cochleosacculotomy procedure, in which a fracture is purposely produced in the bony spiral lamina of the cochlea, with the hope that it will result in a permanent perilymph–endolymph fistula. Given the apparent physiologic "inertia" of the endochondral bone in its response to injury, the dramatic new bone formation seen with otosclerosis is all the more remarkable.

In contrast to endochondral bone, the periosteal bone is capable of new bone formation in response to a variety of traumatic and inflammatory stimuli. The most impressive clinical example is seen in the bony endolabyrinthine obliteration that follows infectious or radiation labyrinthitis. The new bone seen in this condition (labyrinthitis ossificans), which often fills the entire endolabyrinthine space, most likely originates in the thin inner periosteal bone lining the labyrinth (Fig. 7).

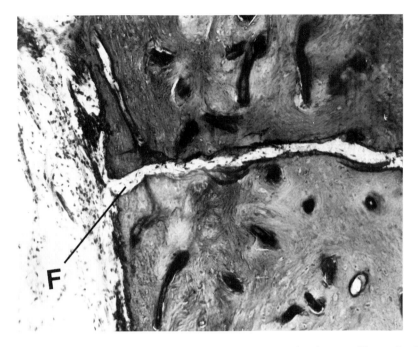

FIG. 6. Microfracture. This high-power photograph illustrates a microfracture (F) crossing the otic capsule. Note the absence of a bony callous and the plugging of the fracture line by fibrous connective tissue.

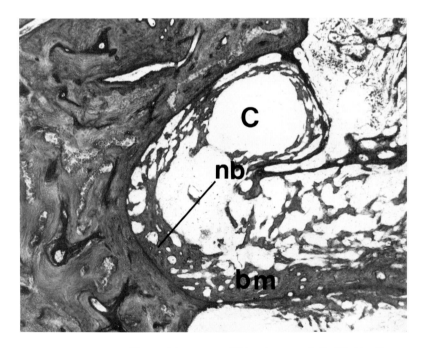

FIG. 7. Ossifying labyrinthitis. The cochlear space (C) has been partially filled by fibrous connective tissue and new bone (nb). Note the deposition of the new bone peripherally and extending across the basilar membrane (bm).

AGING CHANGES IN THE OTIC CAPSULE

The microscopic signs of aging in the otic capsule are more subtle than in skeletal bone. Since the basic processes of turnover and metabolism are minimal, the factors in aging that modulate these processes to produce decreased bone turnover and osteoporosis are not in evidence here. The features that distinguish the aged otic capsule are not readily apparent. Although a gradual replacement of cartilage remnants by bone has been shown, histologists have been unable to demonstrate a significant reduction in overall cartilage content with aging. There appears to be a general decrease in cellularity of the cartilage rests with age and also in the cellularity of chondroid bone (12). There may be more calcification of cartilage remnants and plugging of vascular canals in the endochondral bone. The canals are plugged with calcified matter, a process termed micropetrosis (13). The overall decrease in vasculature probably results in a decrease in bone metabolism although the process is so subtle even when fully operative that a decrease in old age would be difficult to document. Although the exact rate of new bone formation with age is not known, the tetracycline-labeling studies mentioned earlier certainly suggest that active new bone formation continues until death (16).

An age-associated bony change of particular interest is seen at the fundus of the internal auditory canal. In 1958 Sercer and Krmpotič-Nemanič (44) found that with aging there was increased osteoid deposition at the tractus spiralis foraminosus, the point of entrance from the modiolus to the internal auditory canal. He hypothesized that gradual compression of the arteries and nerve fibers of the cochlea may contribute to presbycutic hearing loss. Subsequently Krmpotič-Nemanič (21) restudied this material in detail. She found that sleeves of osteoid were laid down around the vessels and nerve fibers, leading to compression and at times complete closure of the foramina. The new bone appears to compress the peripheral fibers more, a finding coherent with the high frequency hearing loss seen. In very old individuals, she also found osteoid deposits in the saccular area, compressing the vestibular nerve. Similar osteoid deposits were seen with advancing age around other cranial foramina, such as the stylomastoid foramen and foramen rotundum (22). The etiology of these osteoid deposits is uncertain; they may be related to the constant movement of the vessels and nerves associated with CSF and cardiovascular pulsations. Although the etiology and implications are not clear, the findings are plainly documented.

BONE PHYSIOLOGY OF THE OSSICLES

In both histology and physiology, the auditory ossicles occupy an intermediate position between the otic capsules and the rest of the temporal bone. They are embryologically derived from the mesenchyme of the first and second branchial arches, with the exception of the medial aspect of the stapes footplate, which, as previously described, demarcates from the labyrinthine capsule (lamina vestibularis). The cartilage precursors of the ossicles are seen early; the stapes blastema may be distinguished as early as three weeks after conception (18). Ossicular remodeling in the embryo involves changes in shape as well as size; the fetal stapes is ring-like, its shape determined by the stapedial artery around which it forms. Later, with involution of this artery and excavation along the obturator surface of the stapedial crura, the ossicle achieves its adult form (7).

The ossification of the ossicles reflects the origins of their cartilage precursors. The malleus and incus undergo endochondral ossification with centers of ossification and cellular changes similar to the long bones. The stapes footplate, by contrast, resembles the endochondral layer of the otic capsule, with a nonzonal pattern of ossification and persistent viable cartilage cells (12,34). A labeling study of postnatal ossicular growth in dogs suggests that appositional (periosteal) growth in the malleus and incus leads to an increase in external dimensions and is complete within the first month of postnatal life. Internal (Haversian or osteonic) growth continues, but at a lower rate than in long bones (37). Subsequent remodeling of the malleus and incus leads to the formation of a rudimentary medulla and cortex, although the medullary cavities never contain marrow. Like the otic capsule, these ossicles demonstrate persistent cartilage islands into adult life; unlike endochondral bone, these are gradually completely replaced by bone over the individual's lifetime (49).

Injury and Repair

Based on their histologic appearance, ossicles should be capable of forming bony union. (That this is seldom seen clinically with the malleus and incus is probably because the points of mechanical weakness are at the joints rather than within the ossicles themselves.) The stapes is again the exception; fractures of the stapedial crura usually heal by fibrous union if at all. This, however, may be more a matter of inadequate bony mass rather than the inability to mount an osteogenic response. Fractures of the footplate, on the other hand, never heal properly. This is probably owing to the endochondral derivation of this structure, possibly aggravated by persistent perilymph leakage or mucosal ingrowth.

Aging Changes

Clinical interest in ossicular aging has focused on the ossicular joints and specifically on the question of whether a stiffening of these joints may contribute to age-associated hearing loss. The joint changes in ossicles appear to consist of fraying and fibrillation, with subsequent thinning and calcification. Hyaline material and occasional calcium deposits were seen within the joints, and degeneration led rarely to bone effusion of the articulating surfaces (10). These changes appear to have no clinical significance and overall the ossicular joints appeared to be less prone to degenerative or inflammatory arthritis than other joints. An unpublished personal study at the University of Toronto of 30 temporal bones from patients with rheumatoid arthritis failed to disclose any significant joint pathology or significant conductive hearing loss.

FUTURE DIRECTIONS

Research interest in bony metabolism of the ear is directed along three lines. These are studies of bone destruction, bony repair, and the possible autoimmune response exhibited toward endochondral bone.

Studies of bone destruction have been carried out in the context of cholesteato-matous erosion of bone. Although the role of collagenolytic enzymes has been demonstrated and appears to be significant in bone destruction, it is currently thought that mechanical pressure from the expanding cholesteatoma may also play a part. This is a partial reversion to an earlier theory that suggested that mechanical pressure was the main factor in bony resorption. Bone destruction by otosclerosis has also been an area of intense interest and numerous studies have advocated the use of sodium fluoride to harden the otic capsule. There are numerous theoretical objections to this hypothesis, which, although intriguing, is not generally accepted (19). It is hoped that the experimental studies in other bone systems will yield new drugs for the prevention of bone resorption (45).

The study of new bone formation in the mastoid and the middle ear has gained clinical impetus with the use of bone replacement implants. The most biocompatible of these appear to be the porous hydroxylapatite implants and ceramic glass implants. A number of clinical papers have been written examining the bone implant interface and the osteogenic response adjacent to these implants.

A rebirth of interest in the physiology of the otic capsule was initiated by Yoo and co-workers (50), who in 1982 demonstrated in animal models an induced autoimmunity to Type II collagen, the form of collagen present within the cartilage rests of the endochondral bone. They hypothesized that this autoimmunity in humans may account for otosclerosis and Meniere's disease. Yoo's findings have been questioned by Harris and co-workers (14), who were unable to confirm the histologic changes described. Although the issue is not yet resolved, it represents an exciting new direction in the study of the otic capsule, one that will perhaps yield concrete answers to clinical questions posed by these "idiopathic" disorders.

REFERENCES

1. Anson, B. J. (1969): The labyrinths and their capsule in health and disease. *Trans. Am. Acad. Ophthalmol.*, 73:17–38.
2. Anson, B. J., and Winch, T. R. (1974): Vascular channels in the auditory ossicles in man. *Ann. Otol. Rhinol. Laryngol.*, 83:142–158.
3. Aoki, K., Esaki, S., and Honda, Y. (1986): Effect of middle ear infection upon the pneumatization of the mastoid. *Laryngoscope*, 96:430–437.
4. Bonucci, E. (1984): The structural basis of calcification. In: *Ultrastructure of the Connective Tissue Matrix*, edited by A. Ruggeri and P. M. Motta. Martinus Nijhoff, The Hague.
5. Costa, O. A., and Covell, W. P. (1965): Variations in the endochondral bone of the otic capsule. *Laryngoscope*, 75:1462–1476.
6. Daniel, H. J., Schmidt, R. T., Oishan, A. F., and Swindler, D. R. (1982): Ontogenetic changes in the bony labyrinth of *Macaca mulatta*. *Folia Primatol. (Basel)*, 38:122–129.
7. Dass, R., and Makhni, S. S. (1966): Ossification of the ear ossicles. *Arch. Otolaryngol.*, 84:306–312.
8. Eby, T. L., and Nadol, J. B. (1986): Postnatal growth of the human temporal bone. *Ann. Otol. Rhinol. Laryngol.*, 95:356–364.
9. Eggston, A. A., and Wolff, D. (1947): *Histopathology of the Ear, Nose, and Throat*. Williams & Wilkins, Baltimore.
10. Etholm, B., and Belal, A. (1974): Senile changes in the middle ear joints. *Ann. Otol. Rhinol. Laryngol.*, 83:49–54.
11. Gussen, R. (1967): Globuli interossei as a manifestation of bone resorption. *Acta Otolaryngol (Stockh.)*, 63:411–423.
12. Gussen, R. (1968): Articular and internal remodelling in the human otic capsule. *Am. J. Anat.*, 122:397–417.
13. Gussen, R. (1969): Plugging of the vascular canals in the otic capsule. *Ann. Otol. Rhinol. Laryngol.*, 78:1305–1315.

14. Harris, J. P., Woolf, N. K., and Ryan, A. F. (1986): A reexamination of experimental Type II collagen autoimmunity: Middle and inner morphology and function. *Ann. Otol. Rhinol. Laryngol.*, 95:176–180.
15. Hawke, M., Farkashidy, J., and Jahn, A. F. (1975): Nonlamellar new bone formation in the anterior attic recess. *Arch. Otolaryngol.*, 101:117–119.
16. Hawke, M., and Jahn, A. F. (1975): Bone formation in the normal human otic capsule. *Arch. Otolaryngol.*, 101:462–466.
17. Hawke, M., and Jahn, A. F. (1987): *Diseases of the Ear: Clinical and Pathologic Aspects.* Lea and Febiger, Philadelphia.
18. Jahn, A. F. (1972): Embryological development of the human ear. *Univ. Toronto Med. J.*, 50:16–20.
19. Jahn, A. F., and Vernick, D. (1986): *Otosclerosis: Diagnosis and Management.* Am. Acad. Otol. Head and Neck Surg., Washington, DC.
20. Kakizaki, I., and Altmann, F. (1970): The interglobular spaces in the human labyrinthine capsule. *Ann. Otol. Rhinol. Laryngol.*, 79:666–679.
21. Krmpotič-Nemanič, J. (1972): Ueber die Morphologie des inneren Gehoerganges bei der Alters-schwerhoerigkeit. *HNO*, 20:246–459.
22. Krmpotič-Nemanič, J., Nemanic, J., and Kostovic, I. (1972): Macroscopical and microscopical changes in the bottom of the internal auditory meatus. *Acta Otolaryngol.*, 73:254–258.
23. Langman, J. (1969): *Medical Embryology.* Williams & Wilkins, Baltimore.
24. Laros, G. S. (1976): Normal structure of bone: Light and electron microscopy. In: *Bones and Joints*, edited by L. V. Ackerman, H. J. Spjut, and M. R. Abell, pp. 16–24. Williams & Wilkins, Baltimore.
25. Manasse, P. (1897): Ueber knorpelhaltige Interglobularraume in der menschlichen Labyrinthkapsel. *Z. Ohrenheilkd.*, 31:1–22.
26. Marovitz, W. F., and Shapiro, L. J. (1969): The distribution of phosphorylase activity in the otic capsule and ossicular chain of fetal and newborn rats. *Ann. Otol. Rhinol. Laryngol.*, 78:587–597.
27. Meyer, M. (1927): Ueber eine eigentümliche Art von Knochengewebe beim erwachsenen Menschen den lamellenlosen, feinfaserigen-strähnenartigen-Markknochen und über den embryonalen Markknochen. *Z. Anat. Entwicklungsgesch.*, 83:734–751.
28. Montes, G. S., Bezerra, M. S. F., and Junqueira, L. C. U. (1984): Collagen distribution in tissues. In: *Ultrastructure of the Connective Tissue Matrix*, edited by A. Ruggeri and P. M. Motta, pp. 65–88. Martinus Nijhoff, The Hague.
29. Parry, D. A. D., and Craig, A. S. (1984): Growth and development of collagen fibrils in connective tissue. In: *Ultrastructure of the Connective Tissue Matrix*, edited by A. Ruggeri and P. M. Motta. Martinus Nijhoff, The Hague.
30. Pedziwiatr, Z. (1971): Morphological data for the theory of temporal bone vibrations. *Pol. Med. J.*, 10:547–563.
31. Rarey, K. F. (1985): Morphology of the temporal bone. *Ear Nose Throat J.*, 64:282–291.
32. Rasmussen, H., and Bordier, P. (1974): *The Physiological and Cellular Basis of Metabolic Bone Disease*, p. 22. Williams & Wilkins, Baltimore.
33. Rauchfuss, A. (1980): Some morphologic details of the endochondral layer of the labyrinthine bone. *Arch. Otorhinolaryngol.*, 226:239–250.
34. Rauchfuss, A. (1981): Ein Beitrag zur Entwicklung der Gehörknochelchen und des Ringbandes. *Arch. Otorhinolaryngol.*, 233:77–87.
35. Rauchfuss, A. (1981): Zur enchondralen Ossifikation der Labyrinthkapsel: Die Enstehung der ossei und der Interglobularräume. *Arch. Otorhinolaryngol.*, 233:237–250.
36. Reddi, A. H. (1981): Cell biology and biochemistry of endochondral bone development. *Coll. Res.*, 1:209–226.
37. Roberto, M. (1978): Quantitative evaluation of postnatal bone growth in the auditory ossicles of the dog. *Ann. Otol. Rhinol. Laryngol.*, 87:370–379.
38. Robles-Marin, D., Smith-Agreda, V., Marti-Faus, M., Berlanga-Hernandez, J. L., et al. (1984): Histochemical and enzymatic changes in the chondrocytes next to the vascular invasion during endochondrial ossification. In: *Bone Circulation*, edited by J. Arlet, R. P. Ficat, and D. S. Hungerford, pp. 23–27. Williams & Wilkins, Baltimore.
39. Schuknecht, H. F., and Gulya, A. J. (1986): *Anatomy of the Temporal Bone with Surgical Implications.* Lea and Febiger, Philadelphia.
40. Schulter, F. P. (1976): A comparative study of the temporal bone in three populations of man. *Am. J. Phys. Anthropol.*, 44:453–468.
41. Schmidt, H. M., and Dahm, P. (1977): Die postnatale Entwicklung des menschlichen Os temporale. *Gegenbaurs Morphol. Jahrb.*, 123:689–698.
42. Sercer, A. (1958): L'etiopathogenie de l'otospongiose et les facteurs anthropologiques. *Arch. Ital. Otol. Rinol. Lar.*, 769:1–92.
43. Sercer, A. (1966): Versuch einer biomechanischer Erklärung, warum die Labyrintkapsel aus unreifem Knochen gebaut ist. *Laryngol. Rhinol. Otol.*, 45:74–81.

44. Sercer, A., and Krmpotic-Nemanic, J. (1958): Ueber die Ursache der progressiven Altersschwer-hoerigkeit (presbyacusis). *Acta Otolaryngol. [Suppl.] (Stockh.)*, 143.
45. Torbinejad, M., Clagett, J., and Engel, D. (1979): A cat model for the evaluation of bone resorption: Induction of bone loss by simulated complexes and inhibition by indomethacin. *Calcif. Tissue Int.*, 29:207–214.
46. Urist, M. P., editor (1980): *Fundamental and Clinical Bone Physiology*, p. 31. J. B. Lippincott, Philadelphia.
47. Urist, M. P., editor (1980): *Fundamental and Clinical Bone Physiology*, p. 33. J. B. Lippincott, Philadelphia.
48. Weaver, D. S. (1979): Applications of the likelihood ratio test to age estimation using the infant and child temporal bone. *Am. J. Phys. Anthropol.*, 50:263–270.
49. Wustrow, F. (1956): Die knochenbildung in der Gehoerknochelchen. *Z. Laryngol. Otol.*, 35:487–498.
50. Yoo, T. J., Stuart, J. M., Kang, A. H., Townes, A. S., et al. (1982): Type II collagen autoimmunity in otosclerosis and Meniere's disease. *Science*, 217:1153–1155.
51. Zechner, G. (1971): Ueber knorpelreste in der menschlichen knoerchernen Labyrinthkapsel. *Arch. Klin. Ohr. Nas. Kehlk. Heilk.*, 198:317–324.
52. Zechner, G., and Altmann, F. (1969): Ground substance of the otic capsule. *Arch. Otolaryngol.*, 90:418–428.

Physiology of the Ear,
edited by A. F. Jahn and J. Santos-Sacchi.
Raven Press, New York © 1988.

An Anatomical Tour of the Cochlea

Robert V. Harrison and Ivan M. Hunter-Duvar

*Department of Otolaryngology, The Hospital for Sick Children,
Toronto, Ontario, Canada M5G 1X8*

Anatomical studies of the inner ear have progressed hand in hand with the development of microscopic techniques. The names of many early explorers of cochlear anatomy are very familiar to us, e.g., Corti (7), Claudius (6), Hensen (13), Böttcher (5), Retzius (26), and Held (12). The introduction of the transmission electron microscope allowed more detailed ultrastructural descriptions of the cochlea; comprehensive studies have been made, for example, by Engström and Wersäll and their colleagues (8,9), Spoendlin (27), Iurato (18), Bredberg (3), Kimura (20), and many others since then.

The development of the scanning electron microscope allowed different visualization of the cochlea. The first of such studies were made by Barber and Boyle (1), followed by many detailed studies including those by Lim (24), Bredberg and colleagues (4), Hunter-Duvar (15–17), Harada (11), and many others. It is with the scanning electron microscope that we now take this anatomical tour of the cochlea.

THE COCHLEA

The spiral canal of the cochlea lies anterior to the vestibule. In humans its total length is about 35 mm, coiled into a little over $2\frac{1}{2}$ turns, the basal of which has a diameter of 10 mm. Figure 1 shows the cochlea of the chinchilla with its bony shell removed to reveal the two major perilymph-filled compartments, scala tympani and scala vestibuli. Separating these two scalae, the endolymph-filled scala media, together with the organ of Corti and basilar membrane, collectively make up the membranous cochlear duct. This duct ends blindly at the apical end of the cochlea. At the base, it communicates with the saccule of the vestibule via the ductus reuniens. Sound vibrations from the ossicular chain are admitted to the cochlea by movement of the stapes footplate within the oval window. Pressure changes within the cochlea are released via the round window.

Figure 2 shows the apical turn of the cochlea (chinchilla) as seen from above, after removal of its bony shell. At this point, the helicotrema provides a communication between scala vestibuli and scala tympani. In the human this aperture is approximately 0.05 mm². In this view of the cochlea, both the tectorial membrane and Reissner's membrane have been removed to uncover the surface of the sensory epithelium. On this reticular lamina, the rows of outer and inner hair-cell stereocilia are clearly outlined.

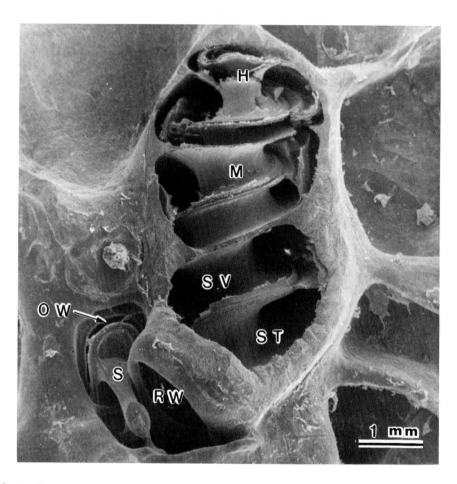

FIG. 1. The (opened) cochlea as seen from a lateral aspect. H, helicotrema; M, modiolus; OW, oval window; RW, round window; S, stapes; SV, scala vestibuli; ST, scala tympani.

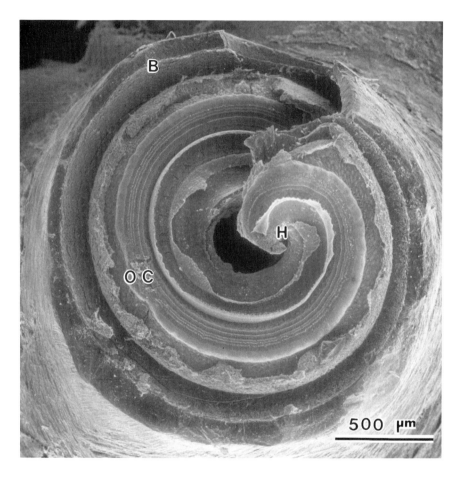

FIG. 2. The apical turn of the cochlea as seen after dissection of bony covering. B, bony wall of cochlea; H, helicotrema; OC, organ of Corti.

A closer view of the cochlear duct is illustrated in Fig. 3. The stria vascularis is shown to the top and left. Here, because of fixation shrinkage of the tissue, the stria and the spiral ligament have separated from the bony wall of the cochlea.

The remains of some of Reissner's membrane are seen to the lower right of Fig. 3. Normally this extends from the inner spiral limbus to the spiral ligament on the vestibular side of stria vascularis. Reissner's membrane consists of two cellular layers: a layer of polygonal epithelial cells on the side of scala media and a flat mesothelial layer facing scala vestibuli.

The tectorial membrane shown here has shrunk (as always in fixed tissue) to reveal the underlying sensory hair cells. The tectorial membrane is an acellular matrix and has been described as being composed of filaments and fibrils in a homogeneous ground substance (19,21,22,28). In the natural state it appears to be a soft gel, with an increasing thickness from the basal to apical cochlear regions. The membrane tends from the interdental cell region of the spiral limbus to the outer margin of the reticular lamina. Its outer zone consists of a marginal band and a marginal net (rand-

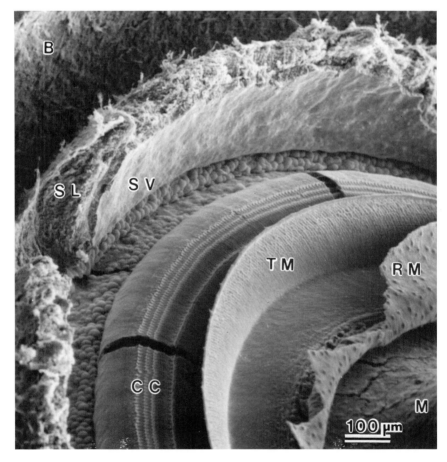

FIG. 3. The cochlear partition. B, bony wall of cochlea; M, modiolus; OC, organ of Corti; SL, spiral ligament; SV, stria vascularis.

fasernetz), which is attached to the outermost rows of Deiters' cells or Hensen's cells (19,23). Figure 4 shows a view of the underside of the tectorial membrane after its detachment. The upper area shows some of the marginal net. Along the central area is Hensen's stripe, which is normally near the position of the inner hair cells. In this region, small trabeculae may serve to anchor the tectorial membrane to the organ of Corti. Between the marginal net and Hensen's stripe is the so-called Hardesty's membrane into which the tallest rows of outer hair-cell stereocilia project forming a good mechanical coupling between the two structures (14). At the inner hair-cell level, it is not clear if such coupling normally exists. If it does, it is much less firm than for the outer hair cells.

THE BASILAR MEMBRANE

The cochlear duct is bounded on the side of the scala tympani by the basilar membrane, which is attached medially to the osseous spiral lamina and laterally at

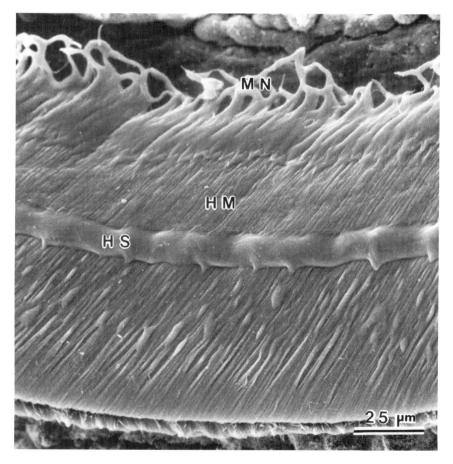

FIG. 4. The under-surface of the tectorial membrane. HM, Hardesty's membrane; HS, Hensen's stripe; MN, marginal net.

the spiral ligament. Two views of the basilar membrane as seen from scala tympani are given in Fig. 5. Figure 5A is from the apical turn of the cochlea and Fig. 5B from the base. In both photomicrographs, gaps in the tympani covering layer of mesothelial cells reveal some of the radial fibrils that make up the substance of the membrane. The fiber bundles are more densely packed at the cochlear base (Fig. 5B) compared with the apex (Fig. 5A). This graded difference along the length of the basilar membrane together with an increased width and decreased thickness toward the apex provide a stiffness gradient along the cochlear length. These are the necessary conditions for the propagation of a traveling wave and the passive mechanical tuning of the basilar membrane, which are consistent with the principles of von Békésy's place theory of frequency coding (2).

THE ORGAN OF CORTI

The organ of Corti is attached to the basilar membrane and consists of the sensory hair cells, the cells that support them, and the nerve fibers that innervate them. The

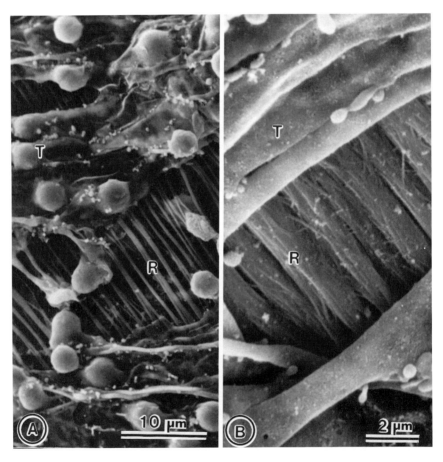

FIG. 5. The basilar membrane as seen from scala tympani at the cochlear apex **(A)** and at the cochlear base **(B)**. R, radial fiber bundles; T, tympanic covering layer.

surface of the sensory epithelium, the reticular lamina, is shown in Fig. 6. Here the familiar arrangement of inner and outer hair cells and supporting cells is evident. Apical regions of the pillar cells and Deiters' cells make up part of the reticular lamina. The latter can be distinguished in Fig. 6 by the abundant microvilli on their surfaces. The pillar cell and hair cell surfaces have, in contrast, fewer microvilli. The pillars of the pillar cells and phalangeal process Deiters' cells contain a rigid substructure of protein fibrils including actin (10), which indicates their important function in the mechanical support of the organ of Corti. An impression of this role is given in Fig. 7, which shows Deiters' cells and their phalangeal processes linking and mechanically coupling the basilar membrane to the reticular lamina. Deiters' cells are about equal in number to the outer hair cells. The spaces between the hair cells and extensions of Deiters' and pillar cells are the perilymph-filled spaces of Nuel.

Lateral to the outer hair cell/Deiters' cell area are Hensen's and Claudius' cells. Their position is shown in Fig. 8, which is the view from scala media of the surface of the organ of Corti. These cells are not highly differentiated but they may have

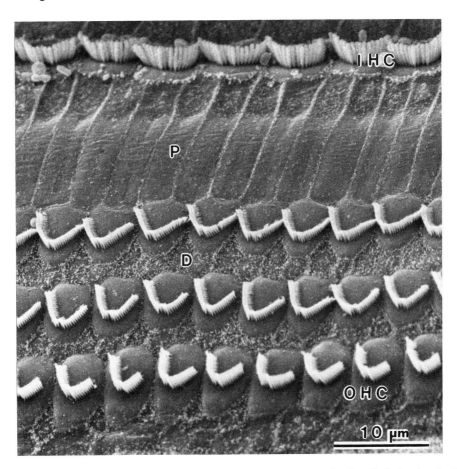

FIG. 6. The sensory epithelium of the organ of Corti—the reticular lamina. D, Deiters' cells; IHC, inner hair cells; OHC, outer hair cells; P, pillar cells.

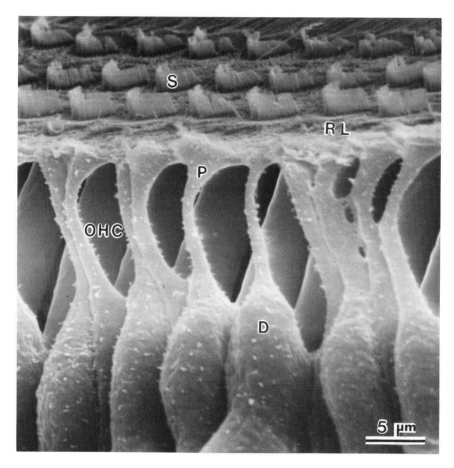

FIG. 7.   The supporting role of Deiters' cells in the organ of Corti. D, Deiters' cells, OHC, outer hair cell; P, phalangeal process of Deiters' cell; RL, reticular lamina; S, stereocilia of outer hair cells.

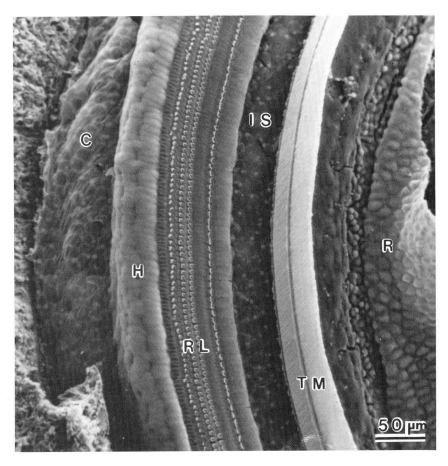

FIG. 8. Surface view of the organ of Corti. C, Claudius cells; H, Hensen cells; IS, inner sulcus cells; R, Reissner's membrane; RL, reticular lamina; TM, tectorial membrane (retracted).

some function in absorbing small particles of debris. At the base of the cochlea the Claudius' cell area also contains a group of Böttcher's cells, which may have a secretion or resorption function.

THE HAIR CELLS

The outer hair cells (OHCs) have a cylindrical shape and are almost totally surrounded by the fluid-filled spaces of Nuel as can be gleaned from Fig. 7. The length of the OHCs depends on their position along the basilar membrane, being longer at the cochlear apex (50 μm) compared with the base (20 μm). The inner hair cells (IHCs) are flask shaped with a relatively narrow neck area leading to the apical stereocilia-bearing surface. The scanning electron microscope has been particularly useful in examining the stereocilia of hair cells, as Figs. 6, 9, and 10 illustrate.

The cuticular plate that covers most of the apical surface of the cell supports the stereocilia. For the OHCs these number 50 to 150 and are arranged in rows that

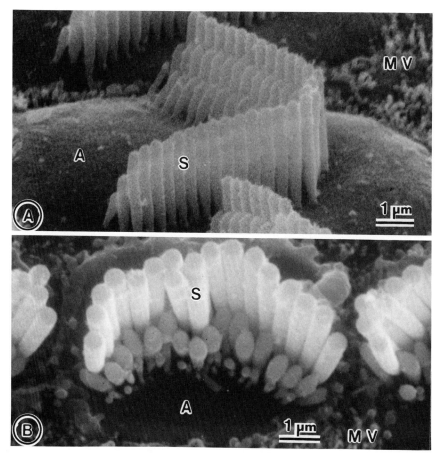

FIG. 9. Stereocilia of outer hair cells **(A)** and an inner hair cell **(B)**. A, apical surface of hair cell; MV, microvilli of supporting cells; S, stereocilia.

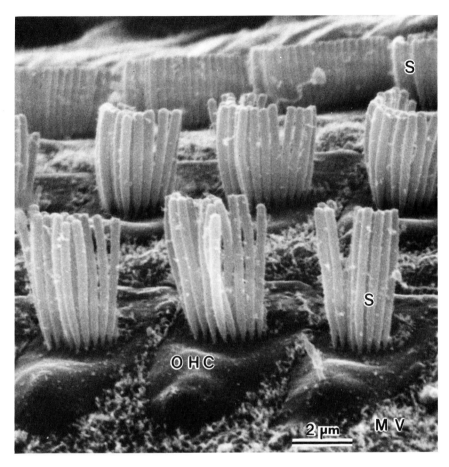

FIG. 10. Hair cells at the cochlear apex. OHC, outer hair cell; MV, microvilli of supporting cells; S, long stereocilia of the cochlear apex.

have a "W" form (Figs. 6 and 9A). The stereocilia are largest in the row facing away from the modiolus; toward the modiolus their length reduces. The average length of the stereocilia depends on cochlear position. Thus, at the apex the longest can be more than 8 μm, whereas at the extreme base, they are only about 1 μm in length. This difference between apical and basal stereociliar length is illustrated by comparing Fig. 9A, taken from a basal to mid-cochlear region, and Fig. 10, showing the cochlear apex.

The stereocilia are normally joined together by a large number of horizontal cross links. In addition, the tip of each shorter sterocilium gives rise to a fine extension that joins it to the taller stereocilium of the next row (25) (these are *not* clearly seen in Fig. 9).

Each IHC supports approximately 60 stereocilia. As with the OHC stereocilia, they are held together with cross links and have a length that is dependent on their position in the cochlea. The IHC stereocilia form rows along the long axis of the hair-cell apex; this is clearly illustrated in Fig. 6.

Normally the stereocilia of both IHCs and OHCs have an erect appearance. Indeed they contain structural proteins such as actin (10), which imparts a rigidity to them that is of great importance to the hair-cell transduction process.

ACKNOWLEDGMENTS

The authors are grateful to Richard Mount, Claudia Fleckeisen, and Brenda Rutledge for their assistance in the preparation of the figures and text for this chapter. One of the authors (R.V.H.) is supported by the Canadian Medical Research Council (PG-13, MA-9330) and the Masonic Foundation of Ontario.

REFERENCES

1. Barber, V. C., and Boyle, A. (1968): Scanning electron microscopic studies on cilia. *Z. Zellforsch.*, 84:269.
2. von Békésy, G. (1960): *Experiments in Hearing*. McGraw-Hill, New York.
3. Bredberg, G. (1968): Cellular pattern and nerve supply of the human organ of Corti. *Acta Otolaryngol. [Suppl.] (Stockh.)*, 236.
4. Bredberg, G., Ades, H. W., and Engstrom, H. (1972): Scanning electron microscopy of the normal and pathologically altered organ of Corti. *Acta Otolaryngol. [Suppl.] (Stockh.)*, 301.
5. Böttcher, A. (1869): Uber Entwicklugn und Bau des Gehörlabyrinths nach Untersuchungen an Säugetieran. *Nova Acta Academiae Cesariae*, 35:1.
6. Claudius, M. (1856): Bemerkungen uber den Bauder hautigen Sprialleiste der Schnecke. *Z. Wiss Zool.*, 7:154.
7. Corti, A. (1851): Recherches sur l'organe de l'ouie des mammifères. *Z. Wiss Zool.*, 3:109.
8. Engström, H., Ades, H. W., and Andersson, A. (1966): *Structural Pattern of the Organ of Corti*. Almquist & Wiksell, Stockholm.
9. Engström, H., and Wersäll, J. (1958): The ultrastructural organization of the organ of Corti and of the vestibular sensory epithelia. *Exp. Cell Res.*, 5:460.
10. Flock, A., and Cheung, H. (1977): Actin filaments in sensory hairs of the inner ear receptor cells. *J. Cell Biol.*, 75:339–343.
11. Harada, Y. (1983): *Atlas of the Ear by Scanning Electron Microscopy*. MTP Press, Lancaster.
12. Held, H. (1926): Die cochlea der Säuger und der Vögel, ihre entwicklung und ihr Bau, 467. In: *Handbuch der Normalen und Pathologischen Physiologie II*, edited by A. Bethe. Springer, Berlin.
13. Hensen, V. (1863): Zur Morphologie der Schnecke des Menshen und der Säugethiere. *Z. Wiss Zool.*, 13:481.
14. Hoshino, T. (1977): Contact between the tectorial membrane and the cochlear sensory hairs in the human and the monkey. *Arch. Otorhinolaryngol.*, 217:53.
15. Hunter-Duvar, I. M. (1978): Electron microscopic assessment of the cochlea. *Acta Otolaryngol. [Suppl.] (Stockh.)*, 351.
16. Hunter-Duvar, I. M. (1977): Morphology of the normal and the acoustically damaged cochlea. *Scanning Electron Microsc.*, II:421.
17. Hunter-Duvar, I. M., and Hinojosa, R. (1984): Sensory epithelia. In: *Ultrastructural Atlas of the Inner Ear*, edited by I. Friedmann and J. Ballantyne, p. 211. Butterworth, London.
18. Iurato, S. (1967): *Submicroscopic Structure of the Inner Ear*. Pergamon Press, New York.
19. Iurato, S. (1960): Submicroscopic structure of the membranous labyrinth I. The tectorial membrane. *Z. Zellforsch.*, 51:105.
20. Kimura, R. (1975): The ultrastructure of the organ of Corti. In: *International Review of Cytology*, edited by G. H. Bourne and J. F. Danielli, p. 42. Academic Press, New York.
21. Kronester-Frei, A. (1978): Ultrastructure of the different zones of the tectorial membrane. *Cell Tissue Res.*, 193:11.
22. Lim, D. J. (1977): Fine morphology of the tectorial membrane. Fresh and development. In: *Inner Ear Biology*, edited by M. Portmann and J.-M. Aran, INSERM Colloque, 68, p. 47. INSERM, Paris.
23. Lim, D. J. (1972): Fine morphology of the tectorial membrane: Its relationship to the organ of Corti. *Arch. Otolaryngol.*, 96:199.

24. Lim, D. J. (1969): Three dimensional observations of the inner ear with the scanning electron microscope. *Acta Otolaryngol. [Suppl.] (Stockh.)*, 255.
25. Pickles, J. O., Comis, S. D., and Osborne, M. P. (1984): Cross-links between stereocilia in the guinea-pig organ of Corti and their possible relations to sensory transduction. *Hear. Res.*, 15:103–112.
26. Retzius, G. (1884): *Das Gehörorgan der Reptilien, der Vögel und der Säugethiere*. Samson and Wallin, Stockholm.
27. Spoendlin, H. (1966): The organization of the cochlear receptor. In: *Advances in Otolaryngology*, p. 13. S. Karger, Basel.
28. Steel, K. P. (1983): The tectorial membrane of mammals. *Hear. Res.*, 9:327.

Physiology of the Ear,
edited by A. F. Jahn and J. Santos-Sacchi.
Raven Press, New York © 1988.

Cochlear Microanatomy and Ultrastructure

Peter A. Santi

*Department of Otolaryngology, University of Minnesota Medical School,
Minneapolis, Minnesota 55455*

Recent advances in the anatomy and physiology of the peripheral auditory apparatus have dramatically increased our understanding of audition. The site of hair-cell transduction appears to be at the distal tips of the stereocilia (21). In addition, the possibility that the outer hair cells mechanically alter the characteristics of the basilar membrane is being seriously considered (5,57,74). At the anatomical level, methods that have a strong biochemical foundation are providing an understanding of the composition of cochlear structures at the molecular level. The purposes of this chapter are to provide a brief, contemporary review of the normal anatomy of the mammalian cochlea and to complement previous anatomical reviews (24–26,31,37,38,64,67).

ANATOMICAL METHODS FOR COCHLEAR TISSUES

The anatomy of the cochlea has been difficult to understand primarily because of its heterogeneity. In many regions of the cochlea, tissues are only a few cell layers thick and surrounded by large fluid spaces embedded in bone. It therefore seems appropriate to begin this review with a brief discussion of the anatomical methods used to investigate cochlear tissues.

One of the first and still most useful methods to investigate inner-ear tissues is to prepare whole-mount surface preparations. This procedure can be successfully applied to several inner-ear tissues (e.g., the organ of Corti/basilar membrane, Reissner's membrane and the tectorial membrane, and the stria vascularis/spiral ligament). Excellent descriptions of cochlear surface preparations were provided by Retzius (45,46) in the late 1800s. A systematic analysis of surface preparations and the representation of hair-cell damage along the length of the basilar membrane was provided by Engström and co-workers (8). They developed a map, called a cochleogram or cytocochleogram, that showed hair-cell damage along the length of the basilar membrane. This map has evolved as the standard representation of hair-cell damage.

A reliable and relatively simple method for examining the complete length of the basilar membrane was provided by Axelsson and co-workers (2) using decalcified, or soft surface preparations. Bohne (3) improved the method and produced plastic-embedded, or hard, surface preparations that could first be examined by light microscopy and then sectioned and examined by transmission electron microscopy. Bohne's method minimized histological processing artifacts and allowed for the detection of even subtle alterations of the hair cells (e.g., stereocilia damage) at the light microscope level (35). Scanning electron microscopy (SEM) provided another method to examine surface preparations of cochlear tissues with increased resolution (22,37,38); however, it is difficult to produce cytocochleograms at the SEM level. Currently, immunocytochemistry is revealing the composition of cochlear structures at the molecular level and holds great promise for improving our understanding of normal and pathological cochlear function.

MICROANATOMY

The mature mammalian cochlea consists of a bony and membranous labyrinth. The central core of the cochlea is called the modiolus and contains nerve fibers, blood vessels, and other connective tissues. A mid-modiolar, radial section through a chinchilla cochlea is shown in Fig. 1. The external bony covering of the cochlea, or the otic capsule, is very thin in some mammals (e.g., chinchilla, guinea pig, and gerbil), which has facilitated their use for cochlear research. The otic capsule has two openings: the oval and round windows. It is through these windows that most sound energy enters and leaves the cochlea. Airborne sound vibrations are converted to mechanical vibrations of the tympanic membrane and transmitted to the oval window of the cochlea through the ossicles (i.e., the malleus, incus, and stapes). Movement of the oval window produces fluid pressure waves within the three fluid-filled canals of the cochlea (Fig. 1). These fluid pressure waves induce a traveling wave whose location of maximum displacement along the basilar membrane is frequency specific. Vibration of the basilar membrane induces mechanoelectrical changes in the hair cells of the organ of Corti, which the brain perceives as hearing.

The two perilymphatic canals are the scala vestibuli (which ends at the oval window) and the scala tympani (which ends at the round window). At the cochlear apex, these two canals communicate directly with one another through an opening called the helicotrema (Fig. 1). The fluid within these canals is called perilymph and resembles extracellular fluid in its composition (i.e., high Na^+, low K^+). The endolymphatic space, or the scala media, lies between the two perilymphatic scalas (Fig. 1). It is blind ended in the cochlear apex but communicates with the vestibular system in the cochlear base through the ductus reuniens. Cochlear endolymph resembles intracellular fluid in its composition (i.e., high K^+, low Na^+). The endolymphatic space of the scala media also exhibits a positive electrical potential relative to the surrounding perilymphatic tissues (63,69). This potential is called the positive endocochlear potential ($+EP$) and is ~80 mV in the cochlear base and decreases toward the apex.

The scala media contains the sensory and supporting cells necessary for converting sound-induced mechanical vibrations to neural responses. The structure of the cells and tissues that comprise the scala media is crucial for our understanding of the function of the normal and pathological inner ear. The remainder of this chapter will describe the anatomy of these cells and tissues from the modiolus to the lateral wall.

SPIRAL GANGLION

The cochlea is innervated by three types of nerve fibers: autonomic, afferent, and efferent. Autonomic nerve fibers appear to be primarily associated with blood vessels

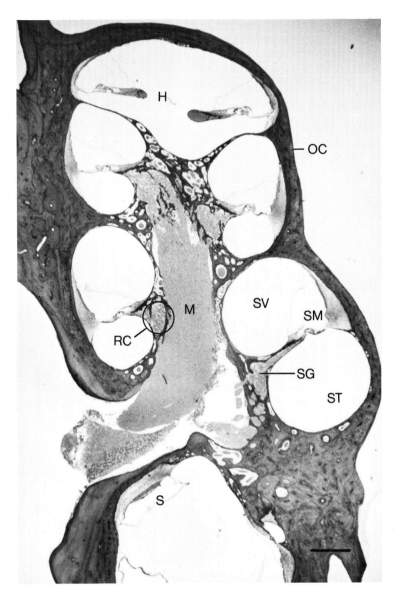

FIG. 1. A mid-modiolar section of a cochlea showing the otic capsule (OC), modiolus (M), helicotrema (H), the three cochlear scalae [scala vestibuli (SV), scala media (SM), and scala tympani (ST)], and the saccule (S) portion of the vestibular labyrinth. Rosenthal's canal (*circled*) contains the spiral ganglion (SG). Bar = 500 μm. (JB4 section courtesy of A. J. Duvall.)

of the modiolus and spiral lamina (39,49,66). Afferent nerve cell bodies are located in a spiral, bony channel called Rosenthal's canal (Fig. 1). The collection of cell bodies within the canal is called the spiral ganglion. In the guinea pig, the canal has an average width of 300 μm in the cochlear base and narrows toward the apex where it divides into a cluster of nerve cell bodies and fibers (9). Efferent nerve fibers are also contained within Rosenthal's canal in a discrete bundle called the intraganglionic spiral bundle. The cell bodies of the efferent nerve fibers are located in the superior

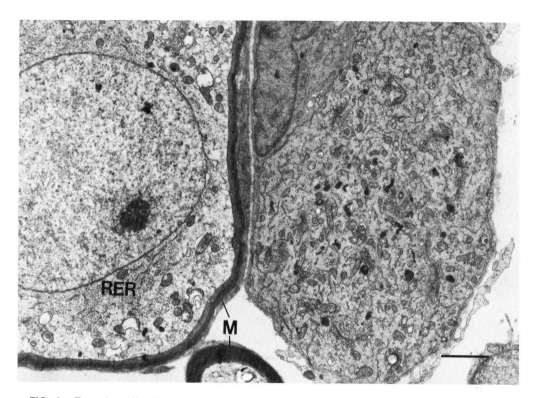

FIG. 2. Types I and II spiral ganglion neurons from Rosenthal's canal. The type I neuron cell body contains a compact myelin sheath (M), abundant rough endoplasmic reticulum (RER), and a prominent nucleus. The type II cell has a more electron-dense, filamentous cytoplasm and a thin myelin sheath. Bar = 2 μm.

olivary nucleus in the brain. Their nerve fibers leave the nucleus and form the crossed and uncrossed olivocochlear bundle (44). The nerve fibers travel through the inferior portion of the vestibular branch of the VIII cranial nerve and enter the cochlea via a nerve-fiber bundle called the anastomosis of Oort. In the guinea pig, the efferent nerve fibers enter Rosenthal's canal, in a single bundle, at ~3 mm from the cochlear base and travel in apical and basal directions (9,44).

In animals, two types of afferent cell bodies can be differentiated (Fig. 2) in the spiral ganglion (27). Type I cell bodies are large, numerous (~95%), and surrounded by a compact sheath of myelin. Their cytoplasm contains a prominent spherical nucleus and abundant rough endoplasmic reticulum. Type II cell bodies are smaller, fewer in number (~5%), and unmyelinated. Their cytoplasm contains a lobulated nucleus and abundant filaments. Evidence suggests that type I neurons innervate the inner hair cells, and type II neurons innervate the outer hair cells (65). However, in humans, the largest and most numerous cell bodies are unmyelinated (41).

SPIRAL LAMINA, SPIRAL LIMBUS, AND INNER SULCUS CELLS

The osseous spiral lamina is a thin channel of bone through which the myelinated nerve fibers pass to and from the organ of Corti (Figs. 1, 3, and 4). In the guinea

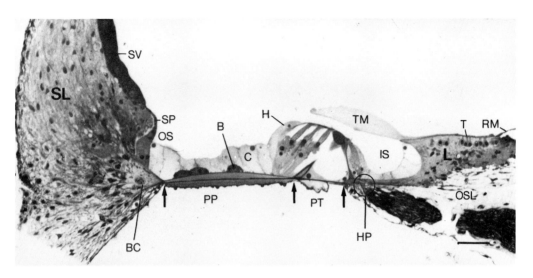

FIG. 3. A radial, plastic-embedded section through the first cochlear turn showing the spiral ligament (SL), stria vascularis (SV), spiral prominence (SP), outer sulcus (OS), basilar crest (BC), pars pectinata (PP) and pars tecta (PT) of the basilar membrane, Claudius' cells (C), Böttcher's cells (B), Hensen's cells (H), tectorial membrane (TM), inner sulcus (IS), spiral limbus (L), T or interdental cells (T), Reissner's membrane (RM), habenula perforata (HP, *circled*), and osseous spiral lamina (OSL). Bar = 50 μm.

pig, the spiral lamina has a maximum width of ~500 μm at ~3 mm from the cochlear base and decreases toward the cochlear apex (10). At its lateral edge, nerve fibers lose their myelination and pass through openings in the bone called the habenula perforata (Fig. 3). The spiral lamina also provides the structural base for the spiral limbus and the inner sulcus cells (Figs. 3 and 4).

The spiral limbus is a vascularized, connective-tissue structure that overlies the lateral portion of the osseous spiral lamina. Reissner's or the vestibular membrane attaches to the most medial edge of the spiral limbus (Figs. 1 and 3). The epithelial surface of the spiral limbus is covered by the medial edge of the tectorial membrane. The apicolateral edge of the spiral limbus forms a wedge-shaped prominence (tooth of Huschke or vestibular lip) and a medially directed cavity called the inner sulcus (Figs. 3 and 4). The basal edge of the spiral limbus is called the tympanic lip. The epithelial cells of the spiral limbus, called T or interdental cells, have flask-shaped bodies and a large, flattened apical process (Fig. 3). The cell bodies are arranged in radial rows that can clearly be seen in surface preparations. The most likely function of the interdental cells is to produce or maintain components of the tectorial membrane. The matrix of the spiral limbus contains capillaries, fibroblast-like cells, and numerous filaments (26). However, the composition of the filaments and the classification of the connective tissue cells is not known.

The inner sulcus is a furrow formed by the lateral edge of the spiral limbus, the medial edge of the organ of Corti, and apically by the tectorial membrane (Figs. 3 and 4). The general consensus is that the inner sulcus communicates with the scala media via the lateral edge of the tectorial membrane and, therefore, contains cochlear endolymph. The inner sulcus cells have a tall, cuboidal shape and are ~20 μm thick and ~16 μm wide. They have a spherical nucleus ~6 μm in diameter and few cy-

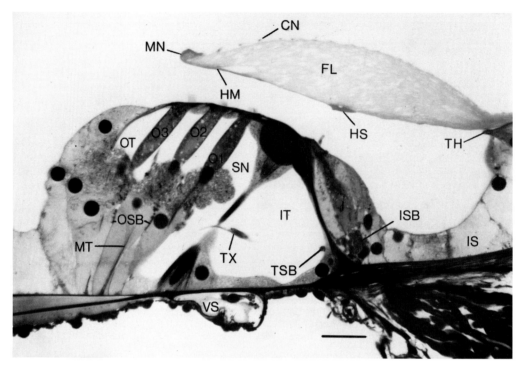

FIG. 4. A radial section showing of the organ of Corti. Note the outer tunnel of Corti (OT), three outer hair cell rows (01, 02, 03), inner hair cell (I), microtubule bundle in Deiters' cells (MT), outer spiral bundle (OSB), space of Nuel (SN), tunnel-crossing fibers (TX), inner tunnel of Corti (IT), tunnel spiral bundle (TSB), vas spirale (VS), inner spiral bundle (ISB), inner sulcus cells (IS), and the tooth of Huschke (TH). The tectorial membrane contains fibrous layer (FL), Hensen's stripe (HS), Hardesty's membrane (HM), marginal net (MN), and the cover net (CN). Bar = 20 μm.

toplasmic organelles, thus, they resemble Claudius' cells. They have short apical microvilli and their borders show the usual tripartite cell junctions.

BASILAR MEMBRANE

The basilar membrane is a connective-tissue structure that forms the floor of the scala media (Figs. 3–5). In humans, its average length is 31.5 mm (16) and its width increases from 150 to 450 μm toward the cochlear apex (72). In the guinea pig, its average length is 18.8 mm and its width increases from 150 to 250 μm toward the cochlear apex (10). This change in width along its length is fundamentally important for its tonotopicity (i.e., high-frequency sounds induce maximal vibrations in its base and low-frequency sounds in its apex). The basilar membrane is attached medially to the spiral lamina and laterally to the spiral ligament at the basilar crest (Figs. 3–5). Its width has been divided into two regions (26): a medial zone (pars tecta or arcuata) and a lateral zone (pars pectinata). The pars tecta extends from the habenula perforata to the lateral edge of the base of the outer pillar cells. The pars pectinata extends from the outer pillars to the basilar crest. The pars pectinata is thicker than

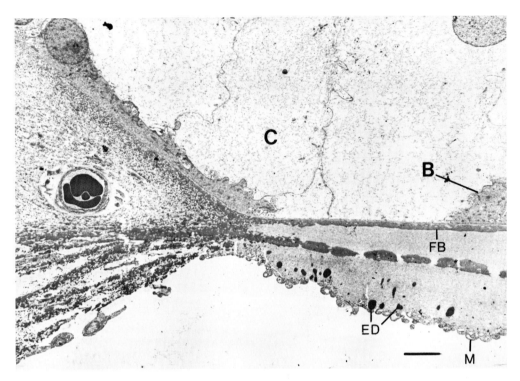

FIG. 5. A transmission electron micrograph showing a portion of the pars pectinata of the basilar membrane and the wedge-shaped basilar crest. Note: Claudius' cells (C), Böttcher's cells (B), two fiber bundles of the basilar membrane (FB), electron-dense deposits (ED), and the mesothelial cells (M). Bar = 0.5 μm.

the tecta and decreases in thickness toward the cochlear apex. The pars tecta consists of a diffuse network of radially arranged filaments (~20 nm in diameter) embedded in an amorphous ground substance. The pars pectinata contains two distinct layers of radial fiber bundles that are organized into upper and middle layers (Figs. 5 and 14). The fiber bundles in the middle layer are ~0.5 μm thick and separated by ~0.5 μm. The thickness of the pectinata is primarily owing to an abundance of ground substance.

The only cellular components of the basilar membrane proper are the mesothelial cells, which contiguously line the scala tympani side of the membrane (Figs. 4 and 5). They are fusiform cells whose long axes are oriented in a spiral direction. Electron-dense materials (Fig. 5) occur just above the mesothelial cells in the ground substance (26). The basilar membrane is primarily acellular and consists of unidentified fibers and ground substance materials. However, it is likely to contain glycoconjugates such as type IV collagen, laminin, and fibronectin since such macromolecules are common in epithelial basement membranes. Additionally, a single blood vessel, called the vas spirale or spiral vessel, may be present beneath the inner tunnel of the organ of Corti (Figs. 3 and 4). This capillary often appears devoid of blood cells and, according to Kimura and Ota (32) is not fenestrated.

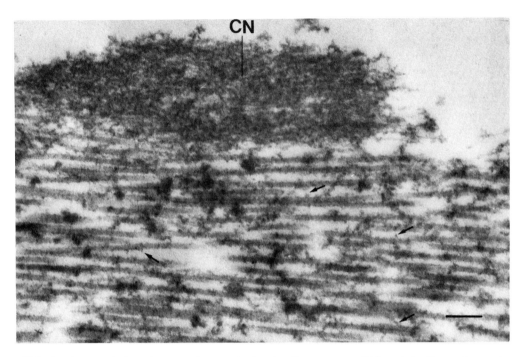

FIG. 6. A transmission electron micrograph showing the cover net (CN) and the fibrous layer of the tectorial membrane. The fibrous layer contains long, straight fibrils that may be collagen type II. The electron-dense deposits (*arrows*) along the thick fibers may be proteoglycans. Bar = 0.1 μm.

TECTORIAL MEMBRANE

The tectorial membrane is an acellular, fibrous structure (Figs. 3, 4, and 6) that has been difficult to histologically preserve in its native state because of its high content of water and soluble components. For this reason, the attachment of the tectorial membrane to the hair-cell stereocilia is controversial. The general consensus is that only the longest row of the outer hair-cell stereocilia are directly attached to the tectorial membrane (30,36,37). After routine fixation, the tectorial membrane is usually not positioned close to the organ of Corti but appears retracted and elevated. However, in fresh and frozen preparations the tectorial membrane appears to be closely applied to the reticular lamina.

Although the tectorial membrane is acellular, several specialized regions can be differentiated within it (24,36) (Fig. 4). These regions are the limbal zone, middle zone (containing the cover net, fibrous layer, and Hensen's stripe), and marginal zone (containing the marginal band, marginal net, and Hardesty's membrane). The limbal zone is the region of the tectorial membrane that covers the spiral limbus. The middle zone contains dense radial strands, called the cover net, that are located on the apical surface of the tectorial membrane. These fibers run in an oblique, apical direction and follow the angle of the outer hair-cell stereocilia bundles. The thick portion of the middle zone is the fibrous layer, which consists of numerous fibrils. The undersurface of the tectorial membrane contains a wedge-shaped band of dense, fibrous material above the inner hair cells known as Hensen's stripe.

Trabeculae, or strands of material, have been observed to extend from Hensen's stripe to the reticular lamina in the region of the inner hair cells (36,37). The marginal zone of the tectorial membrane contains a dense band of material (the marginal band) and a dense network of strands (the marginal net). These strands appear to attach the lateral edge of the membrane to the apical surface of Hensen's cells. In addition, channels through the marginal net may be the primary source of endolymph for the subtectorial space. Another dense layer in the marginal zone, called Hardesty's membrane, is present on the undersurface of the tectorial membrane and overlies the outer hair cells (36,37).

Two types of fibrils have been described within the tectorial membrane and have been classified by Kronester-Frei (33) as types A and B. Type A fibrils are numerous in the fibrous layer of the tectorial membrane and long, straight, and ~10 nm in diameter. Type B are short, coiled, and ~15 to 20 nm in diameter, and occur in the more electron-dense zones of the tectorial membrane. Based on their morphological characteristics, the type A fibrils may be type II collagen. In addition, these fibrils show periodic deposits of material that may be composed of proteoglycans (Fig. 6). Similar materials that have been shown to be proteoglycans have been demonstrated on collagen in other tissues. However, two recent biochemical studies failed to detect significant quantities of uronic acid (a basic unit of most proteoglycans) in the tectorial membrane (29,47). Thalmann and co-workers (70) have recently presented biochemical evidence showing that type II collagen constitutes 50% of total protein of the tectorial membrane. In another study (47), collagen types II, IX, and V were also detected biochemically. However, neither collagens nor proteoglycans have been localized in the tectorial membrane by electron immunocytochemistry. For a more comprehensive review of the structure and composition of the tectorial membrane the reader is referred to a review by Steel (67).

THE ORGAN OF CORTI

The organ of Corti consists of a repeating, geometric array of sensory and supporting cells that lie on the medial portion of the basilar membrane. The organ of Corti contains the following (medial to lateral) components: inner border cells, inner phalangeal cells, inner hair cells, inner pillar cells, inner tunnel of Corti, outer pillar cells, 3 to 4 rows of outer hair cells, space of Nuel, Deiters' cells, outer tunnel of Corti, and Hensen's cells (Figs. 4, 7, and 8). The organ of Corti shows gradual changes along the length of the basilar membrane. These changes include increases toward the cochlear apex in: its radial area, the angle and width of the reticular lamina relative to the basilar membrane, length of the outer hair cell bodies, length of the hair cell stereocilia, and size of Hensen's cells (4,10,25,51). The organ of Corti contains two types of sensory cells (i.e., inner and outer hair cells) that are contained in a complex arrangement of supporting cells (Figs. 4, 7, and 8). In animals, there is usually a single row of inner hair cells and three parallel rows of outer hair cells. The apical portions of the sensory and supporting cells that have direct contact at the endolymphatic surface with the hair cells form a flattened, ridged structure called the reticular lamina (Figs. 7 and 8). The reticular lamina includes the inner border cells, inner phalangeal cells, inner hair cells, inner and outer pillar cells, outer hair cells, and phalangeal processes of Deiters' cells (15). Their relationship is shown in

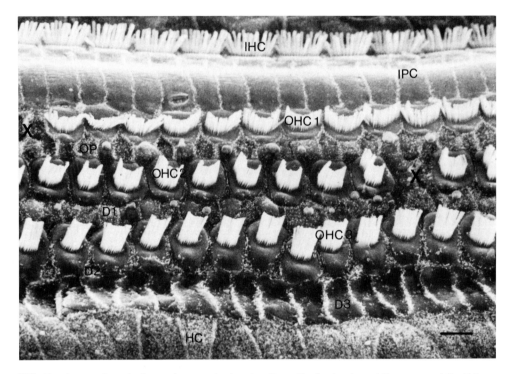

FIG. 7. A scanning electron micrograph showing the reticular lamina of the organ of Corti from the third cochlear turn of the chinchilla. Note the inner hair cell (IHC), inner pillar cell headplate (IPC), outer hair cell row 1 (OHC1), outer pillar cell phalangeal process (OP), outer hair cell row 2 (OHC2), Deiters' cell row 1 phalangeal process (D1), outer hair cell row 3 (OHC3), Deiters' cell row 2 phalangeal process (D2), Deiters' cell row 3 phalangeal process (D3), and Hensen's cell (HC). Two phalangeal scars (X) are present, in row 1 and row 2, indicating loss of an outer hair cell in each row. Bar = 5 μm.

Fig. 7, which is a scanning electron micrograph of the reticular lamina from the first turn of a chinchilla cochlea. A large portion of the reticular lamina is formed by the cuticular plate of the hair cells and their hair-like extensions called stereocilia.

HAIR-CELL STEREOCILIA

The term *stereocilium* comes from the combination of two words: the Greek word *stereos*, meaning solid, and the Latin word *cilium*, meaning eyelid. Stereocilium is an inaccurate term, since cilia are structures that have a complex internal arrangement of axial microtubules. Stereocilia do not contain microtubules and their internal structure closely resembles microvilli, which contain axial microfilaments (actin fibers). Based on their internal structure, it has been proposed (40,53) that the word stereocilium be changed to stereovillus.

Hair-cell stereocilia resemble long, club-shaped microvilli that extend from the cuticular plate of the hair cell (Figs. 7–10). The stereocilia aggregate to form a bundle of three or more rows. They are graded in length between but not within a row. The bundle forms a W-shaped pattern with an increasing acute angle toward the cochlear

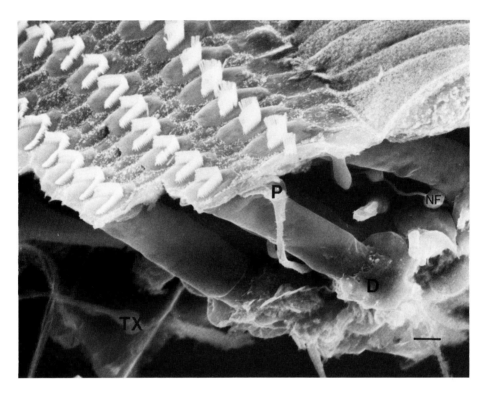

FIG. 8. A scanning electron micrograph showing a critical point drying-induced fracture through the outer hair cell region of the organ of Corti. Note the phalangeal process (P) of Deiters' cell forming a portion of the reticular lamina. The outer hair cells are surrounded by the spaces of Nuel. Their apex is supported by the reticular lamia, and their base is supported by the Deiters' cell (D). Note also the tunnel-crossing fibers (TX) and presumably a spiral efferent nerve fiber (NF) innervating two outer hair cells in the third row. Bar = 5 μm.

apex and the third row of outer hair cells. In inner and outer hair cells, the longest stereocilia are always on the lateral edge of the bundle (i.e., toward the lateral wall of the scala media). Central and adjacent to the longest row of the stereocilia is a clear, spherical region in the cuticular plate. This is the cuticular pore and marks the site of the attachment of a true cilium called a kinocilium. However, this structure is only present during the development of the cochlea. The distal tips of the stereocilia are flattened in the inner hair cells and rounded in the outer hair cells. The stereocilia are thick at their tips and narrow at their base where they enter the cuticular plate. Stereocilia diameter (37,38,73) is greater for inner hair cells (~0.45 μm) than outer hair cells (~0.20 μm). The number of stereocilia/bundles shows a small decrease from the cochlear base to the apex for the inner (77 to 65) and the first and second rows of the outer hair cells (100 to 90). The third row of the outer hair cells shows the greatest decrease in the number of stereocilia (80 to 18). Inner hair-cell stereocilia length increases from the base to the apex (20 to 45 μm) as does outer hair-cell stereocilia length (0.5 to 55 μm). Stereocilia length also increases from the first to the third row (35 to 55 μm).

The external plasma membrane of the stereocilia exhibits an extensive surface coat that has only been recently observed (13,20,38,40,50,59). This is attributed to

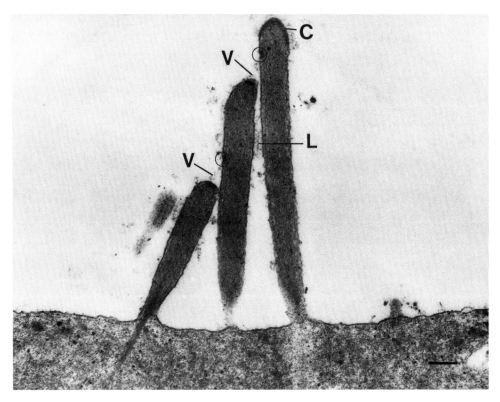

FIG. 9. A radial section through the stereocilia of an outer hair cell showing their internal axial, actin filaments, apical electron-dense cap (C) in the tip of the stereocilia, lateral cross-links (L) showing an intermediate density, vertical cross-links (V), and an electron-dense invagination (*circled*) in the plasma membrane of the stereocilia where the vertical cross-links attach. Bar = 0.2 μm.

the well-known observation that routine fixation and histological processing for transmission and SEM only poorly preserves those carbohydrates that comprise the cell surface coat. Using frozen, unfixed tissue (20) or cationic dyes (38,40,43,50,59) cell surface coats can be preserved and demonstrated. Because of the carbohydrate residues, the surface coat exhibits a strong, negative charge (13). The surface coat on the hair cells appears to be thickest on the stereocilia and the endolymphatic surface of the cuticular plate (38,50). The surface coat probably consists of different components whose functions may include attachment of the stereocilia to one another and to the tectorial membrane, sequestering of cationic chemicals (e.g., Ca^{2+}) and drugs (e.g., aminoglycoside antibiotics), and prevention of stereocilia fusion by repulsion of like negative charges on their carbohydrate residues.

   In addition to a surface coat, other extracellular filaments are also associated with the hair-cell stereocilia. The stereocilia are connected to one another by three sets (42) of extracellular, cross-linking filaments (Figs. 9 and 10). There are two types of lateral cross-links between stereocilia: those within and those between the stereocilia rows. A third type of linkage, the vertical cross-link, consists of a single strand of extracellular material. This strand travels between the tip of a short stereocilium to the shaft of the tall stereocilium in the next row. At the region of its

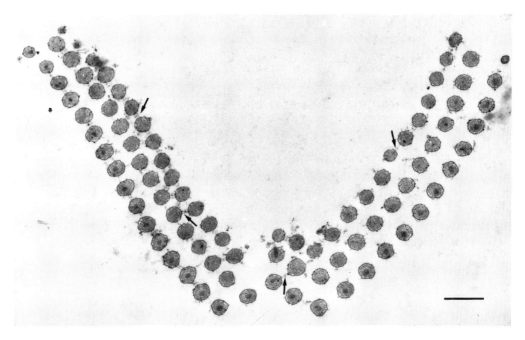

FIG. 10. A horizontal section through an outer hair cell stereocilia bundle near the cuticular plate of the cell. Note the lateral cross-links (*arrows*) between the stereocilia and their internal composition of actin filaments. The dark, central body in the longest row of stereocilia indicates compaction of the actin filaments and formation of the stereocilia rootlets as they insert into the cuticular plate. Bar = 0.5 μm.

insertion into the shaft of the taller stereocilium is an indentation of the plasma membrane and a cytoplasmic accumulation of electron-dense material (Fig. 9). An apical cap of electron-dense material on the cytoplasmic side of the plasma membrane also occurs at the tip of each stereocilium. The electron-dense areas and the vertical cross-links have only been recently reported, since they appear to be preserved only by an aldehyde fixative containing a divalent cation such as calcium or magnesium (14,42). It has been proposed that the vertical cross-links are involved in hair-cell transduction and serve as mechanical devices to open ion channels in the tips of the stereocilia (42). The lateral cross-links appear to connect the stereocilia together so that a mechanical force would be distributed throughout the stereocilia bundle. This is important since it appears that only the tallest row of the stereocilia is attached to the tectorial membrane (30). The composition of the cross-links has not yet been determined. However, these structures may be glycoproteins or proteoglycans since they are positively stained by Alcian blue and ruthenium red (38,50).

The internal structure of the stereocilia consists of axial microfilaments (Figs. 9 and 10). These microfilaments are tightly packed in a hexagonal array (71) and have been identified as F-actin (12). The actin filaments are all polarized toward the cuticular plate (12,61). The actin filaments are also associated with fimbrin, which may cross link the filaments into rigid bundles (11,60). The actin filaments form a compact, electron-dense bundle called the rootlet that extends into the cuticular plate and is associated with tropomyosin (60). *In vitro* experiments have shown that stereocilia deflect as stiff rods even when the cell membrane has been removed with detergent

(12). The stiffness of the stereocilia appears to be owing to their internal actin filaments and their insertion into other cytoskeletal elements in the cuticular plate (12,54).

INNER BORDER CELLS AND INNER PHALANGEAL CELLS

The inner border cell separates the inner sulcus cells from the medial surface of the inner hair cell (Figs. 4 and 11). Its apex forms a thin endolymphatic surface that exhibits numerous, tall microvilli. The cell remains thin as it follows the medial border of the inner hair cell. The apical process of the inner phalangeal cell separates the lateral surfaces of the inner hair cells. At their basal pole, the cytoplasm of the border and inner phalangeal cells envelops the unmyelinated nerve fibers associated with the inner hair cell. Neither inner supporting cell shows the extensive arrangement of microtubules that is present in the cytoplasm of the supporting cells of the outer hair cells (i.e., Deiters' cells).

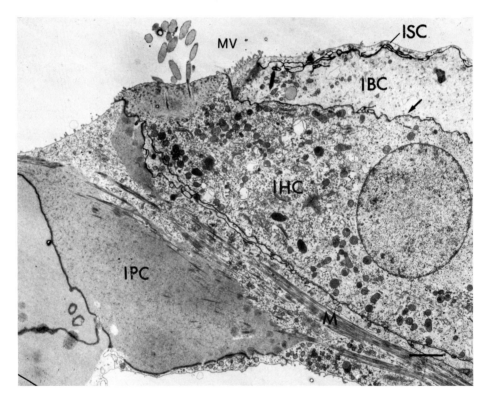

FIG. 11. A radial section through the apex of an inner hair cell (IHC) in a chinchilla that received *in vivo* perilymphatic administration of the protein horseradish peroxidase (shown as an electron-dense reaction product). A single layer of the subsurface cisternae is indicated by the *arrow*. Note the filamentous headplate of the inner pillar cell (IPC) and the prominent bundle of microtubules in the pillar cell cytoplasm (M). The inner border cell (IBC) contains numerous, apical microvilli (MV) and separates the inner hair cell from the inner sulcus cell (ISC). Bar = 2 μm.

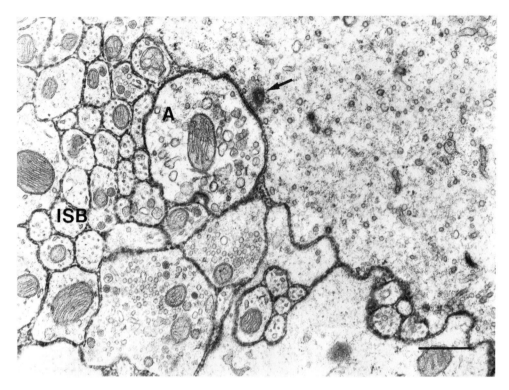

FIG. 12. A radial section through the base of an inner hair cell showing an afferent nerve terminal (A) synapsing on an inner hair cell body. A synaptic body (*arrow*) is present in the hair-cell cytoplasm at the synapse. Numerous radially sectioned nerve fibers, which are part of the efferent inner spiral bundle (ISB), are located next to the afferent terminal. Bar = 0.5 μm.

INNER HAIR CELLS

The inner hair cells form a single row of flask-shaped cells that are surrounded by supporting cells (Figs. 4, 7, and 11). The position of the cell body approximately follows the inclination of the inner pillar cells. The cell apex is wide (in the spiral direction) and exhibits a horizontal array of stereocilia. The cuticular plate is a fibrous network of material in the cell apex that contains a single, lateral cuticular pore. This network contains actin, myosin, fimbrin, and calcium-binding protein (11,60). A striated body has been reported in the infracuticular plate region of the inner, but not the outer, hair cells (58). The inner hair cells contain a large, spherical nucleus (~8 μm in diameter) that contains a single, eccentrically positioned nucleolus. The cytoplasm contains scattered mitochondria, microtubules, and numerous clear-core vesicles. Along the plasma membrane is a single layer of smooth endoplasmic reticulum called the subsurface cisternae (Fig. 11). This layer is more extensive in the outer hair cells (Fig. 13). At the basal pole are efferent and afferent nerve fibers. Efferent nerve fibers form the inner spiral bundle at the basal pole of the inner hair cells (Fig. 12). Numerous small afferent nerve synapses, but few efferent synapses, occur on the cell body of the inner hair cells. Adjacent to the afferent synapses are cytoplasmic bodies, bars, or ribbons (Fig. 12). These structures may serve as a

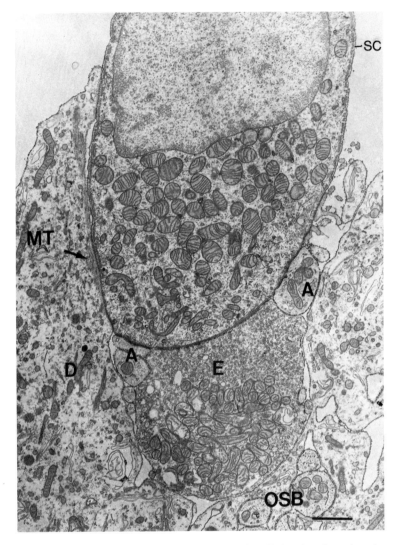

FIG. 13. A radial section through the base of an outer hair cell showing the subsurface cisternae (SC) and numerous mitochondria in the subnuclear pole of the cell. A large vesicle-filled, efferent synaptic terminal (E) and two, adjacent smaller afferent terminals (A) are synapsing with the hair cell. Note the attachment of the Deiters' cell to the side of the hair cell and the presence of microtubules (*arrow*) in the Deiters' cell cytoplasm at the site. Note also a portion of the efferent outer spiral bundle (OSB). Bar = 1 μm.

reservoir of synaptic vesicles. Efferent nerve synapses are commonly found on the afferent nerve fibers.

INNER AND OUTER PILLAR CELLS

The inner and outer pillar cells form the inner tunnel of Corti and portions of the reticular lamina (Figs. 4 and 11). Both pillar cells have a broad base that contains a spherical nucleus ~6 μm in diameter. Their basal pole rests on the basilar membrane, and each cell forms a stout process that extends to the apex of the tunnel. The large rectangular plates, which separate the inner from the outer hair cells, are formed only by the inner pillar cells. The headplates of the outer pillar cells are beneath the inner pillar cells and surface only to form that portion of the reticular lamina between the outer hair cells of the first row. The space between the outer pillar cells and the first row of outer hair cells is called the space of Nuel. However, many investigators use the term spaces of Nuel to include all of the fluid-filled spaces between and around the outer hair cells. The most prominent feature of the cytoplasm of the pillar cells is their rich complement of tubules and filaments. The base of these cells contains a cone-shaped network of F-actin filaments that inserts into a thick bundle of microtubules. These microtubules travel up into a similar filament network in the cell apex. The mediobasal portion of the inner tunnel contains the tunnel spiral bundle, which consists of efferent nerve fibers (Fig. 4). The afferent and efferent nerve fibers cross the tunnel along its base as small bundles, known as the tunnel-crossing fibers, to innervate the outer hair cells.

OUTER HAIR CELLS

The outer hair cells are cylindrically shaped and attach to the organ of Corti at their apex and base (Figs. 4, 8, and 13). Like the inner hair cells, the outer hair cells have an apical bundle of stereocilia that insert into the cuticular plate (Figs. 7–10). A cuticular pore is also present in the outer hair cells. A prominent cytoplasmic component of the outer hair cells is the subsurface cistern. It consists of several layers of smooth endoplasmic reticulum arranged as flattened and tubular cisterns along the shaft of the hair cell body (Fig. 13). In the apical part of the cell, the subsurface cistern forms hollow spheres that have been called Hensen's bodies. Beneath the nucleus, the subsurface cisternae forms a single layer called the subsynaptic cistern. The nucleus is located in the basal end of the cell and is ~6 μm in diameter. Large efferent synaptic terminals are present on the basal end of the outer hair cells (Fig. 13). Smaller afferent synapses are also found on the basal end of the outer hair cells. Adjacent to the Deiters' cells, which support the outer hair cells, is the outer spiral bundle, which contains spirally directed, efferent nerve fibers.

DEITERS' CELLS

Deiters' cells are complex supporting cells that are divided into two parts: the cell body proper and a slender process. The basal pole of the cell attaches to the basilar membrane. The main part of the cell forms a cup-like structure that supports the base of an outer hair cell (Figs. 8 and 13). Deiters' cells are attached to the outer hair cell in their perinuclear region and not at their extreme basal end, where the efferent and afferent synapses occur. A slender process, called a phalangeal process, arises from the body of the Deiters' cell and obliquely extends up through the fluid-filled spaces between the hair cells to form a portion of the reticular lamina (Fig. 8). The apical portion of this process is dumbbell-shaped and makes contact with as many as four different outer hair cells at the reticular lamina (Fig. 7). The second row of the outer hair cells are separated laterally by the phalangeal processes of the

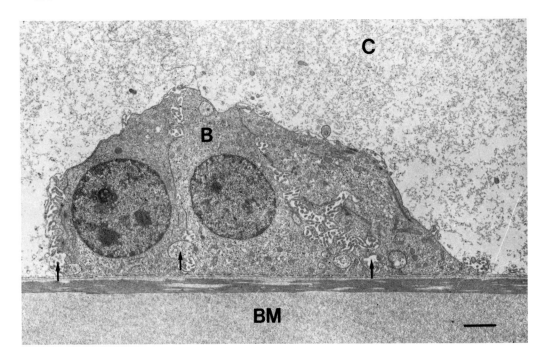

FIG. 14. A radial section through the pars pectinata of the basilar membrane (BM) showing Claudius' cells (C), with their sparse cytoplasmic organelles, and Böttcher's cells (B), with their rich complement of organelles. Note the microvillus-filled channels (*arrows*) associated with the lateral borders of Böttcher's cells. Bar = 2 μm.

first row of Deiters' cell (i.e., those Deiters' cells supporting the base of the first row of outer hair cells). In addition, the Deiters' cells insert into the reticular lamina two cells apically in a crisscross pattern with the basally directed shafts of the outer hair cells (Fig. 8). Deiters' cells contain a prominent strand of microtubules that extends from the basilar membrane to the outer hair cell and up through the phalangeal process to the reticular lamina (Fig. 4). Deiters' cell cytoplasm also contains abundant smooth endoplasmic reticulum.

HENSEN'S CELLS

Hensen's cells mark the lateral border of the organ of Corti and are attached to the reticular lamina by the phalangeal processes of the third row of Deiters' cells (Figs. 3 and 4). Hensen's cells form several layers, not all of which make direct contact with the endolymphatic space. Their nucleus occurs high in their cytoplasm. Hensen's cells increase in size toward the cochlear apex, and in some animals (e.g., the guinea pig) they contain increasing amounts of lipid inclusions toward the upper cochlear turns. The apical surface of those cells that have direct contact with endolymph exhibit numerous microvilli. Adjacent to the medial side of Hensen's cells is the outer tunnel of Corti (Fig. 4), which can be quite prominent in some animals such as the gerbil and kangaroo rat.

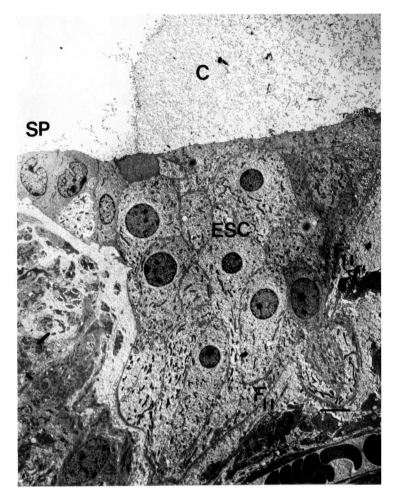

FIG. 15. A radial section through the external sulcus showing a portion of the spiral prominence (SP). Claudius' cells (C) cover the apical surface of the external sulcus cells (ESC). External sulcus cells have a light cytoplasmic density and numerous mitochondria. Fibroblast type II cells (F_{II}) with their dark cytoplasm, and mitochondria-rich, infolded plasma membrane are associated with the root processes of the external sulcus cells. Bar = 5 μm.

BÖTTCHER'S CELLS

Böttcher's cells lie between the basilar membrane and the Claudius' cells (Figs. 3, 5, and 14). They are distributed across most of the width of the basilar membrane in the cochlear base and decrease in number toward the cochlear apex until they are not present at all. They are arranged in a single layer, and toward the apex, they separate into clusters of cells (Fig. 14). They have a cuboidal shape, are ~7 μm on a side, and contain a spherical nucleus ~6 μm in diameter. The cytoplasm of Böttcher's cells contains a rich complement of cell organelles, including microtubules (19). This is in stark contrast to the paucity of organelles characteristic of the surrounding Claudius' cells. Böttcher's cells also exhibit microvillus structures on their lateral cell membranes and spiral intracellular channels (Fig. 14) containing electron-dense

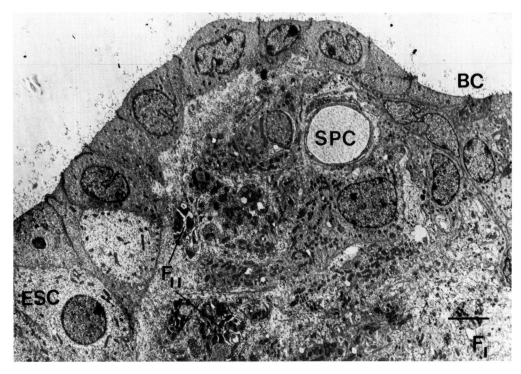

FIG. 16. A radial section through the spiral prominence showing the adjacent external sulcus cells (ESC) and the border cells (BC), which delimit the lateral edge of the stria vascularis. The epithelial cells of the spiral prominence have a polygonal shape and lateral plasmalemma infoldings. Fibroblast type II cells (F$_{II}$) are common in the spiral prominence and intermingle with fibroblast type I cells (F$_I$) in the deeper layers of the spiral ligament. A single spiral prominence capillary (SPC) is shown. Bar = 5 μm.

material (19). The presence of these intracellular processes and the identification of high concentration of acid phosphatase in Böttcher's cells (23) suggest that these cells may have secretory or transport function. The significance of the primarily basal distribution of Böttcher's cells in the cochlea is not clear.

CLAUDIUS' CELLS

Claudius' cells overlie the basilar membrane and extend from Hensen's cells to the spiral prominence epithelium (Figs. 3, 5, 14, and 15). They have a polygonal shape, are ~13 μm thick and ~25 μm wide, and have a spherical nucleus ~6 μm in diameter and few other cytoplasmic organelles. Their apical surface is in direct contact with the endolymph and is covered with short microvilli. The cells are sealed toward the endolymphatic surface by tight junctions. Böttcher's cells are embedded between the base pole of Claudius' cells and the basilar membrane. The primary function of the Claudius' cells appears to provide a paracellular barrier between the endolymphatic space and the cells of Böttcher and the external sulcus.

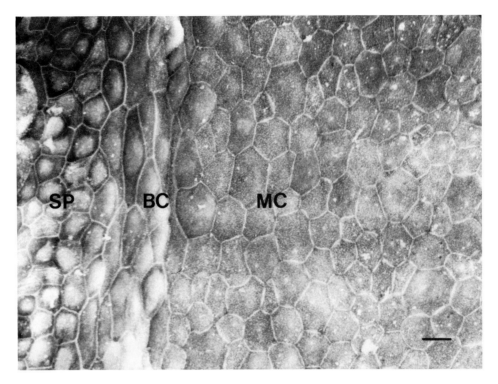

FIG. 17. A scanning electron micrograph showing the spiral prominence epithelia cells (SP), border cells (BC), and the marginal cells (MC) of the stria vascularis. Bar = 10 μm.

EXTERNAL SULCUS CELLS

The open channel or niche formed by the spiral prominence and the Claudius' cells is the external sulcus (Fig. 3). The apical portion of the external sulcus cells is covered by Claudius' cells along most of the length of the scala media (Figs. 15 and 16). However, in the upper cochlear turns, the external sulcus cells have direct apical contact with the endolymph of the scala media. The external sulcus cells form root-like processes that extend into the matrix of the spiral prominence and ligament (6,56). The cells and their processes are separated from the other cell types by a thick basal lamina. The cytoplasm of the external sulcus cells has a rich complement of organelles, including mitochondria, but appears lighter than the surrounding cells. The function of the external sulcus cells is not known.

SPIRAL PROMINENCE

Between the stria vascularis and the basilar membrane is a protuberance of tissue into the scala media known as the spiral prominence (Figs. 3, 15–17). It is a spirally directed tissue that is more prominent in the basal turns. The epithelium of the spiral prominence consists of cuboidal cells. The lateral membranes of these cells show

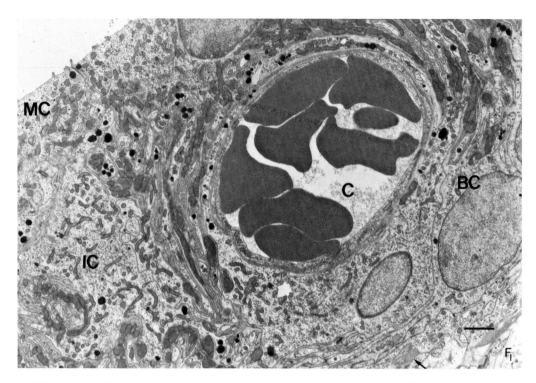

FIG. 18. A radial section of the stria vascularis showing the marginal cells (MC), intermediate cells (IC), intraepithelia capillaries (C), basal cells (BC), fibroblast type I cells (F_1), and the extracellular filaments (*arrow*) of the spiral ligament. Bar = 2 μm.

numerous interdigitations. Within the matrix of the spiral prominence occurs omega-shaped capillary loops (Fig. 19). The matrix of the spiral prominence contains fibroblast-like cells of the spiral ligament (fibroblast type I), dark cells with interdigitating cell membranes that resemble the marginal cells of the stria vascularis (fibroblast type II), and external sulcus cell processes (or roots).

SPIRAL LIGAMENT

The spiral ligament is a connective tissue structure that forms most of the lateral wall of the scala media (Figs. 1 and 3). Its lateral border is the otic capsule and its medial border is the stria vascularis and spiral prominence. The region above the attachment of Reissner's membrane has been called the suprastrial epithelium (17) and may be related to regulation of the lateral wall vessels. The thickness of the spiral ligament decreases toward the cochlear apex and its width extends both above the attachment of Reissner's membrane and below the attachment of the basilar membrane. The matrix of the spiral ligament contains fibroblast-like cells, external sulcus cells, and an abundance of extracellular filaments. Takahashi and Kimura (68) have classified the cells of the spiral ligament into two fibroblast-like cells. The type I fibroblast is most numerous and has few cytoplasmic organelles including lipid inclusions (Figs. 16 and 18). The type II fibroblast shows numerous cytoplasmic

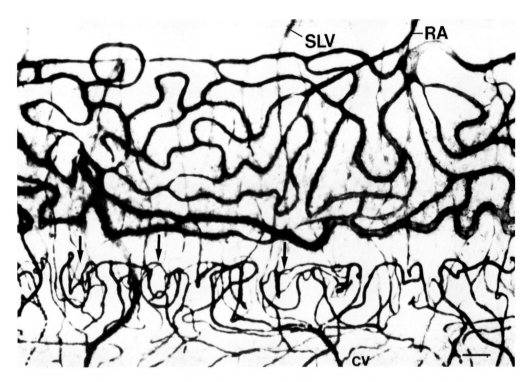

FIG. 19. A soft surface preparation of the lateral wall of the scala media in an animal that received *in vivo* vascular administration of horseradish peroxidase. Radiating arterioles (RA) enter the stria vascularis at its scala vestibuli edge and branch into a capillary network. Relatively unbranched vessels (SLV) travel through the spiral ligament. Capillaries of the spiral prominence (*arrows*) form repeating, omega-shaped loops along its spiral length. Collecting vessels (CV) are shown beneath the spiral prominence. Bar = 50 μm.

organelles and infolding of the plasma membrane that contain mitochondria. These cells are located near surfaces of scala vestibuli, tympani and are adjacent to the spiral prominence and external sulcus cells (Figs. 15 and 16). This second cell type appears to have fluid-transporting characteristics and recently has been shown to contain Na^+, K^+-ATPase, and carbonic anhydrase activity (55). Henson and co-workers (18) have recently described anchoring cells at the medial surface of the otic capsule. Using immunocytochemistry they demonstrated that these cells contain actin, α-actinin, myosin, tropomyosin, and talin. They suggest that these cells and their extracellular filaments may exert tension on the basilar membrane. The spiral ligament is vascularized by relatively unbranched capillaries (Fig. 19) that extend along its width (1).

STRIA VASCULARIS

The stria vascularis is a three-cell-layer, vascularized epithelium that is not bounded by a basal lamina (Figs. 17–19). The stria vascularis is separated from the spiral prominence and Reissner's membrane by spindle-shaped border cells (Figs. 16 and 17). Only one cell type of the stria vascularis has direct contact with the endolymphatic space: the marginal cells. The marginal cells have a lobulated nucleus, a dark-staining cytoplasm, and their laterobasal membranes form highly interdigitated folia containing numerous mitochondria (48,62). Marginal cells also appear to contain microtubules in their apical cytoplasm and cell processes (52). The morphology of these cells strongly suggests active ion transport. Histochemical studies have revealed that these cells are rich in the fluid-transporting enzyme Na^+/K^+-ATPase (28). In the middle layer of the stria vascularis are intraepithelial capillaries and the intermediate cells. The blood supply to the stria vascularis originates from the radiating arterioles at the edge of the scala vestibuli (Fig. 19). The capillaries form an extensive branching network within the stria vascularis and are drained at the scala tympani side by the collecting venules. The capillaries are surrounded by a basal lamina and pericytes, but are not fenestrated. The intermediate cells have a lightly stained cytoplasm and spherical nucleus. Their plasma membranes exhibit interdigitating processes and their cytoplasm is filled with clear vesicles. Intermediate cells also contain lipofuscin and melanin pigment. The basal surface of the stria vascularis is sealed against paracellular transport from the underlying spiral ligament by several layers of fusiform basal cells. These cells have a filamentous cytoplasm and some apically directed processes that interdigitate with marginal and intermediate cell processes.

REISSNER'S MEMBRANE

Reissner's or the vestibular membrane is a thin two-cell-layer membrane that extends from the medial edge of the spiral limbus to the upper (vestibular) edge of

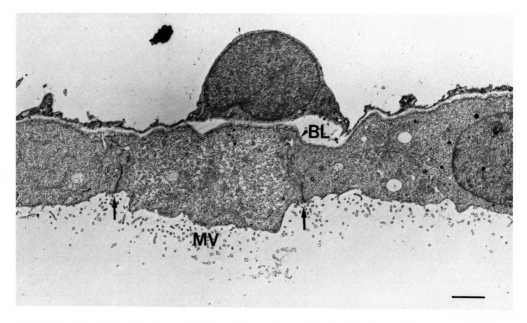

FIG. 20. A radial section through Reissner's membrane showing the two cell types separated by a basal lamina (BL). The cell facing the endolymph exhibits apical microvilli (MV) and tight cell junctions (*arrows*). Bar = 5 μm.

the stria vascularis (Fig. 1). Both cell types have a squamous or low cuboidal shape and are separated by a basal lamina (Fig. 20). The cells that face the endolymphatic side of the membrane exhibit numerous microvilli and are sealed by tight junctions; however, those that face the perilymph are loosely joined together. Although Reissner's membrane appears to be freely permeable to water it prevents penetration of other large molecules [e.g., horseradish peroxidase (7)]. Its cells show a low concentration of ATPase (34) and therefore probably do not have a major role in active ion transport.

ACKNOWLEDGMENTS

I would like to thank Robert Harisson, Wendy Knight, and Susan Nave for their excellent technical assistance in producing these figures. This research has been funded by the NINCDS.

REFERENCES

1. Axelsson, A. (1968): The vascular anatomy of the cochlea in the guinea pig and in man. *Acta Otolaryngol. [Suppl.] (Stockh.)*, 243:1–134.
2. Axelsson, A., Miller, J., and Larsson, B. (1975): A modified "soft surface specimen technique" for examination of the inner ear. *Acta Otolaryngol. (Stockh.)*, 80:362–374.
3. Bohne, B. (1972): Location of small cochlear lesions by phase contrast microscopy prior to thin sectioning. *Laryngoscope*, 82:1–16.
4. Bohne, B., and Carr, C. (1979): Location of structurally similar areas in chinchilla cochleas of different lengths. *J. Acoust. Soc. Am.*, 66:411–414.
5. Brownell, W. E., Bader, C. R., Bertrand, D., and de Ribaupierre, Y. (1985): Evoked mechanical responses of isolated cochlear outer hair cells. *Science*, 227:194–196.
6. Duvall, A. J. (1969): The ultrastructure of the external sulcus in the guinea pig cochlear duct. *Laryngoscope*, 79:1–29.
7. Duvall, A. J., and Sutherland, C. R. (1972): Cochlear transport of horseradish peroxidase. *Ann. Otol. Rhinol. Laryngol.*, 81:705–714.
8. Engström, H., Ades, H., and Anderson, S. (1966): *Structural Patterns of the organ of Corti*. Williams & Wilkins, Baltimore.
9. Fernández, C. (1951): Innervation of the cochlea (guinea pig). *Laryngoscope*, 61:1152.
10. Fernández, C. (1952): Dimensions of the cochlea (guinea pig). *J. Acoust. Soc. Am.*, 24:519–523.
11. Flock, Å., Bretscher, A., and Weber, K. (1982): Immunohistochemical localization of several cytoskeletal proteins in inner ear sensory and supporting cells. *Hear. Res.*, 7:75–89.
12. Flock, Å., and Cheung, H. C. (1977): Actin filaments in sensory hairs of inner ear receptor cells. *J. Cell Biol.*, 75:339–343.
13. Flock, Å., Flock, B., and Murray, E. (1977): Studies on the sensory hairs of receptor cells in the inner ear. *Acta Otolaryngol. (Stockh.)*, 83:85–91.
14. Furness, D. N., and Hackney, C. M. (1985): Cross-links between stereocilia in the guinea pig cochlea. *Hear. Res.*, 18:177–188.
15. Gulley, R. L., and Reese, T. S. (1976): Intercellular junctions in the reticular lamina of the organ of Corti. *J. Neurocytol.*, 5:479–507.
16. Hardy, M. (1938): The length of the organ of Corti in man. *Am. J. Anat.*, 63:291–311.
17. Hawkins, J. E. (1973): Comparative otopathology: Aging, noise, and ototoxic drugs. *Adv. Otorhinolaryngol.*, 20:125–141.
18. Henson, M. M., Burridge, K., Fitzpatrick, D., Jenkins, D. B., Pillsbury, H. C., and Henson, Jr., O. W. (1985): Immunocytochemical localization of contractile and contraction associated proteins in the spiral ligament of the cochlea. *Hear. Res.*, 20:207–214.
19. Henson, M. M., Jenkins, D. B., and Henson, Jr., O. W. (1982): The cells of Boettcher in the bat, *Pteronotus p. parnellii. Hear. Res.*, 7:91–103.
20. Hirokawa, N., and Tilney, L. (1982): Interactions between actin filaments and between actin filaments and membrane in quick-frozen and deeply etched hair cells of the chick ear. *J. Cell Biol.*, 95:249–261.

21. Hudspeth, A. J., and Corey, D. P. (1977): Sensitivity, polarity, and conductance change in the response of vertebrate hair cells to controlled mechanical stimuli. *Proc. Natl. Acad. Sci. USA*, 74:2407–2511.
22. Hunter-Duvar, I. M. (1977): Morphology of the normal and the acoustically damaged cochlea. *SEM*, II: 421–428.
23. Ishii, T., and Balogh, K., Jr. (1966): Acid phosphatase activity in the inner ear. *Acta Otolaryngol. (Stockh.)*, 62:185–192.
24. Iurato, S. (1960): Submicroscopic structure of the membranous labyrinth. I. The tectorial membrane. *Z. Zellforsch.*, 51:105–128.
25. Iurato, S. (1961): Submicroscopic structure of the membranous labyrinth. II. The epithelium of Corti's organ. *Z. Zellforsch.*, 53:259–298.
26. Iurato, S. (1962): Submicroscopic structure of the membranous labyrinth. III. The supporting structure of Corti's organ (basilar membrane, limbus spiralis and spiral ligament). *Z. Zellforsch.*, 56:40–96.
27. Kellerhals, B., Engstrom, H., and Ades, H. W. (1967): Die Morphologie des Ganglion spirale cochleae. *Acta Otolaryngol. [Suppl.] (Stockh.)*, 226:1–78.
28. Kerr, T., Ross, M., and Ernst, S. (1982): Cellular localization of Na + ,K + -ATPase in the mammalian cochlear duct. *Am. J. Otolaryngol.*, 66:386–398.
29. Khalkhali-Ellis, Z., Hemming, F. W., and Steele, K. P. (1978): Glycoconjugates of the tectorial membrane. *Hear. Res.*, 25:185–192.
30. Kimura, R. S. (1966): Hairs of the cochlear sensory cells and their attachment to the tectorial membrane. *Acta Otolaryngol. (Stockh.)*, 61:55–72.
31. Kimura, R. S. (1975): The ultrastructure of the organ of Corti. *Int. Rev. Cytol.*, 42:173–222.
32. Kimura, R. S., and Ota, C. Y. (1974): Ultrastructure of the cochlear blood vessels. *Acta Otolaryngol. (Stockh.)*, 7:231–250.
33. Kronester-Frei, A. (1978): Ultrastructure of the different zones of the tectorial membrane. *Cell Tissue Res.*, 193:11–23.
34. Kuijpers, W., and Bonting, S. (1969): Studies on the (Na + -K +)-activated ATPase. XXIV. Localization and properties of ATPase in the inner ear of the guinea pig. *Biochem. Biophys. Acta*, 173:477–485.
35. Liberman, M. C., and Beil, D. G. (1979): Hair cell condition and auditory-nerve response in normal and noise-damaged cochleas. *Acta Otolaryngol. (Stockh.)*, 88:161–176.
36. Lim, D. J. (1972): Fine morphology of the tectorial membrane: Its relationship to the organ of Corti. *Arch. Otolaryngol.*, 96:199–215.
37. Lim, D. J. (1980): Cochlear anatomy related to cochlear micromechanics. A review. *J. Acoust. Soc. Am.*, 67:1686–1695.
38. Lim, D. J. (1985): Functional structure of the organ of Corti: A review. *Hear. Res.*, 22:117–146.
39. Lorente de Nó, R. (1926): Études sur l'anatomie et la physiologie du labyrinthe de l'oreille et du VIII:e nerf. *Trab. Inst. Cajal Invest. Biol.*, 24:53.
40. Neubager, D.-C. (1986): The vestibular stereovillus membrane: An illustration of the "Greater Membrane" concept. *ORL*, 48:87–92.
41. Ota, C. Y., and Kimura, R. S. (1980): Ultrastructural study of the human spiral ganglion. *Acta Otolaryngol. (Stockh.)*, 89:53–62.
42. Pickles, J. O., Comis, S. D., and Osborne, M. P. (1984): Cross-links between stereocilia in the guinea pig organ of Corti, and their possible relation to sensory transduction. *Hear. Res.*, 15:103–112.
43. Prieto, J. J., and Merchan, J. A. (1986): Tannic acid staining of the cell coat of the organ of Corti. *Hear. Res.*, 24:237–242.
44. Rasmussen, G. L. (1946): The olivary peduncle and the other fiber projections of the superior olivary complex. *J. Comp. Neurol.*, 84:141.
45. Retzius, G. (1881): *Das Gehörorgan der Wirbeltiere. Morphologisch-histologische Studien. I. Das Gehörorgan der Fische und Amphibien.* Samson & Wallin, Stockholm.
46. Retzius, G. (1884): *Das Gehörorgan der Wirbeltiere. Morphologisch-histologische Studien. I. Das Gehörorgan der Reptilien, der Vögel und der Säugetiere.* Samson & Wallin, Stockholm.
47. Richardson, G. P., Russell, I. J., Duance, V. C., and Bailey, A. J. (1987): Polypeptide composition of the mammalian tectorial membrane. *Hear. Res.*, 25:45–60.
48. Rodríguez-Echandía, E. L., and Burgos, M. H. (1965): The fine structure of the stria vascularis of the guinea pig inner ear. *Z. Zellforsch.*, 67:600–619.
49. Ross, M. (1971): Fluorescence and electron microscopic observations of the general visceral, efferent innervation of the inner ear. *Acta Otolaryngol. [Suppl.] (Stockh.)*, 286.
50. Santi, P. A., and Anderson, C. B. (1987): A newly identified surface coat on cochlear hair cells. *Hear. Res.*, 27:47–65.
51. Santi, P. A., Mitchell, W. J., and Harrison, R. G. (1986): A computer-assisted morphometric analysis of the organ of Corti. *Hear. Res.*, 24:189–201.

52. Santos-Sacchi, J. (1978): Cytoplasmic microtubules in strial marginal cells. *Arch. Otorhinolaryngol.*, 218:297–300.
53. Satir, P. (1977): Microvilli and cilia: Surface specializations of mammalian cells. In: *Mammalian Cell Membranes, Vol. 2, The Diversity of Membranes*, edited by G. A. Jamieson and D. M. Robinson, pp. 323–353. Butterworths, London.
54. Saunders, J. C., Schneider, M. E., and Dear, S. P. (1985): The structure and function of actin in hair cells. *J. Acoust. Soc. Am.*, 78:299–311.
55. Schulte, B. A., and Adams, J. C. (1987): Immunocytochemical localization of (Na + + K +)-ATPase and carbonic anhydrase in the lateral wall of the cochlea. 10th Midwinter Meeting of the Association for Research in Otolaryngology, Clearwater Beach, FL, p. 60.
56. Shambaugh, G. E. (1908): On the structure and function of the epithelium in the sulcus spiralis externus. *Arch. Otolaryngol.*, 37:538–546.
57. Siegel, J. H., and Kim, D. O. (1982): Efferent neuronal control of cochlear mechanics? Olivocochlear bundle stimulation affects cochlear biomechanical nonlinearity. *Hear. Res.*, 6:171–182.
58. Slepecky, N., and Chamberlain, S. C. (1982): Distribution and polarity of actin in the sensory hair cells of the chinchilla cochlea. *Cell Tissue Res.*, 224:15–24.
59. Slepecky, N., and Chamberlain, S. C. (1985): The cell coat of inner ear sensory and supporting cells as demonstrated by ruthenium red. *Hear. Res.*, 17:281–288.
60. Slepecky, N., and Chamberlain, S. C. (1985): Immunoelectron microscopic and immunofluorescent localization of cytoskeletal and muscle-like contractile proteins in inner ear sensory hair cells. *Hear. Res.*, 20:245–260.
61. Slepecky, N., Hamernik, R. P., and Henderson, D. (1980): A re-examination of a hair cell organelle in the cuticular plate region and its possible relation to active processes in the cochlea. *Hear. Res.*, 2:413–421.
62. Smith, C. A. (1957): Structure of the stria vascularis and spiral prominence. *Ann. Otol. Rhinol. Laryngol.*, 66:521–536.
63. Smith, C. A., Davis, H., Deatherage, B., and Gessert, C. (1958): DC potentials of the membranous labyrinth. *Am. J. Physiol.*, 193:203–206.
64. Smith, C. A. (1975): The inner ear: Its embryological development and microstructure. In: *The Nervous System, Vol. 3, Human Communication and Its Disorders*, edited by D. B. Tower, pp. 1–18. Raven Press, New York.
65. Spoendlin, H. (1971): Degeneration behavior of the cochlear nerve. *Arch. Klin. Exp. Ohren Nasen Kehlkopfheilk.*, 200:275–291.
66. Spoendlin, H., and Lichtensteiger, W. (1966): The adrenergic innervation of the labyrinth. *Acta Otolaryngol. (Stockh.)*, 61:422.
67. Steel, K. P. (1983): The tectorial membrane of mammals. *Hear. Res.*, 9:327–359.
68. Takahashi, T., and Kimura, R. S. (1970): The ultrastructure of the spiral ligament in the rhesus monkey. *Acta Otolaryngol. (Stockh.)*, 69:46–60.
69. Tasaki, I., and Spyropoulos, C. (1959): Stria vascularis as source of endocochlear potential. *J. Neurophysiol.*, 22:149–155.
70. Thalmann, I., Thallinger, G., Comegys, T. H., and Thalmann, R. (1986): Collagen—The predominate protein of the tectorial membrane. *ORL*, 48:107–115.
71. Tilney, L. G., DeRosier, D. J., and Mulroy, M. J. (1980): The organization of actin filaments in the stereocilia of cochlear hair cells. *J. Cell Biol.*, 86:244–259.
72. Wever, E. G. (1938): The width of the basilar membrane in man. *Ann. Otol. Rhinol. Laryngol.*, 47:37–47.
73. Wright, A. (1984): Dimensions of the cochlear stereocilia in man and the guinea pig. *Hear. Res.*, 13:89–98.
74. Zenner, H. P., Zimmerman, U., and Schmitt, U. (1985): Reversible contraction of isolated mammalian cochlear hair cells. *Hear. Res.*, 18:127–133.

Physiology of the Ear,
edited by A. F. Jahn and J. Santos-Sacchi.
Raven Press, New York © 1988.

Neural Anatomy of the Inner Ear

Heinrich Spoendlin

ENT Department, University Hospital Innsbruck, A-6020 Innsbruck, Austria

THE COCHLEA

The innervation of the cochlea consists essentially of three components (Fig. 1): (a) the afferent neurons, which have their perikarya as all centripetal systems outside the central nervous system in the spiral ganglion in the cochlea; (b) the efferent neurons, which have their perikarya in the central nervous system as all centrifugal systems, originating in the superior olivary complex and reaching the periphery with the vestibular nerve and the vestibulocochlear anastomosis of Oort (38,39); (c) an adrenergic autonomic innervation originating in the superior cervical and the stellate ganglion (57,64).

Afferent Neurons

The number of primary afferent neurons that connects the cochlea with the brain stem varies considerably in different species, with approximately 16,000 in the bat (16), 36,000 in the human (35), 50,000 to 60,000 in the cat (45,51) and more than 200,000 in the whale (15). In the cochlear nerve, the overwhelming majority of nerve fibers are myelinated, with diameters ranging from 4 to 6 μm in a unimodal distribution. Each fiber has a regular myelin sheath of approximately 50 lamellae as a structural basis of a uniform conduction velocity, probably a very important basic functional feature of the cochlear nerve. The nerve fibers are tonotopically arranged within the cochlear nerve according to their area of origin in the cochlea (44). The innervation density as expressed in number of nerve fibers per unit length of the organ of Corti is highest in the middle and lower basal turn in the cat and in the upper basal turn in the human, with a gradual decrease toward the apex and hook area (4,54). All fibers lose their myelin sheath before they enter the organ of Corti through the habenular perforata.

In all mammalian species studied so far, i.e., the cat, guinea pig, rat, rabbit, chinchilla, gerbil, monkey, and human, two distinct types of ganglion cells are found in the normal spiral ganglion (20,29,34,43,53,58): a great majority (90%–95%) of large bipolar type I cells and approximately 5% to 10% of smaller pseudomonopolar type II cells with a number of distinctive features. The most common feature of type II cells in all species is their smaller size and a lighter, more filamentous cytoplasm with fewer ribosomes or Nissl substance than type I cells (Fig. 2). The lack of myelin sheath is a frequent but not constant finding. In humans there are just as many myelinated as unmyelinated small cells (34), and in the cat, some type II cells may

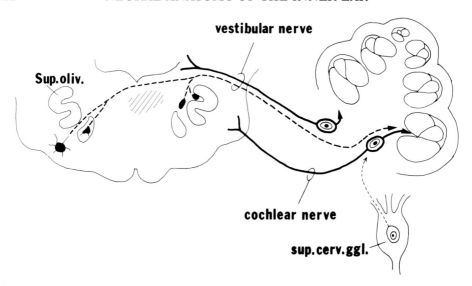

FIG. 1. Schematic representation of the three innervation components of the cochlea: afferent neurons (*solid lines*), olivocochlear efferent neurons (*bold broken line*), and autonomic innervation (*broken line*). Sup. oliv., superior olivary complex; sup. cerv. ggl., superior cervical ganglion.

have a thin myelin sheath. The eccentric position and lobulation of the nucleus are typical in the cat, but absent in rodents and humans. The suspicion that type II cells might be spontaneously degenerating type I cells can be refuted by the fact that two types of ganglion cells are already present in the newborn kitten (42,58). The myelin sheath around the type I neurons of the cat is relatively thin with an inner layer of loose myelin and an outer layer of compact myelin. In the vicinity of the cell body, the central process of type I cells is much larger (diameter: ~2 μm) than the peripheral process (diameter: ~1 μm) (21). Up to the first node of Ranvier, the axon is surrounded by the same type of myelin as the perikaryon. Beyond that, the central, as well as the peripheral, axon is surrounded by the typical compact myelin of peripheral nerves with approximately 50 lamellae (Fig. 2). The axons of type II cells are unmyelinated and have a relatively large caliber close to the cell body, but they thin down considerably with increasing distance from the cell.

The peripheral distribution of afferent neurons is best studied after elimination of efferents by wallerian degeneration following transsection of the olivocochlear efferent fibers within the vestibular nerve. The remaining fibers are afferent fibers, i.e., the inner radial fibers, basilar fibers, and outer spiral fibers (Fig. 3). The basilar fibers are the only afferent fibers reaching the area of the outer hair cells. They can be counted as they pass between the base of the outer pillars in tangential section through this area. Evaluated over long distances in the cochlea of the cat, there is an average of one basilar fiber penetrating between two pillars, which amounts to approximately 2,500 afferent fibers for the outer hair cells. This is an extremely small number compared with the entire population of approximately 50,000 cochlear neurons in the cat cochlea. It means that only approximately 5% of all afferent cochlear neurons are associated with the outer hair cell system, which represents more than three-quarters of the receptor cells of the cochlea. More evidence for this surprising 20:1 ratio of afferent innervation of inner and outer hair cells can be obtained by

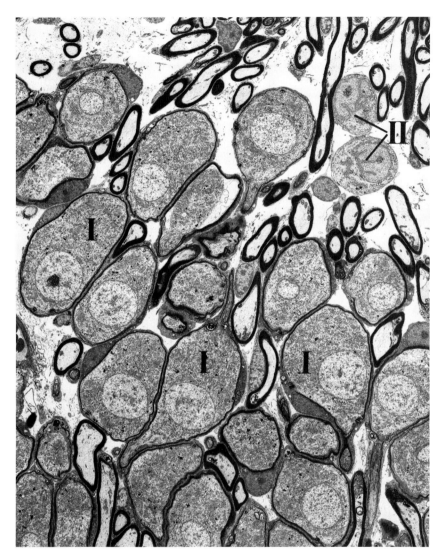

FIG. 2. Electron micrograph (EM) survey of a portion of the spiral ganglion of a cat showing the majority of large myelinated type I ganglion cells (I) and a few smaller type II ganglion cells (II).

reconstruction of the area of the inner hair cells after elimination of efferent inner-vation. The majority of all nerve fibers entering the organ of Corti leads directly, unbranched, to the base of the nearest inner hair cell. Only about one of 20 fibers turns outward to the outer hair cells (51). Similar ratios between neurons associated with the outer and inner hair cells have been found in guinea pigs (29,51) and humans (33) (Fig. 4).

Within the habenula, fibers associated with the outer hair cells cannot be distin-guished from other fibers, but they are usually situated in the most distal portion of the habenular opening. In contrast to the fibers for the inner hair cells, they take an independent spiral course above the habenula for approximately five pillars before

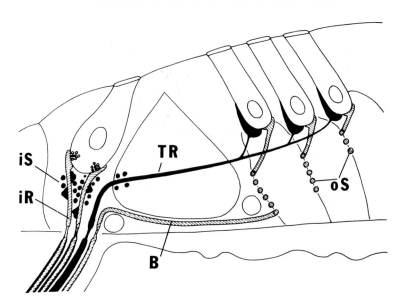

FIG. 3.   Radial innervation schema of the organ of Corti. *Solid lines* are afferent nerve fibers and *hatched lines* are efferent nerve endings. iR, inner radial fibers; iS, inner spiral fibers; TR, tunnel radial fibers; B, basilar fibers; oS, outer spiral fibers.

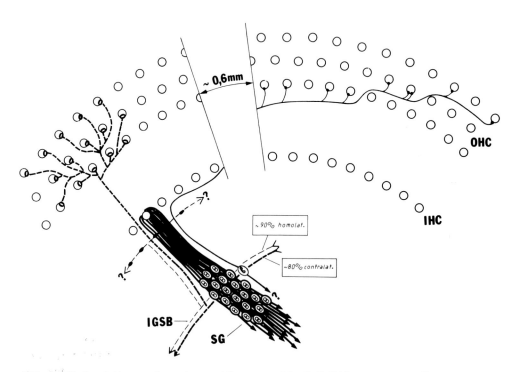

FIG. 4.   Horizontal innervation schema of the organ of Corti. *Solid lines* represent afferent neurons; *broken lines* represent efferent neurons, SG, spiral ganglion; IGSB, intraganglion spiral bundle.

they penetrate between the inner pillars to cross the bottom of the tunnel as basilar fibers. Upon reaching the area of the outer hair cells, they form the outer spiral fibers, which course in a basalward direction and gradually climb up toward the base of the outer hair cells. In its terminal portion, each fiber gives off collaterals, which end with afferent nerve endings at the base of outer hair cells. Each fiber sends collaterals to approximately 10 outer hair cells, and each outer hair cell receives collaterals from several outer spiral fibers according to the principles of multiple innervation. The average spiral extension of the outer spiral fibers in the basalward direction amounts to approximately 0.6 mm (46,50). This peripheral innervation pattern has essentially been confirmed in a recent Golgi study (7). In the cat, there are approximately 100 outer spiral fibers at any given place, but in humans they are much more numerous, running as compact bundles between the Deiters' cells. Accordingly, their spiral extension is probably much larger in humans than in cats.

The ultrastructural organization of the axoplasm varies to some extent between afferent fibers to outer and inner hair cells. The fibers for the outer hair cells contain mainly neurocanaliculi in their axoplasma, whereas the fibers for the inner hair cells contain predominantly neurofibrils. Each afferent ending at the inner hair cell usually forms one synaptic complex with a presynaptic bar of varying size (Fig. 5). In the human, several synapses can be observed in one nerve ending (31). The afferent endings at the base of the outer hair cells, on the other hand, have no synaptic ribbons in the cat (Fig. 6) and only a few relatively small ones in the guinea pig and human (6,30,41,52). In more than 50% of the outer hair cells, Nadol (30,32) describes reciprocal synapses where a single nerve ending of the nonvesiculated type presents two types of synaptic specialization of opposite polarity.

On the basis of location, caliber, and content of mitochondria, Liberman (25) distinguishes at the level of the inner hair cells different types of dendrites, which he can correlate to the spontaneous discharge rate of the neurons by means of single-neuron labeling. The large fibers tend to have their endings at the distal circumference of the inner hair cells, whereas the smaller fibers end mostly on the modiolar side of the basal circumference of the inner hair cells. The average diameter of the radial fiber terminal is highly correlated with the spontaneous discharge of the unit. All 56 recorded and labeled neurons from 14 cats were type I neurons associated with the inner hair cells. This strongly suggests that the activity of outer hair cell innervation has never been sampled in any of the single-unit recordings from the auditory nerve, which is possibly because the central axons of type II neurons are probably not recordable, being unmyelinated and less than 0.5 μm in diameter.

The caliber of the fibers varies considerably along their course through the organ of Corti (Fig. 3). Their diameter is considerably reduced and the axoplasm rather empty, especially where the fibers pass mechanically important supporting structures, such as the basilar membrane at the habenular region or the pillars. Within the organ of Corti, the afferent dendrites to the inner hair cells, the inner radial fibers, are large and very rich in mitochondria, indicating their high metabolic activity (Fig. 5).

In the spiral ganglion of the cat no synaptic contacts between neurons could be found. However, in the spiral ganglion of the human and the monkey, synaptic contacts between small neurons and small unmyelinated fibers from the intraganglionic spiral bundle have been described (2,22).

The neurons of the inner and outer hair cells differ not only in number, arrange-

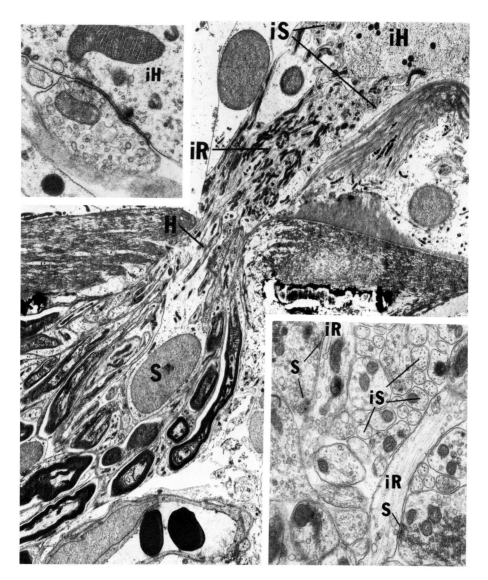

FIG. 5. Electron micrograph (EM) survey of habenula and area below inner hair cells. iH, inner hair cell; iR, inner radial fibers; H, habenula; S, satellite cell; iS, inner spiral fibers. *Upper left inset:* detail of afferent nerve ending at an inner hair cell with synaptic complex. *Lower right inset:* detail of inner spiral plexus with inner spiral fibers making synaptic contacts (S) with afferent inner radial fibers.

ment, and structure, but also in their metabolic behavior. The radial fibers to the inner hair cells are very susceptible to hypoxia in contrast to the outer spiral fibers, and aging changes are found predominantly within type I neurons (9). Pronounced swelling of the radial fibers to the inner hair cells is the first morphological sign of even slight hypoxia and not optimal or somewhat delayed fixation. All this suggests that the neurons of the inner and outer hair cells represent two different systems.

There is general agreement that type II neurons provide the afferent innervation

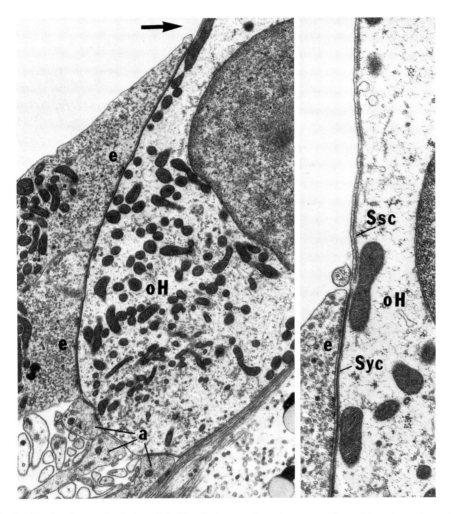

FIG. 6. Basis of an outer hair cell (oH) with large efferent nerve endings (e) and much smaller afferent nerve endings (a), *arrow* points to the area shown in detail on the right-hand side, where we see the subsurface cisternae (Ssc) and the subsynaptic cisternae (Syc) between efferent nerve ending (e) and outer hair cell.

of the outer hair cells and type I neurons the afferent innervation of the inner hair cells. The first suspicion of such a relationship came from the observation that the type II neurons and the afferent fibers to the outer hair cells represent approximately 5% of the entire cochlear nerve population. Following transsection of the eighth nerve in the inner acoustic meatus, most type I neurons degenerate within several months, whereas type II neurons remain morphologically unchanged in normal numbers. At the same time, the afferent nerve supply of the outer hair cells also remains entirely unchanged. This led to the conclusion that type II neurons provide the afferent innervation of the outer hair cells, whereas type I neurons give rise to the radial fibers leading to the inner hair cells (51,56). More recently, these correlations were directly demonstrated by horseradish peroxidase (HRP) labeling of cochlear nerve fibers (21). Additional support for the association of type I neurons to the inner hair cells and type II neurons to the outer hair cells is provided by the fact that retrograde degeneration of type I cochlear neurons starts only after destruction of the inner hair cells but not after selective loss of the outer hair cells.

That type II axons are small in caliber and remain unmyelinated throughout their entire course is functionally important, but difficult to prove, since it is practically impossible to follow them over long distances in normal animals (56). To a limited extent, this is possible with electron microscopic serial sections or with interference contrast microscopy of extra-thick sections following retrograde degeneration of type I cells. In areas of the cochlea where only type II cells remain following transsection of the eighth nerve, we find almost exclusively unmyelinated nerve fibers in the osseous spiral lamina, which indicates that the peripheral axons of type II neurons remain unmyelinated throughout their entire peripheral course.

To follow the central axon of type II neurons is more difficult. Electron microscopic serial sections are only possible for limited distances. In light microscopic preparations the unmyelinated axons become extremely thin at a certain distance from the perikarya and are usually lost at the entrance of the modiolus. Being so small at this level, they will most probably remain very small and unmyelinated in their further centralward course within the cochlear nerve.

Unmyelinated fibers on the other hand are very rare within the normal cochlear nerve. There are two types of unmyelinated fibers. One type has a diameter of 0.2 to 0.5 μm, usually runs alone in its own Schwann-sheaths, and represents only 0.5% of the entire population. The other type is extremely small with a diameter approximately 0.1 μm, usually runs in groups of several fibers in one Schwann-sheath, and represents between 2% and 5% of the entire nerve population. These fibers resemble autonomic fibers very much (Fig. 7). It is more likely that the first small group of somewhat larger unmyelinated fibers represent central axons of type II neurons. Their extremely small number and size is consistent with the inability to obtain single-fiber recordings from them (25). A complete and efficient connection of type II neurons to the central nervous system seems questionable. The fact that type II neurons undergo secondary retrograde degeneration after destruction of the organ of Corti but do not show any degeneration after transsection of the cochlear nerve shows that the central axons are peculiar and unusual.

A number of studies have been undertaken to inject HRP by various means into the cochlear nucleus or nerve, where the histochemically demonstrable tracer is taken up by the axons and transported down to the nerve endings within the organ of Corti. The results of such experiments differed to some extent. In our own experiments, we found the radial fibers to the inner hair cells strongly labeled but not the outer spiral fibers nor the afferent nerve terminals at the outer hair cells (23,58,60). Leak-Jones and Snyder (23), on the other hand, were able to demonstrate some nicely labeled outer spiral fibers and nerve endings at the base of the outer hair cells in cats. Similar results were obtained by Kiang et al. (21). Ruggero et al. (42a) found in similar studies in chinchillas that type II neurons were labeled but much less than the radial fibers of type I neurons. Morest (28) could show by autoradiography that d-aspartate was transported from the cochlear nucleus to type II ganglion cells in cats.

These experiments suggest that the central axon of some type II neurons do indeed project into the cochlear nerve or even into the cochlear nucleus, but it does not say anything about the functional significance of these central connections. The

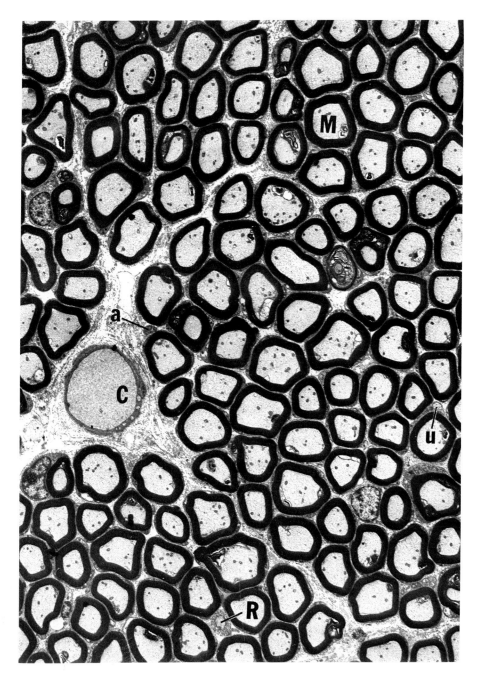

FIG. 7. Portion of a cross section through the cochlear nerve in the inner acoustic meatus showing the densely packed myelinated nerve fibers (M) and very few unmyelinated fibers (u), some of which might be the central axons of some type II neurons, whereas other very small ones probably are autonomic fibers (a). R, Ranvier; C, capillary.

extremely small number and size of the central axons of afferent neurons of the outer hair cell system constitutes a poor information transmission system. In the small unmyelinated axons, saltatory action-potential conduction is not possible, so that the propagation of nerve potentials is presumably very slow with considerable decrement. There seems to be a direct correlation between fiber size, spontaneous activity, and sensitivity (25). After section of the cochlear nerve in the cat, almost all type I neurons degenerate and disappear and only type II neurons, which represent the afferent innervation of the outer hair cell system, remain unchanged in normal numbers. In electrocochleographic recordings of such animals, no compound action potentials can be found, in spite of the remaining normal type II neurons (62). On the rare occasions when electrophysiological recordings could be made from identified type II neurons, they were silent (40). All this suggests that the main information transfer to the central nervous system relies on the inner hair cell system. Furthermore, the outer hair cell system, which represents a great majority of all cochlear hair cells, may have its main functional role at the cellular level; that is, the outer hair cell system possibly monitors the receptor organ electrically or mechanically rather than participates in direct neural information transmission to the central nervous system. The extensive efferent innervation of the outer hair cells supports this concept.

Efferent Neurons

Efferent innervation of the cochlea has been known since Rasmussen (38,39) demonstrated a homo- and contralateral efferent olivocochlear bundle in the cat, rat, and opossum. Efferent innervation of the acoustic system originating in the brain stem is found in practically all species from fish to mammals (65).

With the application of HRP techniques, a clear and direct demonstration of the origin of the cochlear efferents was possible in the kitten (67,68), the adult cat (59,61) and the rat (W. B. Warr, *personal communication*). With HRP labeling, between 1,400 and 1,600 efferent neurons were identified in the cat, more than double the number originally indicated by Rasmussen (38,39). There are at least four different types of neurons. The so-called lateral group is located in the lateral superior olivary nucleus (LSO) and consists of very small fusiform cells deep in the hilus with diameters of approximately 10 μm and somewhat larger cells medial to it. The so-called medial group consists of medium-sized oval-shaped cells in the medial nucleus of the trapezoid body (MNTB) and of very large multipolar cells with diameters as large as 20 μm in the periolivary nucleus (PON). In the cat, 85% to 90% of the neurons in the LSO are homolateral, whereas 70% to 80% of the larger neurons in the MNTB and PON are contralateral (Fig. 1).

The contralateral fibers cross the midline at the floor of the fourth ventricle. They join the homolateral bundle within the vestibular root and run with the vestibular nerve into the periphery before they cross over to the cochlear nerve deep in the inner acoustic meatus through the anastomosis of Oort (vestibulocochlear anastomosis). The totality of efferent fibers can, therefore, be selectively transected best in the vestibular nerve without damage to the cochlear nerve. Within the modiolus, the efferent nerves form the intraganglionic spiral bundle as one or several nerve bundles in the peripheral portion of the spiral ganglion from where the fibers radiate

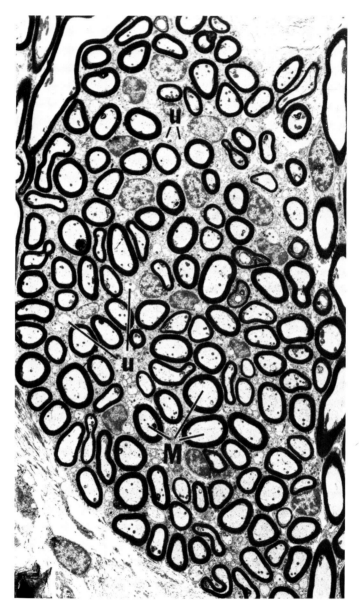

FIG. 8. Intraganglionic spiral bundle with myelinated (M) and numerous unmyelinated (u) fibers of various calibers.

to the organ of Corti. The efferent fibers are best identified in the anastomosis of Oort (1) or in the intraganglionic spiral bundle (61) where we found about two-thirds of the fibers were unmyelinated and of varying sizes (Fig. 8).

By means of degeneration studies with selective transsections of the olivocochlear fibers in the vestibular nerve or at the floor of the fourth ventricle, their peripheral distribution has been mapped in the rat (17), the guinea pig (47,48,70), the cat (49,51), and the chinchilla (19). According to such studies, the large nerve endings at the outer hair cells, the upper tunnel radial fibers, and the inner spiral fibers belong to the efferent innervation (Fig. 3).

The most striking finding is the enormous efferent innervation of the outer hair cells (Fig. 6). On the basis of transmission electron microscopic observation of serial sections (49), or high-voltage electron microscopic observation of a series of extra-thick sections (66), 6 to 10 large efferent endings at the base of each outer hair cell are found. The distribution of the efferents to the outer hair cells is essentially radial, and the tunnel-crossing fibers are relatively large with an average diameter of 1 μm. The efferent innervation of the outer hair cells decreases from base to apex and is less abundant in the second and third rows of outer hair cells. The efferent nerve endings have enormous contact areas with the outer hair cell, about 10 times as large as the contact area of the afferent nerve endings with the hair cell. They have numerous synaptic contacts, in the cat almost exclusively with the hair cell and only exceptionally with an afferent dendrite. This certainly reflects the potential influence the efferents can have on the outer hair cells.

At the area of contact with efferent nerve endings, the plasma membrane of the outer hair cells is regularly paralleled by a subsynaptic cisterna, which seems to be a continuation of the subsurface cisternae typical for outer hair cells (Fig. 6). Similar subsurface cisternae are found in smooth muscle cells, a structural similarity that might be related to the capacity of the outer hair cells to contract.

The efferents at the level of the inner hair cells are quite different. They form the inner spiral fibers and tunnel spiral fibers. They are small, with diameters between 0.1 and 0.6 μm, and the majority is about 0.2 μm. Their number increases from base to apex of the cochlea, in contrast to the efferents of the outer hair cells. Their number is usually approximately 200 at any place in the middle turn of the cat cochlea. The spiral extension and final terminals are unknown. They form a plexus with the afferent dendrites, which penetrate through the spiral bundles on their way to the inner hair cells. Along their course, these inner spiral fibers form various enlargements filled with synaptic vesicles partly surrounding the afferent dendrites. They have almost exclusively synaptic contacts, mostly *en passant*, with afferent dendrites and only exclusively with the inner hair cells (Fig. 5). In rodents, one finds some exceptions to this rule.

In reconstruction of this area, Liberman (24) found that each afferent dendrite from the inner hair cell has up to 20 synaptic contacts with efferent inner spiral fibers. Even some afferents and efferents from the outer hair cells occasionally synapse with inner spiral efferents, and rarely some synaptic contacts between ef-ferents and afferents are found just above the habenula.

There is evidence that the efferents for the inner and outer hair cells belong to two different systems. Morphologically, the efferents of the outer hair cells are large and radial and synapse predominantly with the receptor cells, whereas the efferents of the inner hair cell system have a spiral distribution and synapse exclusively with dendrites but not with the receptor cell (Figs. 3 and 4). In addition, they degenerate much more slowly than the efferents of the outer hair cell system. The most important evidence was provided by a study of Warr and Guinan (69). Radioactive leucine or methionine was injected into the area of either LSO or MNTB using auditory evoked potential recordings for orientation of the pipette. After 11 to 36 hr, the cochleas were evaluated by autoradiographic techniques, and the silver grains in the area below the inner hair cells and at the base of the outer hair cells were counted. After

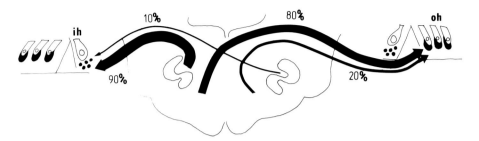

FIG. 9. Origin of the efferent fibers for the outer hair cells (oH) and the inner hair cells (iH).

injection in the LSO, silver grains were found almost exclusively in the inner hair cell area, predominantly homolateral but also some contralateral. After injection in the MNTB, most grains were found in the area of the contralateral outer hair cells, and only approximately 10% in the inner hair cell region, which might be due to passage of the outer hair cell efferents through this area (Fig. 9).

These results are consistent with degeneration studies in which a midline lesion leads to degeneration of the majority of efferents of the outer hair cells, but has no effect (18) or only a partial effect (52) on the efferents of the inner hair cell area. After midline lesion, most unmyelinated large fibers of the intraganglionic spiral bundle degenerate and the majority of the remaining nerve fibers are unmyelinated. This indicates that the large myelinated efferent fibers belong to the contralateral system associated to the outer hair cells, and the small unmyelinated fibers to the homolateral efferents, associated with the inner hair cell system. The situation might, however, be more complex if one considers that the olivocochlear efferent system consists of a number of different neural groups. The inner hair cell efferents are probably slow with a more general influence on the sensory organ, whereas the outer hair cell efferents are presumably fast, tonotopically organized, and well suited for a more differentiated influence on the receptor organ. They have been shown to be as sensitive and sharply tuned as the primary afferents with the same characteristic frequencies (26).

Although there are definite electrophysiologically measurable efferent effects on the cochlear potentials (5,10,13), there is sparse and conflicting evidence concerning the physiological significance of the efferents in the hearing process.

The striking discrepancy between the extensive anatomical representation of the efferents in the organ of Corti and the physiological effects has not yet been solved. A number of negative findings and the clinical observation that transsection of the vestibular nerve in cases of Meniere's disease did not induce any measurable changes of hearing led to the conclusion that the efferent system under normal conditions has no function (37). Such a situation, however, seems unlikely since the efferent system is anatomically so well represented and highly developed that it is hardly conceivable that it would not have any functional significance.

The role of efferents has to be considered in connection with the new concepts of the role of the outer hair cell system. There is morphological and functional evidence that the outer hair cells can contract like muscle cells (12,71) and therefore can influence the micromechanics of the cochlea. Recent experiments also indicate that outer hair cell contraction can be induced by efferent stimulation (14) so that the efferents would have an important monitoring function in the cochlear receptor.

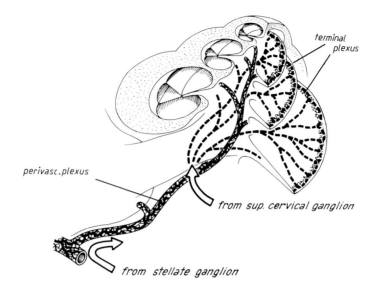

FIG. 10. Schematic representation of the autonomic nerve supply of the cochlea.

Autonomic Innervation

The presence of an autonomic nerve supply to the inner ear has always been assumed. An unequivocal demonstration has thus far been achieved only for the sympathetic or adrenergic system, which can be best identified by means of the histochemical demonstration of its specific transmitter, noradrenaline. On the other hand, cholinergic parasympathetic fibers can hardly be differentiated from somatic cholinergic fibers. In the ear they are possibly part of the olivocochlear efferent system, if they are present at all.

The best way to show adrenergic innervation is by histochemical demonstration of noradrenaline of Falck et al. (8). Using this technique, two types of adrenergic innervation are found—a perivascular and a blood vessel independent innervation (63,64) (Fig. 10).

A dense continuous perivascular adrenergic plexus exists in the adventitia of the basilar artery, the inferior anterior cerebellar artery, and the labyrinthine artery and its greater modiolar branches. Further peripherally, the perivascular network disappears and is no longer present in the osseous spiral lamina and membranous labyrinth.

On the other hand, a rich adrenergic nerve plexus is found independent of blood vessels. The most striking adrenergic nerve plexus is seen within the osseous spiral lamina in its peripheral zone, just before the habenula perforata. A large number of green fluorescent fibers with varicosities run between the other nerve, fibers independent of the blood vessels (63,64). Whether those fibers sometimes penetrate the habenula cannot be decided, but they never appear to cross the tunnel of Corti to reach the outer hair cells. Most likely, the majority of them turns before entering the habenula to form the arcades of the terminal plexus. In combined preparations of ink perfusion of the blood vessels and histochemical demonstration of noradrenaline, such a plexus of adrenergic fibers is unquestionably shown in all turns (Fig.

10). The adrenergic fibers in the osseous lamina are most conspicuous in the apical turn, where they can be followed through the entire length of the osseous spiral lamina. This seems to correspond with the special autonomic innervation of the cochlear apex described by Palumbi (36). There is, however, no adrenergic innervation in the other parts of the membranous labyrinth, especially not in the spiral ligament and stria vascularis.

In the osseous spiral lamina, the adrenergic nerve fibers run predominantly between the myelinated fibers of the cochlear neurons without any closer relation to them. In the tympanic lip, they run usually at a certain distance from the blood vessels, the wall of which consists only of endothelium and some pericytes. These adrenergic fibers are of small size and have various enlargements filled with numerous dense core vesicles of diameters between 600 and 1,200 Å. Such accumulations of dense core vesicles are typical for the adrenergic system, and they can be enhanced by the administration of 6-hydroxydopamine, which accumulates very quickly in adrenergic neurons.

The perivascular adrenergic innervation consists of several fascicles of small nerve fibers in the adventitia and a few larger myelinated nerve fibers. All these fibers have no direct contacts to the smooth muscle cells of the vessel and no definite nerve endings, so that any sympathetic influence can only occur over distance by diffusion of the transmitter noradrenaline. The fact that there are some large unmyelinated fibers indicates that fast saltatory nerve conduction is also possible in this system (55).

As shown by lesions in the cervical sympathetic chain, the adrenergic fibers of the cochlea, which are independent from blood vessels, originate in the superior cervical ganglion. The perivascular fibers, on the other hand, have their origin in the stellate ganglion from where they reach the labyrinthine artery via perivascular nerve plexus of vertebral and basilar artery. There are, therefore, two different types of adrenergic innervation of the inner ear, one strictly perivascular and the other independent from blood vessels (Fig. 10). The functional significance of both systems is not yet clear.

THE VESTIBULAR LABYRINTH

As in the cochlea, the vestibular apparatus is provided with afferent, efferent, and autonomic innervation.

Afferent Neurons

The vestibular afferent neurons that connect the vestibular sensory epithelium with the vestibular nuclei in the brain stem are bipolar neurons. The perikaryons are located in Scarpa's ganglion within the inner acoustic meatus. The vestibular nerve is divided into two major portions: (a) the superior division, innervating the lateral and superior crista, and the macula utriculi and (b) the inferior division, innervating the macula sacculi and the posterior crista via singular nerve.

The superior division is composed of approximately 12,000 neurons and the inferior division, approximately 6,500 neurons. The diameter of the nerve fibers varies from 1 to 15 μm. The ampullary nerves contain more large fibers than the macular nerves. On the basis of the size of the ganglion as well as the size and position of the nucleus, two types of neurons can be distinguished: numerous large neurons and a few small neurons. The latter contribute approximately 5% of the neural population in the superior division and 12% in the inferior division. Both types of neurons show various degrees of myelination, from entirely missing to thick myelin sheaths.

All fibers lose their myelin sheaths when they enter the sensory epithelium through the basement membrane. Above the basement membrane, they form a horizontal plexus with considerable branching before they contact the sensory cells.

Two types of sensory cells are found in the vestibular sensory epithelia: (a) The phylogenetically younger type I cells, found only in higher vertebrates, are bottle-shaped and surrounded by a nerve chalice. (b) A phylogenetically older type II cell, found in all vertebrates, is connected with 10 to 20 individual small nerve endings. Type II cells are usually associated wtih small nerve fibers and type I cells with large nerve fibers. The innervation ratio of sensory cells/nerve fiber is 2:6 for the superior cristae, 3:1 for the posterior crista, 4:6 for the macula sacculi, and 5:6 for the macula utriculi (3).

The sensory cells of the cristae obviously have a richer innervation than those in the maculae. In the cristae, there are approximately 60% type I cells, whereas in the maculae, type I and type II cells are equally represented. It is assumed that fibers innervating many hair cells show a regular spontaneous firing rate and fibers innervating only a few hair cells show an irregular activity. Most fibers from the maculae have regular discharge patterns, whereas fibers from the cristae frequently show irregular firing. Since thin fibers, innervating type II cells, have more ramifications and innervate a greater number of hair cells than thick fibers, associated with the type I cells, it is assumed that irregular firing units are type I associated fibers.

The receptoneural junction between nerve endings and type II cells are characterized by typical synaptic complexes with membrane thickening and synaptic bars of variable forms. In type I cells, there are two types of contacts between sensory cells and nerve chalice:

1. Areas with an irregular empty intercellular space with an average width of 200 Å and fusion of the unit membranes at certain spots. This type of receptoneural contact is mostly found in the supranuclear portion of the sensory cells. It is rather unspecific and resembles very much contacts between supporting cells.

2. Areas with a very regular intercellular space of 270 Å width, filled with a dense amorphous material. The dense zones are very specific for the receptoneural contacts between type I cells and nerve chalice and represent approximately 30% of the cell surface. Associated with these dense zones, one frequently finds very large synaptic bars of various forms within the cytoplasm of the sensory cell. These specific dense zones probably provide more efficient synaptic transmission and might be responsible for the degree of spontaneous activity, which is directly related to the sensitivity of the unit. The generally higher spontaneous activity of units in mammals compared with the more primitive vertebrates could be owing to the presence of type I cells in mammals.

Efferent Neurons

In type I units, the efferent endings sit exclusively at the nerve chalice with evidence of synaptic contacts. Usually, several efferent nerve endings are associated with one afferent nerve. They are never in direct contact with the sensory cell of type I. In type II units, the efferent nerve endings may contact the sensory cell directly, but even here synaptic contacts are predominantly with the afferent nerve endings and nerve fibers. Thus, in the vestibular sensory epithelium, the efferent contacts are almost exclusively axodentritic and not with the sensory cells, in contrast to the organ of Corti.

Functionally, the efferents of the vestibular system might be able to change the electrical polarization of the afferent neurons. As shown by Löwenstein (27), spontaneous activity of the afferent neurons can be changed by changing the electrical polarization. It would therefore be possible that the efferents, by changing the polarization of the afferent neurons, change the level of spontaneous activity and therefore the sensitivity of the units. Such an efferent control might be responsible, in part, for the phenomenon of vestibular adaptation (11).

Autonomic Innervation

Below the vestibular sensory epithelia, adrenergic nerve fibers can be demonstrated by the histochemical method of Falck et al. (8). They do not penetrate the basilar membrane and do not have direct contacts with the sensory cells. Also in the vestibular ganglion, numerous adrenergic nerve fibers are found. As in the cochlea, there are perivascular adrenergic fiber systems and blood-vessel-independent adrenergic nerve fibers. They seem to have the same origin as the autonomic fibers for the cochlea, where the blood-vessel-independent nerve fibers originate in the superior cervical ganglion and the perivascular fibers originate in the stellate ganglion. Nothing is known about their functional significance.

REFERENCES

1. Arnesen, A. R., and Osen, K. K. (1984): Fibre population of the vestibulocochlear anastomosis in the cat. *Acta Otolaryngol. (Stockh.)*, 98:255–269.
2. Arnold, W., and Wang, J. B. (1983): Das Spiralganglion des Rhesusaffen. *Laryngol. Rhinol. Otol. (Stuttg.)*, 62:371–377.
3. Bergström, B. (1984): The primary vestibular neurons. In: *Ultrastructural Atlas of the Inner Ear*, edited by I. Friedmann and J. Ballantyne, p. 270. Butterworth, London.
4. Bohne, B. A., Kenworthy, A., and Carr, C. D. (1982): Density of myelinated nerve fibers in the chinchilla cochlea. Abstracts for the Association for Research in Otolaryngology.
5. Desmedt, J. E., and Monaco, P. (1961): Mode of action of the efferent olivocochlear bundle on the inner ear. *Nature*, 192:1263.
6. Dunn, R. A., and Morest, D. K. (1975): Receptor synapses without synaptic ribbons in the cochlea of the cat. *Proc. Natl. Acad. Sci. USA*, 72:3599–3603.
7. Dunn-Ginzberg, R., and Morest, D. K. (1983): A study of cochlear innervation in the young cat with the Golgi method. *Hear. Res.*, 10:227–246.
8. Falck, B., Hillarp, N. A., Thieme, G., et al. (1962): Fluorescence of catecholamines and related compounds condensed with formaldehyde. *J. Histochem. Cytochem.*, 10:348.
9. Feldmann, M. (1984): Morphological observations on the cochleas of very old rats. Abstracts for the Association for Research in Otolaryngology, p. 14.
10. Fex, J. (1959): Augmentation of cochlear microphonics by stimulation of efferent fibers to the cochlea. *Acta Otolaryngol. (Stockh.)*, 50:540.
11. Flock, A. (1973): Efferent nerve fibers: Postsynaptic action on hair cells. *Nature (New Biology)*, 243:124–189.
12. Flock, A. (1986): Mechanical properties of hair cells. *Hear. Res.*, 22:293.
13. Galambos, R. G. (1956): Suppression of auditory nerve activity by stimulation of efferent fibers to cochlea. *J. Neurophysiol.*, 19:424–437.

14. Guinan, J. J., Jr. (1986): Effect of efferent neural activity on cochlear mechanics. *Scand. Audiol.* [*Suppl.*], 25.
15. Hall, J. G. (1966): Hearing and primary auditory centers of the whales. *Acta Otolaryngol.* [*Suppl.*] (*Stockh.*), 224:224–250.
16. Henson, O. W., Jr., Jenkins, D. B., and Henson, M. M. (1982): The intercellular relationships and ultrastructural features of the cells of Boettcher. Abstracts for the Association for Research in Otolaryngology, p. 24.
17. Iurato, S. (1962): Efferent fibers to the sensory cells of Corti's organ. *Exp. Cell Res.*, 27:162–164.
18. Iurato, S. (1964): Fibre efferenti dirette e crociate alle cellule acustiche dell'Organo del Corti. *Monit. Zool. Ital.* [*Suppl.*], 72:62–63.
19. Iurato, S., et al. (1978): Distribution of the crossed olivocochlear bundle in the chinchilla's cochlea. *J. Comp. Neurol.*, 182:57–76.
20. Kellerhals, B., Engström, H., and Ades, H. W. (1967): Die Morphologie des Ganglion spirale cochleae. *Acta Otolaryngol.* [*Suppl.*] (*Stockh.*), 226:1–78.
21. Kiang, N. Y. S., Rho, J. M., Northrup, C. C., et al. (1982): Hair cell innervation by spiral ganglion cells in adult cats. *Science*, 217:9.
22. Kimura, R. S., and Ota, C. Y. (1981): Nerve fibers synapses on primate spiral ganglion. Abstracts for the Association for Research in Otolaryngology, p. 82.
23. Leak-Jones, P. A., and Snyder, R. L. (1982): Uptake transport of horseradish peroxidase by cochlear spiral ganglion neurons. *Hear. Res.*, 8:199–223.
24. Liberman, M. C. (1980): Efferent synapses in the inner hair cell area of the cat cochlea: An electron microscopic study of serial sections. *Hear. Res.*, 3:289–304.
25. Liberman, M. C. (1982): Single neuron labeling in the cat auditory nerve. *Science*, 216:1239–1241.
26. Liberman, M. C., and Brown, M. C. (1986): Physiology and anatomy of single olivocochlear neurons in the cat. *Hear. Res.*, 24:17–36.
27. Löwenstein, O. (1956): Peripheral mechanisms of equilibrium. *Br. Med. Bull.*, 12:2–114.
28. Morest, D. K. (1982): Retrograde axonal transport of D-aspartate from cochlear nucleus to type II spiral ganglion cells in the cat. Abstracts for the Association for Research in Otolaryngology, p. 90.
29. Morrison, D., Schindler, R. A., and Wersäll, J. (1975): Quantitative analysis of the afferent innervation of the organ of Corti in guinea pig. *Acta Otolaryngol. (Stockh.)*, 79:11–23.
30. Nadol, J. B. (1981): Reciprocal synapses at the base of outer hair cells in the organ of Corti. *Ann. Otol. Rhinol. Laryngol.*, 90:12–17.
31. Nadol, J. B. (1983): Serial section reconstruction of the neural poles of hair cells in the human organ of Corti: I. Inner hair cells. *Laryngoscope*, 93:599.
32. Nadol, J. B. (1984): Incidence of reciprocal synapses on outer hair cells of the human organ of Corti. *Ann. Otol. Rhinol. Laryngol.*, 93:247–250.
33. Nomura, Y. (1976): Nerve fibers in the human organ of Corti. *Acta Otolaryngol. (Stockh.)*, 82:317–324.
34. Ota, C. Y., and Kimura, R. S. (1980): Ultrastructural study of the human spiral ganglion. *Acta Otolaryngol. (Stockh.)*, 89:53.
35. Otte, J., Schuknecht, H. F., and Kerr, A. G. (1978): Ganglion cell populations in normal and pathological human cochleae: Implication for cochlear implantation. *Laryngoscope*, 88:1231.
36. Palumbi, G. (1950): Particolare apparato nervoso recettore nella regione apicale della chiocciola dell'orechio humano. *Boll. Soc. Ital. Biol. Sper.*, 26:136.
37. Pfaltz, R. K. J.: Absence of a function for the cross olivocochlear bundle under physiological conditions. *Arch. Klin. Exp. Ohr. Nas. Kehlk. Heilk.*, 193:89–100.
38. Rasmussen, G. L. (1942): An efferent cochlear bundle. *Anat. Rec.*, 82:441.
39. Rasmussen, G. L. (1946): The olivary peduncle and other fiber projections of the superior olivary complex. *J. Comp. Neurol.*, 84:141–219.
40. Robertson, D. (1985): Brainstem location of efferent neurons projecting to the guinea pig cochlea. *Hear. Res.*, 20:79–84.
41. Rodrigues, E. E. L. (1967): An electron microscopic study on the cochlear innervation: I. The receptoneural junctions at the outer hair cells. *Z. Zellforsch.*, 78:30–46.
42. Romand, R., and Romand, M. R. (1984): The otogenesis of pseudomonopolar cells in spiral ganglion of cat and rat. *Acta Otolaryngol. (Stockh.)*, 97:239–249.
42a. Ruggero, M. A., Santi, P. A., and Rich, N. C. (1982): Type II cochlear ganglion cells in the chinchilla. *Hear. Res.*, 8:339–356.
43. Ryan, A. F., and Schwartz, I. R. (1983): Preferential amino acid uptake identifies type II spiral ganglion neurons in the gerbil. *Hear. Res.*, 9:173–194.
44. Sando, I. (1965): The anatomical interrelationships of the cochlear nerve fibers. *Acta Otolaryngol. (Stockh.)*, 59:417.
45. Schuknecht, H. F. (1962): Neuroanatomical correlates of auditory sensitivity and pitch discrimination in the cat. In: *Neural Mechanisms of the Auditory and Vestibular Systems*. Rasmussen and Windle, Springfield, IL.

46. Smith, C. A. (1975): Innervation of the cochlea of the guinea pig by use of the Golgi stain. *Ann. Otol. Rhinol. Laryngol.*, 84:443.
47. Smith, C. A., and Rasmussen, G. L. (1963): Recent observations on the olivocochlear bundles. *Ann. Otol. Rhinol. Laryngol.*, 78:489–506.
48. Smith, C. A., and Rasmussen, G. L. (1965): Degeneration in the afferent nerve endings in the cochlea after axonal section. *J. Cell Biol.*, 26:63–77.
49. Spoendlin, H. (1966): The organization of the cochlear receptor. *Adv. Otorhinolaryngol.*, 13:1–231.
50. Spoendlin, H. (1968): Ultrastructure and peripheral innervation pattern of the receptor in relation to the first coding of the acoustic message. In: *Hearing Mechanisms in Vertebrates*, edited by A. V. S. DeReuck and J. Knight, pp. 89–119. Churchill, London.
51. Spoendlin, H. (1969): Innervation patterns in the organ of Corti of the cat. *Acta Otolaryngol. (Stockh.)*, 67:239–254.
52. Spoendlin, H. (1970): Structural basis of peripheral frequency analysis. In: *Frequency Analysis and Periodicity Detection in Hearing*, edited by R. Plomp and F. G. Smoorenbur, pp. 2–36. Sijthoff, Leiden.
53. Spoendlin, H. (1971): Degeneration behavior of the cochlear nerve. *Arch. Klin. Exp. Ohr. Nas. Kehlk. Heilk.*, 200:275–291.
54. Spoendlin, H. (1972): Innervation densities of the cochlea. *Acta Otolaryngol. (Stockh.)*, 73:235–248.
55. Spoendlin, H. (1973): Autonomic nerve supply to the inner ear. In: *Vascular Disorders and Hearing Defects*, edited by Darin de Lorenzo, pp. 93–111. University Park Press, Baltimore.
56. Spoendlin, H. (1979): Neural connections of the outer hair cell system. *Acta Otolaryngol. (Stockh.)*, 87:381–387.
57. Spoendlin, H. (1981): Autonomic innervation of the inner ear. *Adv. Otorhinolaryngol.*, 27:1–13.
58. Spoendlin, H. (1981): Differentiation of cochlear afferent neurons. *Acta Otolaryngol. (Stockh.)*, 91:451–456.
59. Spoendlin, H. (1981): HRP-studies on primary cochlear neurons. Poster Inner Ear Biology Workshop, Montpellier.
60. Spoendlin, H. (1982): The innervation of the outer hair cell system. *Am. J. Otol.*, 3:274–278.
61. Spoendlin, H. (1984): Efferent innervation of the cochlea. In: *Comparative Physiology of Sensory Systems*, edited by L. Bolis, R. D. Keynes, and S. H. P. Maddrell, pp. 163–188. Cambridge University Press.
62. Spoendlin, H., and Baumgartner, H. (1977): Electrocochleographic and cochlear pathology. *Acta Otolaryngol. (Stockh.)*, 83:130–135.
63. Spoendlin, H., and Lichtensteiger, W. (1966): The adrenergic innervation of the labyrinth. *Acta Otolaryngol. (Stockh.)*, 61:423–434.
64. Spoendlin, H., and Lichtensteiger, W. (1967): The sympathetic nerve supply to the inner ear. *Arch. Klin. Exp. Ohr. Nas. Kehlk. Heilk.*, 189:346.
65. Strutz, J. (1983): Der Ursprung der akustischen und vestibulären Efferenz bei Vertebraten. Habilitationsschrift, Universität Freiburg.
66. Takasaka, T., Shinkawa, H., Watanuki, K., et al. (1983): High-voltage electron microscopic study of the inner ear. *Ann. Otol. Rhinol. Laryngol.*, 92(Suppl. 101):1–12.
67. Warr, W. B. (1975): Olivocochlear and vestibular efferent neurons of the feline brainstem: Their location, morphology and number determined by retrograde axonal transport and acetylcholinesterase histochemistry. *J. Comp. Neurol.*, 161:159–182.
68. Warr, W. B. (1978): The olivocochlear bundle: Its origins and terminations in the cat. In: *Evoked Electrical Activity in the Auditory Nervous System*, edited by N. F. Naunton and C. Fernandez, pp. 43–65. Academic Press, New York.
69. Warr, W. B., and Guinan, J. J., Jr. (1979): Efferent innervation of the organ of Corti: Two separate systems. *Brain Res.*, 173:152–155.
70. Wright, C. G., and Preston, R. E.: Degeneration and distribution of efferent fibers in the guinea pig organ of Corti. A light and scanning microscopic study. *Brain Res.*, 58:37–59.
71. Zenner, H. P. (1985): Motile responses in outer hair cells. *Hear. Res.*, 22:83–90.

Physiology of the Ear,
edited by A. F. Jahn and J. Santos-Sacchi.
Raven Press, New York © 1988.

Structural and Functional Development of the Ear

Joseph R. McPhee and Thomas R. Van De Water

Laboratory of Developmental Otobiology, Albert Einstein College of Medicine, Bronx, New York 10461

The ear is one of the first sensory structures to appear in the developing embryo. The initial step in the formation of the inner ear occurs in the human during the third week of gestation as a thickening of the surface ectoderm lying adjacent to the rhombencephalon. This otic placode then invaginates to form first an otic cup (27 days in the human) and later, separating from the surface ectoderm, a fluid-filled vesicle, the otocyst. At this stage there is little evidence of the formation of any other related outer or middle ear structures. However, shortly thereafter, through the condensation and thickening of surrounding cephalic mesenchyme, migration of the neural crest from the rhombencephalon, and the outpocketing of endodermal tissue from the primitive pharynx, the complex structures of the external and middle ear begin to form. By the fifth month in human embryonic development, most of the features that will persist throughout the life of the individual have almost completely formed. The developmental process that brings this about consists of a series of interactions involving all three embryonic germ layers including neural crest cells. A fairly complete review of the developmental anatomy of the external and middle ear can be found in the papers of Anson et al. (3,5,6) and in the reviews of Jaskol and Maderson (22) and Rubel (40). Only minor additions to the already extensive body of research on these parts of the ear have been made since these reviews have been published. On the other hand, research on the development of the inner ear has continued intensively, particularly with regard to the sensory structures of the cochlea and vestibular apparatus. The one factor that appears to underlie all that we will discuss here is the myriad number of inductive interactions that must be carefully regulated and timed to produce normally functioning acoustic and vestibular senses. Many of the recent discoveries concerning inner ear development focus on these interactions.

THE OUTER EAR

The outer ear consists of the auricle (pinna), external acoustic meatus (external ear canal), the cuticular and fibrous layers of the tympanic membrane. These structures arise from contributions of the first (Meckel's or mandibular) and second (Reichert's or hyoid) branchial arches, which are located posterior to the developing mandible and inferior to the squama of the temporal bone.

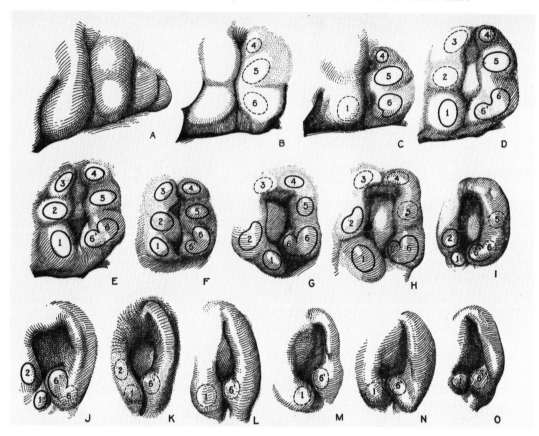

FIG. 1. Illustrations **A** through **O** represent the stages of derivation of the human auricle from components of the mandibular and hyoid arches. Numbers indicate the presumptive (*dashed circles*) and actual (*solid circles*) hillocks first noted by His and later interpreted by Streeter as transitory condensations of mesenchymal primordium of the auricle. A to C, embryos 5 to 11 mm (4–5 weeks); D to G, embryos 13 to 14 mm (6 weeks); H to K, embryos 15 to 18 mm (6.5 weeks); L to O, embryos 18 to 33 mm (7–8 weeks). (From ref. 54.)

The auricle develops from a mixed population of neural crest cells and mesenchyme contained within the first and second branchial arches (Fig. 1). Both arches contribute to the development of six separate prominences or hillocks, three from each arch (20). Streeter (54) has suggested that not too much significance should be placed on these hillocks because of their apparent transitory nature. These hillocks, he states, reorganize to form a posterior portion derived from the second branchial arch and an anterior portion from the first branchial arch. In either case, the posterior portion gives rise to the auricle, whereas the anterior portion forms the tragus (54).

As fetal development continues, the external ear changes its position with respect to the other craniofacial features, moving from a region lateral to the hyoid bone to a more superior and lateral position. This process occurs as a result of mandibular enlargement and lateralization of the temporal bone. Malformation of the craniofacial skeleton can therefore result in considerable displacement of both the pinna and external auditory meatus, as is observed in the congenital micrognathia of Robin's anomaly (38) and other temporomandibular malformation syndromes. In addition,

Smith and Takashima (51,52) have found that the formation of the characteristic plicae of the auricle can be attributed, to a considerable extent, to the normal organogenesis of the auricular muscles. These muscles, although relatively inactive in the adult, can be shown, when defective, to be responsible for producing many of the observed congenital auricular anomalies. Chiu et al. (11) denervated the auricle of postnatal rats and found the resultant auricles to be totally lacking in normal plicae. Smith and Takashima (51) were able to show that one form of protruding auricle was the result of a posterior auricular muscle defect and later that lop ear syndrome can result from a defect of the superior auricularis muscle. Both the auricle and tragus are fully formed by the 28th week of development in the human, although both continue to increase in size until about the ninth year of postnatal development (36). As a result, subsequent disturbances in the postnatal continuation of pinna growth can result in microtia.

The external acoustic meatus forms by 8 weeks gestation in the human as a result of an invagination and ingrowth of ectodermal and mesenchymal components of the first branchial cleft (Fig. 2). Many drugs, including streptomycin (23), the salicylates (56), and thalidomide (25), can result in agenesis or atresia of both the pinna and external auditory meatus if administered during the first trimester. Apposing peridermal surfaces of the invaginating first branchial cleft ectoderm are forced together into what appears as a single strand of epithelial cells (meatal plate) that terminates in a disk-like swelling near the ventral wall of the developing tympanic cavity. These two ectodermal layers later separate to form the cuticular portion of the tympanum and the walls of the external acoustic meatus (16.5 weeks gestation in the human). At 28 weeks the separation of the layers of cells forming the meatal plate produces a lumen that becomes a medial extension of the lumen of the primary external acoustic meatus. Subsequent fetal development consists of continued enlargement of this meatus (4). The proper position of the external meatal opening is on a line extending laterally from the ala nasi of the head in normal anatomical position. At birth, the wall of the meatus is supported by a thin layer of cartilage that is extremely compliant. Ossification does not take place until the 11th month when the ossified tympanic ring finally fuses with the proximal bony walls of the meatus (5). Rubel (42) reported that the persistence of a cartilaginous wall in the meatus probably contributes only minimally to limiting the auditory capacity of the neonates, since most of the transmission effect will be on high frequencies that are the last to develop in the neurosensory structures of the cochlea. The canal is approximately 22 mm long in the newborn and has a narrower and more oval shape than is observed in the adult (32). Growth and development of the canal continue through the seventh year when it attains its maximum length of 25 to 27 mm (63).

The development of the cuticular and fibrous portion of the tympanum and its associated tympanic ring was reported in detail by Anson et al. (6). Briefly, the tympanic ring first appears at about the eighth week of human fetal development as a region of mesenchymal condensation, just inferior to Meckel's cartilage of the second branchial arch. The ring then forms a number of ossification centers over the next 2.5 weeks and shifts its position to a region lying between the first and second branchial arches, just deep to the developing pinna and closely associated on its deep surface with the head of the developing malleus. By 16.5 weeks, the manubrium of the malleus has attached itself to the fibrous stratum of the three-layered tympanic membrane [the cuticular portion having been derived from the

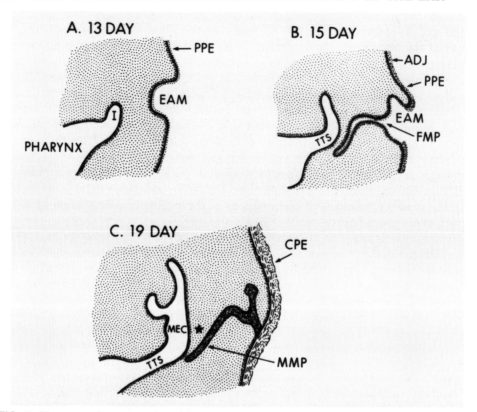

FIG. 2. Diagrammatic presentation of the development of the external auditory meatus and meatal plate in a 13-day-old (**A**), 15-day-old (**B**), and 19-day-old (**C**) mouse embryo. Initially (A), the epidermal histology of the adjacent, nonotic skin (ADJ) is the same as that lining the external auditory meatus (EAM) and over the presumptive pinnal tissues (PPE). By the 15th day (B), the tubotympanic sulcus (TTS) has grown dorsally as an outpocketing of the pharyngeal pouch (I); its endodermal lining approaches the presumptive meatal plate (FMP). By 19 days, the lumen of the external meatus and the enlarged meatal plate (MMP) have become completely occluded. The epidermis of the pinna and the adjacent skin show the first signs of cornification [cornified peridermal epithelium (CPE)]. The *starred area* indicates the approximate location of the presumptive tympanic tissues that lie between the meatal plate and the developing middle ear cavity (MEC).

ectodermal plate that forms the external acoustic meatus, the fibrous layer from cephalic mesenchyme, and the mucosal layer from the epithelial (endoderm) lining of the tympanic cavity]. At 18.5 weeks, ossification of the ring is complete, although osteoblastic activity continues throughout its structure. At 19 weeks, the shape of the ring has become truly annular with a sulcate groove forming along its interior border where the tympanic membrane will attach itself, although still remaining free at this time. At 35 weeks, the ring has achieved a size of 9.5 mm in diameter (compared with 9.75–10.00 mm at term). A deficiency in the ring persists that later becomes the incisura tympanica where the attachment of the pars flaccida segment of the tympanum occurs. Most of the ring at this stage is still not attached to the surrounding temporal bone. Only the posterolateral segment has fused. Final fusion of the ring to the temporal bone occurs at term with continued outgrowth of bone occurring over the next 11 months, joining the ossifying wall of the external acoustic meatus and forming a portion of its ventral wall. The tympanum of the newborn is not as responsive to higher frequencies as it is in the adult. During the first 3 months, the admittance of the neonatal tympanum increases, indicating continued maturation of the tympanum (41).

THE MIDDLE EAR

The middle ear includes the mucosal layer of the tympanum, ossicular chain with accompanying muscular and connective tissue structures, tympanic cavity, auditory (eustachian or pharyngotympanic) tube and the middle ear cleft. The auditory tube and tympanic cavity are endodermal in origin, whereas the ossicular chain and associated structures form from cephalic mesenchyme (including neural crest) that surrounds the pouch. The mucosal layer of the tympanum is also derived from the endoderm of the first pharyngeal pouch (Fig. 2). The tympanic cavity and auditory tube form together as an outpocketing of the first pharyngeal pouch. As a result, the entire tympanic cavity is lined with endoderm-derived epithelium. The pharyngeal pouch itself forms during the third and fourth weeks of human embryonic development. By the 10th week, this outpocketing, called the tubotympanic sulcus, approaches the distal portion of the first branchial cleft (anlage of the external acoustic meatus). The expanded terminal portion of the tube remains narrow and slit-like until the fifth month of fetal development. As it expands, the enveloping membrane is converted into true, ciliated epithelium. During the sixth month, the developing ossicles are incorporated into the enlarging cavity, each ossicle enclosed in its own layer of tympanic epithelium. The clearing and pneumatization of the tympanic cavity does not occur until the eighth and ninth months. In their studies, Jaskoll and Maderson (22) reported that clearance of the tympanic cavity in mammals is primarily the result of programed cell necrosis. Shimizu et al. (48) have stated that the formation of the tympanic cavity is derived from a number of interacting processes including the epithelial invasion of the auditory tube, resorption of fetal connective tissue, thinning of the adjacent wall of the otic capsule, outward proliferation of the temporal bone owing to cartilaginous and fibrous bone formation, and active bone formation of the mastoid cavity.

It has long been held that the ossicular chain forms from the mesenchyme of the first and second branchial arches with the malleus and incus being derived wholly from the first arch and the stapes, with the exception of its footplate, being derived from tissue of the second arch. However, a second, more recently proposed theory (6,19) states that only the head of the malleus and the body of the incus are of first arch origin; whereas the manubrium of the malleus, the long process of the incus, and the superstructure of the stapes are of second arch origin (Fig. 3). Studies of genetic disorders seem to favor this latter theory over the earlier one, since malformation of the stapes usually involves the long crus of the incus (6). Initially, the ossicles are poorly defined with only vague separations between them. They first appear in the sixth week of human embryonic development as condensations of mesenchyme and rapidly chondrify over the next 2 weeks.

As chondrification progresses, the outlines of the malleus, incus, and stapes become progressively more distinct, with the primordial manubrium of the malleus and the long crus of the incus readily apparent. The stapes is already juxtaposed with the developing oval window of the otic capsule. As stated earlier, the stapes is formed from both the second branchial arch tissue [head, crura and stapedial

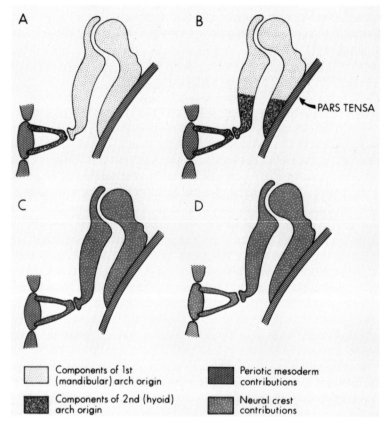

FIG. 3. Diagrammatic presentation of various theories of the embryonic origin of the ossicular chain in mammals. **A** shows the oldest theory, which states that the malleus and incus are derived completely from contributions of the mandibular arch. **B** is the alternate theory, which suggests that only portions of malleus and incus are derived from mandibular arch tissue. **C** and **D** illustrate two alternate theories regarding the migration and incorporation of neural crest cells into the ossicles, including or not including the stapedial footplate.

footplate (partial)] and the mesodermal mesenchyme of the developing otic capsule [stapedial footplate (partial)]. Perhaps this heterologous origin of the stapes is reflected in DiGeorge malformation complex, a congenital malformation that is partially manifested by the failure of embryonic development associated with the third and fourth branchial arch. This failure, in many instances, also produces a stapes that has a completely formed head and crus but entirely lacks the formation of a footplate (39).

Ossification of the ossicular chain begins at approximately 16 weeks and continues throughout the remainder of fetal development. Adult size of the ossicles is achieved by the fifth month of development. Prior to this, the borders of the stapedial footplate form the annular ligament, a flexible fibrous connective tissue attachment to the rest of the otic capsule. A branch of the fetal circulation, the stapedial artery passes through the obturator foramen of the stapes during early development. This vessel sists in the adult mouse and as an anomalous structure in some humans, apparently without affecting the normal function of either the stapes or oval window. The persistence of this vascular structure in humans has been known to occur in certain genetic abnormalities such as trisomy 13 (45). The formation of the annular ligament is critical to the function of the stapes. Failure of the ligament to form properly can result in fixation of the stapedial footplate during the ossification of the bony labyrinth. This type of malformation is associated with a number of anomalies (47).

The tympanic tensor muscle is derived from the first branchial arch and the stapedius muscle from the second branchial arch. By 8 weeks, the mesenchymal tissue that will give rise to each of these middle ear muscles can be identified. At the end of the 16th week, these muscles and their tendons are morphologically distinct.

THE INNER EAR

The inner ear is derived from the thickened surface ectoderm that formed the otic placode. After the invagination and vesiculation of this primordial structure to form the otocyst, the latter elongates dorsoventrally to form a dorsal vestibular (pars superior) portion and a ventral cochlear (pars inferior) portion. The intermediate region gives rise to the utricle and saccule (29). One of the earliest recognizable structures to develop at this initial stage is the anlage of the endolymphatic duct. At first, the duct appears as a short finger-like extension of the dorsomedial surface of the otocyst. Later, the duct extends a considerable distance from the developing inner ear, ending in a large pouch, the future endolymphatic sac. During the early stages of fetal development the duct and pouch extend straight out from the inner ear. The curving of the duct occurs only during the later stages of fetal development and continues during postnatal development until it achieves an angle of 30° to 60° downward. At 5 weeks, the pars superior (vestibular) portion of the otocyst produces two ridge-like structures that, over the next 2 weeks, form the semicircular ducts. At the same time, the pars inferior (cochlear) portion begins to elongate and curl in on itself. At approximately 8 weeks this cochlear duct has coiled on itself one full revolution; at 10 weeks, two revolutions; and at 25 weeks, the duct has completed approximately 2½ turns and has virtually achieved adult size and shape. The proximal narrowing (ductus reuniens) of the cochlear duct where it communicates with the saccule becomes progressively more attenuated during this period of cochlear development (5).

The bony labyrinth first appears as a condensation of mesodermal mesenchyme in the periotic region (6 weeks gestation in the human). This condensed mesenchyme has the ability to synthesize the necessary extracellular matrix components *in situ* for the formation of a fully chondrified, otic capsule (8 weeks gestation) that serves as a template for the subsequent formation of the bony labyrinth (Fig. 4). There is evidence that the developing otocyst plays an important role in the induction and subsequent morphogenesis of its capsule (33,34). Experiments in embryonic mice have indicated that both the chondrogenesis of the capsule and its eventual shape are dependent on the presence and normal development of the neuroectodermal otocyst. Studies on genetic mutant mice (18,44,61) have confirmed this. Consequently, factors that influence the normal development of the neuroepithelial structures of the otocyst can have a significant influence on those structures derived from the capsule, i.e., the bony labyrinth and stapedial footplate. Conversely, abnormal capsule development can adversely affect the development of the sensory structures of the inner ear (59). The cartilaginous capsule persists in its entirety until the 16th week of fetal development, at which point a small portion of the capsule begins to

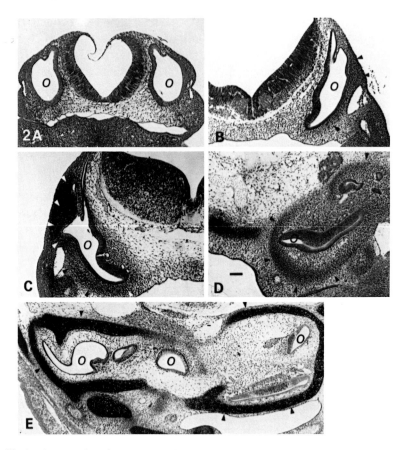

FIG. 4. Photomicrographs of a cross section of the head of a mouse embryo at 11 days (**A**), 12 days (**B**), 13 days (**C**), 14 days (**D**), and 16 days (**E**) of gestation. The developing otocyst (O) undergoes a series of complex morphogenetic stages as the periotic mesenchyme first condenses (*arrows* in B and C) and later chondrifies (*arrows* in D and E). Note the close contouring of the cartilaginous capsule around the otocyst in E, particularly around the semicircular duct on the left-hand side. Ossification begins shortly after 16 days, using the cartilaginous capsule as a template.

ossify, first in the region at the base of the cochlea and utriculus and later in the distal portion of the cochlea, and lastly in the region of the semicircular canals. The pattern of ossification appears to be related to the pattern of membranous labyrinth development in achieving adult size. Final ossification occurs at 23 weeks.

Bone formation is carried out in an unusual manner in the otic capsule. An outer periosteal layer, a middle endochondral, spicular layer, and an inner periosteal layer appear to develop almost independently of each other. The outer layer has the most normal structure, closely resembling the periosteum of long bones. The inner layer is abnormally thin and poorly developed. The middle layer retains much of the original capsule cartilage (globular ossei) in a partially calcified form. Surrounding it are regions of true endochondral bone that have replaced the capsule cartilage. This combination of intrachondral and endochondral bone is unique to the bony labyrinth (5) and perhaps is the cause of highly localized formation of otosclerotic lesions in this tissue and that of the incompletely ossified structures surrounding the

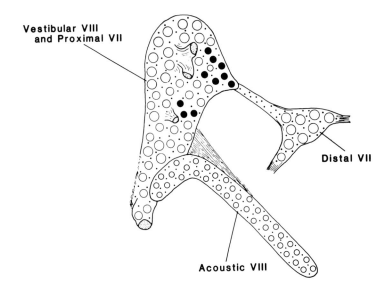

FIG. 5. A diagrammatic reconstruction of the right VIIth and VIIIth cranial nerve ganglion complex of a 12-day-old chick embryo, indicating the tissue origins of the neurons, satellite cells, and Schwann sheath cells. These results are based on orthotopic transplantation of neural crest cells from quail embryos to chick embryo host. (○), placodal neurons; (●), neural crest neurons;⋮, neural crest satellite cells and Schwann cells. (Reproduced with the permission of D. Noden.)

stapedial footplate (in particular, the fissula ante fenestrum and fissula post fenestrum).

The statoacoustic ganglion develops as an aggregation of cells medial and rostral to the otocyst. The neurons that arise from this placodally derived tissue originate primarily from a portion of the medial wall of the otocyst that will later form the macula utriculus (59). This initial cluster of neurons has been found to consist of two different portions, a lateral portion located close to the developing geniculate ganglion, composed of large cells and demonstrating significant alkaline phosphatase activity, and a medial portion composed of smaller cells that does not exhibit any alkaline phosphatase reactivity. Bretos (9) reported that the former cells eventually migrate and form both the partes magnocellulares of the vestibular ganglion and the spiral ganglion of the cochlea. The smaller cells from the medial portion of the developing statoacoustic ganglion eventually form the partes parvocellulares of the vestibular ganglion. In general, the neurons of the statoacoustic ganglion are markedly smaller in size (6–10 μm versus 12–20 μm) than other placode-derived cranial afferent ganglia such as the distal trigeminal (V), geniculate (VII), and petrosal (IX) ganglia. Also, their period of terminal mitoses extends through a later stage of incubation (7 days versus 5 days for other ganglia in the chick). D'Amico-Martel and Noden (14), using chick/quail chimeras, reported that neural crest cells invade the toacoustic ganglion at an early stage, extending along the branches of the VIIIth cranial nerve to the brain stem, crista ampullaris, and macula utriculus as prospective Schwann cells. One or two small clusters of crest-derived neurons remain within the statoacoustic ganglion, perhaps contributing to the vestibular afferent network (Fig. 5).

The sensory structures of the inner ear are derived from the same neuroectoderm that gives rise to the statoacoustic ganglion and the membranous labyrinth. In the utricle, beginning in the seventh to the eighth week, the maculae form from the inner neuroepithelial lining. Within these developing maculae two basic cell types form. One form, the supporting cells, produces a gelatinous substance that forms the otolithic membrane that overlies the sensory epithelium and contains numerous calcareous deposits, the otoconia (Fig. 6). The second, the sensory cells, produces tufts of sensory hairs (stereocilia) at their luminal surface and are invaded around their bases by ingrowing dendrites from the statoacoustic ganglion. The sensory cells, in turn, are separated into types I and II based on the morphology of their sensory hairs and patterns of innervation. Type I sensory cells produce one extremely long kinocilium and very tall stereocilia that extend up through the gelatinous otoconial layer with their cell bodies enveloped by calyx-type nerve endings, whereas type II sensory cells only produce short sensory hairs and are contacted by button-type nerve endings at their bases (Fig. 6). Type I cells are found mostly in the central zone and innervated mainly by thick fibers and are static receptors (displacement of cupula) with a regular discharge pattern. Type II cells, found mainly in the peripheral zone, are innervated by small fibers and are dynamic receptors (movement of endolymph) with an irregular discharge pattern. In the mouse (31), at a very early stage of cytodifferentiation, these developing sensory cells have been observed to form a regular pattern of microvilli covering the site of future hair-cell formation. Some of these microvilli become short, transitional stereocilia that initially number about 200. Only approximately 60 of these microvilli complete their development into fully mature stereocilia having an organ pipe arrangement oriented toward the kinocilium. The vestibular sensory epithelia have a mature configuration in the mouse at about 6 to 14 days post-natally. However, types I (tall cilia) and II (short cilia) sensory cells in mouse vestibular sensory organs can be distinguished as early as gestation day 16 in the mouse (approximately 8 weeks gestation in the human), based on the surface morphology of their sensory hairs. In the human, the superficial appearance of the maculae is similar to that seen in the adult by the 14th to the 16th week of gestation. Apparently the differentiation of these sensory cell types is intrinsic and not under the influence of the ingrowing nerve fibers since synaptic contacts do not occur in the mouse embryo until about 17 days of gestation (55), 24 hours after their differentiation is apparent. Sans and Chat (46) analyzed the temporal and spatial patterns of the terminal mitoses of types I and II hair cells in both macula and crista. They observed that these two types of sensory cells are produced on different days of gestation and their differentiation does not appear to result from the influences of different neuronal contacts.

Although much of the innervation and differentiation is completed early in fetal development, both the crista and the macula utriculus undergo continued development post-natally. In the rat (24), the cristae change their shape and increase in size as late as 13 days post-natally and the utricle undergoes major morphological changes as late as 32 days postnatally. Cristae hair bundles are less developed than those of the maculae utriculi on postnatal day 1 (rat), with evidence of ciliogenesis still present in the cristae. Hair-bundle length increases in both organs with maximum length achieved by postnatal day 32. These observations are in correspondence with the studies by Killackey and Belford (24), which have shown that rat afferent neurons have immature response characteristics at birth, exhibiting only slow, irregular spon-

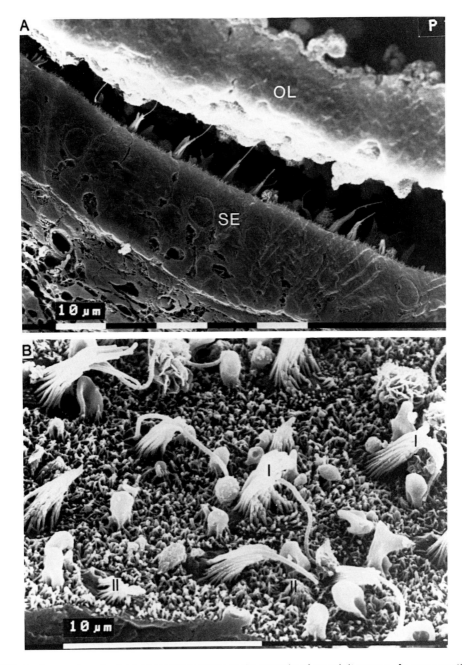

FIG. 6. A scanning electron photomicrograph of the macula of an adult mouse. **A**: cross section through the macula with the otolithic layer (OL) and sensory epithelial layer (SE) indicated. Note the sensory hairs extending up into the otolithic layer. **B**: the arrangement of types I and II sensory hairs and hair cells on the macular surface. Note the single, long kinocilium in each of the type I bundles. (Reproduced with the permission of D. Lim.)

taneous activity. Mature responses are first detected 4 to 5 days post-natally and increase to full mature response by 22 days post-natally.

Development of the otoconia is somewhat variable from species to species. In the mouse, otoconia form before the gelatinous otoconial membrane. In the rat, the otoconia are formed in the amorphous otoconial membrane material itself, similar to what has been observed in the human. It has been hypothesized that certain proteins in the otoconial membrane facilitate the formation of the otoconia by binding calcium. Using energy dispersive X-ray microanalysis, Anniko (1) reported an accumulation of calcium occurring in the apical part of the epithelium of the maculae utriculi as early as the 16th gestation day in the mouse and saturating the organic matrix during otoconial formation. No such accumulation was observed in the otolithic membrane of adult mice.

The cristae ampullaris form from the epithelial lining of the ampullar swelling at the base of each of the semicircular canals. They first appear in the human embryo as localized thickenings of the sensory epithelium at about 8 weeks gestation. The cells forming the crista are also differentiable into two basic types, supporting and sensory. Their development and function are similar to that seen in the maculae. Each of the sensory cells is eventually connected to a dendrite of one of the ampullary branches of the vestibular nerve. In the development of the vestibular apparatus in the mouse (31), the cupula first appears as a thin amorphous membrane that later becomes compact and fibrous as its mass increases. By 6 days of postnatal development, well-developed cupular canals are present in the cupullary membrane. These canals also have been observed in the cupula of the human. In the central zone of the crista, the tall stereociliary bundles are in contact with a part of the cupular canal wall, but short stereociliary bundles are freestanding in the subcupular space. This insertion of the tall ciliary bundles into the cupular canals with shorter ones remaining freestanding also has been observed in human fetal specimens (55). In the periphery of the crista, the cupular canals are smaller and disappear altogether at the extreme periphery. Consequently, only the tall ciliary bundles are in direct contact with the cupula. Cupular material is largely secreted by the supporting cells of the sensory epithelium and the transitional cells of the crista ampullaris (31). In human embryos (16) as late as 7 weeks, no receptor surfaces were delineated and only scattered, poorly formed hair bundles could be seen. Between the 7th and 8th weeks, the receptors began to appear with fairly well-established surfaces in both the utricular macula and cristae. The sensory surface areas not occupied by hair bundles during this period were found to be covered with numerous microvilli, which persisted through the 14th week. By 23 weeks gestation (human), the cristae have attained adult form (16).

Anniko and Hultcrantz (2,21) studied the effects of prenatal gamma-irradiation on mouse inner ear development and found that exposure of the mother to 50 to 200 rad during the 12- to 13-day period of gestation resulted in malformed cristae ampullaris and maculae utriculi. The cuticular plate of the sensory cell was defective as were the sensory hairs with numerous fusions. The efferent nerve endings were reduced in number but had a normal ultrastructure when observed 1 to 2 months post-natally. The most severe damage to otoconia occurred when irradiation took place on the 16th day of gestation with many otoconia malformed and disarrayed. Hair-cell damage was also variable, with type I hair cells proving to be far more susceptible than type II hair cells. These authors concluded that low-dose irradiation of undifferentiated cells at different stages of development would result in a number of abnormalities that were related to the stage of development at which the exposure to radiation occurred. Their results further corroborate the observation of early hair-cell differentiation, since the variation in susceptibility of types I and II cells could only occur if those cell types had already differentiated at the time of exposure. These results also suggest an early critical stage for the formation of the otoconia, occurring shortly after the sensory and support cells have differentiated.

The sensory receptor of the cochlear duct is derived from placodal ectoderm. Starting at about the eighth week of human fetal development, the thickened posterolateral wall of the developing cochlear duct begins to differentiate. At the same time, regions adjoining this duct begin to form both the scala vestibuli and scala tympani. These latter structures impinge on the scala media of the cochlear duct, forcing it into a more triangular shape by 16 weeks. Fusion of the anterior wall of the scala media with the scala vestibuli forms the vestibular (Reissner's) membrane; fusion of the posterior wall of the scala media with the scala tympani forms the basilar membrane. This completes the development of adult cochlea.

Differentiation of the organ of Corti parallels the development of the cochlea. Ruben (43), using [³H]thymidine labeling of the hair cells and supporting cells of the mouse organ of Corti, showed the greatest number of terminal mitoses about the 14th through 18th day of gestation (equivalent to 6 to 12 weeks in the human). The pattern of terminal mitoses occurred first at the apex and last at the base (i.e., the oldest sensory cells are located at the apex of the cochlear duct). He noted that these oldest cells of the organ of Corti were the last to differentiate since the pattern of cytodifferentiation in the cochlear duct of the mouse is from base to apex. In the chick (13), the maturation of the sensory epithelium appears to follow an opposite apical to basal pattern, with the stereocilia first appearing at incubation day 6 in the distal portion of the basal papilla and covering the distal two-thirds of the basilar papilla by 7.5 days *in ovo*. The proximal portion is covered with stereocilia only after 9 days *in ovo*. This suggests that the sensory structures of the organ of Corti in mammals are already fully developed and in place at the end of the early to middle stage of gestation with little, if any, replacement taking place subsequently. In the human, development also begins at the base of the duct and proceeds apically. The process is complete at approximately 20 weeks gestation (35). At 11 weeks, the organ appears as a thickened pseudostratified epithelial layer in its most developed region. Lying against it on the luminal surface is a poorly defined extracellular matrix that will eventually form a tectorial membrane. Based on the observations of Lim and Anniko (31) in the mouse embryo, the tectorial membrane starts as an amorphous covering of the medial surface of the greater epithelial ridge. This sensory membrane develops in two parts, the major tectorial membrane (medial) and minor tectorial membrane (distal). The major part is derived from the greater epithelial ridge and forms first. The minor tectorial membrane forms from the primordial supporting cells of the lesser epithelial ridge (Fig. 7). Both inner and outer hair cells are initially not covered by the tectorial membrane. The inner hair cells are covered first by the major tectorial membrane, whereas the outer hair cells are covered by a separate minor tectorial membrane. The tectorial membrane is composed of fibers that can be distinguished as two different fibril types called types A and B. The main portion of the membrane is composed of type A fibrils and type B fibrils form the cover net, marginal band, and Hensen's stripe. The major tectorial membrane fibers are ar-

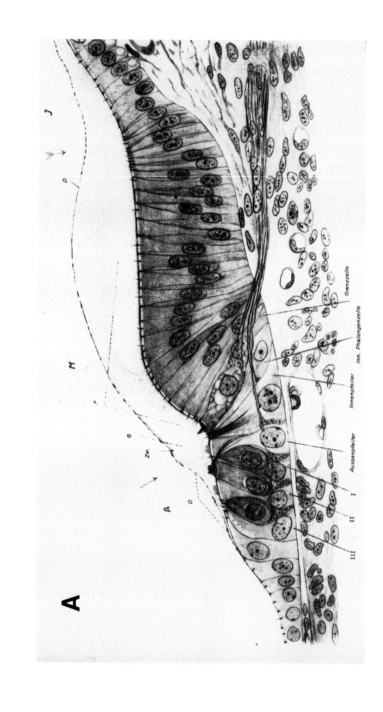

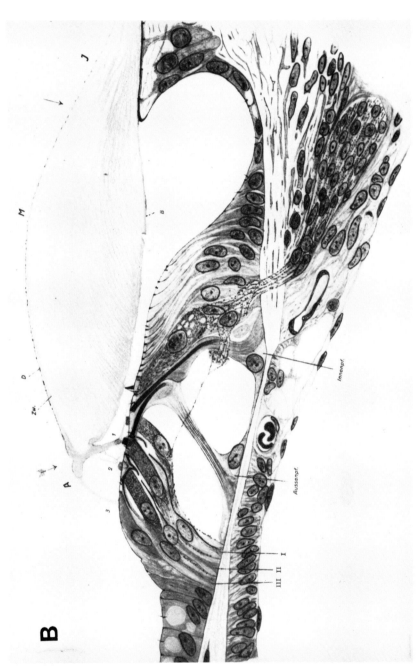

FIG. 7. Drawings of the stages of the development of the organ of Corti in the rabbit at term (**A**) and 6 days post-natally (**B**) showing the major tectorial membrane (M); the minor tectorial membrane (A); and the first (I), second (II), and third (III) ranks of Deiters' cells. (Drawings by H. Held, 1909.)

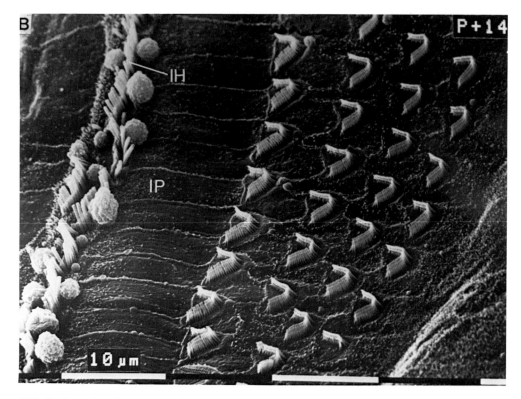

FIG. 8. Scanning electron photomicrograph of the inner and outer hair cell ranks of the organ of Corti in the adult mouse. The outer hair cells are to the right with their stereocilia in four ranks and arrayed in an orderly pattern. The inner hair cells (IH) are separated from the outer hair cells by the inner pillar cells (IP).

ranged radially and those of the minor tectorial membrane are arranged on a slant in the longitudinal direction. This extracellular matrix of the tectorial membrane has been shown to contain a large amount of collagen type II (57,60). The marginal pillars are not an integral part of the tectorial membrane and anchor the marginal band to the third row of Deiters' cells during postnatal days 2 to 16 in the cat (30). Henson's stripe may be a developmental anlage that derives from the attachment zone of the tectorial membrane to the regressing greater epithelial ridge epithelium. Hensen's stripe separates from the tectorial membrane in the kitten 10 to 15 days after birth.

The inner hair cells are derived from the greater epithelial ridge and the outer hair cells from the lesser epithelial ridge of Kölliker's organ. In the mouse, basal turn inner and outer hair cells can be recognized by gestation day 15 (Fig. 8) (31). The future hair cell stereocilia at this early stage can barely be distinguished from cell surface microvilli (27,28). In the human, the tunnel of Corti forms and hair cells appear at the basal end of the organ by the 16th week. The presence of large nerve bundles crossing the tunnel at a higher level [interpreted to be tunnel radial fibers, therefore efferent (53)] and the large number of fibers contacting the upper part of the outer hair cell body found in the organ of Corti in the 14- to 21-day-old mouse may be interpreted as signs of developmental plasticity of the nervous system at this stage. At 25 weeks gestation in humans, the organ of hearing resembles that of an adult (5). As the sensory cell matures, the initial, numerous, short, thin stereocilia are reduced in number, with the remaining ones growing progressively taller. As in most mammalian systems, the mouse auditory sensory cells have kinocilia only during development. The stereocilia form in stepped rows on the surface of the inner hair cells and in the shape of a "W" on the surface of the outer hair cells with the tallest row located at the periphery. As these sensory cells mature, the short, transitional stereocilia gradually disappear (28). Kinocilia are still present in the 14-day-old mouse neonate, even though the organ of Corti is morphologically mature (31). Observation of the 21-day postnatal mouse reveals no remaining kinocilia, suggesting that full sensory maturation in this species is delayed until at least 21 days. Study of cochlear microphonics in the mouse has revealed a mature response pattern at 14 to 15 days post-natally and mature behavioral patterns in response to auditory stimuli occurring 16 to 20 days post-natally, in agreement with the morphological maturation data (49,50).

A highly vascularized region of the cochlea, lining a portion of the scala media is referred to as the stria vascularis. It can first be identified as a protrusion of strial marginal cells on the luminal surface of the scala media. As the marginal cells mature, this protrusion disappears and the luminal cell surface enlarges because of increased number of microvilli. The typical flat hexagonal cell surface with numerous microvilli and distinct cell margins, characteristic of the mature strial marginal cell, first becomes defined at about 6 days after birth in the mouse (31). The specific ionic composition of the endolymph, containing relatively high levels of potassium ion, is reached at 4 to 6 days post-natally. The external sulcus cells reach their mature form at 6 to 14 days post-natally when the cuboidal cells covering the external sulcus area degenerate to expose the newly formed external sulcus cells. At present, the function of the external sulcus cells is unknown. In the gerbil, only small sections of capillaries can be observed in the stria vascularis at birth (7). Adult vasculature in the gerbil stria vascularis is not achieved until 8 to 10 days after birth. The rapid development of the stria vascularis during this period immediately precedes development of cochlear function. This pattern suggests that a fully developed stria vascularis may be related in some way to the ionic composition of the endolymph and the onset of auditory function.

The development of vascularization of the cochlea begins predominantly with the external wall vascularization of the scala tympani, with few vascular structures on the medial surface. Such a pattern suggests that the vessels of the basilar membrane originate from external wall vessels, not from the spiral lamina. Peripheral vascular connections rapidly degenerate after birth (15 to 20 days post-natally in the gerbil for complete degeneration). In general, postnatal vascular development appears to be synchronized with the development of Corti's organ (7).

Morphogenesis of the cochlear ganglion cell peripheral processes begins in the chick otocyst at 3 to 5 days of incubation (13). Fibers emerge from the ganglion and grow in a uniform fashion toward the undifferentiated receptor neuroepithelium. By 6 to 7 days *in ovo*, some of the peripheral fibers directly invade the basal lamina of the otocyst, whereas others first travel beneath this structure and then enter the basal lamina. At 8 to 9 days *in ovo*, numerous branches of the nerve fibers extend in columnar zones oriented radially toward the surface (early synaptogenesis); at this time, the target hair cells first become distinguishable from the surrounding epithelium. By 11 to 13 days of incubation (mid-synaptogenesis), the fibers develop large bulbous preterminal swellings located below the bases of the hair cells. Surplus branches atrophy and withdraw, and the efferent axons are observed for the first time in the sensory epithelia. By 14 to 17 days of incubation (late synaptogenesis), the preterminal swellings disappear and the endings transform into mature foot-shaped extensions at the base of each of the hair cells. The synchrony between hair-cell differentiation and synaptogenesis may reflect a nerve-target cell recognition and interaction (64). Van De Water and Ruben (62) have proposed that differentiating sensory receptors of the inner ear provide a chemotactic stimulus that encourages the growth of neurites from statoacoustic ganglion neurons to their respective target sites. Dechesne et al. (15,17) have reported that neuron-specific enolase (NSE) may serve as such a means of communication between the nerve fibers and their target cells. NSE (gamma-gamma form) is found localized within differentiated neurons, whereas NSE (alpha-alpha form) is exclusively associated with undifferentiated neurons. In the mouse, the first appearance of NSE (gamma-gamma) occurred at 15 gestation days, concomitant with the formation of contacts between the afferent fibers and the sensory neuroepithelium; NSE was found in the hair cells at 17 gestation days during the formation of the first synaptic structures. However, recent results obtained from the study of aneural otic explants (Dragone and Van De Water, *unpublished data*) and isolated statoacoustic ganglion cultures have shown that sensory cells but not neurons can express NSE in the absence of synapses. These results suggest that the expression of NSE within the inner ear sensory receptor cells depends on intrinsic information contained within the genome and not on extrinsic stimuli such as would be provided by synaptogenesis. Parks (37) studied the effects of axonal attachments of afferent sensory neurons from the otocyst to the cells of the nucleus magnocellularis in the developing chick embryo and concluded that these early contacts do not influence the maturation of magnocellularis neurons. The normal loss of long dendrites, observed to occur in these cells during the later stages of embryonic development, occurs normally, even when the otocyst is destroyed and no cochlear afferents are formed. Van De Water (58) has also shown that the hair cells of the inner ear are capable of cytodifferentiation without the extrinsic stimulus that might be provided by the neuronal elements of the statoacoustic ganglion neurons.

Apparently some auditory neurons possess the ability to modify and expand terminal arbors post-natally. The population of sensory hair cells in the macula neglecta of the sea skate increase from 500 to 3,000 post-embryonically, but at the same time the number of neurons innervating the structure does not appreciably increase (12). Instead, the terminal arbors of the auditory neurons expand to include more hair cells. These neurons shift their arbors, breaking contact with the older centrally located hair cells as they branch out to include the younger hair cells that differentiate at the periphery of the macula. Further studies on the chick exposed to postnatal acoustic trauma have shown that the organ of Corti retains the ability to regenerate new hair cells and nerve endings in response to acoustic trauma well beyond the posthatching period (D. A. Cotanche and J. T. Corwin, *personal communication*).

CONCLUSION

As seems to be the case in any study of development, the formation of the ear involves a far more complex set of interactions than was originally theorized. Con-

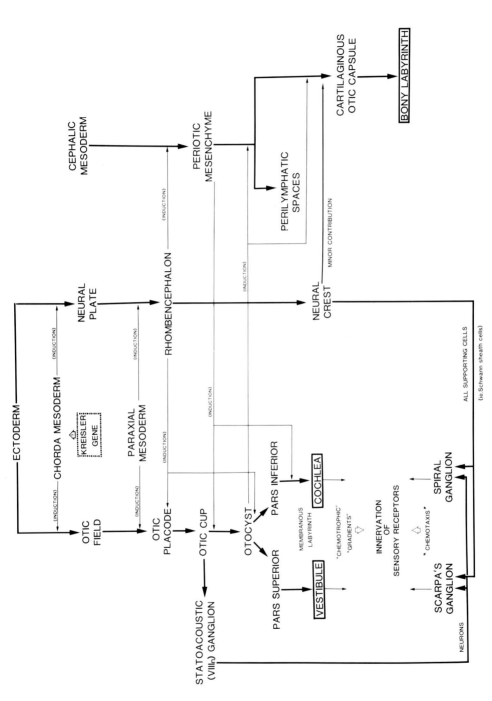

FIG. 9. Chart of the currently known interactions that occur between the organs and tissues involved in the normal formation of the mouse inner ear.

tributions from each of the primary germ layers, under a number of influences (local mesodermal mesenchyme, neural crest, otic and rhombencephalic neuroepithelium, and statoacoustic ganglion neurons) undergo a series of intricate developmental steps leading to the eventual formation of the ear and its associated structures. Figure 9 illustrates some of the interactions that have been identified during the early stages of otic development in the mouse, a mammal that has been shown to have a pattern of ear development closely related to that of humans.

One observation of particular clinical interest that has recently been made is the considerable mutability in the innervation of the sensory hair cells, a characteristic that results in a number of observed postnatal changes on exposure to both physical and chemical factors. Studies on rodents have shown that certain drug and noise levels, relatively innocuous in the adult, can cause severe defects in the cochlea of neonates at certain developmental stages (8,10,26). These hypersensitive periods have been shown to correspond to the final stages of cochlear development. The corresponding period in human fetal development would begin at 26 to 28 weeks of gestation and extend through the first 3 months of neonatal development (36,40). Such studies point up the difficulty in making general statements concerning the developmental mechanisms involved in the specific pathologies mentioned in this chapter, since both temporal and spatial variables are at work. It is valid to say, however, that those factors that are known to influence hearing and vestibular function in the adult will almost undoubtedly have a far more profound effect on the embryo and neonate.

REFERENCES

1. Anniko, M. (1980): Development of otoconia. *Am J. Otolaryngol.*, 1:400–410.
2. Anniko, M., and Hultcrantz, M. (1984): Vestibular hair cell pathology following low-dose irradiation during embryonic development. *Acta Otolaryngol. (Stockh.)*, 98:292–301.
3. Anson, B. J., and Bast, T. H. (1946): The development of the auditory ossicles and associated structures in man. *Ann. Otol. Rhinol. Laryngol.*, 55:467–493.
4. Anson, B. J., Bast, T. H., and Richany, S. F. (1955): The fetal and early postnatal development of the tympanic ring and related structures in man. *Ann. Otol. Rhinol. Laryngol.*, 64:802–823.
5. Anson, B. J., and Donaldson, J. A. (1981): *Surgical Anatomy of the Temporal Bone*. W. B. Saunders, Philadelphia.
6. Anson, B. J., Hanson, J. S., and Richany, S. F. (1960): Early embryology of the auditory ossicles and associated structures in relation to certain anomalies observed clinically. *Ann. Otol. Rhinol. Laryngol.*, 69:427–447.
7. Axelsson, A., Ryan, A., and Woolf, N. (1986): The early postnatal development of the cochlear vasculature in the gerbil. *Acta Otolaryngol. (Stockh.)*, 101:75–86.
8. Bock, G. R., and Saunders, J. C. (1977): A critical period for acoustic trauma in the hamster and its relation to cochlear development. *Science*, 197:396–398.
9. Bretos, M. (1980): La morphogénèse primordial du ganglion stato-acoustique et de l'oreille interne chez l'embryon de souris II. Etude de l'évolution des ébauches chez l'embryons de 10 ½ à 12 jours. *Arch. Belg.*, 91:77–113.
10. Carlier, E. and Pujol, R. (1980): Supranormal sensitivity to ototoxic antibiotic of the developing rat cochlea. *Arch. Otorhinolaryngol.*, 226:129–133.
11. Chiu, D. T., Crikelair, G. F., and Moss, M. L. (1979): Epigenetic regulation of rodent auricular shape of position. *Plast. Reconstr. Surg.*, 63:411–417.
12. Corwin, J. T. (1985): Auditory neurons expand their terminal arbors throughout life and orient toward the site of postembryonic hair cell production in the macula neglecta in elasmobranchs. *J. Comp. Neurol.*, 239:445–452.
13. Cotanche, D. A., and Sulik, K. K. (1984): The development of stereociliary bundles in the cochlear duct of the chick embryo. *Dev. Brain Res.*, 16:181–193.
14. D'Amico-Martel, A., and Noden, D. M. (1983): Contributions of placodal and neural crest cells to avian cranial peripheral ganglia. *Am. J. Anat.*, 166:445–468.

15. Dechesne, C. J., and Pujol, R. (1986): Neuron-specific enolase immunoreactivity in the developing mouse cochlea. *Hear. Res.*, 21:87–90.
16. Dechesne, C. J., and Sans, A. (1985): Development of vestibular receptor surfaces in human fetuses. *Am. J. Otolaryngol.*, 6:378–387.
17. Dechesne, C. J., Sans, A., and Keller, A. (1985): Onset and development of neuron-specific enolase immunoreactivity in the peripheral vestibular system of the mouse. *Neurosci. Lett.*, 61:299–304.
18. Deol, M. S. (1964): The abnormalities of the inner ear in Kreisler mice. *J. Embryol. Exp. Morphol.*, 12:475–490.
19. Hanson, J. R., Anson, B. J., and Strickland, E. M. (1962): Branchial sources of the auditory ossicles in man. *Arch. Otolaryngol.*, 76:200–215.
20. His, W. (1885): Die formentwickelung des ausseren Ohres. *Anat. Mensch. Embryo.*, III:211–221.
21. Hultcrantz, M., and Anniko, M. (1984): Malformations of vestibular organs following low-dose gamma irradiation during embryonic development. *Acta Otolaryngol. (Stockh.)*, 97:7–17.
22. Jaskoll, T. F., and Maderson, P. F. A. (1978): Study of the avian middle ear and tympanum. *Anat. Rec.*, 190:177–200.
23. Kern, G. (1962): On the problem of intrauterine streptomycin damage. *Schweiz. Med. Wochenschr.*, 92:77–83.
24. Killackey, H. P., and Belford, G. R. (1979): The formation of afferent patterns in the somatosensory cortex of the neonatal rat. *J. Comp. Neurol.*, 183:285–304.
25. Knapp, K., and Lenz, W. (1963): Die formen der thalidomide embryopathie. *Roentgen. Europ.*, 5:105–113.
26. Lenoir, M., and Pujol, R. (1980): Sensitive period to acoustic trauma in the rat pup cochlea: Histological findings. *Acta Otolaryngol. (Stockh.)*, 89:317–322.
27. Lewis, E. R., and Li, C. W. (1967): Evidence concerning the morphogenesis of saccular receptors in the bullfrog (Rana catesbeiana). *J. Morphol.*, 139:351–361.
28. Li, C. W., and Ruben, R. J. (1979): Further study of the surface morphology of the embryonic mouse cochlear sensory epithelia. *Otolaryngol. Head Neck Surg.*, 87:479–485.
29. Li, C. W., Van De Water, T. R., and Ruben, R. J. (1978): The fate mapping of the eleventh and twelfth day mouse otocyst: An "in vitro" study of the sites of origin of the embryonic inner ear sensory structures. *J. Morphol.*, 157:249–268.
30. Lim, D. J. (1977): Fine morphology of the tectorial membrane: Fresh and developmental. In: *Inner Ear Biology*, vol. 68, edited by M. Portmann and J.-M. Aran, pp. 47–60. INSERM, Paris.
31. Lim, D. J., and Anniko, M. (1985): Developmental morphology of the mouse inner ear: A scanning electron microscopic observation. *Acta Otolaryngol. [Suppl.] (Stockh.)*, 422:1–69.
32. McLellan, M. S., and Webb, C. H. (1957): Ear studies in the newborn infant. *J. Pediatr.*, 51:672–677.
33. McPhee, J. R., and Van De Water, T. R. (1985): A comparison of morphological stages and sulfated glycosaminoglycan production during otic capsule formation: In vivo and in vitro. *Anat. Rec.*, 213:566–577.
34. McPhee, J. R., and Van De Water, T. R. (1986): Epithelial-mesenchymal tissue interactions guiding otic capsule formation: The role of the otocyst. *J. Embryol. Exp. Morphol.*, 97:1–24.
35. Nakai, Y. (1970): An electron microscopic study of the human fetus cochlea. *Pract. Oto-Rhino-Laryngol.*, 32:257–267.
36. Northern, J. L., and Downs, M. P. (1974): *Hearing in Children*. Williams and Wilkins, Baltimore.
37. Parks, T. N. (1979): Afferent influences on the development of the stem auditory nuclei of the chicken: Otocyst ablation. *J. Comp. Neurol.*, 183:665–678.
38. Randall, P., Krogman, W., and Jahins, S. (1965): Pierre Robin and the syndrome that bears his name. *Cleft Palate J.*, 2:237–246.
39. Robinson, H. B. (1975): DiGeorge's or III-IV pharyngeal pouch syndrome: Pathology and a theory of pathogenesis. *Perspect. Pediatr. Pathol.*, 2:173–206.
40. Rubel, E. W. (1978): Ontogeny of structure and function in the vertebrate's auditory system. In: *Handbook of Sensory Physiology, Vol. IX: Development of Sensory Systems*, edited by M. Jacobson, pp. 135–237. Springer-Verlag, New York.
41. Rubel, E. W. (1984): Ontogeny of auditory system function. *Annu. Rev. Physiol.*, 46:213–229.
42. Rubel, E. W. (1985): Strategies and problems for future studies of auditory development. *Acta Otolaryngol. (Stockh.)*, 421:114–128.
43. Ruben, R. J. (1967): Development of the inner ear of the mouse: A radioautographic study of terminal mitoses. *Acta Otolaryngol. [Suppl.] (Stockh.)*, 220:1–44.
44. Ruben, R. J. (1973): Development and cell kinetics for the Kreisler (kr/kr) mouse. *Laryngoscope*, 83:1440–1468.
45. Sando, I. (1980): Discussion of inner ear anomalies—reply to Dr. Schuknecht In: *Morphogenesis and Malformation of the Ear. March of Dimes Birth Defects Foundation Original Article Series, Vol. XVI, No. 4*, edited by R. J. Gorlin, pp. 73–82. Alan R. Liss, New York.

46. Sans, A., and Chat, M. (1982): Analysis of temporal and spacial patterns of rat vestibular hair cell differentiation by tritiated thymidine radioautography. *J. Comp. Neurol.*, 206:1–8.
47. Shambaugh, G. E., Jr. (1952): Developmental anomalies of the sound conduction apparatus and their surgical correction. *Ann. Otol. Rhinol. Laryngol.*, 61:873–883.
48. Shimizu, S., Aoki, K., and Honda, Y. (1984): A study of the correlative relationship about the development of mucosa and of the tympanic cavity in the human middle ear. *Ear Res. Jpn.*, 15:178–181.
49. Shnerson, A., and Pujol, R. (1982): Age-related changes in C57BL/6J mouse cochlea. I. Physiological findings. *Dev. Brain Res.*, 2:65–75.
50. Shnerson, A., and Willott, J. F. (1979): Development of inferior colliculus response properties in C57BL/6J mouse pups. *Exp. Brain Res.*, 37:373–385.
51. Smith, D. W., and Takashima, H. (1978): Protruding auricle, a neuromuscular sign. *Lancet*, 1:747–748.
52. Smith, D. W., and Takashima, H. (1980): Ear muscles and ear form. In: *Morphogenesis and Malformation of the Ear. March of Dimes Birth Defects Foundation Original Article Series, Vol. XVI, No. 4*, edited by R. J. Gorlin, pp. 299–302. Alan R. Liss, New York.
53. Spoendlin, H. (1984): Primary neurons and synapses. In: *Ultrastructural Atlas of the Inner Ear*, edited by I. Friedmann and J. C. Ballantyne, pp. 133–164. Butterworths, London.
54. Streeter, G. C. (1922): Development of the auricle in the human embryo. *Contr. Embryol. Carneg. Inst.*, 14:111–138.
55. Tanaka, T., Ozeki, Y., Aoki, T., and Ogura, Y. (1975): Morphological relation of the vestibular sensory hairs to the otolithic membrane and cupula. A scanning electron microscopic study. In: *The Proceedings of the 5th Extraordinary Meeting of the Barany Society*, edited by M. Marimoto, pp. 403–409. Barany Society, Kyoto.
56. Taylor, M. (1937): Prenatal medication and its relation to the fetal ear. *Surg. Gynecol. Obst.*, 64:542–549.
57. Thalmann, I., Thallinger, G., Comegys, T. H., and Thalmann, R. (1986): Collagen—the predominant protein of the tectorial membrane. *ORL*, 48:107–115.
58. Van De Water, T. R. (1984): Developmental mechanisms of mammalian inner ear formation. In: *Hearing Science*, edited by C. Berlin, pp. 49–108. College Hill Press, San Diego.
59. Van De Water, T. R. (1986): Determinants of neuron-sensory receptor cell interaction during development of the inner ear. *Hear. Res.*, 22:265–277.
60. Van De Water, T. R., and Galinovic-Schwartz (1987): Collagen type II in the otic extracellular matrix: Effect on inner ear development. *Hear. Res.*, 30:39–48.
61. Van De Water, T. R. and Ruben, R. J. (1974): Organ culture of the mammalian inner ear: A tool to study inner ear deafness. *Laryngoscope*, 84:738–751.
62. Van De Water, T. R., and Ruben, R. J. (1983): A possible embryonic mechanism for the establishment of innervation of inner ear sensory structures. *Acta Otolaryngol. (Stockh.)*, 95:470–479.
63. Wever, E. G., and Lawrence, M. (1954): *Physiological Acoustics*. Princeton University Press, Princeton, NJ.
64. Whitehead, M. C., and Morest, D. K. (1985): The development of innervation patterns in the avian cochlea. *Neuroscience*, 14:255–276.

Physiology of the Ear,
edited by A. F. Jahn and J. Santos-Sacchi.
Raven Press, New York © 1988.

Cochlear Signal Processing

Jont B. Allen

AT&T Bell Laboratories, Murray Hill, New Jersey 07974

This chapter describes the mechanical function of the cochlea, or inner ear, the organ that converts acoustical signals into neural signals. Models of the cochlea are important and useful because they succinctly describe the principles of the operation of the preneural portion of the hearing system. Many cochlear hearing disorders are still not well understood, and if systematic progress is to be made in improved diagnostics and treatment of these disorders, a clear understanding of basic principles is essential. The literature is full of speculations about various aspects of cochlear function and dysfunction. Unfortunately, we still do not have all the facts about many important issues, including how the cochlea attains its frequency selectivity. However, the experimental body of data has been growing at an accelerating pace as greater attention has been focused on this and other important and related issues.

Several topics will be covered here. First, the history and concepts behind the early cochlear models will be described, including extensions that have taken place in recent years. Next, recent modeling efforts in cochlear micromechanics are described. These models are intended to describe the mechanics of the tectorial membrane and the hair cells in greater detail. This leads to a discussion of the difference between basilar membrane, hair cell, and neural tuning. Finally the success of several of the micromechanical models is discussed.

FUNCTION OF THE INNER EAR

The purpose of modeling the cochlea is to help us understand how auditory signal processing is performed. The signals from 30,000 neurons represent the output of the human cochlea. These neurons encode 3,500 cochlear inner hair cell signals, which are filtered versions of the sound pressure at the tympanic membrane. In other words, each hair-cell signal has a limited frequency content, with a frequency spectrum that depends on the hair-cell location along the basilar membrane. In the cat, approximately 20 neurons encode each of these narrow-band hair-cell signals using a neural timing code, whereby the time between neural pulses carries the information being signaled into the auditory central nervous system.

We describe the cochlear signal processing that ensues by two separate means. First, we describe the signal representation at various points in the system. Second, we refer to models of the auditory system. These models are our most succinct means of conveying the results of years of detailed and difficult experimental work on cochlear function. An alternative way of describing our knowledge of the cochlear function (which we try not to use) would be to describe the multitude of experimental results. This body of experimental knowledge has been very efficiently represented (to the extent that it is understood) in the form of mathematical models. When the experimental results are at variance with the model or when no model exists, the model is not a useful description, and the more basic description, using the experimental data base, is necessary. Several good books and review papers are available that make excellent supplemental reading (3,29,36,40,41,46).

For pedagogical purposes the inner ear may be functionally divided into several subcomponents. From Figs. 1 to 3, three major divisions may be defined and are classified here as: (a) macromechanics, (b) micromechanics, and (c) transduction.

Macromechanics describes the fluid motions of the scalae and assumes for analysis purposes that the basilar membrane is frequently treated as a dynamic system having mass, stiffness, and damping. Micromechanics describes the details of the motion of the organ of Corti, the inner and outer hair cells, the tectorial membrane, pillar cells, and the motion of the fluid in the space between the reticular lamina and the tectorial membrane. Transduction describes the electrochemical response of the inner hair cell to basilar membrane motions. This topic, however, is beyond the scope of this chapter.

There is a great deal of diverse opinion in the literature about several critical issues because of experimental uncertainty. For example, it is very difficult to observe experimentally the motion of the basilar membrane in a functionally undamaged cochlea. Furthermore, questions regarding the relative motion of the tectorial membrane to other adjacent structures are largely a matter of conjecture. Such questions are therefore at present best investigated by theoretical means. As a result, a variety of opinions exist as to the detailed function of the various structures.

On the other hand, firm and widely accepted indirect evidence exists on how these structures work. Since this indirect evidence takes on many forms, such as morphological, electrochemical, mechanical, acoustical, biophysical, these data are probably best related via a model.

COCHLEAR MACROMECHANICS

The first widely recognized model of the cochlea, attributed to Helmholtz (14), is described in an appendix of his book *On the Sensations of Tone*, which was first published in 1862. Helmholtz likened the cochlea to a bank of highly tuned resonators that are selective to different frequencies, much like a piano, where each string represents a different place on the basilar membrane. In fact, the model he proposed was unsatisfactory because it omitted many important features, the most important of which is the cochlear fluid that couples the mechanical resonators together.

It was not until the experimental observations of von Békésy in 1928 on human cadaver cochleas that the nature of the basilar membrane traveling wave behavior was unveiled. Typical fluid motions in the cochlea are shown by the arrows in Fig. 1. Figures 2 and 3 show an expanded view with details of the cochlear duct. Von Békésy found that the cochlea is like a linear "dispersive" transmission system in which different frequency components that make up the input signal travel at different speeds along the basilar membrane, thereby isolating those various frequency components at different places along the basilar membrane. He described this dispersive wave as a "traveling wave," which he observed using stroboscopic light in

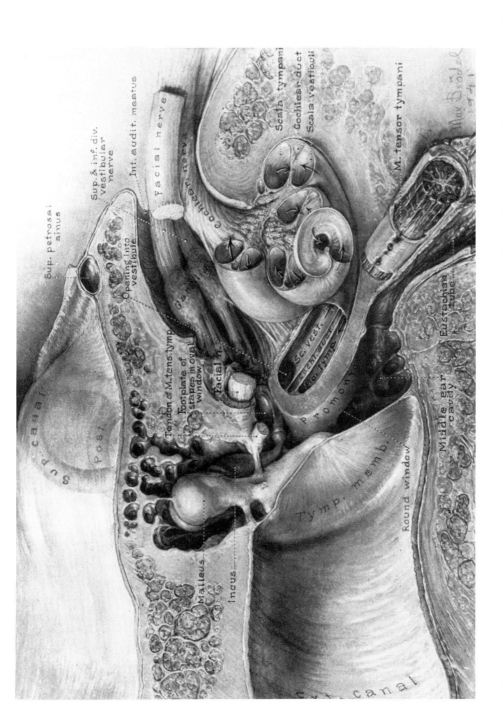

FIG. 1. In this detailed drawing of the human cochlea, most of the major components are identifiable. Sound is directed by the pinna down the ear canal where it becomes a plane wave owing to the ear canal's small diameter. The sound is transmitted to the cochlea via the ossicles. The motion of the stapes displaces the fluid in the vestibular chamber of the cochlea. An equal amount of fluid is displaced at the round window since the net volume of fluid within the cochlea is constant. (© 1941, Max Brödel, "Three unpublished drawings of the anatomy of the human ear." W. B. Saunders, 1946.)

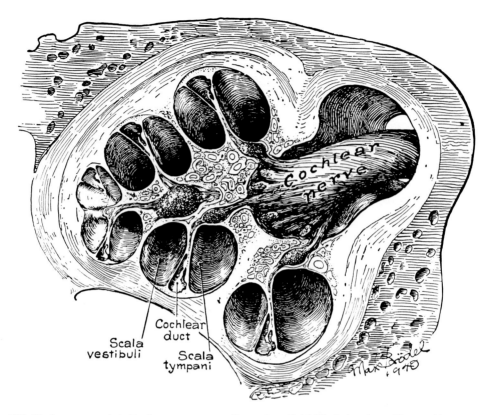

FIG. 2. As we move into the inner ear, we see the various fluid-filled chambers. The cochlear nerve forms the central core of the cochlea and extends into the VIIIth nerve, which also comprises the facial and vestibular nerve bundles. The cochlear duct, defined as the space between Reissner's membrane and the basilar membrane, is at an 80-mV potential This potential is important in the transduction process. (© 1940, Max Brödel from *1940 Year Book of the Eye, Ear, Nose and Throat.*)

a dead human cochlea, at sound levels well above our pain threshold, i.e., 120 dB SPL and above. Sound levels of this magnitude were required to obtain displacement levels that were observable under his microscope. These pioneering experiments were so difficult and important that von Békésy received the Nobel prize in 1961 for his experimental observations.

Through the years these experiments have been greatly improved, but von Békésy's fundamental observation of the traveling wave still stands. His original experimental results, however, are not characteristic of the responses seen in more recent experiments in several ways.

Today we find that the traveling wave has a more sharply defined location on the basilar membrane for a pure tone input than observed by von Békésy. In fact, according to more recent measurements, the response of the basilar membrane to a pure tone can change in amplitude by about five orders of magnitude per millimeter of distance along the basilar membrane. To describe this response, it is helpful to call on one of the early models of macromechanics, the transmission line model, which was investigated by Zwislocki (44,45) and later elaborated by Peterson and Bogert (28). This model is also frequently called the one-dimensional model.

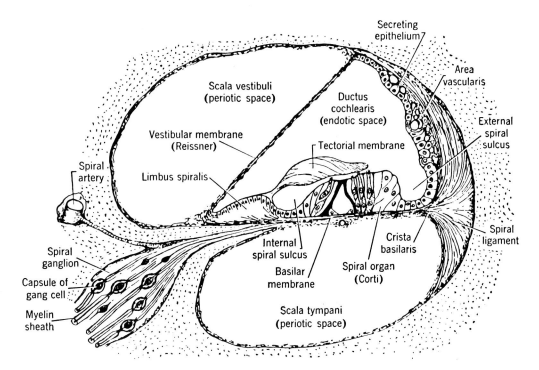

FIG. 3. We show here a more detailed cross section of the cochlear canal with tectorial membrane, cochlear nerve, basilar membrane, and other structures of significance. (© 1943, Rasmussen.)

THE TRANSMISSION LINE MODEL OF THE COCHLEA

Between the years of 1931 and 1950, Ranke (30) formulated the first hydrodynamic models of the cochlea. Ranke's main contribution was his studies of the fluid effects in the cochlea. He came to many important and fundamental findings, but his work remained either greatly misunderstood or ignored and is only now beginning to be appreciated (39,41).

The transmission line model of Zwislocki (45) was first introduced in 1945 as a simplified version of the more complete formulation of Ranke (30). Zwislocki's theory was more easily evaluated, but, as Ranke has pointed out (30), it was not as accurate as the more complete theory. A modern version of the Zwislocki model is shown in Fig. 4. The stapes input pressure p_{in} is at the left, with the input velocity v_{in}, as shown by the arrow, corresponding to the stapes velocity. This model represents the mass of the fluids of the cochlea as electrical inductors. Frequently electrical circuit networks are useful in describing mechanical systems. This is possible because of an electrical to mechanical analog that relates the two systems of equations, and the electrical circuit elements comprise an accepted standard for describing these equations owing to their frequent use. From the circuit of Fig. 4, it is possible to write the equations that describe the system, and many engineers and scientists find it quicker to read these circuit diagrams than to interpret the equations.

Different points along the basilar membrane are represented by the cascaded sec-

BASE   APEX

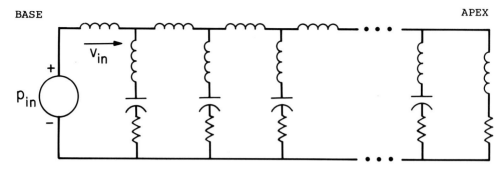

FIG. 4. The most commonly exploited basilar membrane-cochlear model is the transmission line model. In this model the inductors represent the mass of the cochlear fluid (series elements) and the basilar membrane mass (shunt inductors). The inductor values are frequently assumed to be independent of their position along the length of the cochlea. The stiffness of the basilar membrane is represented by the shunt capacitors. The stiffness is position dependent and is usually assumed to vary exponentially with position. The basilar membrane is stiffest (smallest capacitance) near the stapes. Thus the resonant frequencies of the shunt elements, taken in isolation, are largest at the stapes (base) and smallest near the helicotrema (apex). This model, called the transmission line model or one-dimensional model, has been an important research tool since it was introduced by Zwislocki in 1948 (44). The model does not have as sharp a high frequency cutoff as two- and three-dimensional models. However, it does capture many of the essential features of the system in a qualitative way, such as the traveling wave observed by von Békésy.

tions of the transmission line model. Thus the position along the model line corresponds to the longitudinal position along the cochlea. The series (horizontal) inductors represent the fluid inertia along the length of the cochlea, and the elements connected to ground (the common point along the bottom of the figure) represent the mechanical (acoustical) impedance of an element of the corresponding section of the basilar membrane. Each inductor going to ground represents the mass per unit length of the basilar membrane section, whereas the capacitor represents the compliance (stiffness) of the section of basilar membrane. The compliance is believed to vary systematically with a stiffness that decreases exponentially along the length of the cochlea. Thus each piece of basilar membrane is tuned to a different frequency, since the stiffness changes with position. For convenience, we assume here that the mass of the basilar membrane remains constant along its length, which roughly speaking, seems to be the case.

During the following discussion it will be necessary to introduce the concept of impedance, which may be foreign in its most general form, but is actually a simple concept. Impedance is defined under conditions of pure tone stimulation; thus impedance is a function of frequency. For example, the impedance of the tympanic membrane (TM) is defined as the pure tone pressure in the ear canal divided by the resulting TM volume velocity (the velocity × the area of motion). The pressure and velocity referred to here are conventionally described by complex numbers to account for the phase relationship between the two. Other common impedance definitions are the voltage/current ratio in an electrical circuit, and the force divided by the velocity in mechanical systems.

To understand the inner workings of our circuit of Fig. 4, let us assume that we excite the line at the stapes with a sinusoidal current of frequency f. Because of conservation of charge (charge cannot be created or destroyed in this circuit), the total current through the basilar membrane must equal the current at the stapes. The physical law that we are modeling is not conservation of charge, since the cochlea is not an electrical circuit, but conservation of fluid mass or, equivalently, conservation of the fluid volume within the scalae since the fluid is incompressible.

When the stapes is displaced, thereby producing a fluid volume displacement in the upper scala (Figs. 2 and 3), the net volume displacement of the basilar membrane must displace an identical volume. Simultaneously, the round window membrane connected to the scala tympani must bulge out by an equal amount. In practice the motion of the basilar membrane is quite complicated. However, the total volume displacement of the basilar membrane, at any instant of time, must be equal to the volume displacement of the stapes or of the round window membrane.

Consider next where the fluid current v_{in} will flow or where it can flow. For a given input frequency, the basilar membrane impedance has a minimum at one point along the length of the cochlea. The impedance of interest here is that of each group of three elements in the series in Fig. 4, i.e., the inductor-capacitor-resistor combination going to ground at each point along the length of the cochlea. These three elements in this configuration have special significance because at one frequency the impedance of the inductor and capacitor cancel each other, and the only impedance element remaining is the impedance (resistance) of the resistor. Thus, at one point along the length of the cochlea, for a given frequency, the impedance is small, namely that point where the basilar membrane compliance reactance cancels its mass reactance. This point is called the resonant point. At that point the basilar membrane appears to have a hole in it (e.g., the flow resistance is all that remains of the impedance). To the left of the resonant point, the basilar membrane is increasingly stiff (having a large capacitive impedance), and to the right of the resonant point, the impedance is a large mass reactance (inductive impedance). In fact, in this region the impedance is largely irrelevant since little current will flow past the hole. Thus the fluid current has maximum flow basal to where the impedance has its minimum.

Of course the above description is dependent on the input frequency f, since the location of the hole, or impedance minimum, is frequency dependent. If we were to put a pulse of current in at the stapes, the highest frequencies that make up the pulse would be filtered out near the stapes, whereas the lower frequencies would propagate down the line. As the pulse travels down the basilar membrane, the higher frequencies are progressively removed, until almost nothing is left when the pulse reaches the right end of the model (the helicotrema end or the apex of the cochlea).

From this description it is possible to understand why the various frequency components of the signal are mapped out on the basilar membrane.

Let us next try a different mental experiment with this model. Suppose that the input at the stapes were a slowly swept tone or chirp. What would the response at a fixed point on the basilar membrane look like? In Fig. 5, we show the model frequency response magnitude of the basilar membrane. This is the ratio of the basilar membrane displacement at one point along its length (the output) to the stapes displacement (the input), as a function of the frequency f at the input. The response is a bandpass response, with a shallow low-frequency slope and a very sharp high-frequency slope. We see in Fig. 5, that the maximum relative amplitude of vibration for the particular point chosen was at 1 kHz.

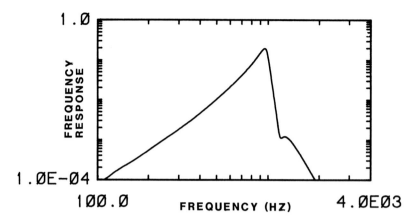

FIG. 5. When we view the model at a given place on the basilar membrane as a function of frequency, the response is found to be a bandpass filter. The slope on the high-frequency side of a real cochlea is place dependent and varies from 50 dB/octave for a low-frequency place, near the helicotrema, to more than 500 dB/octave for a high-frequency place in the base. This latter slope would give a 42-dB change in output for a semitone change in frequency (a change corresponding to going from C to C# on a musical scale). By comparison, the slope for the model on the low-frequency side of the model filters is quite shallow and between 12 to 18 dB/octave.

INADEQUACIES OF THE ONE-DIMENSIONAL MODEL

The transmission line model was a most important development since it was in agreement with the experimental evidence of the day, and it is based on a simple set of physical principles, i.e., conservation of fluid mass and a spatially variable basilar membrane stiffness. In fact, this model was the theory of choice until improved experimental observations were available in the late 1960s and early 1970s.

In 1976 Zweig and colleagues pointed out that accurate, but approximate, solutions for the transmission line equations could be found by the use of a method in physics called the ''WKB'' method (41,43). As further results became available, it eventually became clear that the one-dimensional transmission line theory was not totally satisfactory, since that theory did not agree with the more detailed and complete descriptions derived from a more rigorous analysis. This point was first made by Ranke (30), and again much later by Lesser and Berkley (23). It is now possible to compute the response of a two-dimensional (5) and even the response of a three-dimensional geometry (9). As the complexity of the geometry of the models approached the physical geometry, the solutions tended to display steeper high frequency slopes and therefore increased frequency selectivity.

A great deal of neural data from the VIIIth nerve is available that defines quite precisely the input–output properties of the cochlea at threshold levels. However, since the signals undergo significant transformations between the basilar membrane and neural measurement point, one cannot directly compare neural response curves with the basilar membrane model, at least not without careful consideration. We ultimately seek a model that accurately describes the 3,500 human inner hair cell outputs or the 30,000 neural signals.

What is important is that the frequency response, as computed by the transmission line model of the basilar membrane motion, is quite different from the response as estimated from the nerve fiber measurements. The difference can be on the order of 20 to 40 dB (20 dB is a factor of 10, and 40 dB is a factor of 100) and appears to be even greater under some conditions. Thus, when the two-dimensional models showed sharpened responses relative to the transmission line model, the hope was that these more detailed models would converge to the response measured in the nerve fiber. Although a significant increase in sharpness was found, the desired convergence has not occurred.

NONLINEAR EFFECTS

A second area where the existing one-dimensional theory is inadequate follows from the nonlinear phenomena that have been experimentally observed, such as:

1. the frequency-dependent response-level compression as first observed by Rhode (31,32) in the basilar membrane response;
2. the frequency-dependent response-level compression as observed by Russell and Sellick (34) in the inner hair cell receptor potential;
3. the frequency-dependent response-level compression as observed by Kiang and Moxon (20), Allen and Fahey (4), and others, as measured neurally in response to a second subthreshold tone [this is a form of two-tone suppression (35)];
4. distortion components generated within the cochlea that have been measured by Goldstein and Kiang (12), Fahey and Allen (11), and others.

Since the transmission line theory is a linear theory, many researchers have studied ways of making the cochlear models nonlinear in order to study the numerous nonlinear effects (13,21). These models are still in the developmenal stage; therefore it is necessary to describe some of the data that they are trying to model rather than the models themselves.

The Basilar Membrane Nonlinearity

One of the most interesting of these nonlinear effects was first observed by Rhode (31,32) when he measured the input-output characteristics of the basilar membrane as shown in Fig. 6. He found the basilar membrane displacement to be related to the stapes displacement in a highly nonlinear fashion. For every 4 dB of level increase on the input, the output only changed 1 dB. This compressive nonlinearity was dependent on frequency and only occurred near the most sensitivity frequency for the point on the basilar membrane that he was measuring (e.g., the tip of the tuning curve). For other frequencies the system was linear, that is, 1 dB of input change gave 1 dB of output change for frequencies away from the best frequency. This nonlinear effect was highly dependent on the health of the animal and would disappear or not be present at all if the animal was not in its physiologically prime state. One interpretation of this nonlinear effect is that of a level- and frequency-dependent gain (amplification) that increases as the input level is reduced. From Fig. 6A it would appear that Rhode found approximately 35 dB excess gain at 7 kHz for 55 dB SPL relative to the gain at 105 dB SPL.

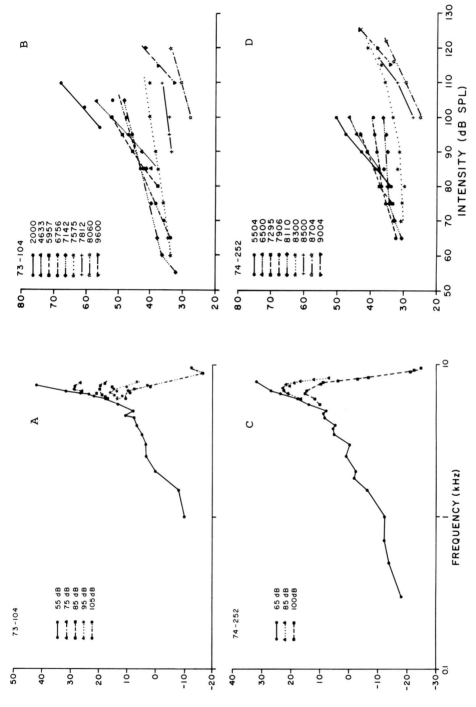

FIG. 6. The measurements shown in this figure are taken from Rhode (32) and show the basilar membrane displacement as a function of frequency normalized by the input level, for different input levels (**A,C**). In (**B,D**) we see the same data in a different format plotted as a function of input sound level with frequency as the parameter. Rhode was the first to find the nonlinear effect shown here (31,32), which may be interpreted as a frequency- and level-dependent gain, with increasing gain with lower levels. This extra gain is maximum near the best frequency of the basilar membrane measurement point.

The Receptor Potential Nonlinearity

In 1977, Russell and Sellick (34) found a similar result in the receptor potential of the inner hair cell of their guinea pig preparation—a frequency-dependent, compressive, nonlinear effect (Fig. 7). These two independently measured findings, at different points in the system, give credibility to the hypothesis that the basilar membrane response is inherently nonlinear and that at low-sound-pressure levels, the basilar membrane displacement is being amplified in a frequency-selective manner, producing the narrow-band tips on the tuning curves of high frequency neurons at low levels (8). If this is the case, then there should be a correlate of this phenomenon in the neural signal. In Fig. 8 we see the effect of adding a low-frequency bias tone, below the neurons threshold, on the frequency response of a neuron (4,11,20). Such a family of neural tuning curves are qualitatively similar to the responses found by Rhode (32) and Russell and Sellick (34).

A Nonlinear Paradox

It is interesting to note here the paradox between the volume conservation law and the nonlinearity found by Rhode (32). The first law says that the volume displacement of the basilar membrane must be equal to the stapes volume displacement at each instant of time. Rhode observed that the basilar membrane displacement is not proportional to the input displacement but appears to have excess gain near the best frequency. This implies that the traveling wave must redistribute along the basilar membrane length, as a function of the input level, in a highly constrained manner. This in turn would require that the neural phase must change with level, which in general is not found below 4 kHz (2). One way out of this paradox is to add an extra degree of freedom between basilar membrane motion and hair cell excitation. A second approach is to note that the experimental evidence for the nonlinear excess gain is all above 4 kHz, and therefore perhaps the excess gain is not present below 4 kHz, where the neural phase data have been measured.

TWO-DIMENSIONAL COCHLEAR MACROMECHANICS

In this section we return to the linear models and try to give a bit of the flavor of the extended hydrodynamic theories of cochlear mechanics, so that the reader may better appreciate how and why they represent an improvement on the transmission line theory.

The first step toward a more manageable theory was taken by Ranke (30) in 1950 in what he called a "short-wave" theory. Short-wave theory is most accurate near the cutoff frequency, whereas long-wave theory (the one-dimensional model is a long-wave theory) is best basal to the cutoff frequency (39,41). Ranke's attempts were historically significant (39,41) but never actually developed into a useful theory for several reasons. For example, it is not known how to optimally interface the long-wave model to the short-wave model, since some sort of matching procedure is required.

Then in 1972, Lesser and Berkley (23) proposed a rectangular box model of the cochlea in which the scalae were straight and the cochlea was assumed to be sym-

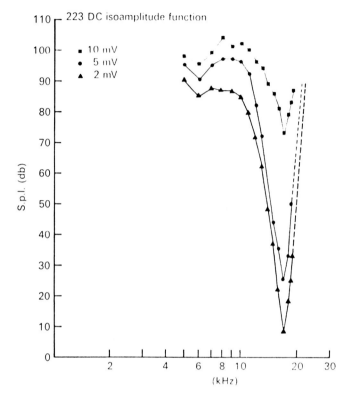

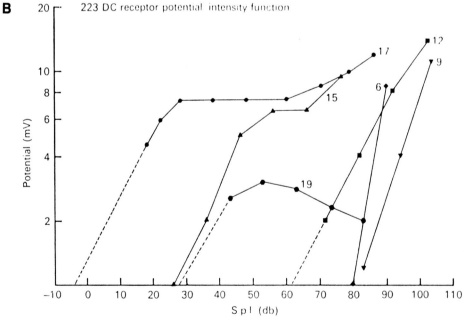

FIG. 7. Russell and Sellick (34) found a nonlinear and frequency-dependent effect in the receptor potential similar to that found by Rhode for the basilar membrane (32). In (**A**) we see the sound-pressure level, in dB, required to obtain 2, 5, and 10 mV of receptor potential in an inner hair cell. The format of this figure differs from that of Rhode in that the response is not normalized by the input sound level. In (**B**) we see curves similar to Rhode's that show nonlinear compression of the response. Not shown are the rectifying effects of the cilia, which produce a large DC component in the inner hair cell response.

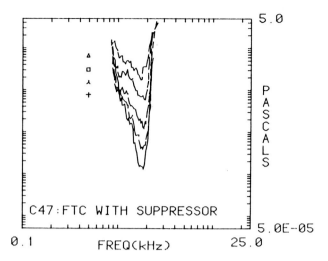

FIG. 8. When the response of a neuron is measured in the presence of a second (suppressor) tone we see that it may have a strong attenuation effect, even though the suppressing tone produces no response when present alone. The symbols define the frequency and level of the suppressor tone that was presented while the tuning curve was measured. When the suppressor-tone level was increased, the threshold of the tuning curve increased in a frequency-dependent way. The lowest threshold tuning curve was measured with the suppressor tone turned off. One interpretation of this effect is that at low levels of input sound pressure, the extra basilar membrane gain (as described, for example, in Fig. 6) is high. When the suppressor tone is present, it suppresses the extra gain, just as a high-level signal does in Fig. 6. According to this model, the suppressor signal does not give rise to an output when presented alone because of the high pass filtering that results from the tectorial membrane resonance model as described in Fig. 18C.

metric about the basilar membrane. This geometry is shown in Fig. 9. A main point of their paper was to demonstrate the importance of extending the models to two dimensions because of the effect of this extension on the solutions, a point that had been made years earlier by Ranke (30). Their line of reasoning inspired research that kept people busy computing for at least 10 years. As mentioned, via numerical methods, we have now moved beyond the two-dimensional formulation into the realm of three-dimensional models. More time is needed to evaluate fully the significance of these more detailed calculations and models, but it presently appears that they alone do not close the gap, as was originally hoped, between model and experiment. Thus the most important problem that still remains unsolved in cochlear theory is explaining the sharpness of tuning of the neurally measured response. Although the two-dimensional models brought the neural data and model calculations into agreement on the high-frequency side of the tuning curve, they did not improve the match on the low-frequency side. The most recent experimental measurements either indicate or are consistent with a 20-dB difference between basilar membrane responses and neural responses on the low-frequency side of the tuning curve. Such a transformation will be discussed next.

Cochlear Micromechanics

Micromechanics refers to the mechanics of the organ of Corti. The most commonly accepted description of the motion of the organ of Corti was proposed by ter Kuile

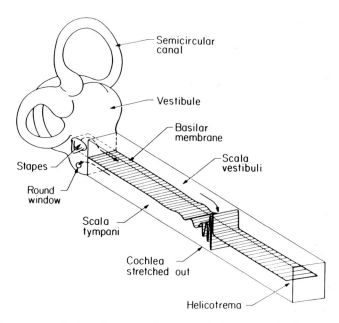

FIG. 9. This figure shows the traveling wave at one point in time on the basilar membrane. Because of the dispersive nature of the basilar membrane, a wake appears behind the main pulse. This pulse also becomes broader as it travels down the basilar membrane owing to the attenuation of the higher frequency components. (From ref. 43.)

in 1900 (22). His concept is shown in Fig. 10 where we see how he proposed that the displacement of the basilar membrane could drive the hair cells in a radial mode of excitation. In Fig. 11 we see a similar description of this mode of excitation from Allen (1). A simple analysis of the model reveals that the vertical motion (the y direction) of the basilar membrane is linearly related to the radial shearing motion (the z direction) seen by the cilia of the inner hair cells, which are known to be the transducers that sense the motions of the basilar membrane. Thus the model of ter Kuile is equivalent to a lever that linearly converts the vertical basilar membrane motion into radial shearing motions appropriate for the excitation of the inner hair cells. (The word motion is used to avoid the important question of whether velocity or displacement is the actual inner hair cell excitatory stimulus.)

The ter Kuile model seemed adequate as a first step, but several important problems remained. First, there have been no direct observations to confirm the ter Kuile model nor are there likely to be any in the near future, because of the inherent difficulty in making observations of such small motions in such difficult places. Second, we cannot yet be sure, given the present experimental data, if the neural and basilar membrane responses are in agreement with each other, as described in the previous section. It was hoped that a simple modification of the ter Kuile model might bring together the various theories and the experimental data. We will argue this possibility here.

Basilar Membrane versus Neural and Hair-Cell Tuning

At this point it is again necessary to remove ourselves from the models and look at some experimental data in order to understand the nature and magnitude of the

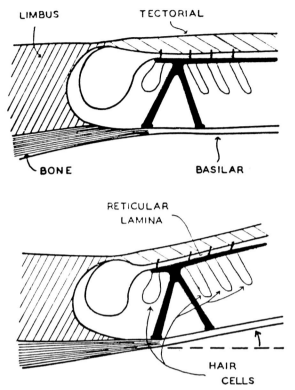

LIMBUS   TECTORIAL

BONE   BASILAR

RETICULAR
LAMINA

HAIR
CELLS

FIG. 10. In 1900, ter Kuile (22) first described his model of how the vertical displacement of the basilar membrane is transformed into a radial shearing required to drive the inner hair cell cilia. At that time it was generally assumed that the tall cilia of each inner hair cell was connected to the tectorial membrane. It is now generally believed that inner hair cells are not driven directly by the tectorial membrane, but are dragged by the surrounding fluid that is in phase with the displacement. This would happen because the viscous boundary layer (a thin fluid layer where viscous forces dominate) is greater than the 6-μm distance between the tectorial membrane and the top surface of the hair cells (this surface is called the reticular lamina). As a result, the relative shear of these two surfaces acts as a mechanical resistor, or dashpot, as it is referred to in mechanical terms. The mechanical equivalent of the entire system is a lever, or electrically, it is a transformer. (From ref. 1.)

discrepancy between the mechanical tuning of the basilar membrane and neural signal. In Fig. 12 we see tuning responses from Sellick et al. (37) of the basilar membrane as compared with a neural measure, where the responses differ by approximately 10 to 20 dB on the low-frequency side of the response.

The voltage in the inner hair cell was first measured by Russell and Sellick (34). This voltage, called the receptor potential, is tuned like the neuron. In a later paper, Sellick et al. (38) show much more detail, as seen in Fig. 13. These results consistently show a difference on the low-frequency side of the characteristic frequency. In the summary of their 1983 paper (38) they stated: "In conclusion, a demonstration of inner hair cell tuning at the level of the basilar membrane continues to elude us."

Robles et al. (33) also have compared basilar membrane tuning with a neural measure. Their summary result is shown in Fig. 14. Again on the low-frequency side of the tuning curve, they find a difference, but in their case, the difference is in the form of a large variance, which they indicate by error bars (see the displacement response at 2.8 kHz). It is interesting to note that in the frequency region near 1.75 kHz the neural signal is less sharply tuned than either of the mechanical measures, an observation unique to all such experiments.[1]

Is the difference between basilar membrane, neural, or hair cell measures signif-

---

[1] The measurements of basilar membrane motion by Khanna and Leonard (18) are not direct comparisons with neural or receptor measures. As a result of the normalization procedure used by them and the ear canal standing wave they report (19), their data are not a direct test of this question. Furthermore, they have not observed the nonlinear compression as seen by Rhode (31,32), Russell and Sellick (34), Sellick et al. (37,38), and Robles et al. (33).

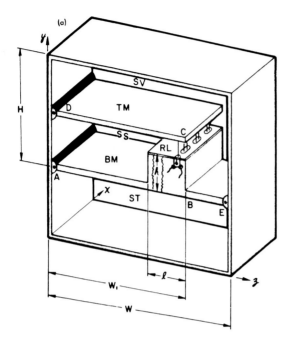

FIG. 11. We show here a labeled three-dimensional representation of the previous figure (**a**) and compare it with a detailed labeled drawing of the organ of Corti (**b**). The inner hair cells seen in (b) are the transducers that signal the central nervous system (CNS). The purpose of the outer hair cells is still unknown other than the obvious structural one. The cilia length of the outer hair cells define ϵ, the subtectorial space. The neurons connected to the outer hair cells are for the most part efferent neurons. It has been shown that the CNS can modify, to some extent, the mechanical properties (e.g., the stiffness) of the outer hair cell cilia. The inner hair cells on the other hand appear to be passive displacement detectors that input to the afferent primary neurons. (From ref. 1.)

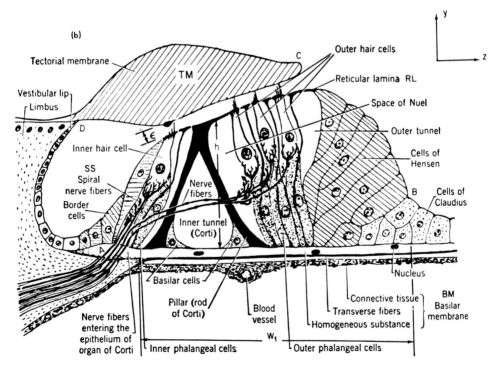

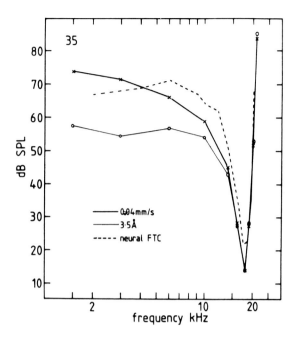

FIG. 12. Basilar membrane isovelocity (x) and isodisplacement curves (○) compared with a neural tuning curve (*broken line*) derived from the guinea pig spiral ganglion with a comparable characteristic frequency to that of the basilar membrane measurement point. The spiral ganglion data were courtesy of D. Robertson. (From ref. 37.)

icant, or is it an artifact of the experimental technique? Unfortunately, we cannot yet be sure of the answer to this important question. At present the Neely and Kim (26) model accounts for neural tuning data, or receptor potential data, for neurons tuned above 5 kHz. This model assumes that basilar membrane tuning is equal to neural tuning. The Allen model (1,3) describes neural data for frequencies below 5 kHz, but in that model, neural and mechanical tuning differs by approximately 20 dB one-half octave or so below the best frequency. Thus two micromechanical models that make quite different assumptions have been shown to fit tuning data in different frequency regions. Until the experimental questions are resolved, it seems that this theoretical question must remain open.

MICROMECHANICAL MODELS

We next discuss two classes of theories that attempt to model the experimentally observed frequency selectivity. The first is based on the idea that the tectorial membrane vibrates at its own resonant frequency, near the resonant frequency of the basilar membrane. In 1980, different versions of this resonant tectorial membrane approach were independently proposed by Zwislocki and Kletsky (48) and Allen (1). The second is the theory of Neely and Kim (26), which calls on the idea of an active, or negative resistance, basilar membrane. Most recently, Neely and Kim (27) have published a more comprehensive theory in which they merge the resonant tectorial membrane model of Allen (1) with their active basilar membrane theory.

Zwislocki's Tectorial Membrane Models

Zwislocki (46) has proposed a number of tectorial membrane models for sharpening the basilar membrane response. In 1979 he and Kletsky (47) proposed a model for

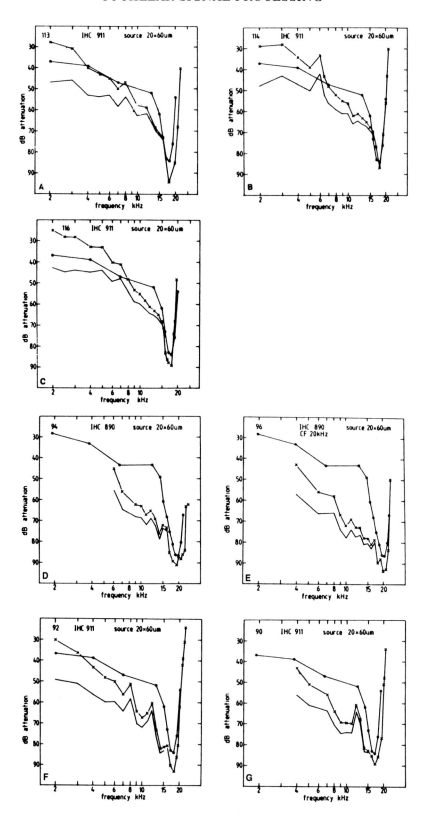

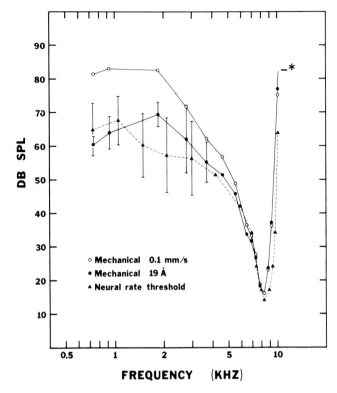

FIG. 14. Comparison of mechanical and neural response measurements. Both the displacement (●) and the velocity (○) are shown for comparison. The neural measurements (*broken line*) and the basilar membrane displacement are shown with error bars that represent one standard deviation of the measurement. What is unusual about this comparison is that the neural response is less sharply tuned than either of the mechanical responses. (From ref. 33.)

sharpening based on longitudinal smoothing by the tectorial membrane, which resulted from the longitudinal mechanical properties of the tectorial membrane, followed by a difference that resulted from the usual ter Kuile shearing motion at the inner hair cells. With some simple analysis, one may show that this model is similar in its effect to the spatial difference model proposed by Hall in 1977 (13). This model is not, however, a resonant tctorial membrane model.

In 1980, Zwislocki and Kletsky (48) proposed two new approaches to this problem, which they called models I and II. Model I is a resonant reed that is mass loaded. The resonant system is meant to represent the tectorial membrane mass and the stereocilia stiffness.

FIG. 13. This figure summarizes one of the major problems in hearing research today, namely the observed difference between the measured basilar membrane frequency response and hair cell measured frequency response. The problem is that most measurements of basilar membrane frequency response are not as sharply tuned as the hair cell responses. **A,B,C:** Measurements of the motion of the small Mossbauer source placed on the edge of the basilar membrane compared with the isoamplitude curve at 0.9 mV inner hair cell d.c. receptor potential (○). Basilar membrane isovelocity curve at 0.04 mm/sec (X). Basilar membrane isodisplacement curve at 3.5 Å (continuous curve). **D,E,F,G:** As for A, B, C but with the small source placed in the middle of the basilar membrane. (From ref. 38.)

This model of excitation distinctly differs from the model of ter Kuile, since there is no analog of the spiral limbus-tectorial membrane coupling. Their model differs from that of Allen (1) in exactly this way, since in Allen's model, the radial stiffness of the tectorial membrane was specifically taken into account in a functionally significant way. In Allen's model, the coupling element plays an important role in the excitation of the cilia. As a result, the shape of the frequency response owing to the radial resonance in Allen's model is quite different from that measured by Zwislocki and Kletsky (compare Fig. 18C with Fig. 2 of ref. 48). In summary, these two systems are *not* isomorphic.

Zwislocki and Kletsky's model II (48) seems to be a partial joining of the spatial smoothing model (47) and model I described above. This model consists of a parallel bank of resonating reeds tuned to slightly different frequencies. The reeds are connected, along the longitudinal axis, with a nonlinear elastic medium that mechanically couples them. Again, as in model I, this system has no spiral limbus analog. The model system is shown in a photograph in the original paper, along with some experimental results showing the suppression effects they saw of one tone on a second. Both models I and II are described as nonlinear models, but only the first is a sharpening model.

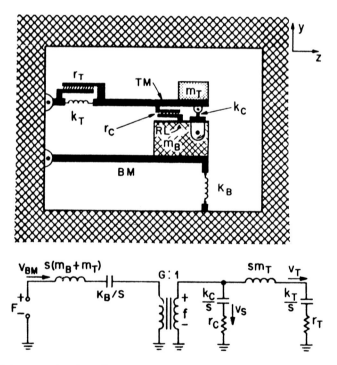

FIG. 15. A model assumption that allows one to match neural tuning data is to introduce a spring, or elastic element, in the tectorial membrane (element k_T of the figure). The addition of this element gives rise to a response cancellation owing to resonance in the response function describing the relation between the basilar membrane and the shear seen by the hair cells. This may be shown by analyzing the electrical equivalent circuit given in the lower part of the figure. (From ref. 1.)

Allen's Tectorial Membrane Model

In Fig. 15 we see a model extension of the ter Kuile model where the tectorial membrane is given a new degree of freedom to vibrate in the radial direction (1), depicted here as the z direction. On the low-frequency side of the tuning curve for this model a partial cancellation of the shear motion occurs at the site of the inner hair cells, relative to the up-down motion of the basilar membrane. This cancellation is a result of the added degree of freedom (the elastic tectorial membrane element labeled k_T). This cancellation could account for the difference frequently observed between basilar membrane motion and neural response below the characteristic frequency. In Fig. 16 we show cat neural tuning data for several neural units, and in Fig. 17, the model result using the linear two-dimensional macromechanical model coupled to the resonant tectorial membrane micromechanical model (3). In the model calculation we have held the model output constant and plotted the resulting input

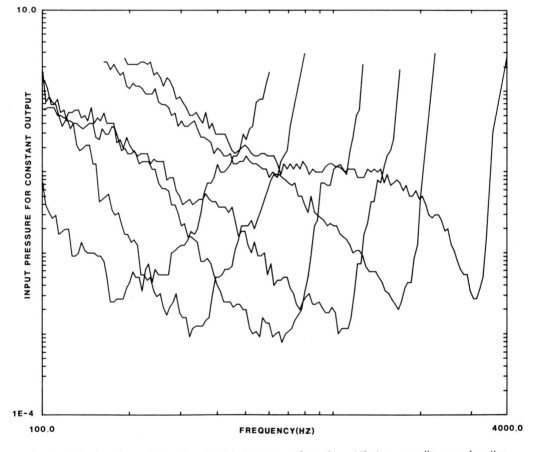

FIG. 16. We show here six low-threshold tuning curves from the cat that are equally spaced on the log-frequency axis. Only units having characteristic frequencies between 100 Hz and 4 kHz are displayed because this is the important frequency range for speech communication. No similar data are available for humans. However, all known mammals give similar results. Note the amplitude range of the plot that covers a 10^5 range or 100 dB.

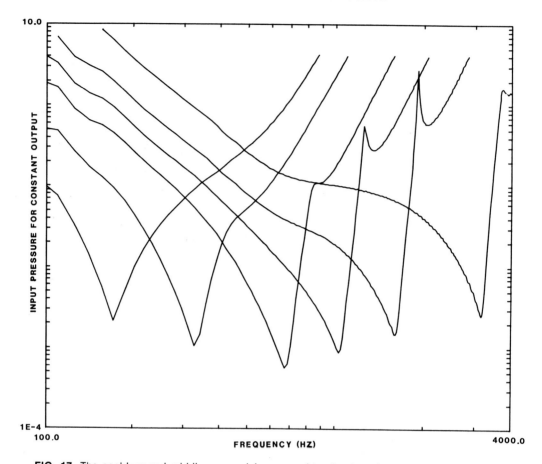

FIG. 17. The cochlear and middle ear models are used to simulate the ear canal pressure for a constant output, which here was assumed to be the shear velocity of the tectorial membrane-reticular lamina. The model calculation was done in the frequency domain with a linear two-dimensional cochlear model. The basilar membrane micromechanical model is that defined in Fig. 15.

pressure in the ear canal. Intermediate model results (not shown) for the cochlear input impedance and the cochlear microphonic also agree with experimentally observed results.

In Fig. 18 we show four measures from the model as a function of position along the basilar membrane, for six different input frequencies: In (A) we see the model neural output, given constant input pressure in the model ear canal; in (B) we show the model neural phase; in (C) we show the model transfer function magnitude relating the basilar membrane to hair cell displacement, which results from the resonant tectorial membrane model; and in (D) we see the basilar membrane impedance magnitude for the resonant tectorial membrane model, which is required when calculating the basilar membrane velocity using the macromechanical model. For these results we assumed that the model neural output was proportional to the TM-RL shear velocity as described in the legend for Fig. 17.

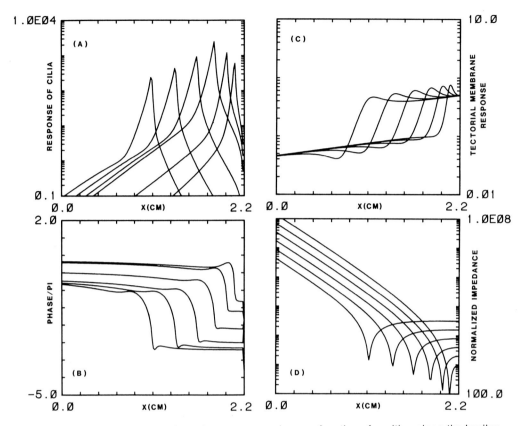

FIG. 18. This figure illustrates how the response varies as a function of position along the basilar membrane, for six different input frequencies. Panel **A** gives the shear velocity; **B** shows the shear phase, **C** shows the basilar membrane to shear transfer function magnitude (this is defined as the ratio of the cilia response to the basilar membrane response), and **D**, the model basilar membrane impedance magnitude. Note particularly the effect of the resonant tectorial membrane on the tuning curve, as shown in (C). The effect of the tectorial membrane in this model is to change the quasi-low-pass basilar membrane transfer function (Fig. 5) into a bandpass filter as seen in Fig. 17.

From Figs. 16 and 17 it is clear that the model does a reasonable, but not perfect, job of describing the neural data. Note that the resonant tectorial membrane transfer function (Fig. 18C) has a 20-dB "sharpening" effect on the response for frequencies below the cutoff frequency, which is close to the difference observed by Sellick et al. (38) as seen in Fig. 13. Our model effort does not at present attempt to account specifically for the Sellick et al. data.

Neely and Kim's Negative Resistance Model

A second and alternative approach to account for sharp neural tuning has been proposed by Neely and Kim (26) and has been worked out in some detail by Neely in his Ph.D. thesis (25). This model calls on the concept of negative damping, or resistance, in the basilar membrane. This model distinguishes itself from the resonant

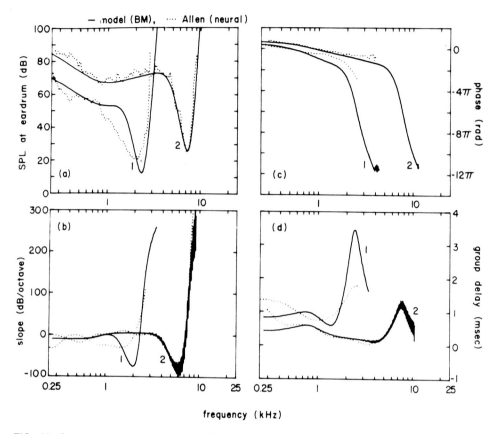

FIG. 19. Comparison of neural data (*dotted lines*) and model results (*solid lines*) from Neely and Kim's active basilar membrane model. (**a**): Threshold tuning curves; (**b**): slope of the tuning curves; (**c**): phase of the response; and (**d**): group delay of the response. The neural phase data in (c) and (d) are plotted after removing 1.2-msec delay attributable to acoustic, synaptic, and neural spike propagation delays. (From ref. 26.)

tectorial membrane models owing to one of its basic assumptions, i.e., the model assumes that the neural and the basilar membrane responses are identical. Therefore the original ter Kuile model was used unmodified in Neely's theory (the tectorial membrane was assumed to be rigid in the radial direction (26) (Fig. 2). One serious problem with this model is the lack of a definable relationship between the model parameters and the cochlear anatomy.

The results of Neely and Kim (26) shown in Fig. 19 are a very impressive match to high frequency neural tuning curves, both magnitude and phase, where phase data are available. In general, the higher the characteristic frequency of the neural data being matched, the better the model fit.

In a recent paper, Neely and Kim (27) join the resonant tectorial membrane model of Allen (1) with an active source that represents active outer hair cells. This model gives the best fit to tuning curve data to date for any of the models, if the entire 100 Hz to 30 kHz hearing range is considered. This paper also improves on the earlier paper (26) by having a definable correspondence between many of the model parameters and the cochlea anatomy, with the important exception of the active source pressure.

The use of a negative resistance is supported by the observations, first made by Kemp (15), of emissions from the cochlea.

Evoked Echoes and Spontaneous Emissions

In 1958 Elliott (10) observed that the threshold of hearing was not a smooth function of frequency, but that it fluctuated in a quasiperiodic manner with a period of a few hundred hertz. Such microstructure could be characteristic of low-level standing waves attributed to slight mismatches at different positions along the basilar membrane (17).

Later it was observed by Kemp in 1978 (15,16) that low-level dispersive reflections may be found in response to a pulse of sound in the ear canal. The delay involved approximately corresponds to a round trip travel time along the basilar membrane. The reflections are nonlinear in their behavior since they grow at less than a linear rate with increasing input pulse level. Because of the nonlinear character of the echoes, it will not be easy to model them until the nonlinear properties of the basilar membrane are better understood.

A third somewhat bizarre observation was then made with the finding that narrow-band tones emanate from the human cochlea (16,42). In animals, similar tones have been correlated with damage to the cochlea. It would be natural to ask if the microstructure in the hearing threshold previously observed correlates to these narrow-band tones, the speculation being that the tones are just biological noise passively amplified by the presumed standing waves mentioned above. Such narrow-band noise would have a Gaussian amplitude distribution, and the amplitude distribution of the tones seems to be closer to that of a pure tone, which is contrary to the standing-wave model.(6).

When these spontaneous emissions were first observed, many researchers were quick to conjecture that the cochlea was an active system that occasionally became unstable (8,16). Hence models that incorporate negative damping, such as Neely's (26), are interesting. The use of negative damping in the model serves the function of sharpening the tuning of the cochlear filters. It also has the capability, in theory, of making the basilar membrane oscillate, thus giving rise to the emissions that were observed by Kemp (15).

The source of the proposed negative damping is still unknown, but we believe we know where to look for it. In 1985 Brownell et al. (7) found that isolated outer hair cells change their length when placed in an electric field. This has led to the speculation that outer hair cells act as linear motors directly driving the basilar membrane. The displacement of the linear motors would probably be a function of the outer hair cell receptor potential, which in turn is modulated by both the position of the basilar membrane (forming a tight feedback loop) and the efferent neurons that are connected to the outer hair cells (forming a very slow feedback loop). The details of this possibility are the topic of present-day research. The work of Liberman and his colleagues gives important constraints on how this system might work. In Fig. 20 we see a figure from Liberman and Dodd (24) that indicates the complex relationships between the state of the inner and outer hair cells and the neurally measured frequency response. Perhaps an improved understanding of this interaction will lead to the breakthrough that we need in describing the cochlear frequency selectivity and the nonlinear characteristics of the basilar membrane.

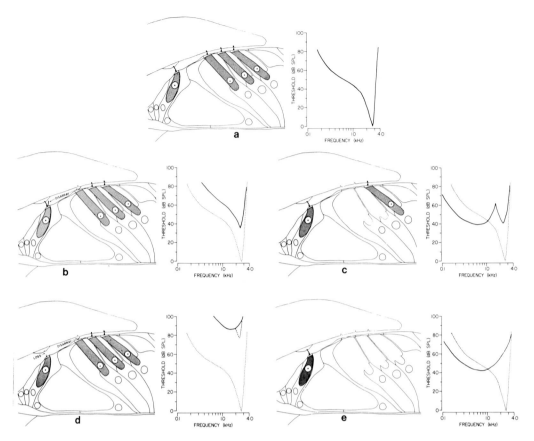

FIG. 20. Schematic representation of a normal organ of Corti (**a**) and four different damage states. Each damaged state is shown with the particular tuning curve abnormality that was found to arise from radial fiber innervation from such a region. From this figure we see that the tuning of the inner hair cell is systematically dependent on the nature of the damage. (**b**): Damage to the inner hair cells raises the threshold of the unit but does not significantly change the shape of the tuning. (**c**): Damage to the first and second rows of outer hair cells enhances the frequency-dependent notch seen just below 2.0 kHz. We interpret this notch as having the same physics as the model effect described in Fig. 18C, which results from the resonant tectorial membrane (Fig. 15). The tip is also missing, which might suggest a loss of basilar membrane gain because of the partial loss of outer hair cells. Note how this loss is accompanied by a lower threshold in the tail region (below 1.0 kHz). This could be interpreted as a loss of the cancellation in that frequency region owing to the shifting of the "zero" of the resonant tectorial membrane. (**d**): Inner hair cell loss uniformly increases the threshold. (**e**): Total outer hair cell loss results in a hypersensitive tail threshold. This is an extension of the result from (c). (From ref. 24.)

REFERENCES

1. Allen, J. B. (1980): Cochlear micromechanics—A physical model of transduction. *J. Acoust. Soc. Am.*, 68:1660–1670.
2. Allen, J. B. (1983): Magnitude and phase frequency response to single tones in the auditory nerve. *J. Acoust. Soc. Am.*, 73:2071–2092.
3. Allen, J. B. (1985): Cochlear modeling. *IEEE ASSP*, 2(1):3–29.
4. Allen, J. B., and Fahey, P. F. (1983): Nonlinear behavior at threshold determined in the auditory canal and on the auditory nerve. In: *Hearing—Physiological Bases and Psychophysics*, edited by R. Klinke and R. Hartmann, pp. 128–133. Springer-Verlag, New York.

5. Allen, J. B., and Sondhi, M. M. (1979): Cochlear macromechanics—Time domain solutions. *J. Acoust. Soc. Am.*, 66:123–132.
6. Bialek, W., and Wit, H. P. (1984): Quantum limits to oscillator stability: Theory and experiments on acoustic emissions from the human ear. *Physics Lett.*, 104a(3):173–178.
7. Brownell, W. E., Bader, C. R., Bertrand, D., and de Ribaupierre, Y. (1985): Evoked mechanical responses of isolated cochlear outer hair cells. *Science*, 227:194–196.
8. Davis, H. (1983): An active process in cochlear mechanics. *Hear. Res.*, 9:79–90.
9. deBoer, E. (1981): Short waves in three-dimensional cochlear models: Solutions for a "block" model. *Hear. Res.*, 4:53–77.
10. Elliott, E. (1958): A ripple effect in the audiogram. *Nature*, 181:1076.
11. Fahey, P. F., and Allen, J. B. (1985): Nonlinear phenomena as observed in the ear canal and at the auditory nerve. *J. Acoust. Soc. Am.*, 77:599–612.
12. Goldstein, J. L., and Kiang, N. (1968): Neural correlates of the aural combination tone 2f1-f2. *Proc. IEEE*, 56:981–992.
13. Hall, J. L. (1981): Observations on a nonlinear model for motion of the basilar membrane. In: *Hearing Research and Theory*, edited by J. V. Tobias and E. D. Schubert, pp. 1–61. Academic Press, New York.
14. Helmholtz, H. L. F. (1862/1954): *On the Sensations of Tone*, pp. 406–410. Dover Publications, New York.
15. Kemp, D. T. (1978): Stimulated acoustic emissions from within the human auditory system. *J. Acoust. Soc. Am.*, 64:1386–1391.
16. Kemp, D. T. (1979): Evidence of mechanical nonlinearity and frequency selective wave amplification in the cochlea. *Arch. Otorhinolaryngol.*, 224:37–45.
17. Kemp, D. T. (1980): Towards a model for the origin of cochlear echos. *Hear. Res.*, 2:533–548.
18. Khanna, S. M., and Leonard, D. (1982): Basilar membrane tuning in the cat cochlea. *Science*, 215:305–306.
19. Khanna, S. M., and Leonard, D. G. B. (1986): Relationship between basilar membrane tuning and hair cell condition. *Hear. Res.*, 23:55–70.
20. Kiang, N., and Moxon, E. C. (1974): Tails of tuning curves of auditory nerve fibers. *J. Acoust. Soc. Am.*, 55:620–630.
21. Kim, D. O., Molnar, C. E., and Peiffer, R. R. (1973): A system of nonlinear differential equations modeling basilar-membrane motion. *J. Acoust. Soc. Am.*, 54:1517–1529.
22. Kuile, E. ter. (1900): Die Uebertragung der Energie von der Grundmanbran auf die Haazellen. *Pflugers. Arch.*, 79:146–157.
23. Lesser, M., and Berkley, D. (1972): Fluid mechanics of the cochlea, Part I. *J. Fluid Mech.*, 51(3):497–512.
24. Liberman, M. C., and Dodds, L. W. (1984): Single-neuron labeling and chronic cochlear pathology. III. Stereocilia damage and alterations of threshold tuning curves. *Hear. Res.*, 16:55–74.
25. Neely, S. T. (1981): Fourth-order partition dynamics of a two-dimensional model of the cochlea. Doctoral dissertation, Washington University, St. Louis, MO.
26. Neely, S. T., and Kim, D. O. (1983): An active cochlear model showing sharp tuning and high sensitivity. *Hear. Res.*, 9:123–130.
27. Neely, S. T., and Kim, D. O. (1986): A model for active elements in cochlear biomechanics. *J. Acoust. Soc. Am.*, 79:1472–1480.
28. Peterson, L. C., and Bogert, B. P. (1950): A dynamical theory of the cochlea. *J. Acoust. Soc. Am.*, 22:369–381.
29. Pickles, J. O. (1982): *An Introduction to the Physiology of Hearing*. Academic Press, London.
30. Ranke, O. F. (1950): Theory operation of the cochlea: A contribution to the hydrodynamics of the cochlea. *J. Acoust. Soc. Am.*, 22:772–777.
31. Rhode, W. (1971): Observations of the vibrations of the basilar membrane in squirrel monkeys using the Mossbauer technique. *J. Acoust. Soc. Am.*, 49:1218–1231.
32. Rhode, W. (1978): Some observations on cochlear mechanics. *J. Acoust. Soc. Am.*, 64:158–176.
33. Robles, L., Ruggero, M. A., Rich, N. C. (1986): Basilar membrane mechanics at the base of the chinchilla cochlea. I. Input-output functions, tuning curves, and response phases. *J. Acoust. Soc. Am.*, 80:1364–1374.
34. Russell, I., and Sellick, P. (1978): Intracellular studies of hair cells in the mammalian cochlea. *J. Physiol.*, 284:261–290.
35. Sachs, M. B., and Kiang, Y. S. (1968): Two-tone inhibition in auditory-nerve fibers. *J. Acoust. Soc. Am.*, 43:1120–1128.
36. Schroeder, M. R. (1975): Models of hearing. *Proc. IEEE*, 63:1332–1350.
37. Sellick, P. M., Patuzzi, R., and Johnstone, B. M. (1982): Measurement of basilar membrane motion in the guinea pig using the Mossbauer technique. *J. Acoust. Soc. Am.*, 72:131–141.
38. Sellick, P. M., Patuzzi, R., and Johnstone, B. M. (1983): Comparison between the tuning properties of inner haircells and basilar membrane motion. *Hear. Res.*, 10:93–100.

39. Siebert, W. M. (1974): Ranke revisited—A simple short-wave cochlear model. *J. Acoust. Soc. Am.*, 56:594–600.
40. Stevens, S. S., and Davis, H. (1938): *Hearing, Its Psychology and Physiology*. John Wiley, New York.
41. Viergever, M. A. (1980): *Mechanics of the Inner Ear: A Mathematical Approach*. Delft University Press, Delft, The Netherlands.
42. Zurek, P. M. (1981): Spontaneous narrowband acoustic signals emitted by human ears. *J. Acoust. Soc. Am.*, 69:514–523.
43. Zweig, G., Lipes, R., and Pierce, J. R. (1976): The cochlear compromise. *J. Acoust. Soc. Am.*, 59:975–982.
44. Zwislocki, J. J. (1948): Theorie der Schneckenmechanik. *Acta Otolaryngol. [Suppl.] (Stockh.)*, 72.
45. Zwislocki, J. J. (1950): Theory of the acoustical action of the cochlea. *J. Acoust. Soc. Am.*, 22:778–784.
46. Zwislocki, J. J. (1980): Five decades of research on cochlear mechanics. *J. Acoust. Soc. Am.*, 67:1679–1685.
47. Zwislocki, J. J., and Kletsky, E. J. (1979): Tectorial membrane: A possible effect on frequency analysis in the cochlea. *Science*, 204:639–641.
48. Zwislocki, J. J., and Kletsky, E. J. (1980): Micromechanics in the theory of cochlear mechanics. *Hear. Res.*, 2:505–512.

Physiology of the Ear,
edited by A. F. Jahn and J. Santos-Sacchi.
Raven Press, New York © 1988.

Cochlear Physiology

Joseph Santos-Sacchi

Laboratory of Otolaryngology, New Jersey Medical School, University of Medicine and Dentistry of New Jersey, Newark, New Jersey 07103-2757

The hair cells of the organ of Corti, the sensory epithelium that rests on the basilar membrane, transduce mechanical movements of the basilar membrane into electrical responses that initiate a complex series of events, ultimately leading to the perception of sound. The purpose of this chapter is to introduce the reader to the basic electrophysiology of the peripheral auditory system. For more detailed information, the reader is referred to more comprehensive reviews of this topic (15–18,34,45,58).

BIO-ELECTRIC POTENTIALS

The basis of our understanding of cochlear function rests heavily on measures of the electrical activity of intracellular and extracellular compartments of the membranous labyrinth. It is essential, therefore, to understand some underlying principles governing the generation of bio-electric potentials.

Electrical potential differences in biological structures are essentially produced by the separation of charged particles [positively (cationic) or negatively (anionic) charged ions] across some barrier. In cells, the plasma membrane provides the barrier across which ions are separated and enables cells to maintain a resting potential difference across the membrane. One can measure the potential difference across a cell's membrane with the aid of an electronic device (voltmeter) and electrodes (Fig. 1). The magnitude of this potential difference varies with cell type and typically lies within the range of 10 to 100 millivolts (mV) at rest. The cell interior is negative relative to the exterior because there is a net negative charge on the inner surface of the membrane. Both the magnitude and polarity of the resting potential are dependent on the properties of the plasma membrane barrier and the concentrations of various ions on either side of the membrane.

The plasma membrane of cells is composed of a phospholipid bilayer, within which float proteins and protein complexes (Fig. 1). Although the phospholipid bilayer is freely permeable to water, ions cannot pass through it. However, some special types of proteins that span the lipid bilayer provide aqueous channels that permit the passage of selected ions across the membrane. These aqueous channels impart a semipermeability to the plasma membrane, i.e., specific ions (e.g., K^+, or Na^+) are able to pass into or out of the cell more readily than others, depending on the relative proportion of conducting ion-selective channels within the plasma membrane.

In cells, the concentrations of the major biological ions (K^+, Na^+, Cl^-, and large organic anions) are distributed differentially across the membrane. The concentration

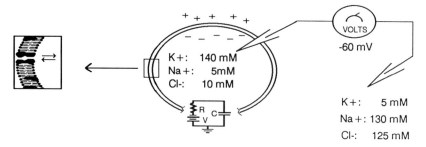

FIG. 1. Schematized hypothetical mammalian cell illustrating typical concentrations of intracellular and extracellular ions. The membrane potential can be recorded by placing an electrolyte-filled glass tube drawn to a fine tip (<0.5 μm) through the membrane and into the intracellular fluid. The difference in potential between this electrode and the extracellular one, measured with a voltmeter, indicates a membrane potential of −60 mV. As described in the text, membrane channels within the lipid bilayer (*insert*) permit the selective passage of ions, which establishes the magnitude and polarity of the membrane potential. The circuit inset in the cell membrane illustrates a simple equivalent circuit of a cell membrane, which consists of (a) a battery of −60 mV whose value is determined from the Goldman equation, (b) a lumped resistance of 30 MΩ representing the sum of individual channel resistances in parallel, and (c) a capacitor of 20 pF, representing the ability of the membrane to separate and store charges of opposite polarity. The product of the resistance and capacitance determines the cell's ability to register rapid changes in membrane potential (see text).

of K^+ and organic anions is high intracellularly, and that of Na^+ and Cl^- is high extracellularly. The maintenance of Na^+ and K^+ concentrations is assisted by a metabolically active pump that translocates potassium ions into the cell and sodium ions out. Although the large organic ions are membrane impermeant, the other ions are capable of crossing the semipermeable membrane and will tend to move either in or out of the cell depending on electrical and chemical forces acting on them. In the steady state, however, these forces are in equilibrium and there is no net movement of charged particles across the membrane.

The electrical and chemical forces alluded to above are, respectively (a) the electromotive force that causes repulsion of particles of like charge and (b) the force associated with concentration gradients that induces movements of particles from areas of high concentration to areas of lower concentration. Thus, if a high concentration of K^+ exists on one side of a permeable membrane (e.g., inside a cell), K^+ will diffuse to the other side (outside the cell). As positively charged potassium ions move across the membrane, a separation of charge across the immediate vicinity of the membrane arises, such that the outside of the membrane is at a positive potential relative to the inside. This developing potential difference provides an electromotive force that counteracts the outward K^+ diffusion brought on by the concentration gradient. The equilibrium potential for a given ion is that potential difference across a semipermeable membrane at which the electrochemical forces are in balance and no net flux of ions occurs across the membrane. Given the concentration of a specific ion on either side of a membrane that is selectively permeable to that ion, the Nernst equation can be used to calculate the equilibrium potential. Thus, for a particular ion X,

$$E_{(X)} = 2.3 \frac{RT}{ZF} \log \frac{[X]_o}{[X]_i} \qquad [1]$$

where $E_{(X)}$ is the equilibrium potential in mV, R is the gas constant, T is temperature in degrees kelvin, Z is the valence of the ion (e.g., $+1$ for K^+), F is Faraday's constant, and $[X]_o$ and $[X]_i$ are the free concentrations of the ion outside and inside the cell, respectively.

In steady state, at 25°C, an artificial cell with potassium concentrations of 5 mM extracellularly and 140 mM intracellularly will have a transmembrane potential of 86 mV (inside negative).

$$E_{(K)} = 60 \text{ mV} \log \frac{[5]}{[140]} = -86 \text{ mV} \tag{2}$$

We know, however, that real cell membranes have channels permeable to ions other than K^+, and these ions could conceivably contribute to the resting potential. Equilibrium potentials for Na^+ and Cl^- according to the concentrations listed in Fig. 1 are $+85$ and -65 mV, respectively. In the case where these three ionic species are present simultaneously, the membrane potential of the cell will depend not only on the concentration of these ions inside and outside the cell, but also on the relative membrane permeability of each ion. The membrane potential in such a case can be quantified by the Goldman equation

$$V_m = 2.3 \frac{RT}{F} \log \frac{P_{(K)}[K]_o + P_{(Na)}[Na]_o + P_{(Cl)}[Cl]_i}{P_{(K)}[K]_i + P_{(Na)}[Na]_i + P_{(Cl)}[Cl]_o} \tag{3}$$

where $P_{(ion)}$ denotes the relative membrane permeability of the individual ionic species. If the permeabilities are different, the more permeable ion will contribute to a greater extent, forcing the membrane potential closer to its equilibrium potential. In the case in which the permeability of any one ion is much greater than the other two, the equation will simplify to the Nernst equation for that ion. In general, the membrane potential mainly depends on the K^+ concentration across the membrane, because the plasma membrane is more permeable at rest to K^+ than to other ions. If, however, the membrane is perturbed by some external force, the membrane's properties may be altered—the permeability to various ions may change. We can appreciate from the Goldman equation that the membrane potential of the cell will be affected by externally induced alterations in the relative membrane permeabilities of ions. It is by this means that cells may electrically signal the effects of external stimuli.

Thus far we have seen that a cell consists of a barrier, the cell membrane, which separates charged particles, ions, on either side. Furthermore, we know that forces exist that can move these charged particles across the membranous barrier. The membrane may be thought of as a resistance that impedes the flow of ions (current) across it. The reciprocal of resistance is conductance, a measure of the ease with which ions flow. The larger the resistance of the membrane, the less current will flow for a constant driving force. In electrical terms this is described by Ohm's law,

$$V = IR \tag{4}$$

where voltage V is the driving force across the resistance R, which induces a flow of charged particles I through the resistive pathway. The units for voltage, resistance, and current are volts (V), ohms (Ω), and amps (A), respectively. One volt across a 1-Ω resistor will produce 1 A of current. One amp is defined as the passage of 1 coulomb (C) (6.28×10^{18} charged particles) across a given point in 1 sec.

In a cell at rest, the net current across the membrane is zero, and the voltage across it is at the resting potential for reasons discussed. If, however, a current is injected into the cell by means of an electrode placed inside the cell, that current will flow across the membrane and alter the resting membrane potential. For example, in a cell whose resting potential is -60 mV, and membrane resistance is 30 MΩ, a negative 0.1 nA of current injected intracellularly, will generate an electrotonic potential of -3 mV across the membrane and hyperpolarize the cell to -63 mV. A positive 0.1 nA current will depolarize the cell to -57 mV. The relation between current and voltage (I–V curve) for an "ohmic" resistive element is linear, as described by Ohm's law. Cell membranes, however, may not necessarily obey this linear relationship. In fact, some membranes may only permit current flow in one preferential direction across the membrane, a process termed rectification. This deviation from linearity is owing to the variable resistive properties of the membrane as a consequence of ionic channel conductance and gating properties.

The cell membrane possesses another quality that can be likened to the electrical property of a capacitor. This property, capacitance, occurs when two electrically conducting materials (intra- and extracellular fluids) are separated by an insulating material (lipid bilayer). A capacitor is able to separate and store charges of opposite polarity on either surface of the insulator. When charges are separated, a voltage is set up across the capacitor, such that

$$V = Q/C \qquad [5]$$

where V is the voltage, Q is the charge in coulombs, and C is the capacitance in farads. A change in Q (delta Q) across the capacitor will produce a change in V (delta V). The magnitude of capacitance indicates how well the capacitor can store a charge.

The capacity of membranes plays an important role in determining time-dependent changes in membrane potential. As discussed previously, the injection of current across a cell membrane produces a change in transmembrane voltage that depends on the value of the membrane resistance, as expressed in Ohm's law. However, the time taken to achieve this voltage change will depend on the magnitude of the membrane capacitance that is in parallel with the resistance across the membrane (Fig. 1). The voltage change is an exponential function of time, with a time constant T, given by

$$T = RC \qquad [6]$$

The time constant of a cell is that time required for delta V to reach 63% of its ultimate value. Delta V essentially will reach steady state after about five time constants. Cell membranes typically have a fixed capacitance of 1μF/cm^2 of surface membrane, so that cell size and membrane resistance will mainly determine the cell's time constant. The time constant will limit the extent to which the cell's membrane potential can follow variations in transmembrane current. In essence, the membrane imparts a low pass filter characteristic, reducing the ability of the cell to register voltage fluctuations above the frequency determined by its time constant.

BASIC HAIR CELL PHYSIOLOGY

The hair cell, a mechanoreceptor, serves as a sensory transducer for a variety of organs in vertebrates that transmit information to the CNS about mechanical forces impinging on the organism. In the organ of Corti, inner hair cells (IHCs) and outer hair cells (OHCs) sense the acoustically induced mechanical vibrations of the basilar membrane on which they rest.

Hair cells are specialized epithelial cells, and as with all surface epithelial cells, the plasma membrane of hair cells is polarized into an apical portion and a basolateral portion. Special membrane structures, called tight junctions, tightly join the apical circumference of hair cells to adjacent supporting cells, thereby preventing the intermixing of ions and molecules of apical and basal compartments (e.g., endolymph and perilymph). The types of ion-selective channels present in the apical and basolateral membranes are different. The apical region contains the hair cell's transduction channels (see below). The basolateral membrane of hair cells has Ca^{2+} channels, a few types of K^+ channels, including a Ca^{2+}-activated K^+ channel, and Cl^- channels, all of which are in a low conducting state at the resting potential of the cell (5,38,46,54,74,75).

The current–voltage relation of the hair cell does not obey Ohm's law but is rectified in the depolarizing direction. In some hair cell types (54), there is evidence that this occurs because of the presence of Ca^{2+} channels, which are voltage sensitive. Depolarization of the membrane opens these channels and allows Ca^{2+} ions to enter the cell. Intracellular Ca^{2+} ions bind to a site on Ca^{2+}-activated K^+ channels, causing them to open and permit an outward flow of K^+ ions. The probability of Ca^{2+}-activated K^+ channels opening is also increased as the membrane potential is depolarized. The result is a preferential increase in total membrane conductance on depolarization—rectification. Consequently, the cell will repolarize toward the resting potential because the increase in K^+ permeability forces the membrane potential toward the equilibrium potential of K^+. Ca^{2+} channels close on this repolarization.

The means by which hair cells respond to mechanical stimuli has been studied in detail in a number of hair cell systems of lower vertebrates (34,35,44,46,47,60). Hair cells from these systems and the organ of Corti have in common structural specializations of the apical plasma membrane, stereocilia, which enable the cells to sense mechanical perturbations (34,47).

At rest, a steady inward current is thought to flow through transduction channels located within the plasma membrane at the apices of the stereocilia (13,44,60). Although these channels appear to be nonspecific in that a variety of positively charged ions can carry the current, micromolar concentrations of calcium are required to sustain the current (13). Since the concentration of K^+ is usually higher in the fluids facing the apical surface of hair cells in these systems (140 mM in endolymph[1]), K^+ is considered to be the physiological charge carrier. Modulation of the resistance of the apical stereociliar membrane by altering the number of closed and open transduction channels is thought to occur during the bending of stereocilia at the axis of insertion into the apex of the cell. This modulation alters the current flowing into the hair cell and induces changes in the membrane potential, i.e., elicits receptor potentials (30). The morphological polarization of these stiff rod-like structures (36) in some manner imparts a physiological response polarity. Movement of the ster-

---

[1]Recently it has been suggested that the fluid that surrounds the stereocilia in the organ of Corti is similar to perilymph (63).

eociliary bundle in a direction toward the tallest stereocilia results in an increase in the transduction current and a depolarization of the cell's membrane potential; movement in the opposite direction reduces the current and hyperpolarizes the cell (Fig. 2) (34,47). Cross-linking of stereocilia at their apical poles by extracellular fibrillar material may provide the physical substrate of this channel-gating mechanism (62).

The magnitude of the receptor potential depends on the degree to which the stereocilia are displaced from their resting position, but the response is not symmetrical for equal displacements in the hyperpolarizing and depolarizing directions. Displacement–response studies in different types of hair cells, including mammalian IHCs and OHCs, have shown that the voltage response for stereociliar displacements in the depolarizing direction is larger (47,65) (Fig. 3).

This rectification is of special interest in cochlear hair cells where a response to frequencies in the kilohertz range is required. At high frequencies, the combination of this response asymmetry and the IHC membrane's low pass filter characteristics (owing to the membrane time constant) functions to produce sustained intracellular depolarizations. If the response to hair bundle displacement were symmetrical, then the voltage response at high frequencies would be attenuated to an imperceptible level by membrane characteristics. Response asymmetry thus ensures that hair cells will register high-frequency stimulation. The polarity of the asymmetry is also significant since it is in the direction of excitation. On depolarization, the hair cell will effect an increase in the activity of sensory nerve fibers that innervate it (Fig. 2C).

In some types of hair cells, the ion channels of the basolateral membrane may contribute to the frequency selectivity of a particular cell (14,54). That is, an interplay between Ca^{2+} and K^+ channels and/or unique kinetic characteristics of individual K^+ channels may underlie a natural electrical resonance of the hair cell (1,45), which would selectively amplify stimuli of a characteristic frequency. In the hair cells of the mammalian organ of Corti, this frequency selectivity at the cell membrane level has not been found to exist, so it is likely that basilar membrane–organ of Corti micromechanics solely provide for the frequency-resolving power of the inner ear.

Hair cells influence neural activity via chemical synapses (35,37). Depolarization of the hair cell membrane increases the conductance of Ca^{2+} channels in the basolateral membrane of the cell (54), and an influx of Ca^{2+} ensues because the intracellular concentration of unbound Ca^{2+} is much lower than the extracellular concentration. The net increase of intracellular Ca^{2+} that occurs during depolarization is thought to promote fusion of intracellular membranous vesicles containing neurotransmitter with the hair cell's presynaptic plasma membrane, as occurs at the neuromuscular synapse (51). This results in a release of neurotransmitter into the extracellular space between the hair cell and nerve terminal. The neurotransmitter molecules bind to receptors located on the postsynaptic membrane of the nerve fiber and alter the ionic conductance of this membrane, resulting in a depolarization. If the depolarization is sufficient, threshold will be crossed and the nerve will initiate an action potential.

COCHLEAR POTENTIALS

Electrical potentials can be measured in the cochlea in various anatomic compartments. These include the cells comprising the membranous labyrinth and the

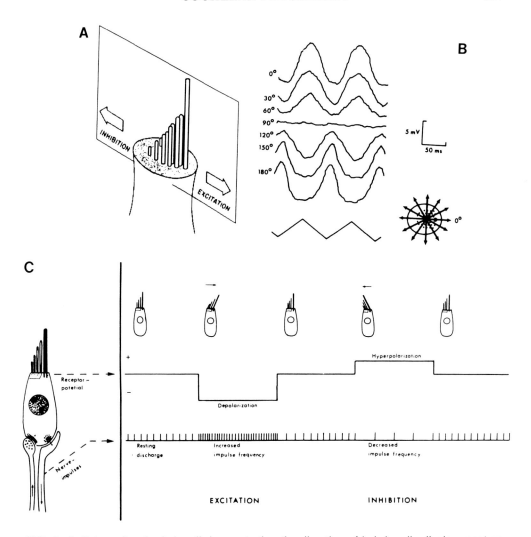

FIG. 2. A: Schematic of a hair cell demonstrating the direction of hair bundle displacement associated with excitation (depolarization) and inhibition (hyperpolarization). Movement toward the kinocilium (the tallest rod-like structure) is excitatory. In mammals the kinocilia are absent in the adult, but movement toward the tallest stereocilia is still excitatory. (From ref. 78, and Flock, Å. Sensory transduction in hair cells, *Handbook of Sensory Physiology*, vol. 1, edited by W. R. Loewenstein, Springer-Verlag, Berlin, 1971.) **B:** Intracellular receptor potentials measured during movements of the hair bundle in various directions. Note that movements of the bundle towards (0°) or away from (180°) the kinocilium produce the largest receptor potentials; movements orthogonal (90°) to that axis produce little or no response, whereas intermediate movements produce smaller responses. (From ref. 77.) **C:** Hair cell afferent nerve activity recorded during displacements of hair bundles in the lateral line organ. Movement toward the kinocilium produces a depolarization of the hair cell membrane accompanied by an increase in afferent spike activity above spontaneous rate. Movement away from the kinocilium produces a hyperpolarization that decreases the spike activity below the spontaneous rate. Effects on afferent activity are thought to be owing to modulation of neurotransmitter release from the hair cell. (From ref. 32.)

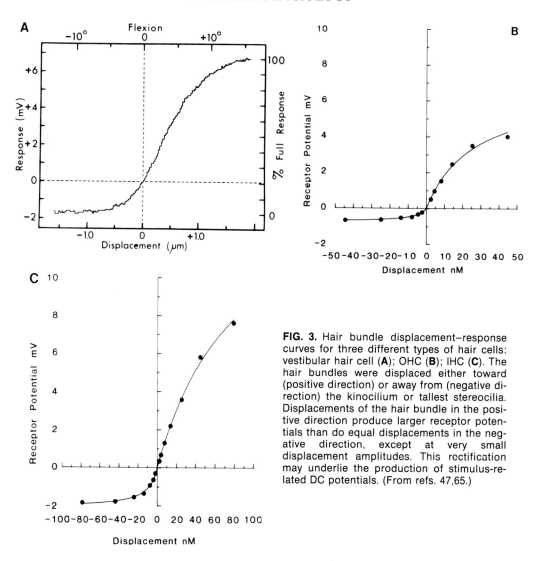

FIG. 3. Hair bundle displacement–response curves for three different types of hair cells: vestibular hair cell (**A**); OHC (**B**); IHC (**C**). The hair bundles were displaced either toward (positive direction) or away from (negative direction) the kinocilium or tallest stereocilia. Displacements of the hair bundle in the positive direction produce larger receptor potentials than do equal displacements in the negative direction, except at very small displacement amplitudes. This rectification may underlie the production of stimulus-related DC potentials. (From refs. 47,65.)

extracellular fluid-filled scalae. Two classes of potentials are distinguishable: those that are stimulus dependent and those that are not. Stimulus-dependent potentials are measured in response to acoustic stimulation. The others are resting potentials that arise because of conditions previously described.

Resting Potentials in the Cochlea

The potential measured in the endolymph of the scala media of the cochlea is positive relative to the perilymph of the scala tympani. The endolymphatic potential (EP) attains values near +80 mV in the base of cochlea, and its magnitude is slightly smaller in the higher turns. The source of this potential is thought to be the stria vascularis (80). The EP is very important for normal sensory function, since it provides an electrical driving force for the movement of positively charged ions through stereociliar transduction channels (64).

The cells within the organ of Corti have negative resting potentials that vary with cell type (6,7,27,39,65,66,79). Supporting cells typically have large potentials ranging from -70 mV to -100 mV. An unusual difference exists between the membrane potentials of IHCs and OHCs. Whereas OHCs have potentials similar to supporting cells, on the average -70mV, IHCs hair cells have potentials near -45 mV. Dallos (21) suggested that these differences are based on electrical characteristics imposed by differing cell morphologies.

Stimulus-Related Potentials

Electrical responses to acoustic stimulation are generated by the hair cells of the organ of Corti. For many years, however, because of the inability to record directly from cochlear hair cells, inferences about these receptor potentials were made by recording responses from areas outside the organ of Corti, e.g., the cochlear scalae (15,17). Such field-potential recordings are averages of responses from many hair cells distributed along the length basilar membrane. However, the response area can be confined to small enough sections of the cochlea duct such that some measure of frequency selectivity at a given location can be evaluated. Figure 4 shows the evoked potential recorded from the third turn of the scala media in response to a pure tone burst of 1,000 Hz. Two components comprise the acoustically evoked response, an alternating current (AC) component whose frequency is the same as the stimulus, and a direct current (DC) component, which displaces the baseline potential, the EP, in a negative direction for the duration of the stimulus. The AC response is the cochlear microphonic (CM) and the DC response is the summating potential (SP).

A typical input–output function displaying the magnitude of the CM versus intensity of the acoustic stimulus is shown in Fig. 5A. For a given frequency, there is a positive linear relationship between the intensity of the acoustic stimulus and the amplitude of the CM. This relation becomes nonlinear at high sound pressure levels, where the response magnitude saturates and eventually decreases, despite increasing stimulus intensity.

At a specific recording location along the cochlear duct, the magnitude of the CM will vary depending on the frequency of the acoustic stimulus. Figure 5B demonstrates the frequency dependence of the CM for three different recording locations along the cochlear duct. It can be seen that the high-frequency cutoff, that point on the high-frequency side of the curves where the response magnitude drops precipitously, differs for each turn. The cutoff is at a progressively lower frequency as one records from base to apex. At one particular recording location, the sharpness of tuning, i.e., the ability to preferentially respond to a narrow range of frequencies, increases as the stimulus intensity approaches auditory threshold levels (Fig. 5C). The frequency that produces the largest response is known as the characteristic or best frequency (BF). This tuning of the CM is a result of the frequency specificity of maximum basilar membrane vibration along the cochlear duct; that is, a me-

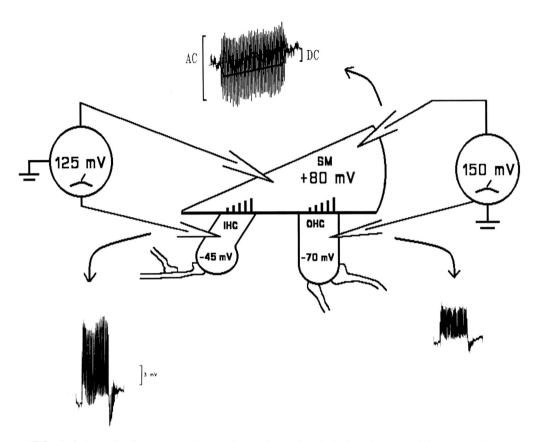

FIG. 4. Schematic of a cross section of the scala media, illustrating the potentials recorded from the extracellular and intracellular compartments of the cochlea. The fluid compartment of the scala media (SM) is at a positive potential relative to the other scalae. The voltage drop across the apical surfaces of the hair cells is therefore enhanced, being about 125 mV for the IHC and 150 mV for the OHC. These voltage drops are thought to be the driving forces responsible for the current flow through the stereociliar transduction channels. Modulation of the resistance of the transduction channels effected by the bending of stereocilia induces alterations in the membrane potentials of the hair cells, i.e., receptor potentials. These potentials can be measured intracellularly and extracellularly. The trace at the top of the figure is the response measured in the third turn scala media of the guinea pig to a tone burst of 1,000 Hz at 80 db SPL (re: 20 μP). Two components can be noted: an AC response (CM) with a peak-to-peak magnitude of 0.563 mV whose frequency is the same as the stimulating frequency and a DC response (SP) whose magnitude is about one-third the AC magnitude and whose polarity is negative (downward) because the recording location has a BF near the stimulating frequency (see text). At the lower left and right are the responses to the same stimulus from a third turn IHC and OHC, respectively. The time scale is compressed a little more than two times compared with that of the extracellular response. Both AC and DC responses are evident; however, the response magnitudes are larger than the extracellular response, and the polarity of the DC components is depolarizing (upward) under these conditions (see text). The peak-to-peak magnitude of the AC component is 4.6 mV for the IHC and 2 mV for the OHC. (From ref. 19.)

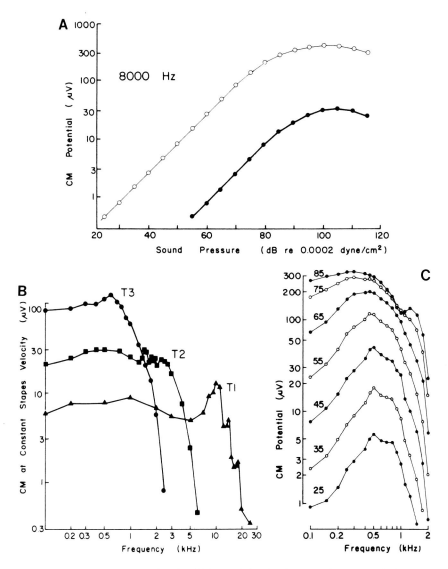

FIG. 5. **A:** Input–output function for the CM at 8 kHz. As the sound pressure is increased, the magnitude of the CM (*open circles*) increases linearly, until at high SPLs the response becomes nonlinear, i.e., saturates and rolls over. The *filled circles* are data taken from a guinea pig whose OHCs had been destroyed in the recording location. Note the shift of the trace to the right, which indicates that more sound pressure is required to obtain response magnitudes comparable to the normal. **B:** Recordings of CM magnitude from three locations along the cochlear duct of the guinea pig: turn 1 (T1), turn 2 (T2), and turn 3 (T3). A constant input stimulus was delivered to the ear, and the responses were measured across the frequency spectrum. The BF differs for each turn as is indicated by the frequency at which the responses fall precipitously. The BF decreases from base to apex. **C:** A family of curves illustrating the CM magnitude versus frequency at several constant sound pressure levels. Note that the sharpness of tuning of the CM increases as the sound pressure is decreased. (From ref. 15.)

chanical filtering underlies the tonotopic nature of the auditory pathway. Measures of CM tuning, however, are not as sharp as recent measures of basilar membrane tuning (53,76), despite the fact that the hair cells, the generators of the CM, are as sharply tuned (27,66,67). This disparity is probably due to the remote recording technique, as the response is from thousands of hair cells whose electrical signals are summed.

The magnitude and polarity of the SP are dependent on the frequency and intensity of the acoustic stimulus (Fig. 6A and B). At the BF, the SP is always negative, when recording in the scala media or differentially between scala vestibuli and tympani (11,29). As we will see, this negativity corresponds to excitatory depolarizing activity of cochlear hair cells. At frequencies below the best, however, the polarity of the SP is positive at low to moderate intensities, but reverses at high intensities. Because of its unique characteristics, the summating potential provides a better measure of frequency tuning along the cochlear partition than does the CM. Figure 6C compares response magnitude versus frequency at a constant sound pressure level for CM and differentially recorded SP in the first turn of the guinea pig cochlea. The negative SP is generated only to a narrow band of frequencies centered on the BF, whereas the frequency extent over which the CM is generated is broad.

Thus far we have seen that electrical responses owing to acoustic stimulation can be recorded in the extracellular compartments of the membranous labyrinth, and indeed they can also be recorded intracellularly from supporting cells (59). These responses are remotely recorded, however, and reflect the electrical activity of hair cells. For some time, the source of these extracellular responses has been thought to be the OHCs, since a dramatic reduction in these responses occurs on selective destruction of these cells (23,24) (Fig. 5A). Further evidence linking IHC and OHC contributions to the remote responses is derived from direct intracellular measures of receptor potentials.

Intracellular receptor potentials recorded from IHCs and OHCs demonstrate some similarities with extracellular stimulus-related potentials (Fig. 4). Both AC and DC responses are measurable, and their input–output functions are similar to gross potentials in showing linear and nonlinear characteristics. Generally, IHCs are more sensitive than OHCs, producing larger responses for a given stimulus intensity. The electrical activity of hair cells has been studied in basal (high BF) and apical (low BF) regions of the cochlea (6,7,20,22,26,27,39,57,65,66,79). Although many similarities between hair cells from these regions exist, notable differences are encountered.

Inner hair cells from both low- and high-frequency regions of the cochlea produce depolarizing DC receptor potentials regardless of stimulus frequency and intensity. AC receptor potentials measured in apical hair cells are larger than their DC counterparts, and eighth nerve fibers innervating these IHCs are capable of phase locking their action potentials to the depolarizing phase of the AC receptor potential. However, AC potentials measured in basal IHCs at their BF are extremely attenuated owing to the cell's membrane time constant (Fig. 7). The DC receptor potential of these cells is responsible for neural excitation, and neural phase locking is absent.

Responses from OHCs in the low- and high-frequency regions of the cochlea differ in some respects. In low-frequency OHCs, AC and DC receptor potentials are generated below and at BF. DC potentials are depolarizing at BF and hyperpolarizing below BF at low intensities, but reverse polarity at higher intensities. This polarity

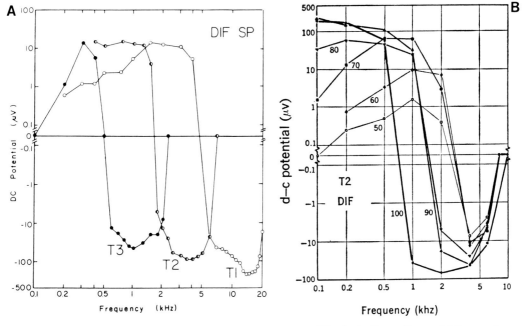

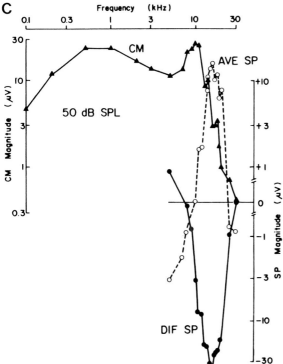

FIG. 6. A: Recordings of SP magnitude from three locations along the cochlear duct of the guinea pig: turn 1 (T1), turn 2 (T2), and turn 3 (T3). Recordings were made differentially with electrodes in the scala tympani and scala vestibuli. A constant input stimulus was delivered to the ear and the responses were measured across the frequency spectrum. The polarity at the BF is negative, and the BF differs for each turn as is indicated by the frequency at which the responses on the low-frequency side reverse polarity, and those on the high-frequency side fall precipitously. (From ref. 17.) **B:** A family of curves illustrating the SP magnitude versus frequency at several constant sound pressure levels. Note that the "sharpness of tuning" of the SP increases as the sound pressure is decreased, as indicated by a narrowing of the breadth of the curves in the hyperpolarizing direction at lower intensities. (From ref. 15.) **C:** Comparison of tuning between CM and SP recorded at the same location along the cochlear duct of the guinea pig. The hyperpolarizing portion of the SP is more sharply tuned than the broad response of the CM. (From ref. 15.)

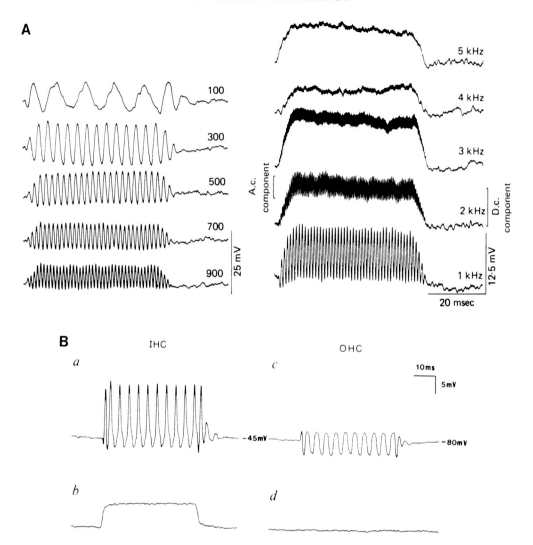

FIG. 7. **A:** Receptor potentials recorded from an IHC located in the basal (high BF) region of the cochlear duct of the guinea pig. Note the disappearance of the AC component in the response as the frequency of stimulation is increased. At high frequencies the AC response is attenuated by the IHC's membrane properties, i.e., the time constant of the membrane limits the ability of the cell to register rapid stimulus variations. Thus the response at BF for cells in this location is essentially DC. (From ref. 67.) **B:** Responses of an IHC and OHC from the basal region of the cochlea to low frequency (a, c) and to high frequency (BF) (b, d) tone bursts. High-BF IHCs produce depolarizing DC potentials regardless of stimulus frequency, however, AC responses at BF are absent. High-BF OHCs produce AC and DC responses at low frequencies, hyperpolarizing DC responses at levels and depolarizing responses at high levels. As with IHCs, OHC AC responses are absent at BF, but so too are DC responses, except at very high intensities. See text for low-BF hair cell response properties. (From ref. 12.)

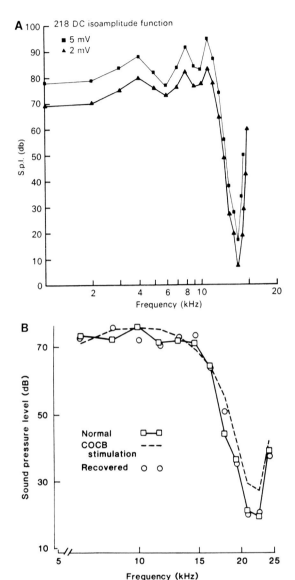

FIG. 8. A: Tuning curve for an IHC located in the basal region of the cochlea. The sound pressure level required to produce a criterion DC response level of 2 or 5 mV is plotted across the frequency spectrum. The more stringent criterion level produces a very sharp tuning curve similar to eighth nerve and basilar membrane tuning curves. (From ref. 66.) **B:** The effect of crossed efferent stimulation on the tuning of IHCs. The tuning curves were obtained as above. During stimulation of the efferent system, the response of the IHC decreased preferentially near BF, thereby detuning the cell. Recovery was full after stimulation. This indicates that stimulation of OHCs by the efferent system can influence the function of IHCs, presumably by altering the mechanical input to the IHCs. (From ref. 7.)

reversal is reminiscent of the polarity reversal of the SP described earlier and further suggests that the SP reflects OHC activity. The production of AC potentials in high-BF OHCs is affected by the cell membrane's time constant, just as occurs with high-BF IHCs. Thus, at BF, the AC response is extremely attenuated, but at frequencies below the BF, AC responses can be measured. DC responses in these cells occur only at frequencies below BF, and similar to OHCs from the apical region, the polarity is hyperpolarizing at low intensities but reverses at higher levels. Since high-BF OHCs do not produce DC responses, the SP measured in the basal portion of the cochlea is thought to be generated by IHCs (65).

The tuning characteristics of IHCs are similar to those of eighth nerve fibers and basilar membrane motion (27,53,61,66,76). Figure 8A shows a tuning curve from an

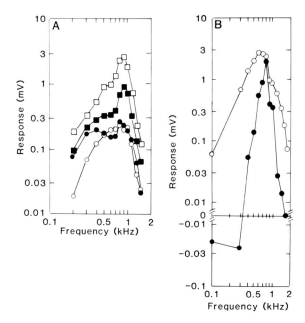

FIG. 9. A: Peak-to-peak AC responses from an IHC (*open boxes*), OHC (*closed boxes*), SM (*closed circles*), and organ of Corti fluid space (*open circles*) as a function of frequency, at a constant sound pressure level of 40 db (re: 20 μP). All records from the third turn of the cochlea. This illustrates several points: IHCs and OHCs from the same region of the cochlea are tuned to the same BF; IHC responses are larger than OHC responses; hair cell responses at BF are larger than the extracellular responses but below BF the response magnitudes are similar. **B:** Comparison of the AC and DC tuning characteristics for a low-BF OHC. Responses were obtained at a constant sound pressure level of 70 db (re: 20 μP). The response magnitude of the DC plot declines more rapidly than the AC plot as the stimulating frequency moves away from the BF, indicating a higher degree of tuning for DC responses. This is similar to the extracellular SP, as noted previously. (From ref. 27.)

IHC from the basal turn of the guinea pig cochlea. The values plotted are the sound pressure levels required to produce a DC receptor potential of 2, or 5 mV across a range of frequencies. The cell is tuned best to a frequency of 16 kHz. Above and below that frequency, more sound pressure is required to produce the response amplitude criterion. In high-frequency OHCs, tuning curves very similar to this are obtained for AC responses, after correcting for attenuation of the response owing to the membrane time constant and recording equipment (65). Best frequency is similar for IHCs and OHCs located in the same region of the organ of Corti. This is also true for IHCs and OHCs in the low-frequency region of the cochlea (Fig. 9A). Measures of tuning in low-BF OHCs indicate that the DC component is more sharply tuned than the AC component (Fig. 9B) (27), analogous to the extracellular responses.

INNER VERSUS OUTER HAIR CELL

There are differences between IHCs and OHCs other than those discussed, including differing ultrastructure and innervation patterns. Notably, the majority of eighth nerve fibers form afferent synapses with the IHCs, indicating that the IHCs are mainly responsible for the activity of the eighth nerve, and thus for the perception of acoustic stimuli. Current concepts envision separate roles for the two cell types. Although the IHC is considered a receptor, the outer is considered a modulator of inner ear mechanics, capable of fine tuning the cochlea's receptive function.

In 1978, Kemp (52) described measurable acoustic emissions in the ear canal of humans following acoustic stimulation. Subsequently, spontaneous otoacoustic emissions were observed in many species, including humans. Indeed, acoustic emissions can be generated by delivering AC current into the scala media—the reverse of normal transduction (43). These observations demonstrated that some structure within the cochlea is capable of driving the basilar membrane to generate acoustic energy. The OHC is considered the prime candidate for this active role. The following observations support this contention: the tuning properties of eighth nerve fibers can be altered by selective destruction of OHCs (25,41) and the tuning properties of IHCs can be altered by (a) stimulation of the crossed efferents that innervate OHCs (6,7) (Fig. 8B), (b) injection of currents into the scala media (57), (c) transient asphyxia (8), and (d) acoustic overstimulation (12). Typically, in these manipulations the effects are preferentially observed around the BF and thought to be mediated via modification of OHC properties. For example, acoustic overstimulation causes a sustained depolarization of OHCs, and this is thought to modify the mechanical input to the IHCs, which show reduced receptor potential amplitudes.

More recently, direct *in vitro* observations have shown that OHCs are capable of both fast motile responses (2–4,9,10,50) and slow motile responses (82). The slow movements may involve the contractile proteins, actin and myosin, found in OHCs (33,81), but the fast movements most likely do not.

Brownell et al. (10) first demonstrated that isolated OHCs will lengthen or shorten depending on the polarity of electrical stimulation; depolarizing currents shorten the cell and hyperpolarizing currents elongate the cell. Neither IHCs nor supporting cells display motile responses. The kinetics of OHC movements are very fast (Fig. 10A). Movement begins within 200 μsec after a current pulse and has been observed up to 8 kHz (3,4).

The molecular mechanism for these movements has not been discovered; however, Brownell (9) proposed an electro-osmotic model for these movements in which the OHC's unique cytoarchitecture (e.g., the lateral subsurface cisternae) plays a crucial role. It is probable that the movements are membrane potential dependent and not current dependent, since blocking the various ionic currents that flow through the OHC membrane does not alter the mechanical response to membrane potential changes (75). The response magnitude versus membrane potential change has been studied and found to be about 20 nm/mV in the linear range of movements (2,3,75); however, movements near the normal resting potential of OHCs (-70 to -90 mV) are rectified, showing larger responses for depolarizations than for hyperpolarizations (Fig. 10B).

The mechanical response is not sensitive to metabolic poisons *in vitro* where extrinsic electrical stimulation drives the hair cells (50). This indicates that metabolic energy is not required for these responses. However, *in vivo*, the driving force would be the OHC receptor potential or extracellular CM/SP—events that are clearly metabolically dependent and linked to the maintenance of the cell resting potential and the EP.

Supporting Cells

Gap junctions are aligned transmembrane channels connecting the cytoplasmic compartments of separate, adjacent cells. In mammalian cells, these channels are known to permit the passage of ions and small molecules (up to 1,000 daltons) among cells (31). In the mid-1970s, it was determined electronmicroscopically that all the

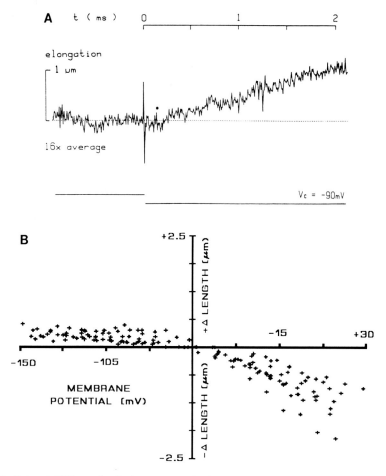

FIG. 10. A: Rate of OHC mechanical response. At time zero the OHC's membrane potential was stepped to −90 mV by a whole cell voltage clamp circuit. Within 200 μsec the cell initiates a change in its length, which reaches a maximum a few msec later. (From ref. 2.) **B:** Pooled data from 9 OHCs. Cells were held at a holding potential near −60 mV and pulsed to a range of new membrane potentials for a period of 200 msec, followed by return to the holding potential. The length changes of the cells were measured from a video monitor using a differential optoresistor. The plot illustrates that when the cells were pulsed to hyperpolarizing potentials very little elongation occurred, as compared with the larger shortening movements upon depolarization. Thus the OHC's mechanical response to membrane potential changes is rectified.

supporting cells of the organ of Corti are joined together by gap junctions (40,48,49). Subsequently, the gap junctions of the supporting cells were shown to be functional, as evidenced by the existence of electrical (ionic) and dye (small molecular) coupling in these cells (68,71,73). That is, injected currents are measurable in cells other than the injected one, and injected dyes spread to adjacent cells (Fig. 11). Various measures have been shown to modulate the conductance of these gap junctions (69,70), and indeed coupling may be different in the intact cochlea as compared with the excised one (72).

With this knowledge, roles for the supporting cells, other than the obvious physical support for the hair cells, can be envisioned. These include metabolic cooperation

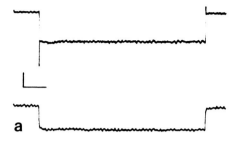

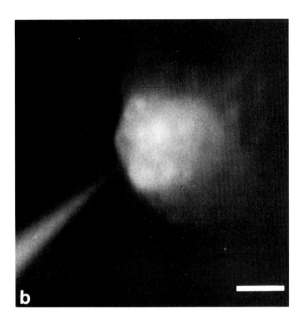

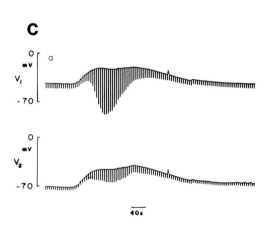

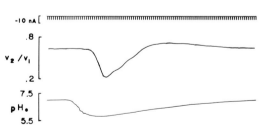

FIG. 11. a: Demonstration of electrical coupling in the Hensen's cells of the organ of Corti. The top trace depicts a voltage pulse measured in one cell in response to a -10 nA current injection. The bottom trace is the voltage pulse measured in an adjacent cell, indicating that current has spread from one cell to the other. The coupling between cells is quite good since the response in the second cell is nearly 80% of that found in the injected one. Vertical scale: 4 mV; horizontal scale: 0.2 sec. (From ref. 71.) **b:** Demonstration of dye coupling in the Hensen's cells. 45 seconds after a fluorescent dye was injected into a single cell, the dye was visible in several adjacent cells. Bar indicates 15 μm. (From ref. 71.) **c:** Effects of cytoplasmic acidification on cell coupling in the organ of Corti *in vitro.* Current pulses of -10 nA were delivered to one cell and the voltage responses were measured in the injected cell (trace 1) and an adjacent cell (trace 2). CO_2-saturated medium was introduced into the perfusion system and caused a drop in the intracellular pH, following the drop in extracellular pH (bottom trace). During the acidification the coupling between cells as determined from the ratio of voltages in cell 2 and cell 1 (trace 4) decreased but returned to normal when intracellular pH recovered. (From ref. 69.)

and potassium sinking. Metabolic cooperation denotes the sharing of important small molecules such as glucose among the cells. This may limit the metabolic burden of individual supporting cells. Potassium sinking denotes the uptake of K^+ by the supporting cells and the movement of these ions through gap junctional channels to distant cells. During intense hair cell and neural activity, K^+ is released into the fluid spaces surrounding the hair cell's basolateral membranes. High external K^+ in these areas can be detrimental to the function of hair cells and the nerve fibers that innervate them because of the ion's depolarizing effects. Removal of K^+ from these spaces is requisite and conceivably could be performed by the supporting cells.

REFERENCES

1. Art, J. J., Crawford, A. C., and Fettiplace, R. (1986): Membrane currents in isolated turtle hair cells. In: *Auditory Frequency Selectivity*, edited by B. C. J. Moore and R. D. Patterson, pp. 81–88. Plenum Press, New York.
2. Ashmore, J. F. (1986): The cellular physiology of isolated outer hair cells: Implications for cochlear frequency selectivity. In: *Auditory Frequency Selectivity*, edited by B. C. J. Moore and R. D. Patterson, pp. 103–108. Plenum Press, New York.
3. Ashmore, J. F. (1987): A fast motile response in guinea-pig outer hair cells: The cellular basis of the cochlear amplifier. *J. Physiol. (Lond.)*, 388:323–347.
4. Ashmore, J. F., and Brownell, W. E. (1986): Kilohertz movements induced by electrical stimulation in outer hair cells isolated from the guinea-pig cochlea. *J. Physiol. (Lond.)*, 377:41P.
5. Ashmore, J. F., and Meech, R. W. (1986): Ionic basis of the resting potential in outer hair cells isolated from the guinea pig cochlea. *Nature*, 322:368–371.
6. Brown, M. C., and Nuttall, A. L. (1984): Efferent control of cochlear inner hair cell responses in the guinea-pig. *J. Physiol. (Lond.)*, 354:625–646.
7. Brown, M. C., Nuttall, A. L., and Masta, R. I. (1983): Intracellular recordings from cochlear inner hair cells: Effects of stimulation of the crossed olivocochlear efferents. *Science*, 222:69–72.
8. Brown, M. C., Nuttall, A. L., Masta, R. I., and Lawrence, M. (1983): Cochlear inner hair cells: Effects of transient asphyxia on intracellular potentials. *Hear. Res.*, 9:131–144.
9. Brownell, W. E. (1986): Outer hair cell motility and cochlear frequency selectivity. In: *Auditory Frequency Selectivity*, edited by B. C. J. Moore and R. D. Patterson, pp. 109–116. Plenum Press, New York.
10. Brownell, W. E., Bader, C. R., Bertrand, D., and de Ribaupierre, Y. (1985): Evoked mechanical responses of isolated cochlear outer hair cells. *Science*, 227:194–196.
11. Cheatham, M. A., and Dallos, P. (1984): Summating potential (SP) tuning curves. *Hear. Res.*, 116:189–200.
12. Cody, A. R., and Russell, I. J. (1985): Outer hair cells in the cochlea and noise induced hearing loss. *Nature*, 315:662–665.
13. Corey, D. P., and Hudspeth, A. J. (1979): Ionic basis of the receptor potential in a vertebrate hair cell. *Nature*, 281:625–627.
14. Crawford, A. C., and Fettiplace, R. (1981): An electrical tuning mechanism in turtle cochlear hair cells. *J. Physiol. (Lond.)*, 312:377–412.
15. Dallos, P. (1973): Cochlear potentials and cochlear mechanics. In: *Basic Mechanisms in Hearing*, edited by A. R. Moller, pp. 335–372. Academic Press, New York.
16. Dallos, P. (1975): Electrical correlates of mechanical events in the cochlea. *Audiology*, 14:408–418.
17. Dallos, P. (1975): Cochlear potentials. In: *The Nervous System: Human Communication and Its Disorders*, edited by D. B. Tower, pp. 69–80. Raven Press, New York.
18. Dallos, P. (1981): Cochlear physiology. *Annu. Rev. Psychol.*, 32:153–190.
19. Dallos, P. (1983): Cochlear electroanatomy: Influence on information processing. In: *Hearing—Physiological Bases and Psychophysics*, edited by R. Klinke and R. Hartman, pp. 32–38. Springer-Verlag, Berlin.
20. Dallos, P. (1985): Response characteristics of mammalian cochlear hair cells. *J. Neurosci.*, 5:1591–1608.
21. Dallos, P. (1985): Membrane potential and response changes in mammalian cochlear hair cells during intracellular recording. *J. Neurosci.*, 5:1609–1615.
22. Dallos, P. (1986): Neurobiology of cochlear inner and outer hair cells: Intracellular recordings. *Hear. Res.*, 22:185–198.

23. Dallos, P., Billone, M. C., Durrant, J. D., Wang, C. Y., and Raynor, S. (1972): Cochlear inner and outer hair cells: Functional differences. *Science*, 218:356–358.
24. Dallos, P., and Cheatham, M. A. (1976): Production of cochlear potentials by inner and outer hair cells. *J. Acoust. Soc. Am.*, 60:510–512.
25. Dallos, P., and Harris, D. (1978): Properties of auditory nerve responses in absence of outer hair cells. *J. Neurophysiol.*, 41:365–383.
26. Dallos, P., and Santos-Sacchi, J. (1983): AC receptor potentials from hair cells in the low frequency region of the guinea pig cochlea. In: *Mechanisms of Hearing*, edited by W. R. Webster and L. M. Aitkin, pp. 11–16. Monash University Press, Clayton, Australia.
27. Dallos, P., Santos-Sacchi, J., and Flock, Å. (1982): Intracellular recordings from cochlear outer hair cells. *Science*, 218:582–584.
28. Dallos, P., Schoeny, Z. G., and Cheatham, M. A. (1970): Cochlear summating potentials: Composition. *Science*, 170:641–644.
29. Dallos, P., Schoeny, Z. G., and Cheatham, M. A. (1972): Cochlear summating potentials: Descriptive aspects. *Acta Otolaryngol. [Suppl.] (Stockh.)*, 302.
30. Davis, H. (1958): A mechano-electric theory of cochlear action. *Ann. Otol. Rhinol. Laryngol.*, 67:789–801.
31. Flagg-Newton, J., Simpson, I., and Loewenstein, W. (1979): Permeability of the cell-to-cell membrane channels in mammalian cell junction. *Science*, 205:404–407.
32. Flock, Å. (1965): Transducing mechanisms in the lateral line canal organ receptors. *Cold Spring Harbor Symp. Quant. Biol.*, 30:133–145.
33. Flock, Å. (1983): Review paper: Hair cells, receptors with capacity?. In: *Hearing—Physiological Bases and Psychophysics*, edited by R. Klinke and R. Hartmann, pp. 2–9. Springer-Verlag, Berlin.
34. Flock, Å., Jorgensen, M., and Russell, I. (1973): The physiology of individual hair cells and their synapses. In: *Basic Mechanisms in Hearing*, edited by A. R. Moller, pp. 273–306. Academic Press, New York.
35. Flock, Å., and Russell, I. J. (1976): Inhibition by efferent nerve fibres: Action on hair cells and afferent synaptic transmission in the lateral line canal organ of the burbot, Lota lota. *J. Physiol. (Lond.)*, 257:45–62.
36. Flock, Å, and Wersall, J. (1962): A study of the orientation of the sensory hairs of the receptor cells in the lateral line organ of fish, with special reference to the function of the receptors. *J. Cell. Biol.*, 15:19–27.
37. Furukawa, T., Hayashida, Y., and Matsuma, S. (1978): Quantal analysis of the size of excitatory post-synaptic potentials at synapses between hair cells and afferent nerve fibres in goldfish. *J. Physiol. (Lond.)*, 276:211–226.
38. Gitter, A., Zenner, H. P., and Fromter, E. (1986): Membrane potantial and ion channels in isolated outer hair cells of the guinea pig cochlea. *ORL*, 48:68–75.
39. Goodman, D. A., Smith, R. L., and Chamberlain, S. C. (1982): Intracellular and extracellular responses in the organ of Corti of the gerbil. *Hear. Res.*, 7:161–179.
40. Gulley, R. S., and Reese, T. S. (1976): Intercellular junctions in the reticular lamina of the organ of Corti. *J. Neurocytol.*, 5:479–507.
41. Harrison, R. V., and Evans, E. F. (1979): Cochlear fiber responses in guinea pigs with well defined cochlear lesions. *Scand. Audiol. [Suppl.]*, 9:83–92.
42. Honrubia, V., and Ward, P. H. (1969): Properties of the summating potential of the guinea pig's cochlea. *J. Acoust. Soc. Am.*, 45:1443–1450.
43. Hubbard, A. E., and Mountain, D. C. (1983): Alternating current delivered into the scala media alters sound pressure at the eardrum. *Science*, 22:510–512.
44. Hudspeth, A. J. (1982): Extracellular current flow and the site of transduction by vertebrate hair cells. *J. Neurosci.*, 2:1–10.
45. Hudspeth, A. J. (1985): The cellular basis of hearing: The biophysics of hair cells. *Science*, 230:745–752.
46. Hudspeth, A. J. (1986): The ionic channels of a vertebrate hair cell. *Hear. Res.*, 22:21–27.
47. Hudspeth, A. J., and Corey, D. P. (1977): Sensitivity, polarity and conductance change in the response of vertebrate hair cells to controlled mechanical stimuli. *Proc. Natl. Acad. Sci. USA*, 74:2407–2411.
48. Iurato, S., Franks, K., Luciano, L., Wermbter, G., Pannese, E., and Reale, E. (1976): Intercellular junctions in the organ of Corti as revealed by freeze fracturing. *Acta Otolaryngol. (Stockh.)*, 82:57–69.
49. Jahnke, K. (1975): The fine structure of freeze-fractured intercellular junctions in the guinea pig inner ear. *Acta Otolaryngol. [Suppl.] (Stockh.)*, 336.
50. Kachar, B., Brownell, W. E., Altschuler, R., and Fex, J. (1986): Electrokinetic shape changes of cochlear outer hair cells. *Nature*, 322:365–367.
51. Katz, B., and Miledi, R. (1967): A study of synaptic transmission in the absence of nerve impulses. *J. Physiol. (Lond.)*, 192:407–436.

52. Kemp, D. T. (1978): Stimulated acoustic emissions from within the human auditory system. *J. Acoust. Soc. Am.*, 64:1386–1391.
53. Khanna, S. M., and Leonard, D. G. B. (1982): Basilar membrane tuning in the cat cochlea. *Science*, 215:305–306.
54. Lewis, R. S., and Hudspeth, A. J. (1983): Voltage- and ion-dependent conductances in solitary vertebrate hair cells. *Nature*, 304:538–541.
55. Mountain, D. C. (1980): Changes in endolymphatic potential and crossed-olivocochlear-bundle stimulation alter cochlear mechanics. *Science*, 210:71–72.
56. Mountain, D. C. (1986): Electromechanical properties of hair cells. In: *Neurobiology of Hearing: The Cochlea*, edited by R. A. Altschuler, D. W. Hoffman, and R. P. Bobbin, pp. 77–90. Raven Press, New York.
57. Nuttall, A. L. (1985): Influence of direct current on dc receptor potentials from cochlear inner hair cells in the guinea pig. *J. Acoust. Soc. Am.*, 77:165–175.
58. Nuttall, A. L. (1986): Physiology of hair cells. In: *Neurobiology of Hearing: The Cochlea*, edited by R. A. Altschuler, D. W. Hoffman, and R. P. Bobbin, pp. 47–75. Raven Press, New York.
59. Oesterle, E., and Dallos, P. (1986): Intracellular recordings from supporting cells in the organ of Corti. *Hear. Res.*, 22:229–232.
60. Ohmori, H. (1984): Mechano-electric transduction currents in isolated vestibular hair cells of the chick. *J. Physiol. (Lond.)*, 359:189–218.
61. Patuzzi, R. B., and Sellick, P. (1983): A comparison between basilar membrane and inner hair cell receptor potential input-output functions in the guinea pig cochlea. *J. Acoust. Soc. Am.*, 74:1731–1741.
62. Pickles, J. O., Comis, S. D., and Osborne, M. P. (1984): Cross-links between stereocilia in the guinea pig organ of Corti, and their possible relation to sensory transduction. *Hear. Res.*, 15:103–112.
63. Runhaar, G., and Manley, G. A. (1987): Potassium concentration in the inner sulcus is perilymphlike. *Hear. Res.*, 29:93–103.
64. Russell, I. J. (1983): Origin of the receptor potential in inner hair cells of the mammalian cochlea—evidence for Davis' theory. *Nature*, 301:334–336.
65. Russell, I. J., Cody, A. R., and Richardson, G. P. (1986): The responses of inner and outer hair cells in the basal turn of the guinea-pig cochlea and in the mouse cochlea grown in vitro. *Hear. Res.*, 22:199–216.
66. Russell, I. J., and Sellick, P. M. (1978): Intracellular studies of hair cells in the mammalian cochlea. *J. Physiol. (Lond.)*, 284:261–290.
67. Russell, I. J., and Sellick, P. M. (1983): Low frequency characteristics of intracellularly recorded receptor potentials in mammalian hair cells. *J. Physiol. (Lond.)*, 338:179–206.
68. Santos-Sacchi, J. (1984): A reevaluation of cell coupling in the organ of Corti. *Hear. Res.*, 14:203–204.
69. Santos-Sacchi, J. (1985): The effects of cytoplasmic acidification upon electrical coupling in the organ of Corti. *Hear. Res.*, 19:207–215.
70. Santos-Sacchi, J. (1986): The temperature dependence of electrical coupling in the organ of Corti. *Hear. Res.*, 21:205–211.
71. Santos-Sacchi, J. (1986): Dye coupling in the organ of Corti. *Cell Tissue Res.*, 245:525–529.
72. Santos-Sacchi, J. (1987): Electrical coupling differs in the in vitro and in vivo organ of Corti. *Hear. Res.*, 25:227–232.
73. Santos-Sacchi, J., and Dallos, P. (1983): Intercellular communication in the supporting cells of the organ of Corti. *Hear. Res.*, 9:317–326.
74. Santos-Sacchi, J., and Dilger, J. P. (1986): Patch clamp studies on isolated outer hair cells. *Advances in Auditory Neuroscience: The IUPS Satellite Symposium on Hearing.* Lone Mountain Conference Center, San Francisco.
75. Santos-Sacchi, J., and Dilger, J. P. (1987): Whole cell currents and mechanical responses of isolated outer hair cells (*submitted*).
76. Sellick, P. M., Patuzzi, R., and Johnstone, B. M. (1982): Measurement of basilar membrane motion in the guinea pig using the Mossbauer technique. *J. Acoust. Soc. Am.*, 72:131–141.
77. Shotwell, S. L., Jacobs, R., and Hudspeth, A. J. (1981): Directional sensitivity of individual vertebrate hair cells to controlled deflection of their hair bundles. *Ann. N.Y. Acad. Sci.*, 374:1–10.
78. Smith, C. A. (1975): The inner ear: Its embryological development and microstructure. In: *The Nervous System. Vol. 3: Human Communication and Its Disorders*, edited by D. B. Tower, pp. 1–18. Raven Press, New York.
79. Tanaka, Y., Asanuma, A., and Yanagisawa, K. (1980): Potentials of outer hair cells and their membrane properties in cationic environments. *Hear. Res.*, 2:431–438.

80. Tasaki, I., and Spyropoulos, C. S. (1959): Stria vascularis as source of endocochlear potential. *J. Neurophysiol*, 22:149–155.
81. Zenner, H. P. (1981): Cytoskeletal and muscle-like elements in cochlear hair cells. *Arch. Otorhinolaryngol.*, 230:81–92.
82. Zenner, H. P., Zimmermann, U., and Schmitt, U. (1985): Reversible contraction of isolated mammalian cochlear hair cells. *Hear. Res.*, 18:127–133.

Physiology of the Ear,
edited by A. F. Jahn and J. Santos-Sacchi.
Raven Press, New York © 1988.

Circulation of the Inner Ear:
I. Comparative Study of the Vascular Anatomy in the Mammalian Cochlea

*Alf Axelsson and **Allen F. Ryan

*Department of Otolaryngology, Sahlgrenska Hospital, 413 45 Göteborg, Sweden; and
**Department of Otolaryngology, University of California Medical Center and Veterans Administration Medical Center, San Diego, California 92103*

The vasculature of the cochlea clearly plays a central role in its function and almost certainly is involved in many pathogenic conditions that result in cochlear damage. Cochlear vessels are the source of metabolites necessary for the maintenance of cochlear tissues. They are one source of the ions and other constituents of cochlear fluids. In addition, they are the primary route by which drugs and other substances enter the cochlea and reach the cochlear tissues. Disturbances of the cochlear vasculature have been implicated in a variety of inner ear disorders, including Meniere's disease, noise damage (13), and sudden hearing loss.

The vasculature of the cochlea is thus intimately related to cochlear function in health and disease. We have studied the vascular anatomy of the cochlea in humans and in several other mammalian species, including the guinea pig, chinchilla, rhesus monkey, rat, rabbit, and gerbil. From such studies it is possible to discern a basic vascular pattern of the inner ear. Differences between species help us to understand which features of the vasculature are necessary for cochlear function. They may also eventually help us to understand some of the inter-species differences that are frequently observed in such aspects of cochlear physiology as sensitivity to noise damage or ototoxic drugs. The purpose of the present study is to determine which aspects of the vascular anatomy of the cochlea are constant across mammalian species and highlight those species differences that have been observed. Detailed descriptions of the vascular anatomy in the human and the guinea pig, including a review of previous literature, vascular measurements, and nomenclature have previously been published (3,7). The more extensive reports on the vascular anatomy in different mammals studied previously are listed in Table 1.

MATERIAL AND METHODS

The methods employed have been presented in detail elsewhere (3,5,11,46). Briefly, experimental animals were anesthetized and an incision was made in the pericardium and in the left ventricle. A plastic tube was inserted in the ascending aorta and ligated. The superior vena cava or right ventricle was then cut, and the animal was left to bleed for a short while. In order to remove the blood from the

TABLE 1. *Previous investigations of the vascular anatomy of the cochlea in mammals*

Guinea pig	Schwalbe (1887), Nabeya (1923), Smith (1951), Wüstenfeld and Kühnert (1964), Hawkins (1968), Nomura and Hiraide (1968), Axelsson (1968, 1971), Maass (1969), Ritter (1978)
Rat	Asai (1908), Nabeya (1923), Hodde et al. (1977), Hornstrand et al. (1980), Tange (1986)
Gerbil	Jones-Mumby and Axelsson (1984), Axelsson et al. (1986)
Chinchilla	Axelsson and Lipscomb (1975)
Rabbit	Nabeya (1923), Axelsson and Lind (1973)
Cat	Nabeya (1923), Smith (1954), Nomura and Hiraide (1968)
Dog	Eichler (1892), Asai (1908), Nabeya (1923)
Pig	Shambaugh (1903)
Monkey	Nabeya (1923), Axelsson (1974)
Man	Eichler (1892), Siebenmann (1894), Nabeya (1923), Scuderi and Del Bo (1952), Smith (1954), Charachon (1961), Levin (1964), Nomura and Hiraide (1968), Axelsson (1968), Kirikae et al. (1969), Johnsson (1972)
Other mammals	Ibsen (1881), different mammals including humans

vessels, the animal was perfused with physiological saline of body temperature for 4 to 7 min under hydrostatic pressure. The animal was then perfused with contrast, 2.5% Berlin blue in water, at the same constant pressure. This perfusion was terminated when the contrast solution no longer entered the vascular system spontaneously. The temporal bones were then removed and the bulla opened. In some species the stapes was removed and small openings were made in the round window and the cochlear apex to allow an injection of fixation solution (2% glutaraldehyde). In most species, however, the cochleas were intact during the 24-hr fixation. The cochleas were then decalcified in 8% ethylenediaminetetraacetic acid (EDTA) (pH 7.4) until the bone was softened, washed in tap water, dehydrated, and stored in glycerine. After the accomplishment of this procedure the cochleas were ready to be dissected.

The cochlea was bisected by a midmodiolar section with a razor blade. Using a combination of fine blades and probes, the tissues of the cochlea were removed and mounted on slides as surface preparations for detailed examination by light and phase-contrast microscopy of all capillary areas.

In some cases, the vascular anatomy was studied in noncontrast-injected cochleas in order to assess the distribution of red blood cells within the vessels (12).

The procedure used for human temporal bones was similar to that used for experimental animals, with the following exceptions. Cadavers were obtained as soon as possible after death, preferably within 24 hr. The vasculature was perfused via the basilar or vertebral arteries. Temporal bones were fixed for 48 hr in 10% formalin, and thereafter treated as were the animal cochleas.

The nomenclature used is that of Axelsson (3). A compilation of the commonly observed vessels and abbreviations used in the text is presented in Table 2.

RESULTS

Modiolus

The major vessels of the modiolus are illustrated schematically in Fig. 1, using the guinea pig as a typical example.

TABLE 2. *Regularly occurring vessels of the mammalian cochlea*

Modiolus	External wall
Spiral modiolar artery (SMA)	Scala vestibuli
Spiral modiolar vein (SMV)	Radiating arterioles (RALs-SV)
Radiating arterioles (RALs-MOD)	Collecting venules (CVLs-SV)
Collecting venules (CVLs-MOD)	Capillaries (CAPs-SV)
Capillaries of the spiral ganglion (CAPs-SGN)	The vessel at the vestibular membrane (VSVM)
Capillaries of the acoustic nerve (CAPs-N VIII)	Scala media
Capillaries of the modiolus wall (CAPs-MOD)	Stria vascularis (SVS)
Lamina spiralis	The vessel of the spiral prominence (VSSP)
Radiating arterioles (RALs-SL)	Arterio-venous anastomoses (AVAS)
Collecting venules (CVLs-SL)	Scala tympani
The vessel of the basilar membrane (VSBM)	Collecting venules (CVLs-ST)
The vessel of the tympanic lip (VSTL)	The venules at the basilar membrane (VLBM)
The limbus vessels (LVS)	

The abbreviations are those used in the text.

The major arterial supply to the cochlea is provided by the spiral modiolar artery (SMA), which is a branch of the common cochlear artery and ascends spirally around the modiolus from the base to the apex.

In humans, a SMA quite similar to that seen in animals supplies the apical portion of the cochlea. However, a separate branch of the common cochlear artery, the vestibulo-cochlear artery (VCA), supplies the lower basal turn as illustrated in Fig. 2. The size and importance of the VCA are more significant in humans than in the other mammals studied.

The SMA almost invariably runs between the spiral ganglion and the main body of the VIIIth nerve fibers. The artery is typically serpentine in its course, as are the radiating arterioles (RALs) in the modiolus (Fig. 3).

Many primary RALs leave the SMA and soon divide into secondary and further ramifications. In the guinea pig, these RALs are tightly wound to form structures that have been termed spring coils.

The cochlea is drained by the spiral modiolar vein (SMV), which originates as the confluence of the venules from the capillary regions in the apical turn and descends in a simple, spiral course from the apex to the base in the bone at the lower medial corner of scala tympani (Fig. 1). The SMV is much less serpentine than the SMA. It empties into the vein of the cochlear aqueduct (vein of Cotugno) at the lower basal turn. The SMV receives collecting venules (CVLs) from the scala tympani of the external wall, the spiral lamina, and the capillary areas in the modiolus.

The appearance and the level at which the SMV is found differ little among the experimental animals examined. In humans, however, the venous system in the modiolus consists of two separate vessels: (a) the vein of the scala vestibuli (VSV) draining the spiral lamina and CVLs of the scala vestibuli and (b) the vein of the scala tympani (VST) draining the spiral ganglion and the external wall of scala media and scala tympani, as illustrated in Fig. 2.

Separate capillaries (CAPs-MOD) supply and drain the modiolar wall, the spiral

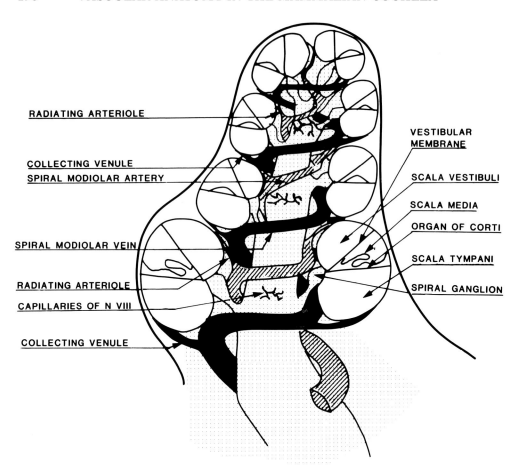

FIG. 1. Schematic view of mammalian cochlea, longitudinal section, showing the major vessels, the spiral modiolar artery, and the spiral modiolar vein in relation to anatomical structures. The spiral modiolar artery is situated in the interspace between the acoustic nerve centrally and the spiral ganglion peripherally at the level of the scala vestibuli. Its primary branches run a serpentine course forming radiating arterioles in the spiral lamina and in the external wall. Ramifications from radiating arterioles supply the capillaries of the modiolus. The spiral modiolar vein is situated in the central angle of the scala tympani immediately below the spiral ganglion.

ganglion (CAPs-SGN), and the VIIIth nerve (CAPs-NVIII). These capillaries form irregular nets and are similar in the mammals examined.

External Wall

The commonly occurring vessels of the external wall are illustrated schematically in Fig. 4.

Scala Vestibuli

RALs of scala vestibuli (RALs-SV) originate as branches of the primary RALs in the modiolus. They supply all of the arterial flow to the external wall vessels. RALs

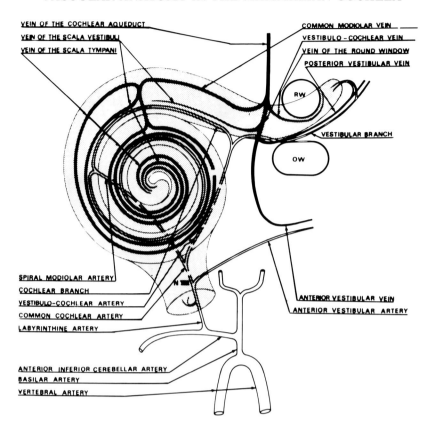

VEIN OF THE COCHLEAR AQUEDUCT
VEIN OF THE SCALA VESTIBULI
VEIN OF THE SCALA TYMPANI

COMMON MODIOLAR VEIN
VESTIBULO - COCHLEAR VEIN
VEIN OF THE ROUND WINDOW
POSTERIOR VESTIBULAR VEIN

RW

VESTIBULAR BRANCH

OW

SPIRAL MODIOLAR ARTERY
COCHLEAR BRANCH
VESTIBULO-COCHLEAR ARTERY
COMMON COCHLEAR ARTERY
LABYRINTHINE ARTERY

ANTERIOR VESTIBULAR VEIN
ANTERIOR VESTIBULAR ARTERY

ANTERIOR INFERIOR CEREBELLAR ARTERY
BASILAR ARTERY
VERTEBRAL ARTERY

FIG. 2. Schematic view of human cochlea, transverse section. The major supplying arterial and draining venous vessels are shown in relation to anatomical structures.

run a fairly straight course radially over scala vestibuli. They typically ramify above the attachment of the vestibular (Reissner's) membrane, and their branches join all the various types of vessels found in the external wall (Figs. 5 and 6).

Above the attachment of the vestibular membrane, capillaries of the scala vestibuli (CAPs-SV) form a capillary net in the scala vestibuli in several species (Fig. 6). It is made up of the finest branches from RALs and CVLs in this region. Typically, this capillary net is sparse. Spirally running capillary segments make up a spiral vessel, the vessel at the vestibular membrane (VSVM), which forms a basal border of this capillary net (Fig. 5). The VSVM occurs regularly in the basal turn as rather long, spiral segments. It becomes irregular and shorter in the apical turns. In the rhesus monkey, only a few capillary loops are observed above VSVM, which are too sparse to be designated a true capillary net. In the chinchilla, neither CAPs-SV nor VSVM are observed.

In the guinea pig and to a lesser extent in the gerbil, there is a tendency for capillaries to form an apical border of the capillary net in scala vestibuli, i.e., a second spiral vessel that is parallel to the VSVM. This second spiral vessel has been termed the vessel of the scala vestibuli (VSSV). Never continuous, it is most prominent in the basal turn.

Venous drainage of the scala vestibuli varies widely across species. In several of

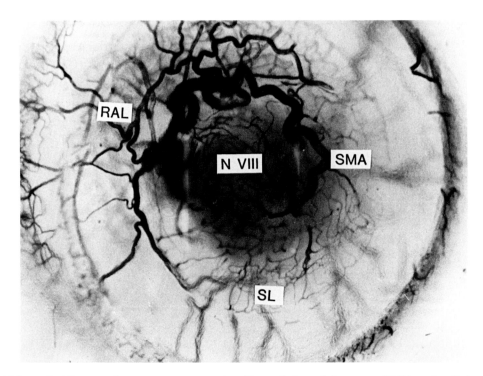

FIG. 3. Gerbil, second turn, transverse section. The spiral modiolar artery (SMA) and radiating arterioles (RAL) run a winding course. There are many delicate capillaries in the N VIII and the spiral lamina (SL).

the animals studied there are no CVLs in scala vestibuli (CVLs-SV) and all venous drainage of the external wall runs through scala tympani. In such animals the CVLs of the scala tympani drain the capillary net of the scala vestibuli and the VSVM by ramifications running externally to the stria vascularis (Fig. 6). However, in the human, rhesus monkey, and guinea pig, true CVLs-SV are seen in scala vestibuli, although they are more delicate and much fewer in number than those in the scala tympani. These CVLs drain the CAPs-SV and the VSVM and travel up the scala vestibuli wall, parallel to the RALs. In the monkey and guinea pig, these CVLs drain into the spiral modiolar vein of the next most apical turn. In humans, they drain into the unique vein of the scala vestibuli.

Scala Media

The external wall of the scala media is dominated by the stria vascularis (SVS), which forms a rich network of capillaries of varying caliber. In most mammals there are, at least in the apical turns, well-defined, spirally running apical and basal marginal vessels. The SVS is supplied by relatively few but large radiating arterioles and drained by relatively few but large collecting venules. It has no connection with other vessels in the external wall (Figs. 5 and 6).

The vessel of the spiral prominence (VSSP) is formed by spirally running vascular

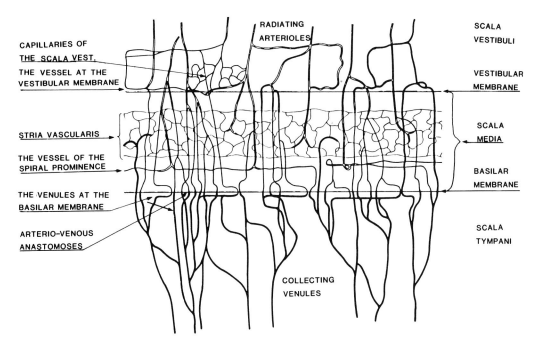

FIG. 4. Schematic view of external wall of the mammalian cochlea. Radiating arterioles predominate in the scala vestibuli and supply the spiral vascular systems: the vessel at the vestibular membrane, capillaries of the scala vestibuli, stria vascularis, the vessel of the spiral prominence. Collecting venules predominate in the scala tympani and drain all capillary vessels. The venules at the basilar membrane, parts of the collecting venules, form a spiral vessel basally to the attachment of the basilar membrane. Radiating arterioles and collecting venules connect with one another by arterio-venous anastomoses external to stria vascularis.

segments of varying length in the spiral prominence. For short sections the VSSP might ramify into two or even three vessels. For other short sections the VSSP might be totally missing. It is supplied by relatively large RALs and drained by many CVLs. The VSSP has no vascular connections with the SVS (Figs. 5 and 6).

Externally to the stria vascularis, some ramifications of RALs supplying the SVS and the VSSP are found. Other ramifications that do not supply any external wall capillaries connect with CVLs of the same caliber from scala tympani. These vessels, termed arterio-venous anastomoses (AVAS), consequently offer a bypass possibility, where the arterial blood in scala vestibuli can be shunted directly to the venous blood in scala tympani thus bypassing the vessels in scala media (Figs. 5 to 8). In most species the number of these anastomoses is large in the basal turn but decreases apically. However, in the rabbit the number of AVAS is small throughout the cochlea.

Scala Tympani

CVLs of the scala tympani (CVLs-ST) drain all capillary areas in the external wall and also have direct anastomotic connections to RALs-SV. Immediately above the

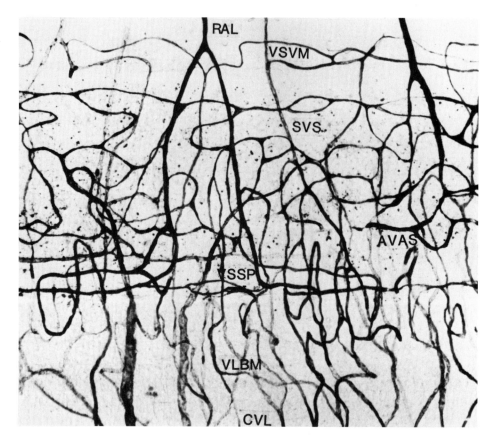

FIG. 5. Guinea pig, basal turn, external wall, apico-basal section. The vascular pattern is demonstrated with a main blood flow over radiating arterioles (RAL) in the scala vestibuli, arterio-venous anastomoses (AVAS) external to stria vascularis, and collecting venules (CVL) of the scala tympani. Capillaries are shunted in perpendicularly and spirally: the vessel at the vestibular membrane (VSVM), stria vascularis (SVS), the vessel of the spiral prominence (VSSP). Collecting venules turn spirally below the attachment of the basilar membrane forming the venules at the basilar membrane (VLBM).

attachment of the basilar membrane to the spiral ligament, the CVLs, which are running almost exclusively apico-basally, turn spirally and make an omega-shaped loop through the thickest portion of the ligament, at the point of basilar membrane attachment. Just below this loop, the CVLs again turn spirally to form distinct spiral sections, vessels that are called the venules at the basilar membrane (VLBM). VLBM are apparent as a vascular margin in all species studied (Figs. 5, 7, and 8).

CVLs between the VSSP and the VLBM, with their pronounced loops in between, make up a second organized vascular bed in the external wall, which runs below and lateral to the capillaries of the stria vascularis but which parallels stria vascularis throughout the cochlea. In some species, such as the guinea pig and human, this bed is not highly defined. In others, such as the gerbil, monkey, rabbit, and chinchilla, it is clearly recognizable as an organized unit in which the density of capillary-caliber vessels is as high as it is in the SVS. In most animals, these vessels have anastomosing, spiral interconnections. In the rat, however, this arrangement is replaced by a true capillary net between the VSSP and the VLBM.

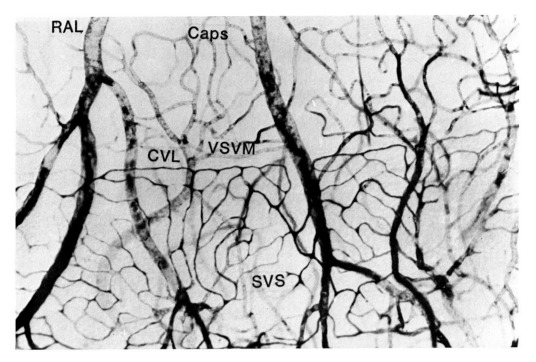

FIG. 6. Rabbit, basal turn, external wall, apico-basal section. Stria vascularis (SVS) has unusually many delicate capillaries. An equally unusual well-formed net of capillaries (Caps) in scala vestibuli is mainly drained by collecting venules (CVL) protruding to scala vestibuli externally to stria vascularis. The vessel at the vestibular membrane (VSVM) forms a basal border of the capillary net. Radiating arterioles (RAL).

Below the VLBM, CVLs typically run radially to empty into the spiral modiolar vein in the modiolus. In the chinchilla, rat, and gerbil, delicate peripheral CVLs unite into larger so-called veins of the scala tympani, which run spirally for some distance before emptying into the spiral modiolar vein (Fig. 8).

In the guinea pig and less so in the rat, CVLs are occasionally observed to run through the perilymph between the external wall of scala tympani and the modiolus. These vessels have been termed suspension veins. Similar observations have been made in the cow (30) and in the human (44).

Spiral Lamina

The commonly occurring vessels of the spiral lamina are illustrated schematically in Fig. 9. RALs of the spiral lamina (RALs-SL) originate as branches of the spiral modiolar artery. From a very serpentine course in the central spiral lamina, they gradually straighten as they course laterally (Fig. 3). Centrally, RALs are located on the apical side of the lamina. Some RALs remain on this side, where they supply the capillary bed in the spiral limbus. Others cross to the basal side of the spiral lamina at about the level of the limbus, where they proceed radially to supply the spiral capillary arcades below the organ of Corti.

CVLs of the spiral lamina (CVLs-SL), which drain the capillaries of the spiral

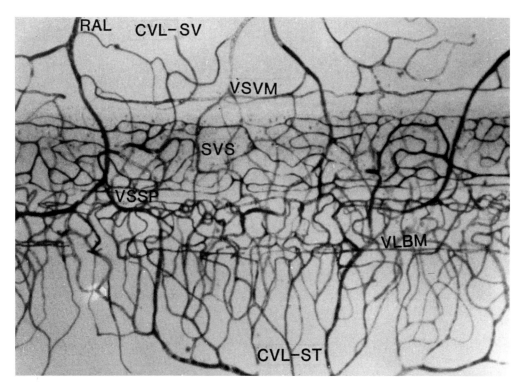

FIG. 7. Rhesus monkey, basal turn, external wall, apico-basal section. The vascular pattern is similar to other mammals. Radiating arterioles (RAL), collecting venules of scala vestibuli (CVL-SV), the vessel at the vestibular membrane (VSVM), stria vascularis (SVS), the vessel of the spiral prominence (VSSP), the venules at the basilar membrane (VLBM), collecting venules of the scala tympani (CVL-ST).

lamina, typically run centripetally on a radial course to empty into the spiral modiolar vein (Fig. 10), In the chinchilla, CVLs show a tendency to merge into quite large CVLs before joining the spiral modiolar vein. In the basal turn of the guinea pig and gerbil, CVLs unite to form a spirally running vein, termed the vein of the spiral lamina (VSL) before emptying into the spiral modiolar vein (Fig. 10). The spiral limbus is supplied by a net of capillaries termed the limbus vessels (LVS). They are independent of the vessels supplying the organ of Corti region, originating from separate RALs and being drained by separate CVLs. In most species this net is quite irregular (Fig. 11). In some species such as the rat, chinchilla, and human, LVS are sparse. In the gerbil, they are somewhat more organized than in other species, with RALs supplying the capillary net at its peripheral edge and CVLs draining its medial edge.

RALs give rise to a spiral vessel on the basal side of the spiral lamina, the vessel of the tympanic lip (VSTL), at the level of the habenula perforata and the edge of the osseous spiral lamina. Typically, the VSTL is composed of discontinuous arcadic bows or loops in the basal and apical turns and a more continuous vessel in the middle turn(s) (Fig. 10). In the myomorph rodents, the rat and gerbil, the VSTL in the middle turn is often a double vessel. In humans, the VSTL is somewhat less continuous than in other species. In several of the mammals studied not only a double

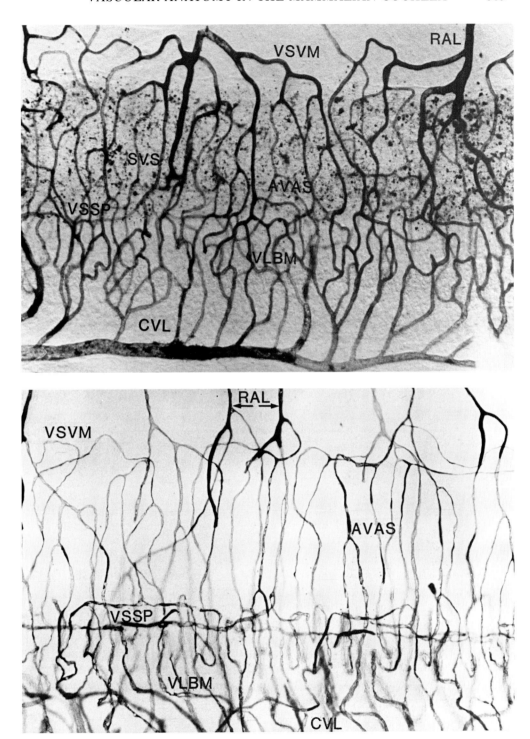

FIG. 8. Guinea pig, external wall, apico-basal section (**bottom**) with stria vascularis dissected away and gerbil (**top**) with stria vascularis (SVS) poorly contrast injected. The ramifications of radiating arterioles (RAL) form direct connections with collecting venules (CVL) as arterio-venous anastomoses (AVAS). The vessel at the vestibular membrane (VSVM), the vessel of the spiral prominence (VSSP), the venules at the basilar membrane (VLBM).

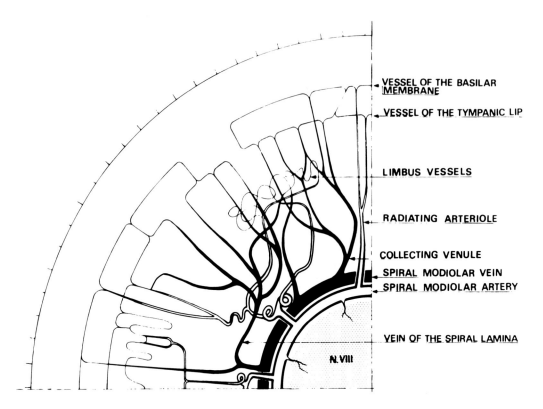

FIG. 9. Schematic view of the spiral lamina, mammalian cochlea, transverse section. The radiating arterioles supply and collecting venules drain the three spirally running capillary arcades, one in the spiral limbus, the limbus vessels, one in the tympanic lip, the vessel of the tympanic lip, and one under the tunnel of Corti, the vessel of the basilar membrane.

VSTL is found but also arcades central to the VSTL connecting RALs with CVLs and also even more central loop formations and anastomoses more centrally in the spiral lamina.

In most species, RALs supply a spiral vessel, the vessel of the basilar membrane (VSBM), which runs beneath the tunnel of Corti. This vessel shows the most interspecies variability of any cochlear vessel. At one extreme, in the human the VSBM is observed almost continuously throughout the cochlea. In the guinea pig, it is continuous in the basal turn (Fig. 10) but occurs more irregularly in the apical turns. In the gerbil and rat, it is observed occasionally in the basal turn and rarely in the apical turns. In the monkey, it is rarely observed in basal turn, but small segments are found infrequently in the second and third turns. In the chinchilla, it is unusual in the basal and second turn and occurs only occasionally in the apical turn. At the opposite extreme from the human, in the adult rabbit the VSBM is completely absent.

Additional Vessels

The vestibular (Reissner's) membrane is avascular in most species. However, in the rabbit sparse and delicate capillaries are observed on the apical side of the

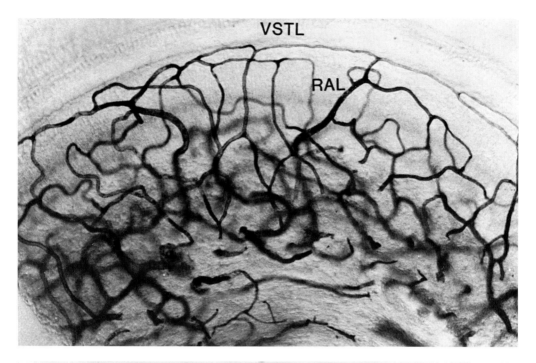

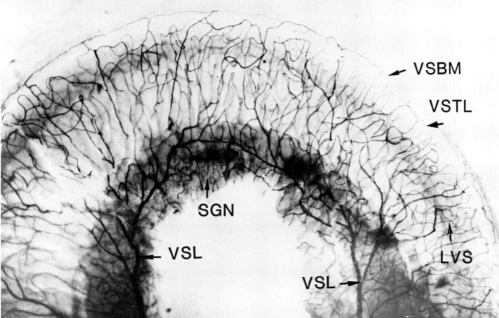

FIG. 10. Spiral lamina, basal turn, transverse section, guinea pig (**bottom**) and gerbil (**top**). In the guinea pig there is a well-developed vessel of the basilar membrane (VSBM) and a less well-developed inner spiral vessel formed by capillary arcades, the vessel of the tympanic lip (VSTL). The collecting venules merge to form spirally running veins of the spiral lamina (VSL). Spiral ganglion (SGN), limbus vessels (LVS). In the gerbil there is no regularly occurring VSBM but a well-developed single or double VSTL. Radiating arterioles (RAL).

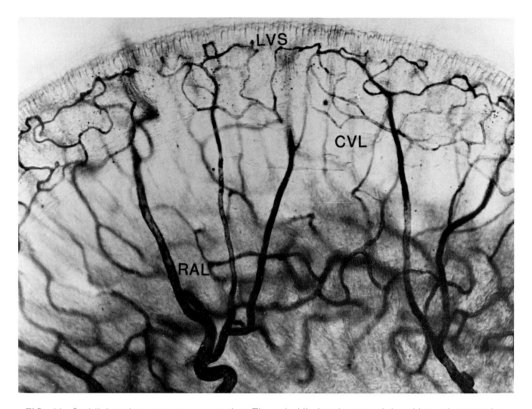

FIG. 11. Gerbil, basal turn, transverse section. The spiral limbus has a peripheral irregular vascular margin, the limbus vessels (LVS), supplied by radiating arterioles (RAL) and drained by collecting venules (CVL).

membrane, connecting RALs-SL to the VSVM in the external wall. Similar observations have been made in the squirrel monkey (22), in the sheep and cow (30), and in humans, particularly embryos (36,41).

In some human cochleas, occasional connections between the vessels of the spiral lamina and those in the external wall have been observed. In these cases, isolated branches from radiating or marginal spiral lamina vessels continue through the normally avascular region between the VSBM and the external wall vessels to form connections with the venules at the basilar membrane.

Apical and Basal Variations in Cochlear Vessels

In all species studied, there is a general tendency for the cochlear vascularization to decrease in a more or less regular fashion from base to apex, least so in the chinchilla. In this process, there is generally not a loss of vessel types, however, the number of vessels within a given area decreases, and the number of ramifications of those vessels is also lessened, from the base to the apex. In the apical turn, this simplification can be quite striking. In particular, a simplification of the stria vascularis capillary net to a few, relatively large looping vessels is observed, along with

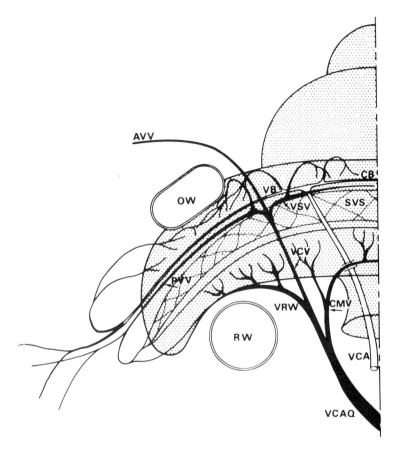

FIG. 12. Schematic view of the basal end of the mammalian cochlea, apico-basal section. The complicated pattern of the arterial and venous system in the region between the oval (OW) and round windows (RW) is illustrated.

a great reduction in the number of arterio-venous anastomoses external to stria vascularis.

The vasculature of the extreme basal end of the cochlea, in the region of the round and oval windows and the "hook," not surprisingly shows some variations from the rest of the cochlea. Essentially, all of the regularly occurring vessels are found here. However, the RALs from the SMA are forced by the geometry of this area to travel in an obliquely spiral direction to reach the region between the windows (Figs. 12 and 13). In addition, the CVLs-ST unite to form a separate vein, the vein of the round window (VRW), which unites with the spiral modiolar vein and the vestibulo-cochlear vein from the vestibulum to form the vein of the cochlear aqueduct (VCAQ) (vein of Cotugno). In all experimental animals, the basal-most portion of the extreme base is supplied by RALs from the vestibulo-cochlear artery (VCA) rather than from the SMA. RALs from VCA meet those from the SMA in the region between the windows to form an anastomosing net (Figs. 12 and 13). In humans, as discussed earlier, a considerably greater portion of the base is supplied by VCA.

The capillary net of the stria vascularis narrows to some degree in the region

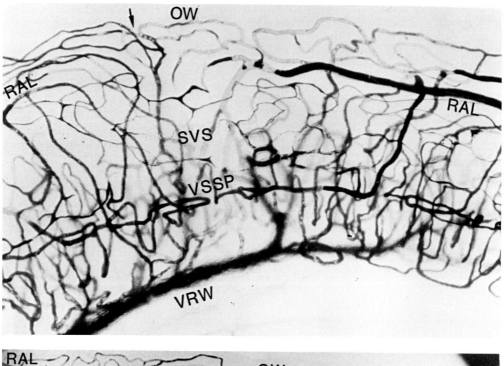

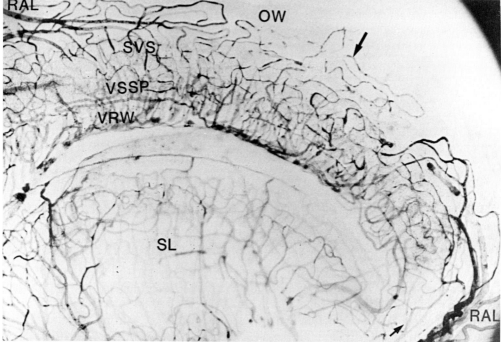

FIG. 13. Basal end, guinea pig (**bottom**), gerbil (**top**). Radiating arterioles (RAL) from two directions merge at the level at the oval window (OW) and form a capillary net in this region. The short collecting venules soon empty into the vein of the round window (VRW) that drains the capillary areas in the stria vascularis (SVS) and the vessel of the spiral prominence (VSSP). Spiral lamina (SL).

between the round and oval windows in all species. This constriction appears to be related to the restricted space between the windows and also to the presence of the anastomosing net formed at the confluence of the RALs from the VCA and the SMA. In most species, the capillary net of stria vascularis remains well organized in this region, however, in humans it becomes poorly organized at this point and remains so in the extreme base. In the rabbit, the stria vascularis loses its organization between the windows but recovers its normal pattern in the extreme base.

Vascular Development in the Cochlea

In the gerbil, the cochlea is not functional at birth. Electrophysiological responses can first be observed at 10 to 12 days after birth (DAB), and they achieve maturity at 18 to 20 DAB (47–49). At birth, the capillaries of the stria vascularis are almost completely undeveloped. They mature rapidly between 8 to 12 DAB, about the time at which the endocochlear potential first appears (10). The VSBM is present throughout the cochlea at birth, is very large, and has many connections with the vessels of the external wall, whereas few connections are apparent between the VSBM and other spiral lamina vessels. The VSBM degenerates after birth, disappearing except for basal turn remnants by 14 to 18 DAB.

In the guinea pig, no substantial changes are observed in the cochlear vasculature postnatally (4). This reflects the mature state of the cochlea at birth in this precocious species, which achieves adult cochlear function well before birth.

DISCUSSION

In addition to the observations already described, there is a considerable body of data from other investigators concerning the vascular anatomy of the cochlea (Table 1). Many observations of very high quality were obtained in the 19th and early 20th centuries. In particular, the work of Eichler (18) and Siebenmann (41) on the human cochlea, and Nabeya (34) on several animal species is noteworthy. Their work differs primarily from that of more recent investigations in the lack of photographic documentation and in some cases in lesser attention to the details of capillary beds. A detailed review of this early literature on the vascular anatomy of the cochlea as well as comparisons with more recent findings has been published (3). A recent development in technique has been the analysis of vascular injection casts by scanning electron microscopy (23,33), which has provided excellent representation of the three-dimensional organization of cochlear vessels. In many cases, these other studies have covered the same species described in the present investigation. The results are in substantial agreement with our own observations and need not be described here. However, the vascular anatomy of several additional animal species has been described in varying degrees of detail. These studies provide additional observations on interspecies variation of cochlear blood supply.

With respect to the existence of vessels in areas that are typically avascular, the existence of capillaries on the apical surface of the vestibular (Reissner's) membrane has been reported in the squirrel monkey (22), cow and sheep but not in the cat (43), pig, hamster, or mole (30). Occasional connections between the vessels of the spiral

TABLE 3. *Regularly occurring cochlear vessels and divergencies*

| | Modiolus | | | Scala vestibuli | | | | External wall | | |
| | | | | | | | | Scala media | | |
	SMA	SMV	CAPs	RALs	CVLs	CAPs	VSVM	SVS	VSSP	AVAS
Human	+[a]	+[b]	+	+	+	+	+	+	+	+
Rhesus monkey	+	+[c]	+	+	+	(+)	+	+	+	+
Rabbit	+	+	+	+	−	+	+	+	+	+
Guinea pig	+	+	+	+	+	+	+	+	+	+
Chinchilla	+	+	+	+	−	−	(+)	+	+	+
Rat	+	+	+	+	−	+	+	+	+	+
Gerbil	+	+	+	+	(+)	+	+	+	+	+

[a] May be absent and replaced by VCA, ramus cochlearis.
[b] Different system with VSV, VST, CMV, and variations.
[c] Variable location in basal turn.
[d] Some extend-protrude to scala vestibuli.
[e] Spirally running collecting vein basal turn, VSL.

lamina and those of the lateral wall have been observed in the squirrel monkey (22), cow (30), and humans (3,44).

In the cat there does not appear to be a VSSP comparable with that seen in other animals. Instead, the data of Smith (43) clearly show a compact looping network of vessels at this location. This is not a technical difference from the present study, since a typical VSSP is clearly shown in Smith's studies of the guinea pig (42).

The cat, like many other mammals, does not regularly exhibit a VSBM. Smith (43) observed this vessel only occasionally and only in two of the eight cats studied.

A number of previous authors speak of one or more capillary beds associated with the spiral ligament and/or the spiral prominence (19). With the exceptions of the rat, as previously described, and the cat as described by Smith (43), the capillary vessels of the spiral ligament do not appear to form a true capillary net. However, the capillaries of the lower portion of the spiral ligament are clearly organized as a bed of high density in all species, and it can be assumed that this organization serves some functional purpose.

It is clear from the data of the current study and from that presented earlier that there is a high degree of similarity between the vascular anatomy of the cochlea of various mammals. This is perhaps to be expected, since all are placental mammals with similarly structured cochleas. However, considering the broad range of species covered, from rodents to humans, the degree of uniformity of the great majority of cochlear vessels is somewhat surprising.

In some vessels, however, a high degree of variation across species was noted. This variability is summarized in Table 3. In particular, the degree of venous drainage of the scala vestibuli varied widely, with most species showing no CVLs in this scala, the guinea pig and rhesus monkey showing some CVLs, and the human showing a substantial number of CVLs and the unique VSV. In the external wall, the degree of development of the vascular bed in the spiral ligament varied from rather

| Scala tymp. | | Spiral lamina | | | | |
VLBM	CVLs	RALs-CVLs	LVS	VSTL	VSBM	Remarks
+	+	+	+	+	+	VCA supplies $\frac{1}{2}$ basal turn
+	+	+	+	+	(+)	
+	+[d]	+	+	+	−	CAPs on Reissner's membrane
+	+	+[e]	+	+	+	VSSV present
+	+[f]	+	+	+	(+)	Vasculature well maintained apically
+[g]	+	+	+	+	(+)	
(+)	+[f]	+	+	+	(+)	VSSV sometimes present

[f] Spirally running veins of scala tympani.
[g] Pronounced capillary net.
+, occurs regularly; (+), occurs infrequently; −, nonexistent.
For abbreviations of blood vessel nomenclature, see Table 2.

simple in the guinea pig and human, to a true capillary net in the rat. Finally, the VSBM varied from uniform presence throughout the cochlea in the human to complete absence in the rabbit. Other occasional differences between species were also noted.

Some of these differences in vascular anatomy may be related to such simple factors as size. The cochlear duct in humans is larger than in the expermental animals studied. This may explain the existence of a separate vein that drains the scala vestibuli.

Another possible explanation for species variations is differential degenerations of vessels that are important embryonically but are not necessary in later life. This may well explain the wide variation seen, for example, in the occurrence of a vessel under the tunnel of Corti since this vessel is known to be large and uniformly present in embryonic life (14–16,20,21,28), and to degenerate rapidly once the organ of Corti achieves maturity (10). Similarly, the existence of connections between the vessels of the spiral lamina and those of the external wall as well as between the modiolus and scala tympani (4,32,50) may reflect occasional survival of vessels that are more commonplace in the immature cochlea (10). VSVMs are presumably a similar phenomenon since they are also reported in the fetal ear of the human (36,41), and the pig (40), as well as adult animals, e.g., squirrel monkey (22), cow, and sheep (30).

It is interesting to note that the degree of relationship of species has relevance to interspecies variability in some cases but not in others. The rat and the gerbil, both myomorph rodents, sometimes show very similar differences from other species, such as a double VSTL in the middle cochlear turn, and a similar pattern of occurrence of the VSBM. However, even more striking is the fact that the vasculature of the rhesus monkey is often more comparable to the rodents studied than to humans.

REFERENCES

1. Asai, K. (1908): Die Blutgefässe im häutigen Labyrinthe des Hundes. *Anat. Hefte,* 36:369–403.
2. Asai, K. (1908): Die Blutgefässe des häutigen Labyrinthes der Ratte. *Anat. Hefte,* 36:711–728.
3. Axelsson, A. (1968): The vascular anatomy of the cochlea in the guinea pig and man. *Acta Otolaryngol.* [*Suppl.*] (*Stockh.*), 243:1–134.
4. Axelsson, A. (1971): The cochlear blood vessels in guinea pigs of different ages. *Acta Otolaryngol.* (*Stockh.*), 72:172–181.
5. Axelsson, A. (1972): The demonstration of the cochlear vessels in the guinea pig by contrast injection. *J. Laryngol. Otol.,* 86:121–128.
6. Axelsson, A. (1974): The blood supply of the inner ear of mammals. In: *Handbook of Sensory Physiology,* edited by W. D. Keidel and W. D. Neff, pp. 214–260. Springer, Berlin, Heidelberg, New York.
7. Axelsson, A. (1974): The vascular anatomy of the Rhesus monkey cochlea. *Acta Otolaryngol.* (*Stockh.*), 77:381–392.
8. Axelsson, A., and Lind, A. (1973): The capillary areas in the rabbit cochlea. *Acta Otolaryngol.* (*Stockh.*), 76:254–267.
9. Axelsson, A., and Lipscomb, D. (1975): The vascular pattern of the chinchilla cochlea. *Acta Otolaryngol.* (*Stockh.*), 79:352–365.
10. Axelsson, A., Ryan, A., and Woolf, N. (1986): The early postnatal development of the cochlear vasculature in the gerbil. *Acta Otolaryngol.* (*Stockh.*), 101:75–87.
11. Axelsson, A., and Vertes, D. (1977): Methodological aspects for the study of cochlear blood vessels. In: *Les colloques de l'Institute de la Santé et de la Recherche Médicale: Inner ear biology XIV Workshop,* edited by M. Portman and J. M. Aran, pp. 265–270.
12. Axelsson, A., and Vertes, D. (1978): Vascular histology of the guinea pig cochlea. *Acta Otolaryngol.* (*Stockh.*), 85:198–212.
13. Axelsson, A., and Vertes, D. (1982): Histological findings in cochlear vessels after noise. In: *New Perspectives on Noise-Induced Hearing Loss,* edited by R. D. Hamernik, D. Henderson, and R. Salvi, pp. 49–68. Raven Press, New York.
14. Baginsky, B. (1886): Zur Entwicklung der Gehörschnecke. *Arch. Mikr. Anat.,* 28:14.
15. Boettcher, A. (1887): Rückblicke auf die neueren Untersuchungen über den Bau der Schnecke, im Anschluss an eigene Beobachtungen. *Arch. Ohr.- Nas.- u. Kehlk-Heilk.,* 24:1–38;160–163;165–166;316–317.
16. Bredberg, G. (1968): Cellular pattern and nerve supply of the human organ of Corti. *Acta Otolaryngol.* [*Suppl.*] (*Stockh.*), 236:1–135.
17. Charachon, R. (1961): *Anatomie de l'Artère Auditive Interne chez l'Homme,* pp. 1–20. Imprimerie Bosc Frères, Lyon.
18. Eichler, O. (1892): Anatomische Untersuchungen über die Wege des Blutstromes im menschlichen Ohrlabyrinth. *Abhandl. math.-phys. Cl königl. sächs Ges Wissensch.,* 18:310–347.
19. Hawkins, J. E., Jr. (1968): Vascular patterns of the membranous labyrinth. In: *Third Symposium on the Role of the Vestibular Organs in Space Exploration,* edited by A. Graybiel, pp. 241–258. NASA, Washington, DC.
20. Hawkins, J. E., Jr., and Johnsson, L. G. (1968): Light microscopic observations of the inner ear in man and monkey. *Ann. Otol.,* 77:608–629.
21. Hilding, D. A., Suguira, A., and Nakai, Y. (1967): Deaf white mink: Electron microscopic study of the inner ear. *Ann. Otol.,* 76:647–664.
22. Hiraide, F., and Inouye, T. (1980): Unusual blood vessels in the cochlea of the squirrel monkey. *Arch. Otorhinolaryngol.,* 229:271–279.
23. Hodde, K. C., Miodoński, A., Bakker, C., and Veltman, W. A. M. (1977): Scanning electron microscopy of microcorrosion casts with special attention on arteriovenous differences and application to the rat's cochlea. *Scanning Electron Microscopy,* II:477–484.
24. Hornstrand, C., Axelsson, A., and Vertes, D. (1980): The vascular anatomy of the rat cochlea. *Acta Otolaryngol.* (*Stockh.*), 79:352–365.
25. Ibsen, L. (1881): *Anatomiske undersögelser over Örets labyrinth,* edited by Prof. Panum, Köpenhamn.
26. Johnsson, L. G. (1972): Cochlear blood vessel pattern in the human fetus and postnatal vascular involution. *Ann. Otol.,* 81:22–41.
27. Jones-Mumby, C., and Axelsson, A. (1984): The vascular anatomy of the gerbil cochlea. *Am. J. Otolaryngol.,* 5:127–137.
28. Kikuchi, K., and Hilding, D. A. (1967): The spiral vessel and stria vascularis in Shaker-1 mice. *Acta Otolaryngol.* (*Stockh.*), 63:395–410.
29. Kirikae, L., Nomura, Y., and Hiraide, F. (1969): The capillary in the human cochlea. *Acta Otolaryngol.* (*Stockh.*), 67:1–8.

30. Kohllöffel, L. U. E. (1977): On the connection membrana Corti—organ of Corti. *Les Colloques de l'Institut National de la Santé et de la Recherche Médicale,* edited by M. Portmann and J. M. Aran, pp. 15–24. Inserm, Paris.

31. Levin, N. A. (1964): Die Vaskularisation des Ohrlabyrinthes beim Menschen. *Anat. Anz.,* 114:337–352.

32. Maass, B. (1969): Quantitative Angaben zur Gefässversorgung der Stria vascularis beim Meerschweinchen. *Z. Laryngol. Rhinol.,* 48:733–753.

33. Miodoński, A., Hodde, K. C., and Kuś, J. (1978): Scanning electron microscopy of the cochlear vasculature. *Arch. Otolaryngol.,* 104:313–317.

34. Nabeya, D. (1923): A study in the comparative anatomy of the blood-vascular system of the internal ear in mammalia and in homo (Japanese). *Acta School Med. Univ. Imp. Kioto,* 6:1–127.

35. Nomura, Y., and Hiraide, F. (1968): Cochlear blood vessel. A histochemical method of its demonstration. *Arch. Otolaryngol.,* 88:231–237.

36. Okano, Y., Sando, I., and Myers, E. N. (1978): Blood vessels on Reissner's membrane. *Ann. Otol.,* 87:170–174.

37. Ritter, K. (1978): Die Gefässe des Innenohres. *Arch. Otorhinolaryngol.,* 219:115–177.

38. Schwalbe, G. (1887): Ein Beitrag zur Kenntniss der Cirkulationsverhältnisse in der Gehörschnecke. *Beitr. Physiol.,* 200–220.

39. Scuderi, R., and Del Bo, M. (1952): La vascolarizzazione del labirinto umanao. *Arch. Ital. Otol.,* Suppl. 11, 63:8–54.

40. Shambaugh, G. E. (1903): The distribution of blood vessels in the labyrinth of the ear of sus scrofa domesticus. *Decennial Public Univ. Chicago,* 10:137–154.

41. Siebenmann, F. (1894): *Die Blutgefässe im Labyrinthe des menschlichen Ohres,* pp. 1–33. J. F. Bergmann, Wiesbaden.

42. Smith, C. A. (1951): Capillary areas of the cochlea in the guinea pig. *Laryngoscope,* 61:1073–1095.

43. Smith, C. A. (1954): Capillary areas of the membranous labyrinth. *Ann. Otol.,* 63:435–447.

44. Tange, R. A., and Bernard, J. L. (1981): A cochlear vascular anomaly in a patient with hearing loss and tinnitus. *Arch. Otorhinolaryngol.,* 233:117–125.

45. Tange, R. A. (1986): The vascular anatomy of the spiral lamina and the spiral limbus in the adult rat. *Arch. Otorhinolaryngol.,* 243:24–26.

46. Vertes, D., and Axelsson, A. (1979): Methodological aspects of some inner ear vascular techniques. *Acta Otolaryngol. (Stockh.),* 88:328–334.

47. Woolf, N. K., and Ryan, A. (1983): Ontogeny of auditory function in the cochlea of the mongolian gerbil. *Neuroscience Abstract,* 9:378.

48. Woolf, N. K., and Ryan, A. (1984): The development of auditory function in the cochlea of the mongolian gerbil. *Hear. Res.,* 13:229–283.

49. Woolf, N. K., Ryan, A., and Harris, J. (1986): Development of mammalian endocochlear potential, normal ontogeny and effect of anoxia. *Am. J. Physiol.,* 250:493–498.

50. Wolff, D. (1935): Anomalous capillary plexus in the scala tympani. *Arch. Otolaryngol.,* 22:44–46.

51. Wüstenfeld, E., and Kühnert, D. (1964): Experimenteller Beitrag zur Frage der Gefässversorgung der Meerschweinchencochlea. *Z. Mikr. Anat. Forsch.,* 71:172–184.

Physiology of the Ear,
edited by A. F. Jahn and J. Santos-Sacchi.
Raven Press, New York © 1988.

Circulation of the Inner Ear:
II. The Relationship Between Metabolism and Blood Flow in the Cochlea

Allen F. Ryan

Department of Otolaryngology, University of California Medical Center and Veterans Administration Medical Center, San Diego, California 92103

A relationship between blood supply and tissue metabolism has long been recognized. Tissues with high levels of metabolism, such as muscle and brain, possess an extensive circulation capable of supplying high levels of metabolites and clearing metabolic end products. Increased metabolism within a tissue also results in an increase in blood flow. The cochlea possesses a rich vascular supply (1), and cochlear metabolism increases during sound exposure (6,11,16). For this reason, it might be expected that the blood flow to the cochlea would increase during acoustic stimulation. However, the bony capsule of the cochlea and the complexity of its vascular supply have made the measurement of cochlear blood flow difficult. Moreover, most investigations of cochlear blood flow and sound stimulation have been conducted using damaging intensities to test the hypothesis that vascular insufficiency plays a role in noise-induced hearing loss. The relationship between cochlear blood flow and physiologic levels of acoustic stimulation remains largely unexplored [see Axelsson and Vertes (2) for a review].

The development of two radiotracer techniques has allowed both metabolism and blood flow to be demonstrated graphically in brain tissue. The 2-deoxyglucose (2-DG) autoradiography technique (20) provides a map of glucose uptake, and thus of glucose metabolism, throughout the brain. 2-DG is a glucose analog that is recognized as glucose by membrane uptake systems and taken into cells in the same manner. Within the cell it is converted to 2-DG-6-phosphate. However, unlike glucose-6-phosphate, 2-DG-6-phosphate is unsuitable for further transformation into substrates for either glycolysis or the pentose shunt. There is also little glucose-6-phosphatase activity in the brain to reverse the reaction. Since the cell membrane is relatively impermeable to 2-DG-6-phosphate, the molecule is then trapped within the cell, with a half-life of approximately 9 hours. If the 2-DG molecule is radiolabeled, the accumulation of labeled 2-DG-6-phosphate within cells provides a record of glucose uptake and thus of glucose metabolism by different tissues. With this method, activation of neural tissue has been shown to result in a dramatic increase in glucose uptake and utilization (18–20).

Radiolabeled diffusion tracers such as iodoantipyrine (IAP) have been used to document blood flow in brain (14). IAP is injected into the bloodstream at a constant rate and diffuses into tissue in proportion to blood flow through that tissue. If the IAP is radiolabeled, the amount of label present in tissue can be demonstrated autoradiographically, providing a map of blood flow rates in various brain regions.

Using and comparing these two methods reveal a close relationship between the level of metabolism and the level of blood flow in normal brain tissue (14,20). Such a parallel relationship is not surprising. The metabolism of neural tissue is almost exclusively mediated by glucose. Tissue storage capacity for this metabolite is virtually nonexistent, and glucose is drawn from serum pools on demand (18). The linkage of metabolism and blood flow in the brain is thought to be mediated by the vasodilatory effects of CO_2 (14), an end-product of glucose metabolism.

Many of the tissues of the inner ear are neural or show similar dependency on glucose as an energy source (22). It therefore seems likely that a similar relationship between glucose metabolism and blood flow might be observed in the tissues of the cochlea, as is seen in the brain. However, there are considerable technical difficulties associated with applying the 2-DG and IAP techniques to the inner ear.

Both 2-DG and IAP are highly diffusible in water and cannot be fixed without displacement (14,20). In the brain, their distribution in tissue is maintained by rapid freezing, frozen sectioning, and immediate drying of sections (20). This methodology is not suitable for the bone-encapsulated, fluid-filled cochlea. Therefore, techniques were developed based on freeze-drying and anhydrous plastic embedding that allow the use of these diffusible radiotracers in the cochlea.

MATERIALS AND METHODS

The methods employed have been described in detail elsewhere (15–17). Briefly, for 2-DG measurement of glucose metabolism, adult mongolian gerbils (*Meriones unguiculatus*) were injected with [^{14}C]-labeled 2-DG and immediately placed into silence, wide-band noise at 85 dB SPL, or a pure tone at the same intensity. After 1 hr, the animals were sacrificed and their cochleas were cryogenically frozen, freeze-dried, and vapor-fixed over osmium and acrolein. The cochleas were embedded in plastic using only nonpolar organic solvents to prevent diffusion of the tracer, halved along the modiolus, and the resultant block faces exposed on X-ray film. The data were quantitated by microdensitometry.

For high-resolution 2-DG autoradiography, the animals were treated as above, with the following exceptions. Subjects were injected with tritiated 2-DG. After plastic embedding, individual cochlear turns were dissected from the block; 5-μm plastic sections were cut and covered with emulsion by a dry-loop technique.

For IAP measurement of cochlear blood flow, gerbils were anesthetized and one cochlea was stimulated with 85-dB SPL wide-band noise. The ossicular chain of the opposite ear was disrupted to reduce bone-conducted stimuli. IAP was infused through a venous catheter for 45 sec, after which the cochleas were cryogenically frozen *in situ* by flooding the bullae with Freon 12 at $-159°C$. The cochleas were then treated in the same manner as for the [^{14}C]-2-DG experiments to produce autoradiographs and densitometric data. Data from the exposed and unexposed cochleas were compared to assess the effects of noise exposure.

RESULTS

2-DG Measurement of Cochlear Metabolism

Representative autoradiographs illustrating the patterns of 2-DG uptake observed in the cochlea in silence and during exposure to 85-dB SPL wide-band noise are

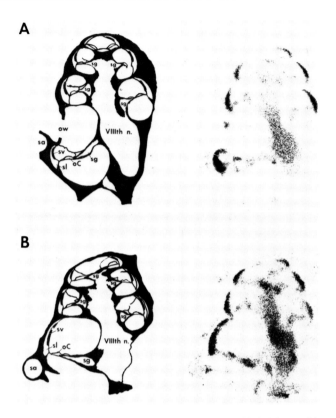

FIG. 1. Typical autoradiographs illustrating the distribution of label in cochleas maintained in silence (**A**) or wide-band noise (**B**) for 1 hr following injection of [^{14}C]-2-DG. The camera lucida drawings show the structures at the surface of each of the sections that were exposed to the film. sv, stria vascularis; sl, spiral ligament; oC, organ of Corti; sg, spiral ganglion; sa, stapedial artery; ow, oval window. (Adapted from ref. 16.)

shown in Fig. 1. In silence, high levels of 2-DG uptake were observed in the external wall structures including the stria vascularis, spiral prominence, and spiral ligament. However, uptake into the sensorineural structures, organ of Corti, spiral ganglion, and VIIIth nerve was very low. The major change observed during exposure to 85-dB noise was an increase in uptake into the ganglion and the VIIIth nerve.

During pure-tone stimulation, this same phenomenon was apparent. However, as shown in Fig. 2, the increases were localized to tonotopically appropriate regions of the ganglion and nerve. Uptake of 2-DG into external wall structures opposite the stimulated region of spiral ganglion did not appear to be higher than in other turns.

These observations were corroborated by the quantitative data based on micro-densitometry and blood curves, which are presented in Fig. 3. Large increases in 2-DG uptake were measured in the spiral ganglion and VIIIth nerve of animals exposed to 85-dB SPL wide-band noise, when compared with silence. However, smaller increases were also noted in the organ of Corti and stria vascularis.

The level of 2-DG uptake into external wall structures also varied along the length of the cochlea. Uptake was highest in the lower basal turn and decreased regularly toward the apex.

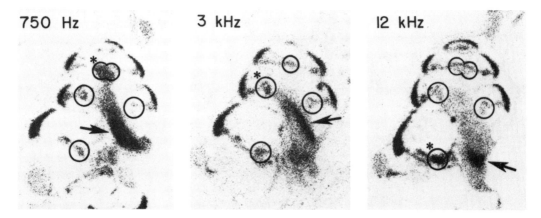

FIG. 2. Autoradiographs obtained from cochleas exposed to one of three pure tones at 85 dB SPL. (From ref. 16.)

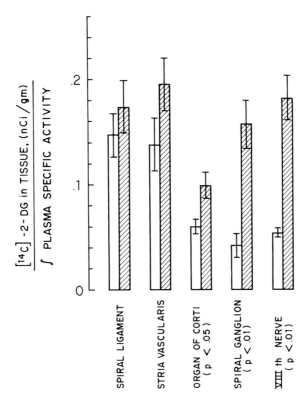

FIG. 3. Mean 2-DG levels in cochlear tissues of the lower basal turn from inner ears in silence (*open bar*) and in 85-dB SPL wide-band noise (*stippled bar*). Tissue levels were normalized for each subject by the integral of the plasma-specific activity curve. Each mean represents six cochleas, vertical bars show one standard deviation about each mean. (From ref. 16.)

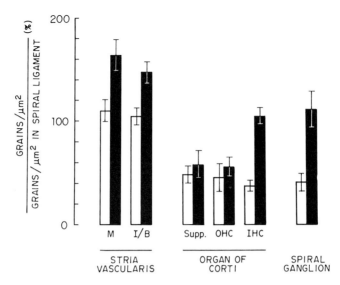

FIG. 4. Level of [^{3}H]-2-DG in individual cells from cochleas exposed to 85-dB SPL wide-band noise (*solid bar*) or maintained in silence (*open bar*). The data are presented as grain counts and were normalized by counts over cells in the spiral ligament, since we have shown that 2-DG uptake in this tissue does not change during sound exposure. Each bar represents 20 cells from two cochleas. Noise exposure was associated with higher levels of 2-DG in both the marginal (M) and intermediate/ basal (I/B) cell regions of the stria vascularis, inner hair cells (IHC), and spiral ganglion cells. In contrast, no stimulus-associated difference was observed in either supporting cells (Supp.) or outer hair cells (OHC).

Using [^{3}H]-labeled 2-DG and high-resolution autoradiography, the effects of acoustic stimulation on the uptake of 2-DG into individual cochlear cells could be assessed. The results are illustrated in Fig. 4. As would be expected from the [^{14}C]-2-DG data, the uptake of [^{3}H]-2-DG into spiral ganglion cells was markedly higher during noise exposure. Within the organ of Corti, although inner hair cells showed higher 2-DG uptake during sound stimulation, neither outer hair cells nor supporting cells showed any stimulus-related differences. In the external wall, noise increased 2-DG uptake in all parts of the stria vascularis.

IAP Measurement of Cochlear Blood Flow

A representative autoradiograph illustrating the distribution of IAP during silence is shown in Fig. 5. The results in many respects parallel the 2-DG data. In silence, high levels of IAP were seen in external wall structures, indicating high levels of blood flow through the vessels of the stria vascularis and spiral ligament. Low levels of IAP were present in sensorineural structures, indicating a much more limited blood flow. During noise exposure, IAP levels were noticeably higher in the spiral ganglion and VIIIth nerve.

A quantitative comparison of optical densities from the exposed and unexposed cochleas is illustrated in Fig. 6. Increased IAP levels were noted during noise exposure in the VIIIth nerve, spiral ganglion, and organ of Corti, suggesting increased blood flow to these structures. In contrast, IAP did not increase in either the stria

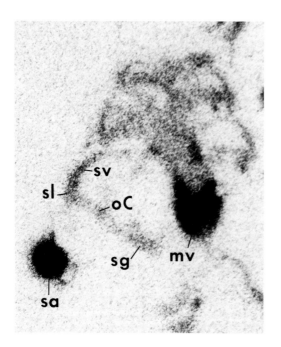

FIG. 5. A typical autoradiograph showing the distribution of [^{14}C]-labeled IAP in an unstimulated cochlea. Note that except for the major vessels of the modiolus (mv) and the stapedial artery (sa), the darkest images correspond to the external wall tissues, the stria vascularis (sv) and spiral ligament (sl). The images of the organ of Corti (oC) and spiral ganglion (sg) are lighter. (From ref. 15.)

vascularis or the spiral ligament, indicating that there was no increase in blood flow to the external wall.

In the external wall structures, the highest levels of IAP were observed in the lower basal turn. A regular decrease along the length of the cochlea was noted.

DISCUSSION

The data illustrated in Figs. 1 to 4 clearly indicate that glucose metabolism increased in certain cochlear structures during exposure to sound. Spiral ganglion cells and VIIIth nerve fibers both showed substantial increases in 2-DG uptake associated with acoustic activation. When the organ of Corti was considered as a whole, stimulation evoked only a modest increase. However, at the cellular level a substantial increase was observed in the inner hair cells, whereas there was little or no effect of stimulation on glucose uptake in outer hair cells or supporting cells. Stimulation also evoked an increase in the glucose metabolism of the stria vascularis but not in the spiral ligament.

The absence of a metabolic increase in the outer hair cells during acoustic stimulation is surprising, especially given the recent demonstration of active mechanical responses in these cells (4), and speculation regarding an active role for outer hair cells in the cochlear transduction process (10). This implies an alternative source of energy. The battery model of Davis (7) hypothesizes a transfer of energy from the stria vascularis to the organ of Corti, mediated by the endocochlear potential and the ionic composition of endolymph. More recently, Brownell and Kachar (5) have suggested that active outer hair cell mechanical responses may be mediated electrochemically rather than by contractile proteins. A sound-induced increase in strial

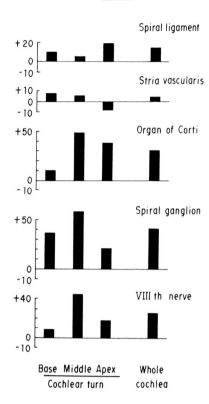

FIG. 6. The effects of wide-band noise stimulation on IAP distribution in the cochlea. Percentage of difference between optical densities from cochleas exposed to 85-dB SPL wide-band noise and those from the opposite, unexposed ears $[(E - V)/V]$. Although there was little difference between the optical densities of the spiral ligament and the stria vascularis, those of the organ of Corti, spiral ganglion, and VIIIth nerve were consistently and significantly higher in the exposed cochleas. This suggests that blood flow was elevated in these structures because of the noise exposure.

metabolism, as indicated by the data presented earlier, is consistent with the Davis model and could provide an indirect method of mediating active mechanical responses in outer hair cells. Alternatively, the outer hair cells may not utilize serum glucose directly as an energy source for mechanical responses. They could rely on an alternative source such as amino acids or stored glycogen.

The similarities between the autoradiographs of Figs. 1 and 5 suggest a close relationship between metabolism and blood flow in the cochlea. The overall patterns of distribution of 2-DG and IAP are quite similar in silence. Changes evoked by noise stimulation are to some extent comparable. The external wall structures also show a similar variation in both tracers along the length of the cochlea.

Such a close relationship between metabolism and blood flow is logical. One would predict that areas displaying an active metabolism would receive a blood flow commensurate with their need for oxygen and for metabolic substrates. Metabolism and blood flow are also well related to the vascular pattern of the cochlea as described in the previous chapter. In areas with rich vascular nets, high blood flow is seen, especially when the cochlea is activated.

It is not surprising that blood flow increases when local metabolism increases. This implies that blood flow in at least some cochlear structures is regulated by the end-products of metabolism, such as CO_2. In support of this hypothesis, Dengerink et al. (8) and Larson and Angelborg (12) have shown that blood flow in the cochlea can be markedly increased by increasing CO_2 concentration in the bloodstream.

However, differences were also apparent in the behavior of metabolism and blood flow. In the stria vascularis, noise stimulation produced an increase in 2-DG uptake but not in blood flow as measured with IAP. This may be related to the function of the stria vascularis, which is thought to be the site of generation of both the cochlear endolymph (9,13) and the endocochlear potential (21). It is possible that blood flow is always high in the strial capillaries to maintain ion exchange and supply metabolites and in turn maintain the resting ionic composition and resting potential of the endolymphatic space. Given such a reserve capacity, strial blood flow may be less sensitive to changes in local metabolism than flow in the neural tissues of the cochlea. Alternatively, strial blood flow may be regulated by the shunting of blood between the strial capillary net and adjacent arterio-venous anastamoses. The resolution of the IAP technique may not be sufficient to resolve such shunting.

Differences in the behavior of 2-DG uptake and IAP distribution also have implications for the determinants of cochlear metabolism. Using a microdissection technique, Canlon and Schacht (6) reported that 2-DG uptake in both the lateral wall and the modiolus increased during sound stimulation. They suggested that a common increase in blood flow to all cochlear tissues might be responsible for the parallel increase in 2-DG uptake. Our IAP and 2-DG data do not support this hypothesis. First, many structures in the cochlea showed no change in blood flow, indicating that flow does not vary in the same manner throughout the cochlea. Second, 2-DG uptake increased in the stria vascularis without a concomitant increase in blood flow. This suggests that the determinant of 2-DG accumulation into cochlear tissues is the rate of uptake by individual cells, not the rate of supply via plasma.

The high levels of glucose metabolism and blood flow that were observed in the spiral ligament and spiral prominence imply that these tissues play an important role in cochlear function. Because neither metabolism nor blood flow changed in these structures during sound stimulation, these tissues may function primarily in cochlear homeostasis. For example, Borghesan (3) suggested that they are involved in maintaining the ionic composition of the cochlear fluids.

ACKNOWLEDGMENTS

This work was supported by grant NS14945 from the United States NIH/NINCDS, by the Research Service of the United States Veterans Administration, and by the Swedish Work Environment Fund. The technical contributions of Charles Graham and Thecla Bennett are gratefully acknowledged.

REFERENCES

1. Axelsson, A. (1968): The vascular anatomy of the cochlea in the guinea pig and in man. *Acta Otolaryngol. [Suppl.] (Stockh.)*, 243:1–134.
2. Axelsson, A., and Vertes, D. (1982): Histological findings in cochlear vessels after noise. In: *New Perspectives On Noise-Induced Hearing Loss*, edited by R. P. Hamernik, D. Henderson, and R. Salvi, pp. 49–68. Raven Press, New York.
3. Borghesan, E. (1967): On the function of the spiral prominence. *Acta Otolaryngol. (Stockh.)*, 63:161–169.
4. Brownell, W. E., Bader, C. R., Bertrand, D., and de Ribaupierre, Y. (1985): Evoked mechanical responses of isolated cochlear outer hair cells. *Science*, 227:194–196.

5. Brownell, W. E., and Kachar, B. (1986): Outer hair cell motility. In: *Peripheral Auditory Mechanisms*, edited by J. B. Allen et al. Springer-Verlag, New York.
6. Canlon, B., and Schacht, J. (1983): Acoustic stimulation alters deoxyglucose uptake in the mouse cochlea and inferior colliculus. *Hear. Res.*, 10:217–226.
7. Davis, H. (1965): A model for transducer action in the cochlea. *Cold Spring Harbor Symp. Quant. Biol.*, 30:181–190.
8. Dengerink, H. A., Axelsson, A., Miller, J. M., and Wright, J. M. (1984): The effect of noise and carbogen on cochlear vasculature. *Acta Otolaryngol. (Stockh.)*, 98:81–88.
9. Engstrom, H., Sjostrand, F. S., and Spoendlin, J. (1955): Feinstruktur der Stria Vascularis beim Meerschweinchen. *Pract. Otorhinolaryngol.*, 17:69–84.
10. Flock, A. (1983): Hair cells, receptors with motor capacity? In: *Hearing—Physiological Bases and Psychophysics*, edited by R. Klinke and R. Hartmann, pp. 2–7. Springer-Verlag, Berlin.
11. Goodwin, P. C., Ryan, A. F., Sharp, F. R., Woolf, N. K., and Davidson, T. M. (1984): Cochlear deoxyglucose uptake: Relationship to stimulus intensity. *Hear. Res.*, 15:215–224.
12. Larsen, H. C., and Angelborg, C. (1987): The vestibular blood flow during CO_2-breathing in rabbits. *Acta Otolaryngol. (Stockh.)*, 103:14–17.
13. Nakai, Y. (1965): Histochemical study of the stria vascularis in the inner ear by electron microscopy. *Ann. Otolaryngol.*, 74:326–339.
14. Rievich, M., Jehle, J., Sokoloff, L., and Kety, S. S. (1969): Measurement of regional cerebral blood flow with antipyrine-[14C] in awake cats. *J. Appl. Physiol.*, 27:296–300.
15. Ryan, A. F., Axelsson, A., Myers, R. R., and Woolf, N. K. (1988): Changes in cochlear blood flow during acoustic stimulation as determined by 14C-iodoantipyrine autoradiography. *Acta Otolaryngol. (Stockh.)*, 105:232–241.
16. Ryan, A. F., Goodwin, P., Woolf, N. K., and Sharp, F. R. (1982): Auditory stimulation alters the pattern of 2-deoxyglucose uptake in the inner ear. *Brain Res.*, 234:213–225.
17. Ryan, A. F., and Sharp, F. R. (1982): Localization of (3H) 2-deoxyglucose at the cellular level using freeze-dried tissue and dry-looped emulsion. *Brain Res.*, 252:177–180.
18. Sokoloff, L. (1977): Relation between physiological function and energy metabolism in the central nervous system. *J. Neurochem.*, 29:13–26.
19. Sokoloff, L. (1981): Localization of functional activity in the central nervous system by measurement of glucose utilization with radioactive deoxyglucose. *J. Cereb. Blood Flow Metab.*, 1:7–36.
20. Sokoloff, L., Reivich, M., Kennedy, C., et al. (1977): The deoxyglucose method for the measurement of local cerebral glucose utilization: Theory, procedure, and normal values in the conscious and anesthetized albino rat. *J. Neurochem.*, 28:13–36.
21. Tasaki, I., and Spyropolous, C. S. (1959): Stria vascularis as source of endocochlear potential. *J. Neurophysiol.*, 22:249–255.
22. Thalmann, R., and Marcus, D. C. (1985): Perspectives in the physiological chemistry of the cochlear duct. In: *Auditory Biochemistry*, edited by D. Drescher, pp. 422–435. Charles C. Thomas, Springfield, IL.

Physiology of the Ear,
edited by A. F. Jahn and J. Santos-Sacchi.
Raven Press, New York © 1988.

Circulation of the Inner Ear:
III. The Physiology of Cochlear Blood Flow: Implications for Treatment

H. A. Dengerink and J. W. Wright

Department of Psychology, Washington State University,
Pullman, Washington 99164-4830

Alterations in cochlear blood flow (CBF) have been implicated in the etiology of a variety of inner ear disorders including Meniere's disease (15,49) and noise-induced hearing loss (5,6,11,12,44). Although the exact contribution of altered CBF in specific disorders is not clear, the viability of the cochlea certainly depends on adequate nutrient perfusion and removal of waste products (21). Variations in CBF may affect the availability of oxygen (27), glucose, which is more rapidly metabolized during sound stimulation (8,52), and other nutrients.

Because of the clinical implications of the possible effects on hearing, a study of CBF is central to the development of possible medical therapy for inner ear disorders. The cochlea, however, is a very small organ and CBF accounts for only about 1/10,000 of the total cardiac output (54). The minute volume of the cochlear vascular bed implies considerable inefficiency when pharmacological treatments meant for the cochlea are given systemically. It also leaves open the possibility of side effects in other organ systems from pharmacological interventions intended for the cochlea. Clearly, pharmacological treatment of cochlear disorders would be optimal if CBF could be increased independent of or with only minimal increases in blood flow to other organ systems.

The goal of altering CBF to maximize perfusion and optimize pharmacological access requires better understanding of the mechanisms that control CBF. A major first step in this understanding is provided by studies of the cochlear vascular anatomy, such as described by Axelsson and Ryan in a previous chapter of this book. This anatomic description outlines many of the limitations to the study of CBF. The intricate interrelationship of the cochlear vessels, the tortuous course of these vessels, and the right angle turns all contribute to the complexity of the system and prevent ready access to the cochlea through its circulation.

Adequate understanding of CBF is also limited by the technical difficulties of measuring CBF, owing in part to the small size of the cochlea. In addition, various segmental networks supply different portions of the cochlea and may be related to different functions. Further, the vessels are embedded in the bony otic capsule precluding direct access.

Several methods have been devised to measure CBF but all have been less than ideal. An ideal measure should be noninvasive (the measurement procedures themselves would not modify the phenomenon being measured) and a direct measure rather than one that assesses phenomena secondary to blood flow. It should be dynamic rather than static and provide a quantitative measure that is linearly related to blood flow. Further, since blood flow involves the volume of blood moving through an area in a given unit of time, the measure should reflect both the volume (number of red blood cells per volume of tissue) and velocity at which the cells move. Finally, the volume of the tissues studied should be discrete enough to permit assessment of blood flow changes in individual turns of the cochlea and in specific vessels of the capillary beds.

Much of the research described in this chapter was carried out using a new measuring technique based on laser Doppler flowmetry. The laser Doppler has been recently developed as a measure of blood flow in various areas of the body and demonstrated in several studies to be a valid measure of CBF (36,37). We have chosen to rely primarily on this method of measurement for several reasons: it is relatively discrete in that measures are limited to cochlear vasculature; it is a dynamic measure, i.e., it reflects changes in CBF that are reversible and occur in real time, as opposed to static or one-time measures that are dependent on death of the animal. It is noninvasive in the sense that the Doppler flowmeter does not interfere with the process measured.

This measure does have limitations however. In its current configuration, use of the laser Doppler flowmeter requires an anesthetized animal, and access to the cochlea must be provided by surgery. Although the laser Doppler is sufficiently discrete to limit measurement to the cochlear vasculature, it cannot measure blood flow in individual cochlear vessels. The Doppler probe is sensitive to reflected light in a volume of 1 mm^3 (22,46). In skin, the depth of penetration is 1.0 mm (42,48). It is not known what the penetration depth is in the more dense cochlea. However, on the basis of its penetration in skin, we assume that, with the Doppler probe placed normal to the basal turn of the cochlea, it measures CBF in the following cochlear vessels collectively: radiating arterioles and capillaries of the scala vestibuli, the vessel at the vestibular membrane, the stria vascularis, the vessels of the spiral prominence, initial segments of the collecting venules and arteriovenous anastamoses.

Numerous other procedures have also been devised to measure CBF. These include microsphere techniques that involve injecting a known number of microspheres into the vascular system and then counting the number that are collected in a chosen vascular bed (3). Histological examination of the blood vessels and red blood cell configurations believed to reflect blood flow has most often been employed to examine the effects of noise on apparent CBF (5). Electrical impedance plethysmography (45) has been used extensively by Snow and Suga (55,56,59,60). It involves passing a small current through the tissue of interest and measuring changes in electrical impedance. It is assumed that changes in blood flow through the cochlea are responsible for changes in impedance. Sonic Doppler measures have been used in one reported investigation (30). Direct visualization of blood flow through the vessels is possible after fenestration of the lateral wall. This approach has been used by Perlman and Kimura (47), Lawrence (34), and more recently by Nuttall (43) who added a computer enhancement technique to improve the apparent visualization. Indirect measures have often been used as an indicator that CBF has changed. These include measures of partial oxygen pressure as well as cochlear microphonic thresholds (49).

In addition to the anatomic limitations on CBF imposed by the physical configuration of the cochlear vascular bed, it is also affected by the dynamic processes that alter blood flow elsewhere in the body. Previous reviews have discussed various aspects of CBF. Snow and Suga (55,56,59,60) provided a list of vasoactive agents that appear to influence CBF as measured by impedance plethysmography. Axelsson and Vertes (5) and Axelsson and Dengerink (4) reviewed studies that examined the histological sequelae of noise exposure. The purpose of this chapter is to consider three dynamic mechanisms that may affect CBF. First, since the cochlear vasculature is supplied by systemic circulation, it is proposed that CBF is subject to changes in systemic pressure. Second, there is growing evidence that CBF may be subject to local or autoregulation. Finally, CBF appears to vary with intravascular fluid volume.

SYSTEMIC AND CBF DYNAMICS

Increases in systemic blood pressure are very clearly associated with increases in CBF. This relationship has been demonstrated by numerous investigators using various measuring techniques and manipulations of blood pressure. Further, as the following demonstrates, the role of blood pressure in controlling CBF is sufficiently dominant to produce a dose–response relationship.

Vasoactive Peptides

The major vasoactive agent that we have chosen to examine with respect to the relationship between CBF and systemic pressures is angiotensin II (AII). AII serves an integrative role with regard to cardiovascular function and electrolyte balance (18). Most important among its effects are its direct inotropic effect on the heart and its ability to increase vascular resistance. The influence of AII on vascular resistance is a consequence of both its direct constricting action on vascular smooth muscle and an indirect action mediated via the central nervous system resulting in activation of the sympathetic nervous system and stimulation of vasopressin and catecholamine release.

The major water balance effects of AII also involve both central and peripheral actions, including increases in thirst, salt appetite, and sodium absorption by the gut, and improved efficiency of water and salt retention by the kidney (28). The multiple cardiovascular and body water balance effects that indirectly influence cardiovascular efficiency suggest that AII plays a fundamental role in the regulation of cardiovascular function, including blood flow to the cochlea.

In the first of these experiments (65) we administered AII randomly to guinea pigs in various doses and measured CBF via a laser Doppler. The results are summarized in Table 1. Both blood pressure and CBF increased with increasing doses of AII. In contrast, skin blood flow decreased in a generally dose-related fashion. Doses employed (0.1–100 pmol/kg) bracketed the levels observed when AII was assayed in the plasma of noise-exposed subjects (14,66). This suggests that the levels of endogenous AII released in the course of normal sound exposure can cause an increase in CBF. The pattern of results, however, suggests that the changes in CBF are secondary to changes in blood pressure. That is, these changes do not necessarily

TABLE 1. *Blood pressure, cochlear and abdominal skin flow changes following intra-arterial injection of angiotensin II*[a]

Dosage of AII	Blood pressure (% of baseline)	Cochlear flow (% of baseline)	Skin flow (% of baseline)
0.1 pmol/kg			
Max. change	+9.6 ± 3.5	+3.6 ± 0.9	−1.9 ± 1.5
1.0 pmol/kg			
Max. change	+12.3 ± 4.7	+3.7 ± 3.1	−4.3 ± 2.8
10 pmol/kg			
Max. change	+32.1 ± 4.7	+10.0 ± 3.1	−7.2 ± 2.3
100 pmol/kg			
Max. change	+79.2 ± 2.5	+20.0 ± 2.8	−12.8 ± 3.2

[a] Values are means ± S.E.
From ref. 12.

indicate that the cochlear blood vessels themselves are responsive to AII stimulation, rather the increase in CBF may be caused by systemic pressure changes.

The ability of AII to increase CBF has also been observed by Laugel (33) in a subsequent study, employing rats instead of guinea pigs. He reported CBF elevations following injection of AII averaged. Vasopressin is another related vasoactive peptide that may be released in response to AII. Laugel (33) reported increases in both blood pressure and CBF in response to injections of vasopressin (542 μmol/kg). Blood pressure increased to an average of 81% above baseline; CBF increased to an average of 61% above baseline.

Catecholamines

Catecholamines have often been implicated in hearing function. Our investigations of catecholamines have been limited to systemic infusions and have separately studied the effects of epinephrine and norepinephrine. Using a procedure similar to the angiotensin study outlined earlier, we infused several doses of epinephrine and norepinephrine. The results are summarized in Table 2. Blood pressure and CBF increased with infusions of epinephrine and norepinephrine in a dose-related fashion. By contrast, skin blood flow decreased with the infusion of these substances and did so in a dose-related manner. In a related study, Laugel (33) has reported that phenylephrine, a relatively pure alpha agonist, also elevated CBF an average of 41% following a dosage of 0.02 mg/kg.

In summary, these findings indicate that substances with vasoconstrictive actions increase CBF in a predictable dose-related fashion. The pattern of these results, however, indicates that the increase in CBF following administration of these agents may be secondary to changes in systemic blood pressure, i.e., secondary to increased cardiac output and peripheral resistance.

LOCAL OR AUTOREGULATION OF CBF

Although these findings suggest that CBF is significantly affected by systemic vascular changes, there are intriguing indications that local regulation or autoreg-

TABLE 2. *Blood pressure, cochlear and abdominal skin flow changes following intra-arterial injection of saline, epinephrine and norepinephrine*[a]

Drug and dose	Blood pressure (% of baseline)	Cochlear flow (% of baseline)	Skin flow (% of baseline)
Saline			
Max. change	+23.8 ± 10.1	+16.2 ± 8.3	+2.1 ± 5.7
Epinephrine			
0.1 μg/kg			
Max. change	+22.0 ± 8.1	+19.8 ± 5.5	−8.8 ± 4.8
1.0 μg/kg			
Max. change	+59.8 ± 12.0	+34.1 ± 6.1	−10.1 ± 10.1
10 μg/kg			
Max. change	+140.4 ± 15.0	+57.6 ± 5.5	−25.1 ± 22.1
Norepinephrine			
0.1 μg/kg			
Max. change	+34.6 ± 5.2	+13.8 ± 3.0	−5.8 ± 5.3
1.0 μg/kg			
Max. change	+122.4 ± 20.0	+22.2 ± 12.1	−13.6 ± 13.4
10 μg/kg			
Max. change	+119.0 ± 32.0	+62.6 ± 5.9	−37.2 ± 14.5

[a] Values are means ± S.E.
From ref. 12.

ulation of CBF also occurs. The phenomenon of autoregulation suggests that CBF may be more closely related to cerebral blood flow than to peripheral blood flow, a not unexpected finding considering that the labyrinthine arteries arise from the vertebrobasilar circulation.

First, the sympathetic nervous system has some influence on CBF. The exact innervation of the cochlear blood vessels is not well understood. However, an adrenergic innervation of cochlear arteries and arterioles has been identified as being separate from that which innervates the vesicles around the afferent nerves (57). Further, Hultcrantz and colleagues (23,24) have reported that sectioning the cervical sympathetic trunk results in increased CBF as measured by their microsphere method. Blood flow in operated ears increased between 133% and 200% of that observed in the unoperated (control) ears. Given this degree of adrenergic control, it should be anticipated that alpha and beta adrenergic agents would restrict CBF. As noted above, however, these agents given intravenously were observed to increase both systemic blood pressure and CBF. It is possible that local release of vasoactive agents may be involved in autoregulation in the cochlea but to a lesser degree, and local regulation is overshadowed by the effects of systemic blood pressure. It would be appropriate to conclude with Snow and Suga (56) that "cochlear vessels appear to be weakly controlled by the adrenergic nervous system. Changes in systemic blood pressure easily overcome this control."

This possibility has been addressed somewhat indirectly by Muchnik. In a series of papers Muchnik and colleagues (38–40) indicated that catecholamines (epinephrine and norepinephrine combined) infused locally (rather than systemically) reduced perilymph PO_2 and cochlear action potentials. When catecholamines were infused systemically, smaller decrements were observed. Given these different degrees of change in cochlear function they inferred that catecholamines cause constriction in the cochlear vasculature, which in turn inhibits cochlear function. They also suggested that systemic catecholamines may increase blood pressure and thus increase CBF, which helps to prevent deterioration of cochlear function.

Unfortunately Muchnik did not measure CBF directly. Similar conclusions, however, may be drawn from another study. Snow and Suga (56) also investigated the effects of AII on CBF. They noted that injection of AII resulted first in a transient decrease in CBF followed by an increase. This increase appeared to parallel an increase in blood pressure. It is possible that the initial effects reflected the constrictive reaction to AII in the blood vessels directly supplying the cochlea and that the later increase resulted from an overriding of this local constriction by increased systemic pressure. Suga and Snow (59) reported the similar biphasic effect of phenylephrine and of methoxamine. These findings suggest that many of the same regulators of systemic blood pressure also are active in the cochlear vasculature. The local effects, however, may not be sufficiently powerful to overcome the systemic effects.

An intriguing implication of these findings is that alpha antagonists would result in both decreased blood pressure and increased CBF, owing to an inhibition of vasoconstriction secondary to loss of sympathetic tone. Precisely such an effect has been reported by Suga and Snow (60), who used the electrical impedance plethysmographic technique. Systematic investigations of such effects have not been carried out, however, and other investigators using laser Doppler measures have simply reported decrements in both CBF and blood pressure following injection of phentolamine hydrochloride (37).

Another implication of this interpretation is that the effects of systemically administered vasoactive agents on CBF would be even greater if local compensatory vasoconstriction did not occur. Such an interaction between systemic and local effects has been suggested by the research on nicotinic acid, which is a vasodilating agent. Snow and Suga (56) reported no effects of nicotinic acid on CBF using electrical impedance plethysmography. Similarly Hultcrantz et al. (24), using microsphere techniques, reported no significant effects of nicotinic acid in intact ears. When nicotinic acid was given following cervical sympathectomy and the distal fibers stimulated, however, nicotinic acid resulted in an increase in CBF. Without nicotinic acid the CBF was 1.78 μl/min; with nicotinic acid the flow rate increased to 2.26 μl/min. Nicotinic acid may interact with sympathetic tone and vasoactive agents but appears not to influence CBF on its own.

A second line of evidence that supports the possibility of local regulation is based on some observations in which blood pressure and CBF have not covaried. Local control may at times override systemic mechanisms in determining CBF. For example, Laugel (33) investigated the interaction of the ovarian steroid progesterone and AII on blood pressure and CBF. He noted that progesterone pretreatment of ovariectomized rats enhanced the blood pressure increases caused by AII. By contrast, the increase in CBF normally seen with AII infusions was reduced by progesterone pretreatment.

The dissociation of CBF from blood pressure is also suggested by the effects of nicotine on CBF. Nicotine is a cholinomimetic agent and specifically a ganglionic-stimulating and blocking agent (61,63). As such, nicotine may be expected to mimic sympathetic effects on the cardiovascular system. Nicotine elevates heart rate, increases blood pressure, and promotes peripheral vasoconstriction (1,2,7,9,16,17,41). Thus, one would anticipate that nicotine would increase CBF. Vatner et al. (62) reported that a 0.2 μg/kg dose of nicotine resulted first in elevated cerebral blood flow and velocity and then in a decrease. They attributed these changes to effects on the carotid chemoreceptors and the sympathetic nervous system. The later decrement in cerebral perfusion, however, was independent of mean arterial pressure, which remained elevated, suggesting the overriding influence of local mechanisms.

In one study (13) nicotine was administered in varying doses to guinea pigs while their CBF and skin blood flow were monitored. Higher doses of nicotine resulted in greater blood pressure increases than the lower doses, which in turn resulted in greater blood pressure increases than did saline. As Fig. 1 indicates, skin blood flow decreased with administration of nicotine and did so more for higher than lower doses. The lower panel of Fig. 1 presents the average CBF as a percentage of baseline as a function of time after infusion. The effects of nicotine on CBF are not as clear as those on skin blood flow. Low doses of nicotine resulted in increased CBF. The highest dose, 0.2 μg/kg (the same dose that Vatner et al. reported as causing a biphasic effect on cerebral blood flow), resulted in a decrease in CBF. Thus, at the higher doses skin blood flow and CBF responded differently to nicotine, raising the possibility of local mechanisms in the control of CBF.

Like nicotine, but even more clearly, carbon monoxide raises the issue of local control of CBF (20). During administration of 5% CO in air, CBF declined to 85% of the average baseline and then rebounded to as much as 159% of baseline with removal of the CO. Although CO resulted in a transient decrease and then a major increase in CBF, blood pressure was decreased and remained suppressed following CO administration.

A third line of evidence for local or autoregulation of CBF comes from the time course of the observed changes. Whereas CBF generally varied with changes in blood pressure, CBF changes typically returned to baseline sooner than did blood pressure. This observation has been frequent in our own research (20) and in the results reported by Suga and Snow (60). Short et al. (54) also reported that exsanguination resulted in steady decreases in both skin blood flow and blood pressure. CBF, however, lagged far behind. For example, when blood was removed at the rate of 1.1 ml/min/kg, blood pressure dropped steadily to 19% of baseline. In contrast, CBF did not decrease until after 18 min of exsanguination and only reached 74% of the baseline when the recording was terminated. This suggests that an effective mechanism for maintaining cochlear perfusion exists, independent of systemic pressure.

A final line of evidence that suggests autoregulation is one that investigates CBF in relation to hypertension. Recently our laboratory employed the spontaneously hypertensive rat (SHR) model of essential hypertension (51,67). In the chronic hypertensive patient (58) and the SHR (53) the upper and lower limits of cerebral autoregulation appear to have shifted to higher levels of blood pressure. The systemic infusion of AII resulted in an impairment of CBF in the SHR, compared with Wistar-Kyoto (WKY) normotensive control rats. This impairment represented a mean flow rate that was 31% of that of the WKY at the high dose of AII (1,000 pmol/50 μl/min for 5 min), 66% at 100 pmol, and 25% at 10 pmol. This difference in CBF could not be explained by strain differences in systemic blood pressure in that the change from baseline blood pressure was significantly greater in the SHR than in

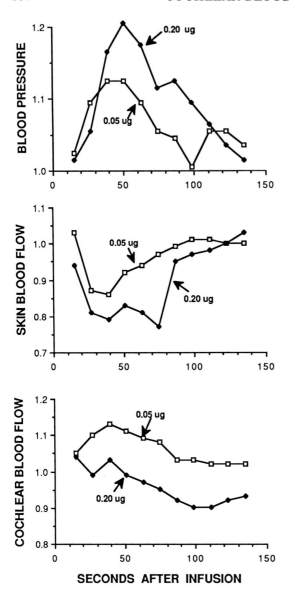

FIG. 1. Blood pressure (*top panel*), skin blood flow (*middle panel*), and cochlear blood flow (*bottom panel*) plotted as proportion of baseline and seconds after infusion. (Adapted from ref. 13.)

the WKY animals at the 100- and 1,000-pmol doses. Pretreatment with the specific angiotensin receptor antagonist Sarile (Sar[1], Ile[8]AII) significantly reduced CBF in both SH and WKY animals when the 1,000- and 100-pmol doses of AII were administered. These results are interpreted as indicating that the SHR demonstrates a form of cochlear autoregulation that decreases the caliber of the cochlear vessels to maintain blood flow at constant rates in the face of increases in perfusion pressure. However, this regulatory response may be deleterious in that it prevents the necessary increase in perfusion of the cochlea when metabolic needs are increased, such as during noise exposure.

Wth long-term antihypertensive treatment in humans (64) and SHRs (10), or acute use of angiotensin receptor antagonists, as currently employed, a shift in cerebral and CBF autoregulation back toward the pattern seen in normotensives may occur.

FLUID VOLUME

The relation between CBF and fluid volume has been less extensively investigated than that between CBF and systemic blood pressure. Understanding this relationship is also hindered by the fact that blood pressure and fluid volume are both interdependent and dependent on related mechanisms.

A positive relationship between CBF and fluid volume was repeatedly found in animals infused with saline. In our studies of vasoactive agents we have routinely used an isotonic saline control. The observed result in these control animals has been a small, transient but consistent increase in CBF. For example, Goodwin et al. (20) reported that a bolus injection of saline had negligible effects on blood pressure but resulted in an average 10% increase in skin blood flow and a similar increase in CBF. Although increase in skin blood flow was maintained for several minutes, the increase in CBF fell to below baseline within 10 minutes after injection.

Osmolytic agents have particular import for CBF. They create an osmotic gradient between the vascular fluid and surrounding tissues causing a diffusion of water into the intravascular space. This results in an increased intravascular fluid volume and creates a temporary hemodilution that decreases viscosity, which in turn enhances blood flow.

Mannitol is an osmotic diuretic (19) that has previously been reported to increase CBF (31,32). When Goodwin et al. (20) injected guinea pigs with 1.5 ml of 20% mannitol, blood pressure increased to 140% of baseline within 3.75 min post-injection and recovered within 20 min. CBF increased to as much as 160% of baseline in less than 1 min following injection and returned to baseline within 10 min post-injection. Skin blood flow increased to as much as 170% of baseline within 1 min of injection and remained elevated for 30 to 40 min. These results confirm the hypothesis that osmolytic agents increase CBF, albeit transiently. Further, the increase seems to not be dependent on increased peripheral resistance: the onset of the increase in CBF occurred prior to the elevation in blood pressure and was paralleled by an increase rather than a decrease in skin blood flow.

Prazma (49), using a different experimental protocol, also concluded that fluid volume may be an important mediator of CBF. He used endolymph PO_2 as an indirect measure of CBF and administered 40% glycerol (1.5 g/kg) to guinea pigs. Glycerol is an osmoactive substance that crosses the vascular membranes slowly. Prazma reported that blood pressure decreased during the 5-min infusion of glycerol, temporarily rebounded after the infusion, and then returned to baseline in approximately 30 min. By contrast, measures of endolymph PO_2 increased during infusion and remained elevated even after blood pressure had returned to baseline. Although PO_2 is an indirect measure of CBF, these findings also suggest that CBF is responsive to changes in fluid volume.

Because of its apparent hemodilution effects, low molecular weight dextran (dextran 40) has been used clinically in the treatment of acoustic trauma (29). The effect of dextran 40 on CBF is most clearly demonstrated in a study by Hultcrantz and

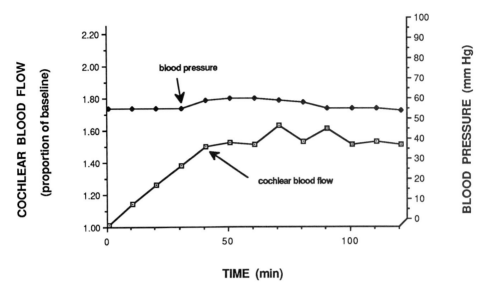

FIG. 2. The change in cochlear blood flow and systemic blood pressure during 1-hr infusion of dextran 40 and for 1 hr following infusion. (From ref. 26.)

Nuttall (26). Using guinea pigs and the laser Doppler to measure CBF, they infused 10% dextran 40 (10 mg/kg) in saline for a 1-hr period. The results are presented in Fig. 2. CBF generally increased during the first 30 min of infusion and reached a plateau averaging 160% of baseline. Isolated observations indicated that this plateau was maintained for at least 1 hr following termination of the infusion. Blood pressure did not change appreciably during dextran 40 infusion. Skin blood flow reflected the same pattern as CBF. Hematocrit decreased from an average of 43% to an average of 32% during the dextran 40 infusion.

Hultcrantz and Nuttall (26) also investigated the effects of normovolemic hemodilution by withdrawing blood and replacing it with isosmotic solutions of 5% dextran 40 or 6% dextran 75. These successive replacements of blood with dextran steadily reduced hematocrit. Blood pressure did not change but cochlear blood flow increased to 180% to 200% of baseline when the hematocrit reached 15%.

At present in our laboratory, Quirk is employing 10-min intra-arterial infusions of 20% mannitol in SHRs and WKY rats, in an effort to elucidate further the mechanisms underlying autoregulation by the cochlear vessels. Thus far Quirk has determined that mannitol infusion results in an initial elevation in CBF in both SHRs and WKY rats during the first few minutes, followed by significant reduction in CBF in the SHR that persists for the remainder of the infusion (Table 3). This reduction does not occur in the WKY rat and it is not reflective of a concomitant reduction in blood pressure; the SHRs show greater mannitol-induced elevations in systemic blood pressure than do the WKY animals. In addition, plasma and blood volume, determined by the Evans blue dye dilution technique, revealed greater fluid expansion in the vasculature of the SHR than in the WKY rat at the conclusion of the mannitol infusion.

TABLE 3. *Mannitol-induced changes in plasma and blood volume, cochlear blood flow, and systemic mean arterial pressure in SHR and WKY rats*

Strain		3 min into infusion (% of change)		10 min into infusion (% of change)		Plasma volume[a] (ml/100 g)	Blood volume[a] (ml/100 g)
		CBF	BP	CBF	BP		
SHR	M	20.4	13.9	11.5	25.6	4.5	11.6
(n = 6)	SEM	4.3	3.2	7.9	4.3	0.7	1.1
WKY	M	21.0	8.8	29.0	10.0	3.5	9.0
(n = 6)	SEM	5.0	2.8	9.5	2.8	0.4	1.1

[a] Plasma and blood volume determinations were made at the conclusion of the 10-min infusion of mannitol (0.2 ml/min) using the Evans blue dye technique.

DISCUSSION

The research that has been described in this chapter permits some tentative conclusions concerning pharmacological alteration of CBF. It is variable and can be manipulated. The available research, however, permits as yet little in the way of firm conclusions regarding clinically applicable techniques for altering CBF.

Although CBF generally appears to rise and fall with systemic blood pressure, this observation does not offer an effective method for treatments that involve increasing CBF. The risks associated with elevated blood pressure are obvious. Further, it appears that local or autoregulation of the cochlear vessels tends to counteract the increased CBF resulting from administration of vasoactive agents. Consequently, the elevations in CBF that have been induced with increased blood pressure are relatively short lived, even shorter in duration than the increases in blood pressure.

The apparent autoregulation of the cochlear vasculature raises the possibility that vasodilating agents may be effective in facilitating CBF since cochlear and other vascular beds appear to be affected by the same vasoactive agents. Further, the neural influences producing cochlear vasoconstriction appear to be somewhat weaker than those producing systemic vasoconstriction. It would therefore appear appropriate to suggest that a weak vasoconstriction antagonist could be used for increasing CBF without compromising systemic profusion. Several vasodilating agents have been tested by previous authors. Although these agents appear to be promising, systematic investigations have not yet been conducted. Consequently, recommendations concerning the clinical use of such agents may be premature.

Autoregulation in the cochlear vasculature is similar to autoregulation of the cerebral blood flow. Some authors (19) have indicated that carbon dioxide may be the most effective agent for increasing cerebral blood flow. A similar possibility exists for CBF (27). However, investigations of CO_2 effects on CBF are sparse and conflicting. Further, systematic and parametric investigations of CO_2 effects on dynamic measures of CBF have not been conducted to date.

Perhaps the most readily available avenue for altering CBF is by changing total intravascular fluid volume. This approach has been clinically used with some justification. Certain osmotic agents appear to increase CBF without increasing systemic blood pressure. Dextran specifically appears to produce an increased CBF that is relatively long lasting—as long as several hours—without increasing systemic blood pressure. Hypervolemic hemodilution, however, may cause other problems such as cardiac overload. Agents such as dextran are eventually excreted along with the excess intravascular water, resulting in dehydration of the tissues and possible renal failure (26,35,68). For this reason Hultcrantz and Nuttall (26) suggest that normovolemic hemodilution may be a more desirable alternative. Normovolemic hemodilution requires partial exsanguination and replacement with isosmotic solutions of osmolytic agents. This normovolemic hemodilution strategy requires further evaluation but may be a promising one, particularly for patients who would be at risk for renal failure with dextran-induced dehydration.

One further caution should be noted concerning the clinical applicability of some osmotic agents for increasing CBF. As summarized in Table 3, plasma and volume increased more for SHR than for WKY rats in response to mannitol infusion. Blood pressure elevations were small for normotensive animals even after 10 min of mannitol infusion, but substantial for hypertensive ones. Within 10 min of initiating the infusion, CBF had reverted to near baseline for the SHRs but continued to rise for the normotensive ones. It appears that autoregulation may play an integral role in CBF even when osmotic agents rather than vasoactive agents are applied. These findings lead to the inference that osmotic agents may be significantly less effective in the hypertensive patient.

REFERENCES

1. Ague, C. (1973): Smoking patterns, nicotine intake at different times of day and changes in two cardiovascular variables while smoking cigarettes. *Psychopharmacologia*, 30:135–144.
2. Ague, C. (1974): Cardiovascular variables, skin conductance and time estimation: Changes after the administration of small doses of nicotine. *Psychopharmacologia*, 37:109–125.
3. Angelborg, C., Hultcrantz, E., and Agerupk, B. (1977): The cochlear blood flow. *Acta Otolaryngol. (Stockh.)*, 83:92–97.
4. Axelsson, A., and Dengerink, H. A. (1986): The effects of noise on histological measures of cochlear blood flow: A review. Paper presented at the meeting of the Association for Research in Otolaryngology, Clearwater Beach, FL.
5. Axelsson, A., and Vertes, D. (1982): Histological findings in cochlear vessels after noise. In: *New Perspectives on Noise-Induced Hearing Loss*, edited by R. Hamernik, D. Henderson, and R. Salvi, pp. 49–68, Raven Press, New York.
6. Axelsson, A., Vertes, D., and Miller, J. (1981): Immediate noise effects on cochlear vasculature in the guinea pig. *Acta Otolaryngol. (Stockh.)*, 91:237–246.
7. Bobbin, R. P., and Gondra, M. I. (1976): Effect of nicotine on cochlear function and noise-induced hair cell loss. *Ann. Otol.*, 85:247–254.
8. Canlon, B., and Schacht, J. (1981): The effect of noise on deoxyglucose uptake into the inner ear of the mouse. *Arch. Otorhinolaryngol.*, 230:171.
9. Cellina, G. U., Honour, A. J., and Littler, W. A. (1975): Direct arterial pressure, heart rate, and electrocardiogram during cigarette smoking in unrestricted patients. *Am. Heart J.*, 89:18–25.
10. Coyl, P., and Heistad, D. D. (1986): Blood flow through cerebral collateral vessels in hypertensive and normotensive rats. *Hypertension*, 8(suppl. II):67–71.
11. Dengerink, H., Axelsson, A., Miller, J., and Wright, J. (1984): The effect of noise and carbogen on cochlear vasculature. *Acta Otolaryngol. (Stockh.)*, 98:81–88.
12. Dengerink, H. A., Wright, J. W., Dengerink, J. E., and Miller, J. M. (1986): A pathway for the interaction of stress and noise influences on hearing. In: *Basic and Applied Aspects of Noise-Induced Hearing Loss*, edited by R. J. Salvi, D. Henderson, R. P. Hamernik, and V. Colletti, pp. 559–569. Plenum Press, New York.
13. Dengerink, H., Wright, J., Goodwin, P., and Miller, J. (1984): The effect of nicotine on cochlear blood flow. *Hear. Res.*, 20:31–36.

14. Dengerink, H. A., Wright, J. W., Thompson, P., and Dengerink, J. E. (1982): Changes in plasma angiotensin II with noise exposure and their relationship to TTS. *J. Acoust. Soc. Am.*, 72:276–278.
15. De Vincentiis, I., Bozzi, L., and Pizzichetta, V. (1964): Sulla terapia medica di alcune gravi ipoacurise. *Valsalua*, 40:16.
16. Elliott, R., and Thysell, R. (1968): A note on smoking and heart rate. *Psychophysiology*, 5:280–283.
17. Erwin, C. W. (1971): Cardiac rate responses to cigarette smoking: A study utilizing radiotelemetry. *Psychophysiology*, 8:75–81.
18. Ganong, W. F. (1983): The brain renin-angiotensin system. In: *Brain Peptides*, edited by D. T. Krieger, M. J. Brownstein, and J. B. Martin, pp. 805–826. John Wiley, New York.
19. Goodman, C. S., and Gilman, A. G. editors (1975): *The Pharmacological Basis of Therapeutics.* Macmillan, New York.
20. Goodwin, P., Miller, J., Dengerink, H., Wright, J., and Axelsson, A. (1984): The laser Doppler: A non-invasive measure of cochlear blood flow. *Acta Otolaryngol. (Stockh.)*, 98:403–412.
21. Hawkins, J. E. (1971): The role of vasoconstriction in noise-induced hearing loss. *Ann. Otolaryngol.*, 80:903.
22. Holloway, G. A., and Watkins, D. W. (1977): Laser Doppler measurement of cutaneous blood flow. *J. Invest. Dermatol.*, 69:306.
23. Hultcrantz, E. (1979): The effect of noise on the cochlear blood flow in the conscious rabbit. *Acta Physiol. Scand.*, 106:29–37.
24. Hultcrantz, E., Hillerdal, M., and Angelborg, C. (1982): Effect of nicotinic acid on cochlear blood flow. *Arch. Otorhinolaryngol.*, 234:151–155.
25. Hultcrantz, E., Linder, J., and Angelborg, C. (1977): Sympathetic effects on cochlear blood flow at different blood pressure levels. *INSERM*, 68:271–278.
26. Hultcrantz, E., and Nuttall, A. L. (1987): Effect of hemodilution on cochlear blood flow measured by laser-Doppler flowmetry. *Am. J. Otolaryngol.*, 8:10–16.
27. Joglekar, S. S., Lipscomb, D. M., and Shambaugh, G. E. (1977): Effects of oxygen inhalation of noise-induced threshold shifts in humans and chinchillas. *Arch. Otolaryngol.*, 103:574–578.
28. Johnson, A. K. (1982): Neurobiology of the periventricular tissue surrounding the anteroventral third ventricle (AV3V) and its role in behavior. In: *Circulation, Neurobiology, and Behavior*, edited by O. A. Smith, R. A. Galosy, and S. M. Weiss, pp. 277–295. Elsevier, New York.
29. Kellerhals, B. (1972): Acoustic trauma and cochlear microcirculation: An experimental and clinical study on pathogenesis and treatment of inner ear lesions after acute noise exposure. *Adv. Oto-Rhino-Laryngol.*, 18:91–168.
30. Kraus, E. M., Badin, R. W., and Riju, J. H. (1982): Pulsed Doppler measurements of cochlear blood flow in response to dopamine in the anesthetized cat: A basis for dopamine treatment of sudden deafness. Paper presented at the research forum of the AAO Head and Neck Surgery, New Orleans.
31. Larsen, H. C., Angelborg, C., and Hultcrantz, E. (1982): The effect of urea and manitol on cochlear blood flow. *Acta Otolaryngol. (Stockh.)*, 94:249.
32. Larsen, H. C., Angelborg, C., and Hultcrantz, E. (1982): Cochlear blood flow related to hyperosmotic solutions. *Arch. Oto-Rhino-Laryngol.*, 234:145.
33. Laugel, G. (1987): Interaction of ovarian steroids and vasoconstrictors on blood pressure and cochlear blood flow. Doctoral dissertation, Washington State University, Pullman, WA.
34. Lawrence, M. (1973): In vivo studies of the microcirculation. *Adv. Oto-Rhino-Laryngol.*, 20:244–255.
35. Matheson, N. (1970): Renal failure after administration of Dextran 40. *Surg., Gynecol. Obstet.*, 131:661–665.
36. Miller, J., Goodwin, P., and Marks, N. (1984): Inner ear blood flow using a laser Doppler system. *Arch. Otolaryngol.*, 110:305–308.
37. Miller, J., Marks, N., and Goodwin, P. C. (1983): Laser Doppler measurement of cochlear blood flow. *Hear. Res.*, 11:385.
38. Muchnik, C., Hildesheimer, M., Nebel, L., and Rubinstein, M. (1983): Influence of catecholamines on cochlear action potentials. *Arch. Otolaryngol.*, 109:530–532.
39. Muchnik, C., Hildesheimer, M., and Rubinstein, M. (1980): Effect of emotional stress on hearing. *Arch. Otorhinolaryngol.*, 228:295–298.
40. Muchnik, C., Hildesheimer, M., and Rubinstein, M. (1984): Effect of catecholamines on perilymph PO2. *Arch. Otolaryngol.*, 110:518–520.
41. Nesbitt, P. D. (1973): Smoking, physiological arousal and emotional response. *Psychophysiology*, 25:137–144.
42. Nilsson, G. E., Tenland, T., and Oberg, P. A. (1980): Evaluation of a laser Doppler flowmeter for measurement of tissue blood flow. *IEEE Trans. Biomed. Eng.*, 27:12.
43. Nuttall, A. L. (1986): Intravital microscopy for measurement of blood cell velocities in the cochlea. Paper presented at the meeting of Association for Research in Otolaryngology, Clearwater Beach, FL.

44. Nuttall, A. L., Hultcrantz, E., and Lawrence, M. (1981): Does loud sound influence the intracochlear oxygen tension? *Hear. Res.*, 5:285.
45. Nyboer, J. (1970): *Electrical Impedance Plethysmography*, 2nd Ed. Charles C. Thomas, Springfield, IL.
46. Oberg, P. A., Nilsson, G. E., Tenland, T., Homstrom, A., and Lewis, D. H. (1979): Use of a new laser Doppler flowmeter for measurement of capillary blood flow in skeletal muscle after bullet wounding. *Acta Chir. Scand. [Suppl.]*, 489:145.
47. Perlman, H. B., and Kimura, R. A. (1955): Observations of the living blood vessels of the cochlea. *Ann. Otolaryngol.*, 64:1176.
48. Powers, E. W., and Frayer, W. W. (1978): Laser Doppler measurement of blood flow in microcirculation. *Plast. Reconstr. Surg.*, 61:250.
49. Prazma, J. (1981): Effect of glycerol on cochlea microcirculation. *Acta Otolaryngol.*, 92:459–461.
50. Prazma, J., Biggers, W. P., and Fischer, N. D. (1981): Effect of ethaverine hydrochloride on cochlear microcirculation. *Arch. Otolaryngol.*, 107:227–229.
51. Quirk, W. S., Wright, J. W., and Dengerink, H. (1988): Angiotensin II-induced changes in cochlear blood flow in normotensive and hypertensive rats. *Hear. Res. (in press)*.
52. Ryan, A. F., Goodwin, P., Woolf, N. K., and Sharp, F. (1982): Auditory stimulation alters the pattern of 2-deoxyglucose uptake in the inner ear. *Brain Res.* 234:213–225.
53. Sadoshima, S., Fujishima, M., Yoshida, F., Ibayashi, S., Shiokowa, O., and Omae, T. (1985): Cerebral autoregulation in young spontaneously hypertensive rats: Effect of sympathetic denervation. *Hypertension*, 7:392–397.
54. Short, S., Goodwin, P. C., and Miller, J. M. (1984): Measuring cochlear blood flow using laser Doppler spectroscopy. Paper presented at the meetings of the Association for Research in Otolaryngology, St. Petersburg, FL.
55. Snow, J. B., and Suga, F. (1972): Control of cochlear blood flow. In: *Vascular Disorders and Hearing Defects*, edited by A. J. deLorenzo, pp. 167–183. University Park Press, Baltimore.
56. Snow, J. B., and Suga, F. (1971): Labyrinthine vasodilators. *Arch. Otolaryngol.*, 97:365–370.
57. Spoendlin, H. H., and Lichtensteiger, W. (1966): The adrenergic innervation of the labyrinth. *Acta Otolaryngol. (Stockh.)*, 61:423–434.
58. Strandgaard, S. (1975): Autoregulation of cerebral blood flow in hypertensive patients: The modifying influence of prolonged antihypertensive treatment on tolerance to acute, drug-induced hypertension. *Circulation*, 53:720–727.
59. Suga, F., and Snow, J. B. (1969): Cochlear blood flow in response to vasodilating drugs and some related agents. *Laryngoscope*, 79:1956–1979.
60. Suga, F., and Snow, J. B. (1969): Cholinergic control of cochlear blood flow. *Amer. J. Otol.*, 78:1081–1090.
61. Taylor, P. (1980): Ganglionic stimulating and blocking agents. In: *The Pharmacological Basis of Therapeutics*, edited by C. S. Goodman and A. G. Gilman, pp. 211–219. Macmillan, New York.
62. Vatner, S. F., Priano, L. L., Rutherford, J. D., and Manders, T. (1980): Sympathetic regulation of the cerebral circulation by the carotid chemoreceptor reflex. *Am. J. Physiol.*, 80:H594–H598.
63. Volle, R. L., and Koelle, G. B. (1970): Ganglionic stimulating and blocking agents. In: *The Pharmacological Basis of Therapeutics*, edited by C. S. Goodman and A. G. Gillman, pp. 585–595. Macmillan, New York.
64. Warshaw, D. M., Root, D. T., and Helpern, W. (1980): Effects of antihypertensive drug therapy on the morphology and mechanics of resistance in arteries from spontaneously hypertensive rats. *Blood Vessels*, 17:257–270.
65. Wright, J., Dengerink, H., Miller, J., and Goodwin, P. (1985): Noise induced increases in inner ear blood flow: The potential role of angiotensin II. *Hear. Res.*, 17:41–46.
66. Wright, J. W., Dengerink, H. A., Thompson, P., and Morseth, S. (1981): Plasma angiotensin II changes with noise exposure at three levels of ambient air temperature. *J. Acoust. Soc. Am.*, 70:1353–1355.
67. Wright, J. W., Quirk, W. S., and Dengerink, H. A. (1987): Angiotension II-induced changes in cochlear blood flow in normotensive and spontaneously hypertensive rats. Paper presented at the meeting of the Association for Research in Otolaryngology, Clearwater Beach, FL.
68. Zaytoun, G. M., Schuknecht, H. F., and Farmer, H. S. (1983): Fatality following the use of low molecular weight dextran in the treatment of sudden deafness. *Adv. Otorhinolaryngol.*, 31:240–246.

Physiology of the Ear,
edited by A. F. Jahn and J. Santos-Sacchi.
Raven Press, New York © 1988.

Cochlear Fluid Dynamics

Alec N. Salt and Ruediger Thalmann

*Department of Otolaryngology, Washington University School of Medicine,
St. Louis, Missouri 63110*

ANATOMY OF COCHLEAR FLUID COMPARTMENTS

Traditionally, the inner ear is described in terms of the bony labyrinth, an intricate series of fluid-filled tubes running through the temporal bone, within which is suspended the membranous labyrinth. The anatomy of the bony and membranous labyrinths is illustrated in Fig. 1. The membranous labyrinth contains a fluid of unique ionic composition, the endolymph, which is separated by cellular structures from the perilymph, a fluid of typical extracellular ionic composition. In the cochlea, these structures divide the system into three chambers: scala tympani (ST), scala media (SM), and scala vestibuli (SV). In humans the three chambers form a spiral of approximately 2¾ turns. ST and SV form the outer chambers, which contain perilymph. Both of these scalae have fenestrae to the middle ear cavity that are closed by the round window membrane and the footplate of the stapes, respectively. ST and SV are connected at the cochlear apex by an opening called the helicotrema. In addition, both compartments are connected to other fluid-filled spaces as shown in the figure. ST perilymph of the basal turn is connected to the cerebrospinal fluid (CSF) of the subarachnoid space by the cochlear aqueduct. SV perilymph of the basal turn has a wide communication with perilymph of the vestibule. SM, containing endolymph, is completely bounded by tissues so that there is no direct fluid connection between endolymph and perilymph. The cells surrounding the endolymphatic compartment constitute an endolymph/perilymph barrier, characterized by specialized tight intercellular junctions (zonulae occludentes) to limit paracellular solute movement (18). In the basal turn, cochlear endolymph is connected to saccular endolymph by the ductus reuniens. Thus all three cochlear scalae have ducts allowing communication with other fluid-filled spaces.

In cross section, SM forms a triangular compartment between the perilymphatic scalae as illustrated in Fig. 2. The three major structures bounding endolymph are Reissner's membrane, stria vascularis, and the organ of Corti. Reissner's membrane is an avascular structure composed of two cell layers that forms the boundary between SM and SV. Stria vascularis is a highly vascular, multilayer epithelium that forms the lateral wall of the scala. The third boundary is the organ of Corti, a complex structure that includes the sensory hair cells of the cochlea. The hair cells are located with their apical surfaces in contact with endolymph, whereas the basolateral membranes are in contact with fluid of perilymph-like composition. This arrangement appears to be a major factor in the remarkable sensitivity of the cochlea as a mechano-

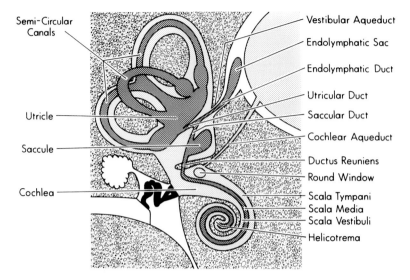

FIG. 1. Anatomy of the inner ear showing the main compartments and interconnecting ducts. Perilymph-filled chambers are lightly shaded and the endolymph-filled membranous labyrinth is heavily shaded.

electric transducer. The cochlear fluids thus play a vital role in cochlear transduction mechanisms.

TECHNICAL ASPECTS OF THE STUDY OF COCHLEAR FLUIDS

The accurate determination of cochlear fluids composition, or study of cochlear fluid dynamics, presents a number of major technical difficulties that are not present

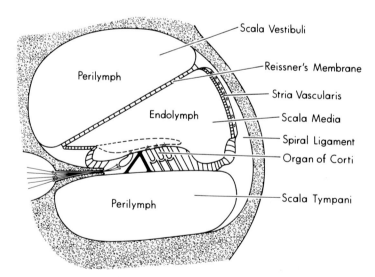

FIG. 2. The cross section of one turn of the cochlea showing the main tissues separating endolymph and perilymph. The acellular tectorial membrane, which overlies the organ of Corti, is represented by a dashed outline.

for most other body fluids (e.g., CSF, plasma, aqueous humor). First, the total volume of cochlear fluids is relatively small. In the guinea pig the volumes of cochlear perilymph and endolymph are approximately 16 μl and 2 μl, respectively. As a result, specialized procedures of sample withdrawal, handling, and analysis are required. Analysis requires a technique that either uses extremely small sample volumes (e.g., helium glow photometry, 2-D polyacrylamide gel electrophoresis, microfluorometry) or is extremely sensitive, allowing the sample to be diluted (e.g., flame photometry, HPLC). An alternative that is available for some ionic substances is the use of ion-selective microelectrodes. These may be inserted directly into the fluids, allowing the composition to be measured without the need to withdraw a sample. A second problem affecting many studies of cochlear fluid physiology in the past concerns the practical difficulty of gaining access to the cochlear fluids without excessive disruption of the normal state. The problem arises from the assumption that a fluid sample withdrawn from one scala represents a pure sample of the intended cochlear fluid, an invalid assumption in some cases (16,68). Under physiological conditions cochlear fluids are maintained at a positive hydrostatic pressure of 2 to 3 mm Hg in guinea pigs (43,81) or 3 to 10 mm Hg in cats (6,55). Perforation of the otic capsule, in order to insert an electrode or withdraw a sample, causes a leakage of fluid as a result of the release of cochlear pressure. The rate of such leakage has been estimated to be as much as 2 μl/min when a perilymphatic scala is perforated (24,53,63). The perilymph is replaced predominantly by CSF entering the basal turn of ST through the cochlear aqueduct. Perilymph composition would thus be expected to change rapidly with time as perilymph becomes replaced by CSF. One alternative technique used extensively is the insertion of electrodes or withdrawal of samples through the round window membrane. A potential problem with this technique arises from the cochlear aqueduct, which enters ST close to the round window. As a perilymph sample is withdrawn, CSF may be pulled into the cochlea with some degree of contamination depending on the volume withdrawn. Using sample glycine levels as an indication of CSF contamination it has been estimated that in guinea pigs samples larger than 200 nl withdrawn through the round window will show significant CSF contamination (16). The hazard of this contamination is that, as will be shown, both perilymph and CSF have a similar ionic composition so that contamination of perilymph samples with CSF is difficult to detect and may often not be realized.

Although endolymph has a smaller total volume, in some respects uncontaminated samples of endolymph can be obtained more easily than perilymph. Unlike the situation for perilymph, the membranous walls of SM are presumed to collapse as the sample is withdrawn so that contamination occurs less readily. A rupture would be detected by loss of endocochlear potential, which can be monitored during sample collection. Contamination of endolymph samples by perilymph is readily detected as endolymph and perilymph have very different ionic composition. Specifically, the low sodium content of cochlear endolymph is a good indicator of sample purity. In some instances it has been argued that the repeatability of findings validates the techniques used and the results obtained. This is not necessarily true if a systematic contamination occurs, such as the case of CSF contamination of samples taken from the round window.

As a consequence of these technical problems, published estimates of fluid composition or turnover/clearance rate depend not only on the measurement system but also on exact procedures used to gain access to fluids. Although some authors have paid considerable attention to this problem and designed sampling procedures to minimize contamination, it is important that these technical limitations be realized by those not actively involved in the study of cochlear fluid physiology. Almost certainly, much of the variation in results among different groups working on cochlear fluids arises from the use of different procedures in the collection of samples as well as differences in analysis procedure, animal species, site of sampling, and so forth.

COCHLEAR FLUIDS COMPOSITION

The ionic composition of perilymph is similar to other extracellular fluids in which Na^+ is the predominant cation. Table 1 summarizes the typical ionic content found for perilymph in ST, SV, and for CSF as found in the guinea pig or rat. Generally similar values would be expected in the human cochlea. The K^+ content of SV perilymph is typically found to be approximately twice that for ST perilymph, and the Na^+ content is somewhat lower in SV. It is therefore incorrect to assume that perilymph composition is homogeneous throughout the cochlea, as different locations show small but systematic differences. The observation that ST perilymph has a composition similar to CSF, whereas SV perilymph differs slightly, raises the question of whether samples of ST perilymph have been contaminated with CSF during the sampling procedures used in many studies. Scheibe and Haupt (69) described a sampling procedure in which CSF pressure was released and the helicotrema perforated before perilymph samples were taken. They found average K concentrations of 6.6 mM and 7.9 mM for ST and SV, respectively, which are higher than previously published values especially for ST. It remains to be determined whether the higher ST value represents less CSF contamination during sampling with this technique or whether the change in composition of the basal turn of ST occurs before sampling as a result of CSF pressure release disturbing the normal state.

The osmolarity of perilymph is similar to that of blood plasma. In guinea pigs, ST perilymph was 292.9 mOsm/kg H_2O and SV perilymph was 293.5 mOsm/kg H_2O, which was not significantly different from plasma that averaged 293.5 mOsm/kg H_2O

TABLE 1. *Cochlear fluids composition*

	ST perilymph	Endolymph	SV Perilymph	CSF
Na^+ (mM)	147	1	141	145
K^+ (mM)	3.4	158	6.7	2.7
Ca^{2+} (mM)	0.68	0.023	0.64	
Mg^{2+} (mM)		0.011		
pH	7.28	7.37	7.26	7.28
Cl^- (mM)	129	136	130	131
HCO_3^- (mM)	19	21	18	19
Osmolarity (mOsm/kg H_2O)	293	304	294	
Electrical potential (mV)	0	90	5	0

ST, scala tympani; SV, scala vestibuli; CSF, cerebrospinal fluid.

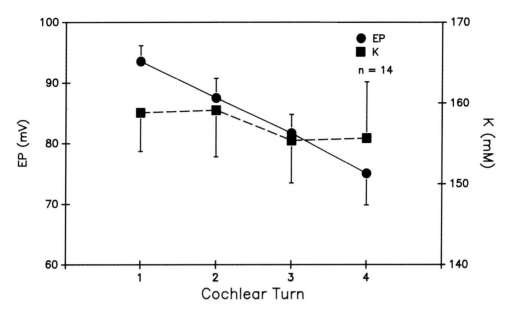

FIG. 3. Longitudinal gradients in scala media of the guinea pig cochlea. The endocochlear potential (EP) declines steadily between turns 1 and 4. Endolymph potassium concentration (K) is also lower in apical turns but shows the greatest change between turns 2 and 3.

(35). In the rat, perilymph osmolarity (average: 289 mOsm/kg H_2O) was found to be a little lower than plasma (298 mOsm/kg H_2O) (75). These results demonstrate that perilymph is close to osmotic equilibrium with blood.

In contrast to perilymph, which is similar to other extracellular fluids, endolymph is a unique extracellular fluid, unlike any other in the body. As shown in Table 1, the predominant cation in endolymph is K, whereas the Na content is exceptionally low. In addition, the endolymph compartment is electrically polarized by +70 to +90 mV, the endocochlear potential (EP). Although numerous early studies of cochlear endolymph suggested that higher Na levels could be found, it is now generally accepted that high Na levels usually reflect contamination problems during sampling procedures. The observation of a higher total solute concentration in endolymph compared with perilymph is in agreement with studies in which endolymph osmolarity was found to be significantly higher than perilymph (35,75), the possible significance of which will be discussed further. In the guinea pig endolymph osmolarity was 304.2 mOsm/kg H_2O, whereas in the rat, basal turn endolymph was 329 mOsm/kg H_2O.

Although it has been documented that cochlear endolymph differs from that found in the vestibular system, where somewhat higher Na and lower K levels are found, it has generally been assumed that cochlear endolymph is homogeneous. A number of studies now show that endolymph composition is not uniform (64,74,75). Sterkers et al. (74,75) found K, Cl, EP, and osmolarity to decrease between turns 1 and 2 in the rat cochlea. As shown in Fig. 3 a similar situation exists in the guinea pig cochlea. In this study EP and endolymph K were measured sequentially in all four turns of the cochlea using ion-selective electrodes. Whereas EP appears to decline steadily with distance, K shows the greatest decline between turns 2 and 3. Although

TABLE 2. *Forces acting on major ions in cochlear fluids*

	Equilibrium potential (mV)	Electrochemical gradient (mV)	Direction of passive flux
Na^+	+134.1	−49.1	IN
K^+	−103.2	+188.2	OUT
Ca^{2+}	+45.5	+39.5	OUT
H^+	−5.6	+79.4	OUT
Cl^-	+1.4	+83.6	IN
HCO_3^-	+2.7	+82.3	IN

Equilibrium potentials are calculated from the concentration data in Table 1 using the Nernst equation. The electrochemical gradient is determined by the difference between the equilibrium potential and the endocochlear potential (+85 mV). The direction of passive ion movement is shown with respect to endolymph.

it is probable that the longitudinal gradients for endolymph are related to the known anatomical and physiological differences along the length of the cochlea, their precise significance is still being considered.

The composition of cochlear fluids plays an important role in passive ionic movements between different compartments of the cochlea. Passive ion movements depend on the permeability of the boundary membrane to a particular ion and on the electrochemical gradient driving ion movement. The driving gradients include contributions from concentration gradients and electric fields. The contribution of the concentration gradient can be calculated using the Nernst equation as shown in Eq. 1 to calculate the equilibrium potential (V_C) for each ion (the voltage that would balance the concentration gradient). The electrochemical gradient is calculated by the difference between the equilibrium potential and the actual potential (V_E) as in Eq. 2. Calculated equilibrium potentials and electrochemical potential differences (V_{EC}) are shown for the major ions in Table 2.

$$V_C = \frac{-RT}{zF} \log_e \frac{(C_e)}{(C_p)} \qquad [1]$$

$$V_{EC} = V_E - V_C \qquad [2]$$

where R is gas constant (8.314 J/mol/°K), T is temperature (kelvin), F is Faraday's constant (96,500 J/V/equivalent), z is algebraic ion valency, and C_e, C_p is ionic concentrations in endolymph and perilymph. Thus V_{EC} represents the electrochemical potential difference that can drive ionic movements between endolymph and perilymph. For sodium, the equilibrium potential is more positive than the endocochlear potential, the difference of which gives an overall gradient of −49 mV tending to drive sodium into endolymph. Sodium must therefore be actively transported out of SM. In contrast, the equilibrium potential for K is far from the endocochlear potential, the difference of which results in a large gradient of 188 mV driving K out of endolymph. The large gradient (over twice that of other ions) is generally believed to drive a standing current of K ions through the hair cells, providing a transducer current according to some variant of the model originally proposed by Davis (10,11). In this model, the hair cells act as passive resistors that modulate an ionic current as a function of mechanical stimulation. On the basis of the electrochemical gradients it is assumed that Ca^{2+} and H^+ would both tend to leak passively out of endolymph whereas both Cl^- and HCO_3^- would tend to leak into endolymph.

ENDOLYMPH DYNAMICS

The maintenance of EP and high endolymphatic K requires active ion transport mechanisms, believed to be localized primarily in stria vascularis. Stria has been demonstrated both to be the source of the EP (78) and to have an extremely high metabolic rate (46,79). If the cochlea becomes anoxic or is treated with Na/K transport inhibitors (e.g., ouabain), then EP falls from its normal value of approximately $+85$ mV, becoming negative within minutes. In the case of anoxia there is a good correlation between the decline of EP and strial ATP content (79). Simultaneous with the decline of EP, endolymph K begins to fall (32) and Na begins to rise (34) as endolymph begins to equilibrate passively with the perilymphatic compartments. The observation of a negative EP when active ion transport is suppressed indicates that the structures bounding SM must have a higher permeability to K^+ than to Na^+. The permeability ratios of K:Na:Cl have been estimated to be 1:0.18:0.23, (32,34,52) from which it is possible to predict the magnitude of the $-EP$ very closely.

The origins of the normal EP have also been investigated. Sellick and Bock (72) perfused endolymph with low K solution and observed the rate of EP recovery and K increase to be closely correlated. On the basis of this result, it is generally accepted that the EP originates from an active secretion of K into endolymph. The cellular mechanisms by which stria vascularis accomplishes this transport have still not been conclusively established. Although the current consensus is that this is achieved by an electrogenic transport of K into endolymph (19,47), recent studies (58,67) have provided evidence that the EP could be generated by conventional Na/K ATPases. Even though the cellular mechanisms are not conclusively known, evidence exists that the K secreted into endolymph probably originates from perilymph rather than blood plasma. Konishi and Kelsey (29) demonstrated that EP declined rapidly when the perilymphatic space was perfused with K-free medium whereas Wada et al. (80) found that EP was maintained when the cochlear vasculature was perfused via the cannulated basilar artery with a K-free artificial blood.

A number of groups have studied endolymph kinetics using radiotracer techniques. Konishi et al. (30) and Konishi and Hamrick (31) perfused the perilymphatic space with solutions containing ^{22}Na, ^{43}K, or ^{36}Cl and measured the rate of uptake of tracers into endolymph. They calculated that these ions turned over with half-times of 33 min, 55 min, and 69 min, respectively. Sterkers et al. (73) measured the rate of uptake of ^{43}K and ^{36}Cl into endolymph following systemic injection of tracer. They reported the uptake into endolymph to be limited by the slower uptake into perilymph. This observation is consistent with the view that endolymph is derived indirectly from perilymph rather than directly from blood.

One of the most controversial aspects of endolymph dynamics is the question of whether endolymph is secreted in one region and resorbed in another, resulting in a volume flow. The existence of endolymph flow was proposed by Guild (15) after iron salts were identified in the endolymphatic sac following their injection into the cochlea. He suggested endolymph was secreted in the cochlea and flowed through the ductus reuniens and the saccule to be resorbed by the endolymphatic sac. Similar results were later obtained using similar histological procedures with a variety of tracer substances including dyes, iron salts, and colloidal silver (2,3,44). All these studies have reported that significant amounts of tracer reach the endolymphatic sac, qualitatively supporting the existence of longitudinal flow. The reported difference in osmolarity between endolymph and perilymph has been suggested as a possible mechanism driving bulk flow (35,75). It is suggested that the resulting influx of water into endolymph would drive endolymph movement toward the sac. However, it cannot be assumed that a net influx of water into endolymph occurs as a result of this gradient. In fact if the endolymph/perilymph boundary has a lower reflection coefficient for K compared with Na, then endolymph could be in osmotic equilibrium with perilymph. Alternatively, if the net water movement associated with ion fluxes tends to be perilymph directed, then the endolymph/perilymph osmolarity difference could represent a steady-state condition, with no net influx or efflux of water. Further investigation is therefore required to establish the significance of the osmotic pressure difference and whether it is associated with endolymph volume flow.

An alternative hypothesis to longitudinal flow was proposed by Naftalin and Harrison (54). They suggested that endolymph flowed radially, secreted by Reissner's membrane and resorbed by stria vascularis. The concept of radial flow was supported by studies of Lawrence et al. (38) and Lawrence (39), which showed that when Reissner's membrane was damaged in one region, the resulting degeneration remained highly localized rather than spreading in a basal direction. Although the possibilities of longitudinal and radial flow have been debated for years, it is also possible that endolymph homeostasis may occur without a concomitant water flow, if endolymph is not secreted in bulk. The ionic composition could be maintained by active ion transport processes in which the total amount of solute transported into or out of endolymph would balance the amount of solute leaking passively across the membranous boundaries. If water equilibrates passively, as in other systems, then endolymph composition would be maintained without volume flow necessarily taking place. Such a process can be called local homeostasis. To add to the complexity of this problem, it is also possible that all three of the mechanisms above (longitudinal flow, radial flow, local homeostasis) could coexist but vary in their contribution to endolymph for different substances and possibly vary in different experimental situations. This is an extension of the dynamic flow theory in which it was speculated that energy and ionic metabolism were by radial mechanisms, whereas a slow longitudinal flow was responsible for removing high molecular weight waste products and cellular debris (45).

From the above ionic turnover data determined by radiotracers it is possible to derive an upper limit for the rate of longitudinal flow assuming all turnover results from longitudinal flow, i.e., if there is no leakage of substance through the tissues at all. Assuming a cochlear endolymph volume of 2 μl, the maximum flow rates calculated from Na, K, and Cl turnover are 30, 18, and 14 nl/min, respectively, for flow that is at a constant rate throughout the length of the cochlea. If, on the other hand, all the stria contribute equally to the flow, then the flow rate would be expected to increase linearly with distance down the cochlea. In this case, basal turn flow rates of 42, 25, and 20 nl/min would give the observed ionic turnover rates. Thus it is highly unlikely that the longitudinal flow rate can be higher than would account for the turnover of the ion with the lowest turnover rate, i.e., approximately 20 nl/min. On the basis of a lower Cl permeability estimate derived from ionic changes occurring during anoxia, Mori and Konishi (52) estimated volume flow could only be as much as 9 nl/min.

One of the strongest indications that longitudinal endolymph flow occurs at some rate comes from studies in which the endolymphatic sac is ablated and the endolymphatic duct blocked. The subsequent development of endolymphatic hydrops (enlargement of the endolymphatic space) (25,27) has been used as evidence that the endolymphatic sac plays a significant role in endolymph resorption. This will be discussed in more detail in a later section.

In view of the importance of ascertaining the fundamental mechanisms of endolymph homeostasis, a number of studies reported attempts to quantify the rate of endolymph flow. Giebel (13) introduced fluorescent rhodamine into scala media, which passed rapidly into the saccule and reached the endolymphatic sac within 10 min of injection. He estimated the rate of flow to be 40 mm/hr (67 nl/min). Proeschel et al. (61) injected ototoxic tracers into endolymph and used the spread of suppression of the compound action potential as an indicator of longitudinal tracer movement. They estimated endolymph flow to be 3.5 mm/min (350 nl/min) and 0.5 mm/min (50 nl/min) in the first and second turns, respectively. The rates derived in both the above studies are extremely high and cannot easily be reconciled with the ionic turnover data. In an attempt to provide a more direct measure of flow, Salt et al. (65) developed a technique in which a minute bolus (2–20 nl) of an ionic tracer tetramethylammonium (TMA) was injected into endolymph. Movement of the tracer was monitored by ion-selective microelectrodes that were capable of detecting extremely low tracer concentrations. They found tracer spread in endolymph to be dominated by passive diffusion rather than volume flow. In order to correct for diffusion, tracer movement down the cochlea (turn 2 to turn 1) was compared with movement in the opposite direction (turn 1 to turn 2). Using a mathematical model combining diffusion and flow, it was shown that the rate of volume flow could be determined by comparing the concentration of tracer recorded in each direction. In animals, higher tracer concentrations were recorded in the former condition by a factor of approximately 2, which was interpreted as corresponding to a volume flow rate of <1 nl/min toward the base. In terms of the major ions, this rate of flow would make a negligible contribution to turnover, suggesting that the majority of turnover occurs through the tissues. For other substances this rate of flow (displacing half the endolymph in 18 hr) could be significant. Similar conclusions were subsequently drawn from studies in which TMA was injected into endolymph by iontophoresis and monitored simultaneously by ion electrodes at two recording sites, one basal and one apical to the injection site (66). The observation of similar TMA concentrations at both recording sites confirmed that endolymph flow was extremely low. The major advantages of this latter technique were that the flow measurements could be made in individual animals and tracer concentrations could be used that were not toxic to the cochlea. In spite of the development of techniques that are extremely sensitive to flow in small compartments, the controversy over the rate of endolymph flow continues. Recently, Syková et al. (77) used similar ionic tracer techniques with tetraethylammonium (TEA) and choline as tracers in the second turn. They observed lower concentrations apically to the injection site than basally, which they interpreted as indicating an endolymph flow rate of 0.2 mm/min (20 nl/min). If flow increases linearly down the cochlea this would correspond to a basal turn flow rate of approximately 40 nl/min, which is well in excess of the maximum turnover suggested by radiotracer measurements. However, the same study reported results of tracer movements between turns 1 and 2, the time courses of which were more consistent with slower flow rates. In addition, they also reported in some instances obtaining similar results for tracer movement in each direction, again suggestive of slower flow rates. In conclusion, although the existence of endolymph flow at some rate is generally accepted there is as yet no consensus on the precise rate of flow or the physiological contribution endolymph flow makes. It must be emphasized that volume flow is not the only mechanism by which solutes in the cochlea can reach the endolymphatic sac (or vice versa). Other mechanisms include passive diffusion (if a concentration gradient exists) and, for charged solutes, electrophoresis under the influence of the potential difference between cochlea and the saccule.

PERILYMPH DYNAMICS

A similar controversy over the fundamental origins of perilymph exists, in part arising from the similar technical difficulties of making meaningful measurements without disturbance of the normal physiological state. Again, two major hypotheses of perilymph origins have developed. First, perilymph is derived from CSF, which enters the cochlea through the cochlear aqueduct. This concept was based on experiments in which various substances were injected into CSF and their spread to the cochlea observed (1,2,14). In nonprimates (guinea pigs, cats, rabbits) these substances could be detected by histological techniques in ST and sometimes in SV. In contrast, tracers do not enter the perilymphatic space in monkeys (40) or humans (62), suggesting that the cochlear aqueduct may not be patent in adult primates. However, movement of tracer from CSF to perilymph does not prove that volume flow exists across the aqueduct, even if the nonphysiological pressures during tracer injection can be ignored. This is illustrated by the study of Kaupp and Giebel (23) in which fluorescent rhodamine was shown to enter CSF of the subarachnoid space after its introduction into perilymph. A possible explanation of the conflicting movements of tracer into and out of perilymph through the aqueduct is that the movements could arise from an oscillation of fluid across the aqueduct. Carlborg (7) and Carlborg and Farmer (8) demonstrated that CSF and perilymphatic pressures are not static in the physiological state but cycle systematically with respiratory cycles. When the cochlear aqueduct was blocked, these cyclical changes were less apparent, suggesting that they arise from small, cyclical volume movements across the aqueduct. The mixing of CSF and perilymph that would result from this oscillation would result in tracers apparently crossing the aqueduct in both directions. In addition, chronic surgical obstruction of the cochlear aqueduct does not alone induce pathological changes in the cochlea, which suggests that the duct is not essential for the maintenance of perilymph composition (26), although there is evidence that the penetration of drugs such as kanamycin into perilymph may be affected by this procedure (28). The alternative view of perilymph origins is that it is produced locally in the cochlea by an ultrafiltration mechanism (9,60,70). Hawkins (17) described capillaries in the SV portion of the spiral ligament close to the attachment of Reissner's membrane, which he believed could be the site of perilymph ultrafiltration. This mechanism could also involve longitudinal perilymph flow, depending on the site of resorption. If, as speculated, perilymph was resorbed in the lower spiral ligament of ST near the basilar membrane, then a volume flow from SV to ST through the helicotrema would be expected. Recent studies (59) have tested these hypotheses of perilymph origins, by using ion-selective electrodes to monitor tracer movements in the perilymphatic scalae. When injection and recording electrodes were both sealed into the scalae, it was demonstrated that longitudinal perilymph movements were extremely slow. In ST, the rate averaged 1.7 nl/min toward the apex in the basal turn, while no significant flow at all could be detected in SV. The effects of such low flow rates on perilymph physiology for the major ions is negligible, since passive diffusion occurs at a much higher rate than volume flow. In comparison, if the cochlea is perforated, then movements of ionic tracers demonstrate that a nonphysiological flow develops at rates up to 2 μl/min, owing to the entry of CSF into the basal turn of ST through the cochlear aqueduct. Thus, within a few minutes of this procedure, perilymph will be displaced by CSF. These results support the earlier studies (53,63) that demonstrated high fluid efflux rates from the perforated cochlea and confirm the speculation that indeed this arises from CSF entry.

These findings suggest that perilymph does not originate by a mechanism involving longitudinal volume flow, such as from CSF entry through the aqueduct or from an ultrafiltration mechanism in SV. The possibility remains that the oscillation of fluid across the cochlear aqueduct may make some contribution of perilymph physiology in the basal turn of ST, but this contribution is likely to be small. Rather, perilymph appears to be maintained by local mechanisms that do not necessarily involve volume secretion at all. Possible alternative mechanisms include passive diffusion, facilitated transport, and active transport of solutes. Exchange is presumed to occur across a blood/labyrinth barrier, comprised of the pericytes, fibrocytes, and endothelial cells associated with the capillaries of the spiral ligament (20).

The characteristics of penetration or exchange of many substances between perilymph and blood have been reported. Juhn and Rybak (20) and Juhn et al. (21) compared the rate of entry of ^{22}Na, ^{36}Cl, and ^{45}Ca into perilymph, CSF, and aqueous humor following systemic injection. They found the rate of penetration of all three substances into perilymph was slower than into CSF or aqueous humor, suggesting the existence of a blood/labyrinth barrier. They found the time for perilymph to reach 50% of the serum activity for ^{22}Na and ^{45}Ca was 190 min and 20 hr, respectively. Using a variety of substances it was shown that the rate of entry into perilymph was related to molecular weight. Sterkers et al. (73) studied the penetration of ^{42}K and ^{36}Cl into endolymph, SV perilymph, ST perilymph, and CSF. They found similar rates of entry into CSF, ST perilymph, and SV perilymph, results that are not in accordance with those of Juhn et al. (21). On the basis of a three-compartment model they derived transfer rate constants between plasma and perilymph of 0.0201 min^{-1} and 0.0239 min^{-1} of K and Cl, respectively. In contrast, Konishi et al. (30) studied the clearance of tracers after perilymphatic perfusion with ^{42}K or ^{22}Na. For both ions, clearance from ST was rapid, falling to less than 10% of the perfused level within 10 min. The decline occurred more slowly in SV, only falling to 90% of the perfused level in 10 min. The difference between the above studies, in suggesting whether CSF, ST perilymph, and SV perilymph have similar kinetics, probably arises from the experimental procedures giving differing degrees of CSF contamination of perilymph that could have been present in some of the studies. In the study of Konishi et al. (30), CSF would not contain tracer, so that CSF influx would cause a rapid tracer decline in ST. In studies in which radiotracer was injected systemically, the tracer would also accumulate in CSF so that the sample contamination would not necessarily be detected and could result in apparently similar kinetics of CSF and perilymph. Using a whole cochlea perfusion technique Jung (22) determined the rate of clearance from the entire perilymphatic system. He estimated clearance half-times of 216, 243, and 93 min for Na, K, and Cl, respectively, which are somewhat slower than the above estimates, possibly owing to less interference by CSF entry. Recently Ferrary et al. (12) compared the penetration of labeled D-glucose and L-glucose into perilymph after intravenous administration. D-glucose entered perilymph relatively rapidly, showing levels only slightly below those in plasma, whereas L-glucose entered perilymph only slowly. These data suggest the existence of a facilitated transport mechanism for glucose across the blood–perilymph barrier.

PATHOLOGICAL DISTURBANCES OF COCHLEAR FLUIDS

Endolymphatic Hydrops/Meniere's Disease

Meniere's disease presents as the three symptoms of (a) tinnitus, (b) fluctuating hearing loss, and (c) periodic attacks of vertigo. Pathologically the disease is characterized by endolymphatic hydrops so it is generally assumed that this represents some dysfunction of the normal mechanisms of endolymph volume regulation, although the precise origins of this dysfunction have not been established. Whereas some authors have described hydrops in terms of an endolymphatic hypertension, measurements by Long and Morizono (43) demonstrate that the hydrostatic pressure difference between endolymph and perilymph in the hydropic cochlea is no greater than in normal animals. They estimated the maximum pressure increase associated with endolymphatic hydrops to be 0.51 mm Hg. This is consistent with the membranous structures bounding SM being very flexible, so that a volume increase can occur without a marked increase in endolymphatic hydrostatic pressure. The most common explanations of the origins of hydrops include (a) a hypersecretion of endolymph, (b) blockage of a duct between the secretion and resorptive areas, and (c) a hypoabsorption of endolymph. The strongest evidence supporting this view comes from the extensive studies of Kimura et al. (27), which showed that in the guinea pig, surgical destruction of the endolymphatic duct and sac resulted in hydrops of the cochlea, saccule, and utricle. On the other hand, destruction of the ductus reuniens resulted in cochlear hydrops and a collapse of a saccule. Although these results are consistent with the cochlea as a source of endolymph and the endolymphatic sac as a site of resorption, there are numerous observations that suggest this explanation may be an oversimplification. First, hydrops may be induced by some conditions that do not involve endolymphatic sac destruction. Hydrops has been reported as a result of otitis media (50), following stapedectomy (71), and following acoustic trauma (41). There is as yet no good explanation of the origin of hydrops under these conditions. In contrast, the observation of hydrops after endolymphatic sac destruction appears to be species dependent, occurring in guinea pigs (25,27), rabbits (4,48), less readily in monkeys (25,42), and chinchillas (76). It is thus difficult to understand how the sac can be essential in one species but not in another. In addition, one may expect that if destruction of the sac results in impaired endolymph resorption, then the chemical composition of endolymph would be changed. On the contrary, endolymph of hydropic guinea pigs has been shown to have an almost identical composition (Na, K, Cl) to normal endolymph (33,51). This demonstrates that near-normal endolymph composition may be maintained in the absence of the endolymphatic sac. This finding, combined with the probable slow endolymph flow rates as discussed earlier, suggests that endolymphatic hydrops does not arise directly from a disturbance of Na, K, or Cl homeostasis. Hydrops arises either from the disturbance of an ion with slower turnover rate (for which volume flow would be a more significant factor in turnover) or from a disturbance in homeostasis of macromolecules. One interesting possibility is suggested by recent studies that have shown that Ca^{2+} homeostasis may be disturbed by endolymphatic sac ablation. In normal endolymph the Ca^{2+} content is exceptionally low (5,56). In hydrops animals, the Ca^{2+} content of both light cells and melanocytes of the vestibular labyrinth was raised (49), and the calcium concentration of cochlear endolymph was increased by an amount that correlated well with the hydrops-induced EP reduction (56). Although it has been speculated that hydrops may be induced by the osmotic pressure increase owing to the Ca^{2+} concentration increase, it is also possible that the elevated Ca^{2+} level may interfere with endolymph volume regulation indirectly. Further studies need to be performed to ascertain whether endolymph Ca^{2+} is regulated locally in the cochlea or only in the vestibular labyrinth/endolymphatic sac.

Perilymphatic Fistulae

Although perilymphatic fistulae would appear superficially to be a straightforward problem, they may be extremely complex, with widely differing pathogenesis, physiological consequences (and clinical symptoms), and prognosis for relief of symptoms. Commonly, fistulae occur between a perilymphatic scala and the middle ear, usually near the stapes or round window membrane (outer membrane break). However, fistulae between endolymph and perilymph (inner membrane break) have also been reported with clinical effects similar to those reported during the Meniere's attack. In addition, a combination of both (double membrane break) may also exist. The origins of perilymphatic fistulae may be extremely varied including congenital defects, bone erosion by cholesteatoma, or from mechanical trauma. This latter category may include fistulae induced by laughing, sneezing, straining, barotrauma (sky diving, scuba diving), acoustic trauma, head trauma, or surgical procedure (e.g., stapedectomy). The clinical symptoms associated with perilymphatic fistulae may be somewhat similar to those of Meniere's disease or may include sudden hearing loss (with or without vestibular symptoms), a mild or sharply localized hearing loss, or isolated mild vestibular disturbances. These symptoms can be triggered by a number of physiological mechanisms. In the case of inner membrane ruptures the intermixture of endolymph and perilymph with associated disruption of cochlear potentials can explain both auditory and vestibular symptoms. For round or oval window breaks, the dysfunction can arise from (a) fluid entering the middle ear, giving a conductive hearing loss; (b) CSF entering the perilymphatic space, disturbing the normal biochemical composition (in this case, the effects will depend on the site of outflow as a greater disturbance will occur the further the fistula is from the cochlear aqueduct); and (c) air entering the cochlea, causing mechanical and chemical disruption of cochlear function.

Investigation of the effects of perilymph fistula is complicated both by the technical problems associated with all studies of perilymph physiology and the differences between experimental animals and humans, especially with respect to the patency of the cochlear aqueduct. Although this subject is now attracting considerable attention with the development of suitable animal models and techniques of fistula induction and monitoring (36,37,57), the interpretation of such results is made complicated by uncontrolled secondary effects, such as CSF leakage and retrograde infection.

ACKNOWLEDGMENTS

The authors thank Arti Vora for technical assistance and typing the manuscript. This chapter was prepared with the support of NIH Program Project P01 NS24372.

REFERENCES

1. Altmann, F., and Waltner, J. G. (1947): The circulation of the labyrinthine fluids. *Ann. Otol. Rhinol. Laryngol.*, 56:684–708.
2. Altmann, F., and Waltner, J. G. (1950): Further investigations on the physiology of the labyrinthine fluids. *Ann. Otol.*, 59:657–686.
3. Andersen, H. C. (1948): Passage of trypan blue into the endolymphatic system of the labyrinth. *Acta Otolaryngol. (Stockh.)* 36:273–283.
4. Beal, D. D. (1968): Effect of endolymphatic sac ablation in the rabbit and cat. *Acta Otolaryngol. (Stockh.)*, 66:333–346.
5. Bosher, S. K., and Warren R. L. (1978): Very low calcium content of cochlear endolymph, an extracellular fluid. *Nature*, 273:377–378.
6. Carlborg, B., Densert, O., and Stagg, J. (1980): Perilymphatic pressure in the cat: Description of a new method for study of inner ear hydrodynamics. *Acta Otolaryngol. (Stockh.)*, 90:208–218.
7. Carlborg, B. I. (1981): On physiologic and experimental variation of the perilymphatic pressure in the cat. *Acta Otolaryngol. (Stockh.)*, 91:19–28.
8. Carlborg, B. I., and Farmer, J. C., Jr. (1983): Transmission of cerebrospinal fluid pressure via the cochlear aqueduct and endolymphatic sac. *Am. J. Otolaryngol.*, 4:273–282.
9. Citron, L., Exley, D., and Hallpike, C. S. (1956): Formation, circulation and chemical properties of the labyrinthine fluids. *Br. Med. Bull.*, 12:101–106.
10. Dallos, P. (1983): Some electrical circuit properties of the organ of Corti. I. Analysis without reactive elements. *Hear. Res.*, 12:89–119.
11. Davis, H. (1965): A model for transducer action in the cochlea. *Cold Spring Harbor Symp. Quant. Biol.*, 30:181–190.
12. Ferrary, E., Sterkers, O., Saumon, G., Tran Ba Huy, P., and Amiel, C. (1987): Facilitated transfer of glucose from blood into perilymph in the rat cochlea. *Am. J. Physiol.*, 253:F59–F65.
13. Giebel, W. (1982): Das dynamische Verhalten der Innenohrflussigkeiten. *Laryngol. Rhinol. Otol.*, 61:481–488.
14. Gisselsson, L. (1949): The passage of fluorescein sodium to the labyrinthine fluids. *Acta Otolaryngol. (Stockh.)*, 37:268–275.
15. Guild, S. R. (1927): The circulation of the endolymph. *Am. J. Anat.*, 39:57–81.
16. Hara, A., Salt, A. N., Varghese, J., and Thalmann, R. (1987): Quantification of cerebrospinal fluid (CSF) contamination of scala tympani (ST) perilymph samples. *J. Acoust. Soc. Am.*, 82:S70.
17. Hawkins, J. E., Jr. (1968): Vascular patterns of the membranous labyrinth. Third Symposium on the Role of Vestibular Organs in the Exploration of Space. Pensacola, FL.
18. Jahnke, K. (1975): The fine structure of freeze-fractured intercellular junctions in the guinea pig inner ear. *Acta Otolaryngol. [Suppl.] (Stockh.)*, 336:1–40.
19. Johnstone, B. M., and Sellick, P. M. (1972): The peripheral auditory apparatus. *Q. Rev. Biophys.*, 5:1–57.
20. Juhn, S. K., and Rybak, L. P. (1981): Nature of blood–labyrinth barrier. In: *Meniere's Disease:*

Pathogenesis, Diagnosis and Treatment, edited by K.-H. Vosteen, H. Schuknecht, C. R. Pfaltz et al., pp. 59–67. Georg Thieme Verlag, New York.

21. Juhn, S. K., Rybak, L. P., and Fowlks, W. L. (1982): Transport characteristics of the blood-perilymph barrier. *Am. J. Otolaryngol.,* 3:392–396.
22. Jung, W. K. (1979): Results in evaluating cochlear kinetics of carbon-14 labelled metabolites. *Rev. Laryngol. Otol. Rhinol.,* 100:207–214.
23. Kaupp, H., and Giebel, W. (1980): Distribution of marked perilymph to the subarachnoid space. *Arch. Otorhinolaryngol.,* 229:245–253.
24. Kellerhals, B. (1979): Perilymph production and cochlear blood flow. *Acta Otolaryngol. (Stockh.),* 87:370–374.
25. Kimura, R. S. (1968): Experimental production of endolymphatic hydrops. *Otolaryngol. Clin. North Am.,* 1:457–471.
26. Kimura, R. S., Schuknecht, H. F., and Ota, C. Y. (1974): Blockage of the cochlear aqueduct. *Acta Otolaryngol. (Stockh.),* 77:1–12.
27. Kimura, R. S., Schucknecht, H. F., Ota, C. Y., and Jones, D. D. (1980): Obliteration of the ductus reuniens. *Acta Otolaryngol. (Stockh.),* 89:295–309.
28. Kimura, R. S., and Maynard, L. B. (1984): Histopathological study of the cochlea with altered perilymph metabolism. *Acta Otolaryngol. (Stockh.),* 97:535–546.
29. Konishi, T., and Kelsey, E. (1973): Effect of potassium deficiency on cochlear potentials and cation contents of the endolymph. *Acta Otolaryngol. (Stockh.),* 76:410–418.
30. Konishi, T., Hamrick, P. E., and Walsh, P. J. (1978): Ion transport in the guinea pig cochlea. I. Potassium and sodium transport. *Acta. Otolaryngol. (Stockh.),* 186:22–34.
31. Konishi, T., and Hamrick, P. E. (1978): Ion transport in the cochlea of guinea pig. II. Chloride transport. *Acta Otolaryngol. (Stockh.),* 86:176–184.
32. Konishi, T., and Salt, A. N. (1980): Permeability to potassium of the endolymph–perilymph barrier and its possible relation to hair cell function. *Exp. Brain Res.,* 40:457–463.
33. Konishi, T., Salt, A. N., and Kimura, R. S. (1981): Electrophysiological studies of experimentally induced endolymphatic hydrops in guinea pigs. In: *Meniere's Disease: Pathogenesis, Diagnosis and Treatment,* edited by K.-H. Vosteen, H. Schuknecht, C. R. Pfaltz et al., pp. 47–58. Georg Thieme Verlag, New York.
34. Konishi, T., and Mori, H. (1984): Permeability to sodium ions of the endolymph–perilymph barrier. *Hear. Res.,* 15:143–149.
35. Konishi, T., Hamrick, P. E., and Mori, H. (1984): Water permeability of the endolymph–perilymph barrier in the guinea pig cochlea. *Hear. Res.,* 15:51–58.
36. Lamm, H., Lehnhardt, E., and Lamm, K. (1984): Instrumental perforation of the round window. Animal experiments using cochleography and ERA. *Acta Otolaryngol. (Stockh.),* 98:454–461.
37. Lamm, K., Lehnhardt, E., and Lamm, H. (1986): Long-term study after perforation of the round window. Animal experiments using electric response audiometry. *Acta Otolaryngol. (Stockh.),* 102:27–30.
38. Lawrence, M., Wolsk, D., and Litton, W. B. (1961): Circulation of the inner ear fluids. *Ann. Otol.,* 70:753–776.
39. Lawrence, M. (1966): Histological evidence for localized radial flow of endolymph. *Arch. Otolaryngol.,* 83:406–412.
40. Lempert, J., Meltzer, P. E., Wever, E. G., Lawrence, M., and Rambo, J. H. T. (1952): Structure and function of the cochlear aqueduct. *Arch. Otolaryngol.,* 55:134–145.
41. Liberman, M. C., and Mulroy, M. J. (1982): Acute and chronic effects of acoustic trauma: Cochlear pathology and auditory nerve pathophysiology. In: *New Perspectives on Noise-Induced Hearing Loss,* edited by R. P. Hamernik, D. Henderson, and R. Salvi, pp. 105–135. Raven Press, New York.
42. Lindsay, J. R. (1947): Effect of obliteration of the endolymphatic sac and duct in the monkey. *Arch. Otolaryngol.,* 45:1–13.
43. Long, C. H., and Morizono, T. (1987): Hydrostatic pressure measurements of endolymph and perilymph in a guinea pig model of endolymphatic hydrops. *Otolaryngol.,* 98:83–95.
44. Lundquist, P. G., Kimura, R., and Wersall, J. (1964): Experiments in endolymph circulation. *Acta Otolaryngol. [Suppl.] (Stockh.),* 188:194–201.
45. Lundquist, P. G. (1976): Aspects on endolymphatic sac morphology and function. *Arch. Oto-Rhino-Laryngol.,* 212:231–240.
46. Marcus, D. C., Thalmann, R., and Marcus, N. Y. (1978): Respiratory quotient of stria vascularis of guinea pig in vitro. *Arch. Otorhinolaryngol.,* 221:97–103.
47. Marcus, D. C., Rokugo, M., Ge, X. X., and Thalmann, R. (1983): Response of cochlear potentials to presumed alterations of ionic conductance: Endolymphatic perfusion of barium, valinomycin and nystatin. *Hear. Res.,* 12:17–30.
48. Martin, G. K., Shaw, D. W. W., Dobie, R. A., and Lonsbury-Martin, B. L. (1983): Endolymphatic hydrops in the rabbit: Auditory brainstem responses and cochlear morphology. *Hear. Res.,* 12:65–87.

49. Meyer zum Gottesberge-Orsulakova, A. M., and Kaufmann, R. (1986): Is an imbalanced calcium-homeostasis responsible for the experimentally induced endolymphatic hydrops? *Acta Otolaryngol. (Stockh.),* 102:93–98.

50. Meyerhoff, W. L., Shea, D. A., and Giebink, G. S. (1980): Experimental pneumococcal media: A histopathologic study. *Otolaryngol. Head Neck Surg.,* 88:606–612.

51. Morgenstern, C., Amano, H., and Orsulakova, A. (1982): Ion transport in the endolymphatic space. *Am. J. Otolaryngol.,* 3:323–327.

52. Mori, H., and Konishi, T. (1985): Permeability to chloride ions of the cochlear partition in normal guinea pigs. *Hear. Res.,* 17:227–236.

53. Moscovitch, D. H., Gannon, R. P., and Laszlo, C. A. (1973): Perilymph displacement by cerebrospinal fluid in the cochlea. *Ann. Otol.,* 82:53–61.

54. Naftalin, L., and Harrison, M. S. (1958): Circulation of labyrinthine fluids. *J. Laryngol.,* 72:118–136.

55. Nagahara, K., Fisch, V., and Diller, N. (1981): Experimental study on the perilymphatic pressure. *Am. J. Otolaryngol.,* 3:1–8.

56. Ninoyu, O., and Meyer zum Gottesberge, A. M. (1986): Changes in Ca^{++} activity and DC potential in experimentally induced endolymphatic hydrops. *Arch. Oto-Rhino-Laryngol.,* 243:106–107.

57. Nomura, Y., and Hara, M. (1986): Experimental perilymphatic fistula. *Am. J. Otolaryngol.,* 7:267–275.

58. Offner, F. F., Dallos, P., and Cheatham, M. A. (1987): Positive endocochlear potential: Mechanism of production by marginal cells of stria vascularis. *Hear. Res.,* 29:117–124.

59. Ohyama, K., Salt, A. N., and Thalmann, R. (1988): Volume flow rate of perilymph in the guinea-pig cochlea. *Hear. Res. (submitted).*

60. Palva, T., and Raunio, V. (1967): Disc electrophoretic studies of human perilymph. *Ann. Otol. Rhinol. Laryngol.,* 76:23–36.

61. Proeschel, U., Sellick, P. M., and Johnstone, B. M. (1984): Measurements of endolymph flow by iontophoresis of ototoxic substances into scala media. In: *Proceeding of the 21st Workshop on Inner Ear Biology,* p. 88. Taormina, Italy.

62. Ritter, F. N., and Lawrence, M. (1965): A histological and experimental study of cochlear aqueduct patency in the adult human. *Laryngoscope,* 75:1224–1233.

63. Salt, A. N., and Stopp, P. E. (1979): The effect of cerebrospinal fluid pressure on perilymphatic flow in the opened cochlea. *Acta Otolaryngol., (Stockh.),* 88:198–202.

64. Salt, A. N., and Konishi, T. (1979): Effects of noise on cochlear potentials and endolymph potassium concentration recorded with potassium-selective electrodes. *Hear. Res.,* 1:343–363.

65. Salt, A. N., Thalmann, R., Marcus, D. C., and Bohne, B. A. (1986): Direct measurement of longitudinal endolymph flow rate in the guinea pig cochlea. *Hear. Res.,* 23:141–151.

66. Salt, A. N., and Thalmann, R. (1987): New concepts regarding the volume flow of endolymph and perilymph. *Adv. Oto-Rhino-Laryngol.,* 37:11–17.

67. Salt, A. N., Melichar, I., and Thalmann, R. (1987): Mechanisms of endocochlear potential generation by stria vascularis. *Laryngoscope,* 97:984–991.

68. Scheibe, F., Haupt, H., and Bergmann, K. (1984): On sources of error in the biochemical study of perilymph (guinea-pig). *Arch. Otorhinolaryngol.,* 240:43–48.

69. Scheibe, F., and Haupt, H. (1985): Biochemical differences between perilymph, cerebrospinal fluid and blood plasma in the guinea pig. *Hear. Res.,* 17:61–66.

70. Schneider, E. A. (1974): A contribution to the physiology of the perilymph. Part I. The origins of perilymph. *Ann. Otol. Rhinol. Laryngol.,* 83:76–83.

71. Schuknecht, H. F., and McNeill, R. A. (1966): Light microscopic observations on the pathology of endolymph. *J. Laryngol. Otol.,* 80:1–10.

72. Sellick, P. M., and Bock, G. R. (1974): Evidence for an electrogenic potassium pump as the origin of the positive component of the endocochlear potential. *Pflugers Arch.,* 352:351–361.

73. Sterkers, O., Saumon, G., Tran Ba Huy, P., and Amiel, C. (1982): K, Cl, and H_2O entry in endolymph, perilymph and cerebrospinal fluid in the rat. *Am. J. Physiol.,* 243:F173–F180.

74. Sterkers, O., Saumon, G., Tran Ba Huy, P., Ferrary, E., and Amiel, C. (1984): Electrochemical heterogeneity of the cochlear endolymph: Effect of acetazolamide. *Am. J. Physiol.,* 246:F47–F53.

75. Sterkers, O., Saumon, G., Tran Ba Huy, P., Ferrary, E., and Amiel, C. (1984): Inter- and intra-compartmental osmotic gradients within the rat cochlea. *Am. J. Physiol.,* 247:F602–F606.

76. Suh, K. W., and Cody, D. T. R. (1977): Obliteration of vestibular and cochlear aqueducts in animals. *Trans. Am. Acad. Ophthalmol. Otolaryngol.,* 84:359–379.

77. Syková, E., Syka, J., Johnstone, B. M., and Yates, G. K. (1987): Longitudinal flow of endolymph measured by distribution of tetraethylammonium and choline in scala media. *Hear. Res.,* 28:161–171.

78. Tasaki, I., and Spyropoulos, C. S. (1959): Stria vascularis as source of endocochlear potential. *J. Neurophysiol.,* 22:149–155.

79. Thalmann, R., Kusakari, J., and Miyoshi, T. (1973): Dysfunctions of energy releasing and consuming processes of the cochlea. *Laryngoscope,* 83:1690–1713.
80. Wada, J., Kambayashi, J., Marcus, D. C., and Thalmann, R. (1979): Vascular perfusion of the cochlea: Effect of potassium-free and ribidium substituted media. *Arch. Otorhinolaryngol.,* 225:79–81.
81. Yoshida, M., and Lowry, L. D. (1984): Hydrostatic pressure measurement of endolymph and perilymph in the guinea pig cochlea. *Am. J. Otolaryngol.,* 5:159–165.

Physiology of the Ear,
edited by A. F. Jahn and J. Santos-Sacchi.
Raven Press, New York © 1988.

The Physiology of the Cochlear Nerve

Robert V. Harrison

*Department of Otolaryngology, The Hospital for Sick Children,
Toronto, Ontario, Canada M5G 1X8*

The cochlear nerve is the only input pathway for auditory information to the central nervous system. This chapter describes the electrophysiological responses of afferent cochlear neurons to acoustic stimulation, the studies of which have been of great importance to determine: (a) how the cochlea normally analyzes and transduces the mechanical vibrations of sound into electrical activity; (b) the pattern of neural input to the central auditory system, in particular, the representation of speech signals; (c) the deficits and degradation of information that result from cochlear damage (such as occurs in sensorineural deafness). In the first section of this chapter the responses of cochlear nerve fibers to simple sounds are described. Building on this we consider the coding of more complex sounds, such as speech, by the ensemble of afferent fibers in the cochlear nerve. Finally, we review some of the changes to cochlear fiber responses that result from cochlear pathology.

THE COCHLEAR NERVE

The cell bodies of afferent cochlear neurons lie in the spiral ganglion of the cochlea. These mostly bipolar cells have one process terminating on the hair cell(s), the other projecting to the cochlear nucleus. The great majority (90%–95%) of cochlear afferent neurons (75,110) terminate on one inner hair cell (inner radial fibers); the other 5% to 10% give rise to the so-called outer spiral fibers, each of which can innervate as many as 20 outer hair cells (83,107). The central axon of these cells are fine, unmyelinated, and probably not sampled using standard microelectrode techniques (60). Therefore, most recordings from cochlear nerve fibers reflect activity of individual inner hair cells. From their origin in the organ of Corti to their termination in the cochlear nucleus, there is no evidence to suggest that cochlear afferents synapse with other neurons or with each other.

The number of axons making up the cochlear nerve varies with species: the kangaroo rat has approximately 16,000 (113), the cat has approximately 50,000 (31), and some large marine mammals have as many as 200,000 (48). Humans have (normally) approximately 30,000 (37).

The axons of the cochlear afferents congregate in the modiolus and form the cochlear nerve keeping an orderly cochleotopic (or tonotopic) arrangement (72,101), which is maintained throughout the whole auditory pathway. Thus, neurons positioned near each other, e.g., in an electrode track, usually reflect activity from adjacent areas of the organ of Corti.

It is appropriate to mention some of the pioneers in single-unit studies of the cochlear nerve. Galambos and Davis (29,30) led the way in making recordings from cochlear nucleus cells in the cat. The first cochlear fiber recordings were made by Tasaki in 1954 (111) and later extended by Katsuki et al. (52). Major advances came later with the introduction of more controlled acoustic stimulation and improved quantitative analysis, notably in the laboratories of Kiang et al. (62,63), Rose and colleagues (7,91,92), and Evans (16; for comprehensive review, see 20). In most studies, single-unit recordings have been made with a microelectrode at the level of the internal auditory meatus, approached via the posterior fossa. Some researchers use an alternative approach and record from cochlear nerve cell soma in the spiral ganglion. In any case, the signal of interest is the action potential spike as it propagates centrally. Almost all studies of cochlear fiber activity have been made in the anesthetized animal. Under these conditions, the middle ear reflex and the influence of efferents on the cochlea are minimal or absent; otherwise, the fiber responses are assumed to be similar to those of awake animals.

FIBER RESPONSES FROM THE NORMAL COCHLEA

Resting Activity

Most afferent cochlear neurons are spontaneously active in the absence of acoustic stimulation, with a range of discharge rates from less than 1 spike/sec to more than 100 spikes/sec. The distribution of these rates is generally bimodal (16,63), with more than half being above 20 spikes/sec (mean: ~60 spikes/sec). Liberman (68) has distinguished three spontaneous rate groups: low (<0.5 spikes/sec), medium (0.5–18 spikes/sec), and high (>18 spikes/sec). He demonstrated that the most sensitive neurons, i.e., with the lowest thresholds of response, are the high spontaneous rate neurons. Figure 1B illustrates this relationship; the open circles represent the minimum thresholds of units with high (>18 spikes/sec) spontaneous rate. The spontaneous discharge is most likely the result of a random release of neurotransmitter from the hair-cell synapse, thus interspike interval histograms of spontaneous activity reveal an approximately Poisson process (63) except that very short intervals do not normally occur because of the refractory period that follows each action potential (this also applies to driven activity; see, for example, the interval histograms of Fig. 6). The reason why cochlear neurons differ in their mean spontaneous rates is unclear. However, anatomical studies by Liberman (69) indicate that 60% of inner radial fibers are larger and have a higher density of mitochondria, and he suggests that these factors might result in higher spontaneous rates.

In response to acoustical stimulation, hair-cell receptor potentials modulate the release of neurotransmitters at the hair cell synapse. Post-synaptically, the membranes of the cochlear afferents depolarize and resulting action potentials are propagated centrally along the nerve axons. Thus, within the limitations of the synaptic process, cochlear fiber responses reflect inner hair-cell receptor potentials.

Response to Pure Tones

Each cochlear nerve fiber responds best to a restricted range of tone frequencies depending on its place of origin along the cochlea. To a single tone alone, the response

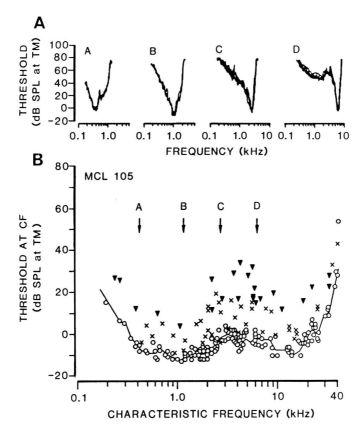

FIG. 1. Spontaneous rates, thresholds, and tuning of normal cochlear nerve fibers. **A**: Representative tuning curves for single units at four CF regions. In each panel three to six tuning curves with similar CF have been superimposed. **B**: The distribution of minimum thresholds for cochlear fibers from a cat born and raised in a low-noise environment. *Open circles* represent units with spontaneous discharge rates of more than 18 spikes/sec. Low spontaneous rate (<0.5 spikes/sec) neurons are indicated by the *closed triangles*. *Cross symbols* represent units with medium spontaneous rate. (From ref. 71.)

is always excitatory—an increase in the mean rate of discharge above spontaneous activity. At the level of the cochlear nerve there is no neural inhibition because there are no inhibitory neurons/synapses to mediate such a process. (Reductions in firing rate do occur, e.g., in two-tone interactions, but these are not the result of neural inhibition; here the term suppression is preferable.)

Figure 2A is reproduced from Evans' studies (22). Here the discharge rate of a cat's cochlear fiber to a tone stimulus is represented by the length of the small bar. The position of the bar indicates the frequency of the stimulus (abscissa) and its intensity (ordinate). Outside the response area, some spontaneous activity is evident. Figure 2C and D represents the same data as isorate and isointensity functions, respectively. In Fig. 2C, the outer curve is the threshold boundary of the response of the fiber, i.e., the frequency and intensity combinations of stimulus that increase the mean firing rate above spontaneous level (which is a little less than 10 spikes/ sec). This is the frequency threshold curve (FTC) or tuning curve for the fiber (61). The other isorate contours describe the supra threshold response of the neuron.

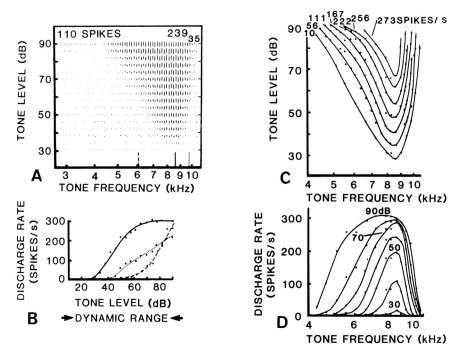

FIG. 2. Response of single cochlear nerve fibers as function of frequency and intensity. **A:** Frequency response map. The length of each vertical line indicates the average number of spikes evoked by a 50-msec duration stimulus at the frequency and intensity indicated by the center of the line. **B:** Vertical sections through A at frequencies indicated by *dashed*, *continuous*, and *dotted lines*, respectively; these are rate versus intensity functions. **C:** Isorate contours. Each contour indicates the tone frequencies and intensities evoking a given discharge rate. These are obtained by taking horizontal sections through a family of rate-level functions as in B. **D:** Isointensity contours, i.e., horizontal sections through A. Note flattening of the contours at the highest levels because of saturation of the response and a shift in frequency of maximum response. (From ref. 22.)

Near its minimum threshold, a fiber usually responds to only one frequency, the best or characteristic frequency (CF). Some studies have reported filter functions with double tip but their origin is obscure (44,74).

The upper parts of Figs. 1 and 3 illustrate tuning curves with different CFs. On a logarithmic frequency scale, high-CF fibers have a sharply tuned tip at low threshold, and a tail—a high-threshold plateau at frequencies below CF (16,63,70). For fibers of lower CF the distinction between tip and tail is progressively lost such that low-CF neurons are more symmetrically "V" shaped (e.g., the fibers tuned to approximately 1 kHz in Figs. 1 and 3). For high-CF fibers the high-frequency cut-off slope of the tip region can have a slope of 600 dB/octave, while that of the low-frequency side of the tip ranges from 50 to 200 dB/octave. The tuning curves for low-CF fibers (<2 kHz) have both high- and low-frequency slopes in the range of 10 to 60 dB/octave. Each cochlear fiber acts like a narrow bandpass filter, the frequency selectivity of which can be quantified by measuring the bandwidth of the tuning curve. For convenience, bandwidths 10 dB above minimum threshold are often used and expressed as a Q factor. Thus, the $Q_{10\ dB}$ is the characteristic frequency divided by the 10-dB bandwidth; the higher the $Q_{10\ dB}$, the sharper the

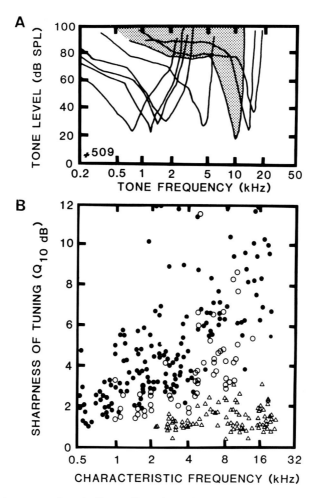

FIG. 3. The tuning properties of afferent fibers from the normal and pathological cochlea. **A**: A sample of FTCs from a normal guinea pig cochlea. **B**: The sharpness of tuning ($Q_{10\,dB}$) of normal cochlear nerve fiber responses (*filled symbols*) and values obtained from damaged cochleas (*open symbols*). $Q_{10\,dB}$ values are plotted as a function of the characteristic frequency of each neuron. *Open circles* represent values from animals with endolymphatic hydrops (45). *Open triangles* are data from kanamycin-treated animals (41,42) where neurons originate in cochlear areas of >90% outer hair-cell loss.

frequency selectivity. In Fig. 3B $Q_{10\,dB}$ values are plotted as a function of CF for cochlear fibers from the guinea pig. The filled symbols represent pooled data from normal animals; slightly higher values are found in the cat (18,19,63) and in those predicted for the human cochlear nerve (41).

It is helpful to use the tip and tail descriptions of tuning curves because these two regions appear to be functionally separate. For example, their thresholds can change independently as a result of metabolic insults such as hypoxia and ototoxic drug damage. In these cases, the tip is much more vulnerable than the tail. In acoustic trauma the tail region sometimes has an improved threshold while the tip threshold is elevated (70,71).

So far, the responses of individual cochlear fibers to a range of stimulus conditions

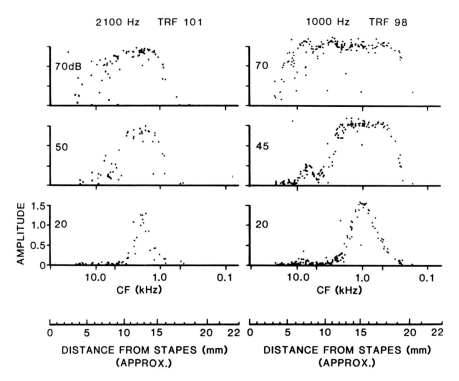

FIG. 4. A population study of cochlear fiber responses to pure tone stimuli. Response amplitudes (fundamental component of Fourier-transformed period histogram) of a population of cochlear neurons to a 2,100-Hz (**left**) and 1,000-Hz (**right**) continuous sine wave, plotted as a function of fiber CF (and also with position of origin along the cochlear length). Stimuli are presented at increasing intensity levels as indicated. The data in each column are from different animals. (From ref. 84.)

have been described and presented in terms of the stimulus parameters. A different approach is to measure the responses of a large population of fibers and determine the spatial distribution of responses across the tonotopic cochlear fiber array. For example, some results from Pfeiffer and Kim (84) are shown in Fig. 4. Each data point represents the response magnitude (see ref. 84 for details) of a separate fiber to pure-tone stimuli of 2.1 kHz (left) and 1 kHz (right), presented at the intensities indicated. Note that CFs of the fibers are represented on the abscissa from high to low frequency such that the equivalent cochlear map in millimeters from the stapes is from left to right. At low stimulus intensity, the pure tones are represented spatially by a narrow band of responding neurons at the appropriate position across the fiber array. At higher stimulus levels there is a spread of activity to adjacent neurons. In the case of 1-kHz stimulus the spread is to both higher and lower CF fibers because of the symmetrical shape of tuning curves for low-CF fibers. For the 2.1-kHz stimulus, the spread of activity is predominantly to higher CF neurons, as would be predicted from the asymmetry of tuning curves of higher CF fibers. These methods have been used to study interactions in tonal complexes (64,66). More examples of such population studies are described later in relation to the neural representation of speech sounds.

Changes in Discharge Rate with Intensity

An increase of a tone stimulus at the CF of a fiber causes an increase in discharge rate up to a level of 40 to 50 dB above threshold where there is a full or partial saturation of discharge rate. A typical example of this sigmoid input/output function is shown in the continuous curve of Fig. 2B. This fiber has a dynamic range (intensity levels over which discharge rate changes) of about 40 dB. The (CF) dynamic range of neurons appears to relate to spontaneous activity such that high spontaneous rate neurons tend to have a narrower dynamic range than low spontaneous rate neurons (27).

Although the majority of neurons show a complete rate saturation at 40 to 50 dB above threshold level (79) there are a small number, those with "sloping saturation" in which discharge rate continues to increase with increasing stimulus intensity over a wide dynamic range (79,94). The rate versus intensity functions for tones away from CF have a different slope—in general, steeper below CF and less steep above CF (17,40,94). These "off-CF" rate functions are illustrated in Fig. 2B by the interrupted curves.

Rate versus intensity functions can be generally described as monotonic and sigmoidal, however, at high levels (~90 dB SPL) the rate may drop (sometimes to spontaneous rate) and within a 10-dB range increase again to a maximum (58). This notch or dip in the rate versus intensity function is accompanied by an abrupt change in the response phase of the neuron (at least for low-CF neurons in which this can be measured). The notch appears to result from a changeover from one process driving the neuron to another; it may be that these two processes are also responsible for the separate tip and tail regions of the FTC.

Intensity Coding

The psychophysical dynamic range, i.e., the intensity range over which we can detect small increments in sound intensity, is greater than 100 dB and much wider than the average dynamic range (45 dB) of individual cochlear neurons to a tone at CF. This discrepancy has raised the question of which mechanisms transmit intensity information in the cochlear nerve (22,23,80). However, studies by Liberman (68) indicated a wider range of thresholds than was previously determined; as shown in Fig. 1, the range can exceed 40 dB in mid-frequency regions. Different neuron populations can code smaller, overlapping segments of the total dynamic range (range fractionation: 8). This, together with the population of neurons with sloping saturation of CF rate versus intensity functions and other factors (23), can probably account for the large psychophysical dynamic range in humans.

Adaptation

At the onset of an acoustical stimulus, e.g., a tone or noise burst, the discharge rate of a cochlear nerve fiber is maximal and then reduces in an approximately exponential fashion. Such adaptation is illustrated in the peristimulus time histograms (PSTH) of Fig. 5. There appears to be a number of stages to the adaptation

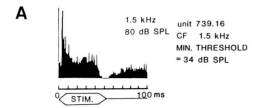

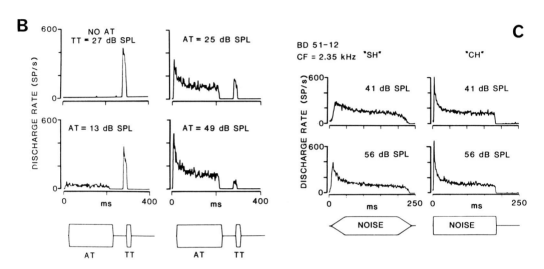

FIG. 5. Adaptation of cochlear-fiber discharge. **A**: Peristimulus time histogram (PSTH) to 50-msec tone presented at 40 dB above threshold. Note rapid initial adaptation followed by a less rapid adaptive process. At stimulus offset, the fiber discharge falls below spontaneous rate; this is termed off-suppression or postadaptation. **B**: Response patterns of a cochlear fiber to a 20-msec test tone (TT) preceded by a 200-msec adapting tone (AT). Both tone bursts have a frequency approximately equal to the fiber CF. The time delay between the two tone bursts is 60 msec. **C**: Response patterns of a fiber to speech-like noise bursts. The stimuli differ only in their rise-fall time, which is 40 msec for the "sh"-like sound and 1 msec for the "ch"-like sound. The bottom panel shows the envelope of the stimuli. (B and C from ref. 11.)

(36,63,108,109,114,116). Over a few milliseconds after stimulus onset, a very rapid adaptation occurs followed by a less rapid one over tens of milliseconds. For longer periods (sec) there appear to be different time constants to the adaptive process.

There is no evidence that hair-cell potentials show adaptation (76,93), and the electrically excited acoustic nerve shows no adaptation (78). Thus, adaptation appears to have its origin at the inner hair-cell synapse and results from various mechanisms that control neurotransmitter release.

When an excitatory sound stimulus terminates, there is a transient decrease of cochlear fiber discharge below spontaneous rate (1,39,108). Such off-suppression or postadaptation can be seen in the PSTH of Fig. 5A. The degree and duration of this off-suppression relate to the amount of adaptation immediately preceding the stimulus offset and are thus determined by the same synaptic mechanisms. Figure 5B illustrates an investigation of postadaptation. A short test-tone burst (TT) is presented after a longer adapting-tone burst (AT). To TT alone there is a large response (Fig. 5B, top left). In the presence of a preceding AT at increasing intensity levels, the response to TT is progressively decreased; the decrease is also dependent on

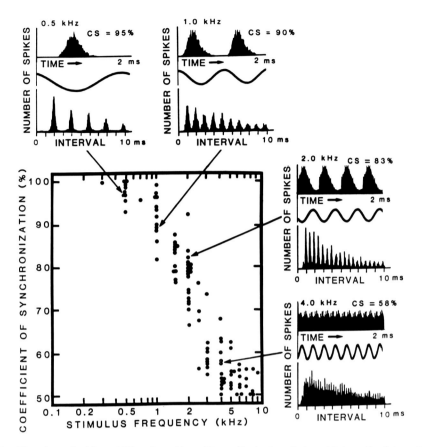

FIG. 6. The phase-locking ability of cochlear fibers. Typical period and interspike interval histograms are shown for fiber responses to pure tone stimuli of 0.5, 1, 2, and 4 kHz. The main graph plots the coefficients of synchronization of responses, i.e., the degree of phase locking to sinusoids as a function of tone frequency. Data are from normal guinea pig cochlear nerve. (From ref. 43.)

the time delay between AT and TT. This phenomenon contributes to psychophysical forward masking phenomena. It is also influential when complex stimuli, such as speech signals, have sequential components (11; see also Responses to Speech Sounds section).

Temporal Coding

In response to a low-frequency sinusoid, a cochlear fiber tends to respond at a particular phase in relation to the stimulus (47,91,92). This phase locking is most evident in response to stimuli below 3 to 5 kHz. In Fig. 6 the response of cochlear neurons to pure tones of 0.5, 1, 2, and 4 kHz is shown in the form of repeated period histograms (a PSTH synchronized to the phase of the stimulus waveform). When a spike occurs it tends to be at a particular phase in relation to the stimulus waveform. A spike does not necessarily occur at every cycle of the stimulus waveform, as can be seen in the analyses of interspike intervals in Fig. 6. In these histograms the bins of the abscissa represent time intervals between spikes. In response to sinusoidal stimuli (0.5, 1, 2, and 4 kHz), the intervals between discharges tend to be integer multiples of the stimulus cycle time.

Phase locking occurs because a cochlear (inner) hair cell is depolarized by deflection of its stereocilia in one direction and this excitation is generated at each cycle of the sound stimulus waveform. This AC receptor potential (93) is thought to directly initiate release of neurotransmitter at the hair-cell synapse. Significant phase locking of fiber responses does not occur at frequencies above 4 to 5 kHz. This is illustrated in Fig. 6, in which the graph shows the fall off in phase-locking ability of cochlear fibers as a function of stimulus frequency. The degree of phase locking is quantified as the number of spikes occurring in the most effective half cycle as a percentage of the total (coefficient of synchronization) (91). Other methods of quantifying phase locking yield similar results (81). A similar fall off in the AC component of the hair-cell receptor potential is also observed at high frequencies (81,93) resulting from the low-pass filtering action of the hair cell. The fall off in phase locking in cochlear-fiber responses thus reflects a limitation of cochlear hair-cell processes.

An important aspect of phase locking is that it can occur without any change in the average rate of discharge of a neuron; it can result from a redistribution of timing of spikes without a change in spike density. Thus, in low-CF fibers phase locking can occur at levels of 20 dB below mean rate threshold and be maintained even when saturation of mean rate has occurred (21–23,26,91).

Response to Broadband Click Stimuli

In response to a broadband acoustical click, a cochlear fiber exhibits a response that depends primarily on cochlear-filtering characteristics. For low-CF fibers the PSTH shows a series of peaks decaying with time in amplitude and having interpeak intervals equal to the reciprocal of the CF. To a first approximation one can consider this pattern to reflect a ringing in the cochlear filter. Because only one phase of basilar membrane movement is effective in exciting the cochlear fiber (more specifically only movement of the stereocilia in one direction is optimal for depolarizing the hair cell), the PSTH histogram represents a half-wave rectified version of the decaying oscillations produced by the filter. For neurons with CF above 4 to 5 kHz, periodic fiber discharge is no longer evident, presumably because of the same limits as for the fall off of phase locking, i.e., the filtering properties of hair-cell membranes. It may also be that the temporal "jitter" associated with the hair-cell synaptic mechanism is also a limiting factor in the maintenance of fine time structure in fiber responses.

For continuous or long-duration, low-frequency tones, the temporal properties of the fiber discharge relate to the stimulus frequency. For impulsive, broadband stimuli, the PSTHs reflect primarily the bandpass characteristics of the cochlear/hair-cell filter. For stimuli that fall between these extreme conditions (e.g., short-tone pips, tones with abrupt onset), responses will reflect contributions of both of these two processes.

Responses to Noise Stimuli

Broadband noise stimuli have been used to investigate the filtering properties of the cochlea using the so-called reverse correlation technique (5,6,21,44,74). In re-

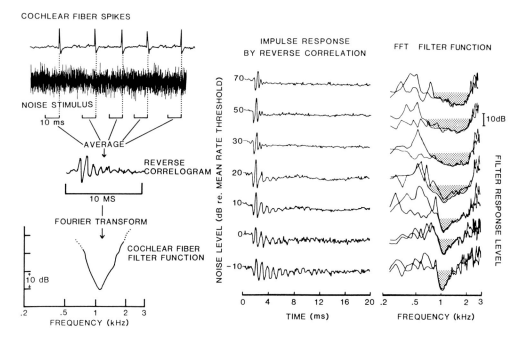

FIG. 7. An analysis of the filtering properties of a cochlear neuron using the reverse correlation technique (6,21,44). The noise stimulus evokes the spike responses in a cochlear neuron as shown in the upper left-hand traces. The frequency components in the noise stimulus that pass through the cochlear filter and evoke a response are assessed by (retro) averaging the 10-msec window of noise preceding each spike. This produces the reverse correlogram that is similar to the impulse response of the system. This response as a function of time can be Fourier transformed to yield the bandpass characteristic of the cochlear-fiber filter. In the middle panel are reverse correlograms derived with noise at −10 dB to 70 dB above the mean-rate threshold for a normal cochlear fiber with a CF of approximately 1 kHz. Fourier transforms are shown to the right, the two superimposed curves are transformed of raw and time-windowed (for smoothing) correlograms. The signal of interest is emphasized by the shaded area.

sponse to a noise stimulus, only the frequency components in the noise that match with (or pass through) the cochlear filter are responsible for spike initiation. A cross-correlation between the noise stimulus waveform and the spike discharge produces a reverse correlogram that is equivalent to the impulse response of the filter. A Fourier transform of this time-domain function yields the filter function of the cochlear fiber. Figure 7 (left) illustrates the stages in a method to derive the reverse correlogram. A sample of the noise stimulus waveform and the spike activity that it evokes are shown in the top diagram. Each spike occurrence triggers an analog average of the noise stimulus in the 10-msec time window directly preceding the spike. This reveals the frequency components passing through the filter that are responsible for spike initiation. Practically, this retro-averaging can be done by recording stimulus and response on magnetic tape and making the average by replaying the tape in reverse. Alternatively, an identical but 10-msec delayed noise can be averaged in real time.

The reverse correlation method depends on the ability of fiber responses to phase lock to low-frequency stimuli, and thus its use is restricted to fibers with CFs below 3 to 5 kHz. Because phase locking is preserved at stimulus levels above the saturation of mean discharge rate (and is also present 10 to 20 dB below mean rate threshold), the reverse correlation method allows investigation of cochlear filtering over a wide dynamic range. Figure 7 (right) shows the filter functions derived with noise stimuli over a 70-dB range. It will be noted that as a function of level, the filtering characteristics change (44,74), being much broader at high levels compared with near threshold. This is also reflected in the increased damping of the oscillations of the reverse correlograms derived at high-stimulus levels (Fig. 7, middle panel).

Noise Masking

If background noise is introduced together with tone or click stimuli, the response of a cochlear neuron to the latter is reduced and eventually abolished. With a broadband masking noise, increments of 10 dB cause threshold changes to the tips of tuning curves by 10 dB, but the tail region is much less elevated in threshold (17). If a low-frequency noise stimulus is used such that only the tail region of a high-CF neuron is stimulated, the threshold of the tail can remain almost unchanged while the tip is raised 10 to 20 dB (58).

Another important effect of background noise is the suppression of the onset peak in discharge rate to tone bursts (63,108). In this case the noise adapts the discharge of the fibers such that additional stimuli cannot effect an increase in discharge. This phenomenon is important in the coding of speech sounds that invariably occur in the presence of background noise (11,13).

Two-Tone Suppression

The firing rate of a cochlear fiber in response to a tone stimulus can be suppressed by a second tone near the CF of the fiber (2,4,50,63,77,96,102). Figure 8 shows the suppressive areas (shaded) for a fiber tuned to 8 kHz. A constant probe stimulus is used to excite the neuron; a second tone whose frequency and intensity combinations fall into the shaded area will reduce the firing rate by 20% or more (4).

In addition to the suppression of mean-discharge rate, this phenomenon has been investigated on a cycle-by-cycle basis to reveal interference with phase locking, a so-called synchrony suppression (3,7,49,51,95). On examination of synchrony suppression it appears that the area of suppression extends throughout the excitatory response area with maximal effects near the CF of the fiber.

There appear to be many similarities between two-tone rate suppression and synchrony suppression and both are thought to reflect nonlinearities in the transduction process. The suppression is not mediated via any inhibitory neural interaction; suppression effects are instantaneous with no neural delay and no neural substrate exists for such interactions.

Combination Tones

Two simultaneously presented tones can give rise to a (psychophysical) sensation of combination tones that are not physically present in the stimulus. Most evident are the difference tone f_2-f_1 and the cubic distortion tone $2f_1-f_2$ in which f_1 and f_2 are

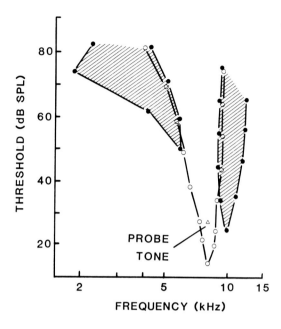

FIG. 8. Two-tone suppression of responses from a normal cochlear fiber. The suppression areas (*shaded*) flank the excitatory tuning curve (*open circles*). A stimulus in the suppression areas was able to reduce the mean firing rate found with the probe by 20% or more. (From ref. 4.)

the primary tone stimuli (and $f_2 > f_1$). When presented such that the combination tone corresponds to the CF of a cochlear fiber (but with the primaries outside the response area) an excitatory response is recorded (35,64,77). Combination tones arise as a result of nonlinear interactions in basilar membrane mechanisms and/or hair-cell transduction. Data on the generation of these distortion products, together with other cochlear nonlinearities (such as two-tone suppression), have been of value for those attempting to model cochlear mechanisms (33,34,38,64,65,88).

RESPONSES TO SPEECH SOUNDS

In recent years attention has been focused on how speech sounds are coded in the cochlear nerve. One approach has been to investigate fiber responses to relatively simple stimuli that are important components of complex speech sounds (11–13,46,54,57,58,86,96,106). For example, rapid amplitude changes together with short, often silent pauses, are common features of speech signals. The intensity of signals can be coded by the rate of discharge, and for the fluctuating amplitude of speech signals it is the onset rate rather than the longer term adapted rate that is most important. The onset rate, being less influenced by adaptation, is a more sensitive indicator of intensity compared with the long-term rate (11).

Because of rapid initial adaptation, the onset response will depend greatly on the envelope rise time for a speech sound. For example, in Fig. 5C PSTH of spike discharge to two noise stimuli with different rise times (sounding like "sh" and "ch," respectively) is illustrated; the time patterns of neural discharge response are very different as are the subjective sounds of these stimuli.

Another important factor is off-suppression or postadaptation. Figure 5B shows that the response to a test tone is significantly reduced by the presence of a preceding adapting tone. Such a situation can often occur in speech signals and is dramatically

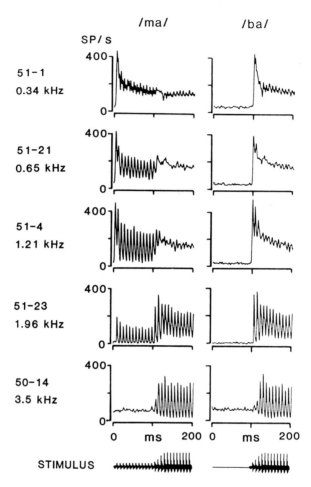

FIG. 9. Response patterns of five single auditory-nerve fibers to /ma/ and /ba/ synthetic stimuli. The stimulus level is approximately 60 dB SPL during the steady-state vowel segment. The histograms are computed from 500 stimulus presentations with a bin width of 1 msec and are three-point smoothed. (From ref. 11.)

demonstrated in Fig. 9. Two synthesized speech sounds, /ma/ and /ba/, stimulate cochlear fibers of different CF. As can be seen from the stimulus waveform (lower trace), the common element is the steady vowel segment /a/, but note how the onset response to this element in the /ba/ sound is much greater because it has not been suppressed by the preceding low-frequency (m) segment.

Representation of Timing Information in Speech

An important aspect of speech coding is the representation of timing information in the temporal discharge of fiber responses. Voiced sounds, including vowels, are generated by low-frequency vibrations of the vocal folds (e.g., 80–160 Hz for adult men). In addition, there are higher frequency formants (see, for example, the amplitude spectrum in Fig. 11), the first three (f_1, f_2, and f_3) being the most important

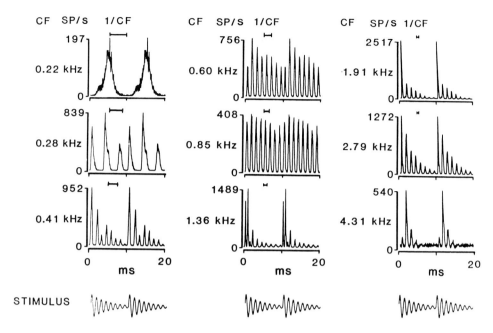

FIG. 10. The temporal coding of vowel-like sounds in the cochlear nerve. Period histograms of nine auditory-nerve fibers to a single-formant stimulus. The stimulus has a fundamental frequency of 100 Hz and a formant of 0.8 kHz. All stimulus levels are between 60 and 63 dB SPL. The unit CFs are about equally spaced on a logarithmic frequency scale. The horizontal marker above each period histogram indicates an interval of 1/CF. (From ref. 11.)

for characterizing a vowel sound. Figure 10 illustrates the responses of nine cochlear fibers to a synthetic, single-formant stimulus (11). The stimulus waveform is shown in the lower traces. It consists of a fundamental frequency (100 Hz) and a single formant at 800 Hz and is presented at approximately 60 dB SPL. The PSTHs (or rather period histograms, because the analysis is time locked to the stimulus phase) clearly show that there are components that correspond to the time structure of the stimulus. Note that when the CF of the fiber is close to the formant frequency (here the fiber tuned to 0.85 kHz), its response pattern is dominated by the formant-frequency component. By contrast, in this fiber's response there is much less evidence of the fundamental component. In other fibers the stimulus fundamental (100 Hz) is well represented. This coding of timing information is an important concept that will be considered later.

Spectral Representation of Speech Sounds

The cochlear nerve can be likened to a bank of overlapping, narrow bandpass filters. The most straightforward neural representation of the spectrum of frequency components in a vowel sound is the discharge rate of a fiber, which is proportional to the energy falling within the bandpass of its tuning curve. This concept and its limitations were examined by Kiang and colleagues (54,55). These authors developed the concept of a neurogram, in which the spectral components of speech sounds are translated into a pattern of neural activity across the tonotopic array of cochlear fibers using a model that incorporates a band of bandpass filters based on real tuning curve data together with other components to stimulate fiber discharge rate saturation and other cochlear nonlinearities.

In the neurogram, spectral energy in speech signals was represented in terms of discharge rate in cochlear fibers, and it was clear that at low-stimulus levels this natural representation was qualitatively similar to the speech spectrogram and therefore an adequately coded version of the speech signal. However, if the stimulus is presented at a high level or in background noise (54,55), this mean-rate representation of the speech was considerably degraded because changes in fiber discharge rates were limited by a saturation of their rate versus intensity functions.

Overall, there are considerable doubts as to whether frequency components in speech sounds can be adequately coded only in terms of mean rate. However, Kiang et al. (54,55) conceded that their model did not include rate-intensity functions with sloping saturation and other factors that might improve the dynamic range of such a mean-rate coding scheme (see also previous section on intensity coding).

Population Studies

Similar conclusions about the inadequacy of a mean-rate coding of spectral components of speech were made (73,82,97,98,117) on the basis of empirical population studies of the representation of speech sounds in the cochlear nerve. These authors recorded the response of many hundreds of cochlear fibers to vowel sounds, in which sounds it is assumed that formant frequency information has to be somehow preserved in the neural code. The lower left-hand panel of Fig. 11 shows the amplitude spectrum of the vowel /e/ that is used as one of the stimuli. The graphs above indicate a measure of the firing rate of approximately 300 cochlear fibers from the cat in response to the stimulus plotted as a function of the fiber CF. Normalized rate expresses the increase in discharge rate of the fiber above spontaneous rate as a function of the maximal (saturation) rate. With the vowel sound presented at 38 dB there is a reasonable representation of the three formant frequencies (arrow symbols) in the mean firing rate. At higher levels this representation is degraded partly because of the saturation of discharge of fibers at high stimulus levels and also because of other nonlinear effects, particularly two-tone suppression (99).

Although the rate-place coding scheme appears to be inadequate, there is considerable information about the frequency content of the stimulus in the temporal pattern of fiber discharges. For example, in Fig. 10, information about the fundamental and formant are clearly present in the period histograms; a histogram of interspike intervals would also contain the same information. Analytically, Fourier transforms of such histograms would reveal large components at frequencies near the formant frequencies present. (An intuitive examination of Fig. 10 should make this evident.) Such Fourier-transform components are a measure of both the firing rate of a fiber and the synchronization of its discharge to frequency components in the (vowel) sound. By averaging Fourier components (for each harmonic of F_0 if the speech sound is voiced) in those neurons whose CF is near each harmonic frequency, one obtains a measure of fiber activity that incorporates rate, timing, and place information. These are called average localized, synchronized rates (13,14,82,99). Similar results are obtained from analysis of interval histograms yielding an average localized

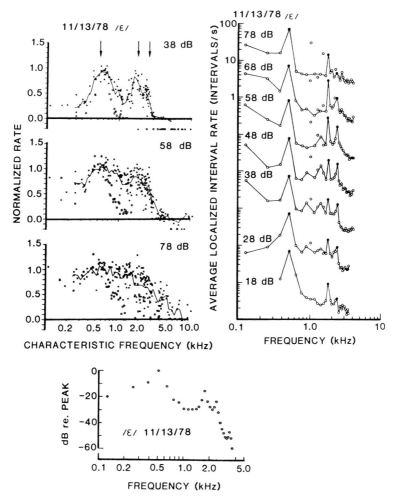

FIG. 11. The representation of vowel sounds in a population of cochlear nerve fibers in the average rate and in temporal aspects of fiber discharge. The lower figure shows the amplitude spectrum of the vowel sound /ɛ/ used as a stimulus. To the left are plots of normalized average rate of discharge for each of a large population of cochlear fibers, plotted as a function of the fibers' characteristic frequencies. The stimulus levels are as indicated in dB SPL. The arrows indicate the frequency positions of the formant frequencies. Note the poor representation of the formant frequencies at high stimulus levels. The right-hand diagram shows the average localized interval rate (ALIR) representation [see text and (99) for details] of the vowel sound, over a range of intensities as indicated in dB SPL. Note the good representation of formant information at high stimulus levels. (From ref. 99.)

interval rate (ALIR) (98,112,117). Such ALIRs are plotted in the right-hand graphs of Fig. 11 as a function of fiber CF. Again the stimulus is the vowel sound /ɛ/; ALIRs were measured in response to stimulus intensities from 18 to 78 dB SPL. A comparison of these data with those on the left, which are based only on discharge rate, indicates how well the representation of formant frequencies is maintained in the timing of fiber responses.

It should be noted that although these internal representations of vowels and other speech sounds are well defined at the level of the cochlear nerve, they all depend on the phase-locking ability of neurons to sound frequency components below 5 kHz. It is not clear whether this phase-locking ability is maintained at higher levels of the auditory pathway, and some evidence (82) suggests that severe degradation occurs at the level of cochlear nucleus even in primary-like neurons. Investigations of the maintenance of neural representation of speech sounds at higher levels of the auditory system and their possible re-representation will be an important area for future research.

FIBER RESPONSES FROM PATHOLOGICAL COCHLEAS

In 1970, Kiang and colleagues published a study (59) on the response properties of neurons from cat cochleas damaged with the ototoxic antibiotic kanamycin. A few years later, Evans (16) reported on fiber responses from mechanically damaged and hypoxic guinea pig cochleas. Since these first studies there have been many investigations of abnormal response properties of neurons from pathological cochleas (9,10,17–19,25,28,36,40–45,56,59,70,71,89,90,100,103,104).

In general, two types of experiment have been described. First, there have been studies of acute (and sometimes reversible) changes in cochlear-fiber response properties, resulting from brief periods of hypoxia, local or systemic drug application, local temperature changes, or short-term noise exposure. These experiments have been designed primarily to dissociate cochlear mechanisms and thus lead to a greater understanding of normal cochlear function. In the second type of experiment chronic damage has been produced in the cochlea, e.g., by poisoning with ototoxic drugs like kanamycin (9,42,59), by overexposure to intense sounds (59,70,100), or by induction of endolymphatic hydrops (45). The main reason for these studies has been to create animal models of cochlear deafness in which detailed electrophysiological recordings from the cochlear nerve in such animals can reveal the functional deficits that we can expect to find in humans with analogously pathological cochleas.

Figure 12 shows the acute effects of systemically injected furosemide, an ototoxic diuretic, on the tuning of a cochlear nerve fiber. The pretreatment FTC is shown by curve A. One minute after injection (B) the low-threshold tip region of the curve is lost (B), but thresholds of the tail region remain relatively unchanged. During a 20-min period the tuning recovers (C–F).

These and similar experiments showed the physiological vulnerability of the sharply tuned tip segment of the FTC and led to the concept of a metabolically active second filter that is responsible for the frequency selectivity of the cochlea, over and above the passive mechanical filter of the basilar membrane. It is now clear that, *in vivo*, the basilar membrane is as sharply tuned as that shown by cochlear fiber responses (53,87,105) but that this tuning depends on some active process at the level of the hair cells, most importantly the outer hair cells to which the basilar membrane is most tightly mechanically coupled. If this coupling is lost or if the cochlea suffers physiological insult, then the sharp basilar membrane tuning is lost.

Figure 13 shows some of the morphological and physiological consequences of poisoning the cochlea with kanamycin (24,42). After 400 mg/kg/day for 8 to 10 days, the basal (high frequency) region of the cochlea has suffered considerable hair-cell degeneration as shown in the lower cochleogram that maps out the hair cells remaining along the total length of the cochlea. The upper diagram of Fig. 13 shows

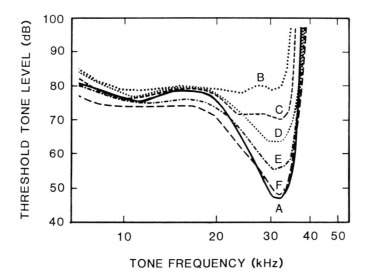

FIG. 12. Physiological vulnerability of cochlear tuning. Effects on the tuning of a single cochlear nerve fiber in cat, from an intra-arterial injection of furosemide, an ototoxic diuretic known to cause reversible hearing loss in humans. A (*solid line*) is the fiber's FTC before injection, B and C are the curves obtained 1 and 2 min, respectively, after injection. Note the progressive loss of the low-threshold, sharply tuned tip segment of the frequency threshold curve until, at C, only a high-threshold, broad curve remains. Curves D, E, and F indicate that the effects on the neural tuning are reversible at this dosage. They were obtained 5, 7, and 20 min after the injection. (From ref. 25.)

tuning curves from a sample of cochlear fibers in this animal. Neurons tuned to high frequency and originating in the damaged region of the cochlea show abnormal response properties. In general, they have elevated thresholds, particularly in the tip region, and have lost their sharp frequency selectivity. In contrast, neurons originating in more intact cochlear regions have more normal tuning curves. The degree to which cochlear fiber tuning deterioration occurs in such kanamycin-treated animals is shown quantitatively in Fig. 3B. Here the open triangles represent $Q_{10\ dB}$ values for fibers originating in cochlear areas where there is more than 90% outer hair-cell loss.

It should be noted that most cochlear fibers originate at, and reflect activity of, inner hair cells. However, in this case of kanamycin poisoning, the loss of outer hair cells is the dominant morphological change. It is possible that the outer hair cells have an important role in the active frequency tuning of the basilar membrane and that their loss has affected the mechanical input to the inner hair cells. It is also possible that the inner hair cells are damaged by the kanamycin poisoning but resist degeneration. Another type of animal model for deafness is one with endolymphatic hydrops (45) as found in Meniere's disease. Cochlear-fiber responses in such an animal indicate a deterioration in tuning but one not usually as severe as in kanamycin-poisoned cochleas. In Fig. 3 the open circles show $Q_{10\ dB}$ values for fiber responses in guinea pigs with endolymphatic hydrops.

Animal Models of Cochlear Deafness

Figure 14 contrasts normal cochlear-fiber responses with those from a cochlea with a 50- to 60-dB threshold elevation across all frequencies caused by kanamycin

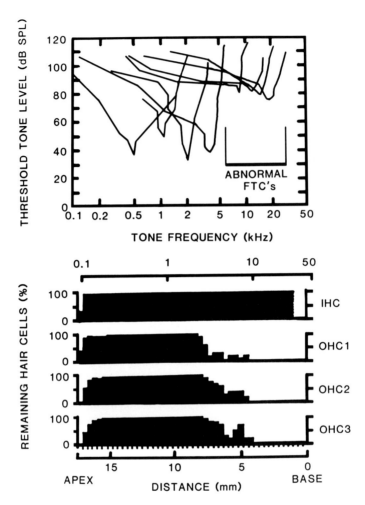

FIG. 13. The effects of hair-cell damage caused by kanamycin poisoning on the thresholds and tuning properties of cochlear neurons. The lower graph indicates the damage to hair cells caused by poisoning with kanamycin (400 mg/kg/day for 8 days). The upper diagrams shows FTCs from this cochlea. Neurons originating in the basal, damaged area of the cochlea show reduced sensitivity (only respond to high levels of sound stimulation) and abnormal tuning. (From ref. 24.)

poisoning. The deterioration of cochlear-fiber tuning results in a degradation of frequency selectivity, which is the ability of the cochlea to resolve the frequency components that are simultaneously present in a complex sound. It is assumed that this will also be the case in human cochlear deafness. Indeed, there are many psychophysical (67,85,115) and evoked potential studies (15,41) in patients that confirm this.

For patients with cochlear hearing loss, poor frequency selectivity should result in a deterioration in speech intelligibility. This is based on the assumption that formant frequency patterns and other spectral cues in speech sounds are coded into a spatial pattern of nerve-fiber excitation that is recognized by higher auditory centers and that a degraded pattern of excitation will be less recognizable. From the limited experimental data available, there is only approximate correlation between speech

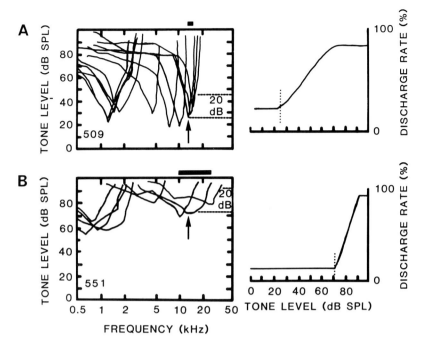

FIG. 14. A comparison of some cochlear fiber response properties from the normal (**A**) and a kanamycin-poisoned pathological cochlea (**B**); on the left are samples of FTCs. To the right are typical discharge rate versus intensity functions for a tonal stimulus at the CF of the fiber. See text for details.

intelligibility and poor frequency selectivity—not as close as some might expect. In addition, a deterioration in the analysis of spectral cues should, theoretically, interfere with sound localization in space.

Apart from the loss of sharp frequency selectivity, cochlear damage also changes the way in which the intensity of sounds is encoded. In the normal cochlea, when a tone at the characteristic frequency is increased in intensity, the changes in cochlear fiber discharge rate are as indicated in the top right of Fig. 14. In damaged cochleas, which result in a loss of the tips to the tuning curves, the rate of spike discharge versus stimulus intensity is as shown in the lower right-hand diagram. It is a much steeper function than that for the normal cochlea (17,40,43); in other words, when a sound stimulus has been increased from threshold to 20 dB above threshold, the cochlear neurons are discharging at maximum rate. One of the most common symptoms of hearing loss of cochlear origin is loudness recruitment. In the animal models we see the steep discharge rate versus intensity functions that may well contribute to the loudness recruitment phenomenon. It must be said that we do not know exactly how loudness is encoded in the brain. However, we can reasonably expect all cues to be used; the two major cues are the spike discharge rate of individual auditory neurons and the total number of neurons active. With regard to the latter, the widening of the response area of neurons in pathological cochleas will mean that for any particular intensity level of stimulation, a larger population of neurons will be stimulated compared with the normal cochlea (16,40,59). In Fig. 14 this spread of excitation is indicated by the bar symbols on the upper abscissae, which represent the cochlear region containing neurons that will be excited by a pure tone stimulus presented 20 dB above its threshold level (see arrow symbols).

This overview of animal models of deafness has shown some of the links between basic physiological research findings and symptoms or problems of cochlear hearing loss in humans. The elucidation of these pathophysiological mechanisms is one purpose of auditory science.

ACKNOWLEDGMENTS

The author is supported by the Canadian Medical Research Council (PG-13, MA-9330) and research grants from the Masonic Foundation of Ontario. R. Mount and B. Rutledge are thanked for their help in preparation of the manuscript.

REFERENCES

1. Abbas, P. J. (1979): Effects of stimulus frequency on adaptation in auditory-nerve fibers. *J. Acoust. Soc. Am.*, 65:162–165.
2. Abbas, P. J., and Sachs, M. B. (1976): Two-tone suppression in auditory-nerve fibers: Extension of a stimulus-response relationship. *J. Acoust. Soc. Am.*, 59:112–122.
3. Arthur, R. M. (1976): Harmonic analysis of two-tone discharge patterns in cochlear nerve fibers. *Biol. Cybern.*, 22:21–31.
4. Arthur, R. M., Pfeiffer, R. R., and Suga, N. (1971): Properties of "two-tone inhibition" in primary auditory neurones. *J. Physiol.*, 212:593–609.
5. de Boer, E., and de Jongh, H. R. (1978): On cochlear encoding: Potentialities and limitations of the reverse correlation technique. *J. Acoust. Soc. Am.*, 63:115–135.
6. de Boer, E., and Jongkees, L. B. W. (1968): On cochlear sharpening and cross-correlation methods. *Acta Otolaryngol. (Stockh.)*, 65:97–104.
7. Brugge, J. F., Anderson, D. J., Hind, J. E., and Rose, J. E. (1969): Time structure of discharges in single auditory nerve fibers of the squirrel monkey in response to complex periodic sounds. *J. Neurophysiol.*, 32:386–407.
8. Cohen, M. J. (1964): The peripheral organization of sensory systems. In: *Neural Theory and Modelling*, edited by R. F. Reiss, pp. 273–292. Stanford University Press, Stanford, CA.
9. Dallos, P., and Harris, D. (1978): Properties of auditory nerve responses in absence of outer haircells. *J. Neurophysiol.*, 41:365–383.
10. Dallos, P., Ryan, A., Harris, D., McGee, T., and Ozdamar, O. (1977): Cochlear frequency selectivity in the presence of haircell damage. In: *Psychophysics and Physiology of Hearing*, edited by E. F. Evans and J. P. Wilson, pp. 249–258. Academic, London.
11. Delgutte, B. (1980): Representation of speech-like sounds in the discharge patterns of auditory-nerve fibers. *J. Acoust. Soc. Am.*, 68:843–857.
12. Delgutte, B. (1984): Speech coding in the auditory nerve II. Processing schemes for vowel-like sounds. *J. Acoust. Soc. Am.*, 75:879–886.
13. Delgutte, B., and Kiang, N. Y. S. (1984): Speech coding in the auditory nerve I. Vowel-like sounds. *J. Acoust. Soc. Am.*, 75:866–878.
14. Delgutte, B., and Kiang, N. Y. S. (1984): Speech coding in the auditory nerve: V. Vowels in background noise. *J. Acoust. Soc. Am.*, 75:908–918.
15. Eggermont, J. J. (1977): Compound action potential tuning curves in normal and pathological human ears. *J. Acoust. Soc. Am.*, 62:1247–1251.
16. Evans, E. F. (1972): The frequency response and other properties of single fibres in the guinea-pig cochlear nerve. *J. Physiol.*, 226:263–287.
17. Evans, E. F. (1974): Auditory frequency selectivity and the cochlear nerve. In: *Facts and Models in Hearing*, edited by E. Zwicker and E. Terhardt, pp. 118–129. Springer, Berlin.
18. Evans, E. F. (1975): The sharpening of cochlear frequency selectivity in the normal and abnormal cochlea. *Audiology*, 14:419–442.
19. Evans, E. F. (1975): Normal and abnormal functioning of the cochlear nerve. In: *Sound Reception in Mammals*. Symp. Zool. Soc. Lond. 197, 37:133–165. Academic, London.
20. Evans, E. F. (1975): The cochlear nerve and cochlear nucleus. In: *Handbook of Sensory Physiology*, vol. 5, pt. 2, edited by W. D. Keidel and W. D. Neff, pp. 1–108. Springer, Heidelberg.

21. Evans, E. F. (1977): Frequency selectivity at high signal levels of single units in cochlear nerve and nucleus. In: *Psychophysics and Physiology of Hearing*, edited by E. F. Evans and J. P. Wilson, pp. 185–192. Academic, London.
22. Evans, E. F. (1978): Place and time coding of frequency in the peripheral auditory system: Some physiological pros and cons. *Audiology*, 17:369–420.
23. Evans, E. F. (1981): The dynamic range problem: Place and time coding at the level of the cochlear nerve and nucleus. In: *Neuronal Mechanisms of Hearing*, edited by J. Syka and L. Aitkin, pp. 69–85. Plenum, New York.
24. Evans, E. F., and Harrison, R. V. (1976): Correlation between outer hair cell damage and deterioration of cochlear nerve tuning properties in the guinea pig. *J. Physiol.*, 256:43–53.
25. Evans, E. F., and Klinke, R. (1974): Reversible effects of cyanide and furosemide on the tuning of single cochlear fibres. *J. Physiol.*, 242:129–131.
26. Evans, E. F., and Palmer, A. R. (1979): On the peripheral coding of the level of individual frequency components of complex sounds at high levels. *Exp. Brain. Res.*, Suppl. II:19–26.
27. Evans, E. F., and Palmer, A. R. (1980): Relationship between the dynamic range of cochlear nerve fibres and their spontaneous activity. *Exp. Brain Res.*, 40:115–118.
28. Evans, E. F., Wilson, J. P., and Borerwe, T. A. (1981): Animal models of tinnitus. In: *Tinnitus* (Ciba Foundation Symposium 85), edited by D. Evered and G. Lawrenson, pp. 108–129. Pitman, Bath.
29. Galambos, R., and Davis, H. (1943): Response of single auditory nerve fibres to acoustic stimulation. *J. Neurophysiol.*, 6:39–57.
30. Galambos, R., and Davis, H. (1948): Action potentials from single auditory nerve fibres? *Science*, 108:513.
31. Gacek, R. R., and Rasmussen, G. L. (1957): Fiber analysis of the acoustic nerve of cat, monkey and guinea pig. *Anat. Rec.*, 127:417.
32. Geisler, C. D., Mountain, D. C., and Hubbard, A. E. (1980): Sound-induced resistance changes in the inner ear. *J. Acoust. Soc. Am.*, 61:1557–1566.
33. Geisler, C. D., and Sinex, D. G. (1980): Responses of primary auditory fibers to combined noise and tonal stimuli. *Hear. Res.*, 3:317–334.
34. Goblick, T., and Pfeiffer, R. R. (1969): Time domain measurements of cochlear nonlinearities using combination click stimuli. *J. Acoust. Soc. Am.*, 46:924–938.
35. Goldstein, J. L., and Kiang, N. Y. S. (1968): Neural correlates of the aural combination tone $2f_1-f_2$. *Proc. IEEE*, 56:981–992.
36. Gorga, M. P., and Abbas, P. J. (1981): AP measurements of short term adaptation in normal and acoustically traumatized ears. *J. Acoust. Soc. Am.*, 70:1310–1321.
37. Guild, S. R. (1932): Correlations of the histological observations and the acuity of hearing. *Acta Otolaryngol. (Stockh.)*, 17:207–249.
38. Hall, J. L. (1980): Cochlear models: Two-tone suppression and the second filter. *J. Acoust. Soc. Am.*, 67:1722–1728.
39. Harris, D. M., and Dallos, P. (1979): Forward masking of auditory nerve fiber responses. *J. Neurophysiol.*, 42:1083–1107.
40. Harrison, R. V. (1981): Rate-versus-intensity functions and related AP responses in normal and pathological guinea pig and human cochleas. *J. Acoust. Soc. Am.*, 70:1036–1044.
41. Harrison, R. V., Aran, J.-M., and Erre, J. P. (1981): AP tuning curves from normal and pathological human and guinea pig cochleas. *J. Acoust. Soc. Am.*, 69:1374–1385.
42. Harrison, R. V., and Evans, E. F. (1977): The effects of hair cell loss (restricted to outer hair cells) on the threshold and tuning properties of cochlear fibres in the guinea pig. In: *Inner Ear Biology*, Coll. INSERM, edited by M. Portmann and J.-M. Aran, pp. 105–124. INSERM, Paris.
43. Harrison, R. V., and Evans, E. F. (1979): Cochlear fibre responses in guinea pigs with well defined cochlear lesions. *Scand. Audiol. [Suppl.]*, 9:83–92.
44. Harrison, R. V., and Evans, E. F. (1982): Reverse correlation study of cochlear filtering in normal and pathological guinea pig ears. *Hear. Res.*, 6:303–314.
45. Harrison, R. V., and Prijs, V. F. (1984): Single cochlear fibre responses in guinea pigs with longterm endolymphatic hydrops. *Hear. Res.*, 14:79–84.
46. Hashimoto, T., Katayama, Y., Murata, K., and Taniguchi, I. (1975): Pitch synchronous response of cat cochlear nerve fibers to speech sounds. *Jpn. J. Physiol.*, 25:633–644.
47. Hind, J. E. (1972): Physiological correlation of auditory stimulus periodicity. *Audiology*, 11:42–57.
48. Jacobs, M. S., and Jensen, A. V. (1964): Gross aspects of the brain and fiber analysis of the cranial nerves in the great whale. *J. Comp. Neurol.*, 123:55–72.
49. Javel, E. (1981): Suppression of auditory nerve responses. I. Temporal analysis, intensity effects and suppression contours. *J. Acoust. Soc. Am.*, 69:1735–1745.
50. Javel, E., Geisler, C. D., and Ravindran, A. (1978): Two-tone suppression in auditory nerve of the cat: Rate-intensity and temporal analyses. *J. Acoust. Soc. Am.*, 63:1093–1104.
51. Javel, E., McGee, J., Walsh, E. J., Farley, G. R., and Gorga, M. P. (1983): Suppression of auditory

nerve responses. II. Suppression threshold and growth, iso-suppression contours. *J. Acoust. Soc. Am.*, 74:801–813.

52. Katsuki, Y., Sumi, T., Uchiyama, H., and Watenabe, T. (1958): Electric response of auditory neurones in cat to sound stimulation. *J. Neurophysiol.*, 21:509–588.

53. Khanna, S. M., and Leonard, D. G. B. (1982): Basilar membrane tuning in the cat cochlea. *Science*, 215:305–306.

54. Kiang, N. Y. S. (1980): Processing of speech by the auditory nervous system. *J. Acoust. Soc. Am.*, 68:830–835.

55. Kiang, N. Y. S., Eddington, D. K., and Delgutte, B. (1979): Fundamental considerations in designing auditory implants. *Acta Otolaryngol. (Stockh.)*, 87:204–218.

56. Kiang, N. Y. S., Liberman, M. C., and Levine, R. A. (1976): Auditory nerve activity in cats exposed to ototoxic drugs and high intensity sounds. *Ann. Otol. Rhinol. Laryngol.*, 85:752–768.

57. Kiang, N. Y. S., and Moxon, E. C. (1972): Physiological considerations in artificial stimulation of the inner ear. *Ann. Otol. Rhinol. Laryngol.*, 81:714–730.

58. Kiang, N. Y. S., and Moxon, E. C. (1974): Tails of tuning curves of auditory-nerve fibers. *J. Acoust. Soc. Am.*, 55:620–630.

59. Kiang, N. Y. S., Moxon, E. C., and Levine, R. A. (1970): Auditory nerve activity in cats with normal and abnormal cochleas. In: *Sensorineural Hearing Loss*, edited by G. E. W. Wolstenholme, and K. Knight, pp. 241–268. Churchill, London.

60. Kiang, N. Y. S., Rho, J. M., Northrop, C. C., Liberman, M. C., and Ryugo, D. K. (1982): Hair-cell innervation by spiral ganglion cells in adult cats. *Science*, 217:175–177.

61. Kiang, N. Y. S., Sachs, M. B., and Peake, W. T. (1967): Shapes of tuning curves for single auditory nerve fibers. *J. Acoust. Soc. Am.*, 42:1341–1342.

62. Kiang, N. Y. S., Watenabe, T., Thomas, E. C., and Clark, L. F. (1962): Stimulus coding in the cat's auditory nerve. *Ann. Otol. Rhinol. Laryngol.*, 71:1009–1026.

63. Kiang, N. Y. S., Watenabe, T., Thomas, E. C., and Clark, L. F. (1965): *Discharge Patterns of Single Fibers in the Cat's Auditory Nerve.* MIT Press, Cambridge, MA.

64. Kim, D. O., Molnar, E. C., and Matthews, J. W. (1980): Cochlear mechanisms: Nonlinear behavior in two-tone responses as reflected in cochlear-nerve-fiber response and in ear-canal sound pressure. *J. Acoust. Soc. Am.*, 67:1704–1721.

65. Kim, D. O., Molnar, C. E., and Pfeiffer, R. R. (1973): A system of nonlinear differential equations modeling basilar membrane motion. *J. Acoust. Soc. Am.*, 54:1517–1529.

66. Kim, D. O., Siegel, J. H., and Molnar, C. E. (1979): Cochlear nonlinear phenomena in two-tone responses. *Scand. Audiol. [Suppl.]*, 9:63–81.

67. Leshowitz, B., and Lindstrom, R. (1977): Measurements of non-linearities in listeners with sensorineural hearing loss. In: *Psychophysics and Physiology of Hearing*, edited by E. F. Evans and J. P. Wilson, pp. 283–292. Academic, London.

68. Liberman, M. C. (1978): Auditory-nerve responses from cats raised in a low-noise chamber. *J. Acoust. Soc. Am.*, 63:442–455.

69. Liberman, M. C. (1980): Morphological differences among radial afferent fibres in the cat cochlea: An electron microscopic study of serial sections. *Hear. Res.*, 3:45–63.

70. Liberman, M. C., and Kiang, N. Y. S. (1978): Acoustic trauma in cats. *Acta Otolaryngol. [Suppl.] (Stockh.)*, 358:1–63.

71. Liberman, M. C., and Mulroy, M. J. (1982): Acute and chronic effects of acoustic trauma: Cochlear pathology and auditory nerve pathophysiology. In: *New Perspectives on Noise-Induced Hearing Loss*, edited by R. P. Hamernik, D. Henderson, and R. Salvi, pp. 105–135. Raven Press, New York.

72. Lorente de Nó, R. (1933): Anatomy of the eighth nerve. The central projection of the nerve endings of the inner ear. *Laryngoscope*, 43:1–38.

73. Miller, M. I., and Sachs, M. B. (1983): Representation of stop consonants in the discharge patterns of auditory-nerve fibers. *J. Acoust. Soc. Am.*, 74:502–517.

74. Moller, A. R. (1978): Frequency selectivity of the peripheral auditory analyser studied using broadband noise. *Acta Physiol. Scand.*, 104:24–32.

75. Morrison, D., Schindler, R. A., and Wersall, J. (1975): A quantitative analysis of the afferent innervation of the organ of Corti in guinea pig. *Acta Otolaryngol. (Stockh.)*, 79:11–23.

76. Mulroy, M. J., Altmann, D. W., Weiss, T. F., and Peak, W. T. (1974): Intracellular electric responses to sound in a vertebrate cochlea. *Nature*, 249:482–485.

77. Nomoto, M., Suga, N., and Katsuki, Y. (1964): Discharge pattern and inhibition of primary and auditory nerve fibers in the monkey. *J. Neurophysiol.*, 27:768–787.

78. Norris, C. H., Guth, P. S., and Daigneault, E. A. (1977): The site at which peripheral auditory adaptation occurs. *Brain Res.*, 123:176–179.

79. Palmer, A. R., and Evans, E. F. (1979): On the peripheral coding of the level of individual frequency components of complex sounds at high levels. *Exp. Brain Res.*, Suppl. II:19–26.

80. Palmer, A. R., and Evans, E. F. (1982): Intensity coding in the auditory periphery of the cat. *Hear. Res.*, 7:305–324.

81. Palmer, A. R., and Russell, I. J. (1986): Phase locking in the cochlear nerve of the guinea pig and its relation to the receptor potential of inner hair-cells. *Hear. Res.*, 24:1–15.

82. Palmer, A. R., Winter, I. M., and Darwin, C. J. (1986): The representation of steady-state vowel sounds in the temporal discharge patterns of the guinea pig cochlear nerve and primary like cochlear nucleus neurons. *J. Acoust. Soc. Am.*, 79:100–113.

83. Perkins, R. E., and Morest, D. K. (1975): A study of cochlear innervation in cats and rats with Golgi methods and Nomarski optics. *J. Comp. Neurol.*, 163:129–158.

84. Pfeiffer, R. R., and Kim, D. O. (1975): Cochlear nerve fiber responses: Distribution along the cochlear partition. *J. Acoust. Soc. Am.*, 58:867–869.

85. Pick, G. F., Evans, E. F., and Wilson, J. P. (1977): Frequency resolution in patients with hearing loss of cochlear origin. In: *Psychophysics and Physiology of Hearing*, edited by E. F. Evans and J. P. Wilson, pp. 273–281. Academic, London.

86. Reale, R. A., and Geisler, C. D. (1980): Auditory-nerve fiber encoding of two-tone approximations to steady state vowels. *J. Acoust. Soc. Am.*, 67:891–902.

87. Rhode, W. S. (1971): Observations of the vibrations of the basilar membrane in squirrel monkeys using the Mossbauer technique. *J. Acoust. Soc. Am.*, 49:1218–1231.

88. Rhode, W. S. (1980): Cochlear partition vibration—recent reviews. *J. Acoust. Soc. Am.*, 67:158–176.

89. Robertson, D., Cody, A. R., Bredberg, G., and Johnston. B. M. (1980): Response properties of spiral ganglion neurons in cochleas damaged by direct mechanical trauma. *J. Acoust. Soc. Am.*, 67:1295–1303.

90. Robertson, D., and Manley, G. (1974): Manipulation of frequency analysis in the cochlear ganglion of the guinea pig. *J. Comp. Physiol. Psychol.*, 91:363–375.

91. Rose, J. E., Brugge, J. F., Anderson, D. J., and Hind, J. E. (1967): Phase-locked responses to low frequency tones in single auditory nerve fibers of the squirrel monkey. *J. Neurophysiol.*, 30:769–793.

92. Rose, J. E., Hind, J. E., Anderson, D. J., and Brugge, J. F. (1971): Some effects of stimulus intensity on response of auditory nerve fibers in the squirrel monkey. *J. Neurophysiol.*, 34:685–699.

93. Russell, I. J., and Sellick, P. M. (1977): Intracellular studies of haircells in the mammalian cochlea. *J. Physiol.*, 284:261–290.

94. Sachs, M. B., and Abbas, P. J. (1974): Rate versus level functions for auditory-nerve fibers in cats: Tone burst stimuli. *J. Acoust. Soc. Am.*, 56:1835–1847.

95. Sachs, M. B., and Hubbard, A. E. (1981): Responses of auditory-nerve fibers to characteristic frequency tones and low-frequency suppressors. *Hear. Res.*, 4:309–324.

96. Sachs, M. B., and Kiang, N. Y. S. (1968): Tow-tone inhibition in auditory nerve fibers. *J. Acoust. Soc. Am.*, 43:1120–1128.

97. Sachs, M. B., Voigt, H. F., and Young, E. D. (1983): Auditory nerve representation of vowels in background noise. *J. Neurophysiol.*, 50:27–45.

98. Sachs, M. B., and Young, E. D. (1979): Encoding of steady state vowels in the auditory nerve: Representation in terms of discharge rate. *J. Acoust. Soc. Am.*, 66:470–479.

99. Sachs, M. B., and Young, E. D. (1980): Effects of nonlinearities of speech encoding in the cochlear nerve. *J. Acoust. Soc. Am.*, 68:858–875.

100. Salvi, R., Perry, J. P., Hamernik, R. P., and Henderson, D. (1982): Relationships between cochlear pathologies and auditory nerve and behavioral responses following acoustic trauma. In: *New Perspectives on Noise-Induced Hearing Loss*, edited by R. P. Hamernik, D. Henderson, and R. Salvi, pp. 165–188. Raven Press, New York.

101. Sando, I. (1965): The anatomical inter-relationships of the cochlear nerve fibres. *Acta Otolaryngol. (Stockh.)*, 59:417–436.

102. Schmiedt, R. A. (1982): Boundaries of two-tone rate suppression of cochlear-nerve activity. *Hear. Res.*, 7:335–351.

103. Schmiedt, R. A. (1984): Acoustic injury and the physiology of hearing. *J. Acoust. Soc. Am.*, 76:1293–1317.

104. Schmiedt, R. A., Zwislocki, J. J., and Hamernik, R. P. (1980): Effects of hair cell lesions on responses of cochlear nerve fibres. I. Lesions, tuning curves, two tone inhibition and responses to trapezoidal-wave patterns. *J. Neurophysiol.*, 43:1367–1389.

105. Sellick, P. M., Patuzzi, R., and Johnstone, B. M. (1982): Measurement of basilar membrane motion in the guinea pig using the Mossbauer technique. *J. Acoust. Soc. Am.*, 72:131–141.

106. Sinex, D. G., and Geisler, C. D. (1983): Responses of auditory-nerve fibers to consonant-vowel syllables. *J. Acoust. Soc. Am.*, 73:602–615.

107. Smith, C. A. (1975): Innervation of the cochlea of guinea pig by use of the Golgi stain. *Ann. Otol. Rhinol. Laryngol.*, 84:443–459.

108. Smith, R. L. (1979): Adaptation, saturation and physiological masking in single auditory-nerve fibers. *J. Acoust. Soc. Am.*, 65:166–178.

109. Smith, R. L., and Zwislocki, J. J. (1975): Short term adaptation and incremental responses of single auditory nerve fibers. *Biol. Cybern.*, 17:169–182.
110. Spoendlin, H. (1970): The structural basis of peripheral frequency analysis. In: *Frequency Analysis and Periodicity Detection in Hearing*, edited by R. Plomp and G. F. Smoorenburg, pp. 2–36. Sijthoff, Leiden.
111. Tasaki, I. (1954): Nerve impulses in individual auditory nerve fibers of the guinea pig. *J. Neurophysiol.*, 17:97–122.
112. Voigt, H. F., Sachs, M. D., and Young, E. D. (1982): Representation of whispered vowels in discharge patterns of auditory nerve fibers. *Hear. Res.*, 8:49–58.
113. Webster, D. B. (1971): Projection of the cochlea to the cochlear nuclei in Merriam's Kangaroo rat. *J. Comp. Neurol.*, 143:323–340.
114. Westerman, L. A., and Smith, R. L. (1984): Rapid and short term adaptation in auditory nerve responses. *Hear. Res.*, 15:249–260.
115. Wightman, F., McGee, T., and Kramer, M. (1977): Factors influencing frequency selectivity in normal and hearing impaired listeners. In: *Psychophysics and Physiology of Hearing*, edited by E. F. Evans and J. P. Wilson, pp. 295–306. Academic, London.
116. Yates, G. K., and Robertson, D. (1980): Very rapid adaptation in auditory ganglion cells. In: *Psychophysical, Physiological and Behavioural Studies in Hearing*, edited by G. van der Brink and F. A. Bilsen, pp. 200–205. Delft University Press, Delft.
117. Young, E. D., and Sachs, M. B. (1979): Representation of steady state vowels in the temporal aspects of the discharge patterns of populations of auditory nerve fibers. *J. Acoust. Soc. Am.*, 66:1381–1403.

Physiology of the Ear,
edited by A. F. Jahn and J. Santos-Sacchi.
Raven Press, New York © 1988.

Neurotransmission in the Inner Ear

*Sanford C. Bledsoe, Jr., **Richard P. Bobbin, and
**Jean-Luc Puel

*Kresge Hearing Research Institute, Department of Otolaryngology, The University of
Michigan, Ann Arbor, Michigan 48109-0506, and **Kresge Hearing Research Laboratory
of the South, Department of Otolaryngology and Biocommunication, Louisiana State
University Medical School, New Orleans, Louisiana 70112-2234*

One area of interest for auditory scientists has been the elucidation of mechanisms of intercellular communication associated with sensory transduction in the inner ear. A major focus to date has been to identify: (a) the neurotransmitters released on the primary afferent neurons at the base of the inner and outer hair cells, i.e., the hair cell transmitters or primary afferent neurotransmitters; (b) the neurotransmitters released on the hair cells and on the afferent endings under the hair cells by efferent neurons originating in the brain stem, i.e., the efferent neurotransmitters in the cochlea; and (c) the neuromodulators that act on the cells in the cochlea. The purpose of this chapter is to review the available evidence concerning the identity of these chemicals in the inner ear. Particular emphasis is given to discussing the hypothesis that the excitatory transmitter released by hair cells is an amino acid (such as glutamate) or structurally related compound. Much of the evidence pertaining to the glutamate hypothesis comes from studies on the amphibian lateral line. Thus, findings in this hair cell system are also discussed and placed in perspective with those in the cochlea and other octavolateralis organs. Many review articles that deal with this topic have been published, and the reader is referred to them for additional material (10,31,33,72,85).

AFFERENT SYNAPTIC TRANSMISSION

Octavolateralis organs comprise a group of sensory structures that includes the inner ear of mammals and lateral-line system of fishes and aquatic amphibia (63,112). The sensory epithelia of these organs contain mechanoreceptive hair cells, supporting cells, and nerve terminals and fibers coming from the central nervous system (CNS). In the cochlea the encoding of sounds is a complex process involving inner and outer hair cells that receive both afferent and efferent innervation. It is generally agreed that the inner hair cells, which receive the bulk of the afferent innervation, are the primary sensory cells of transduction, whereas the outer hair cells, which receive the bulk of the efferent innervation, may modulate transduction through a mechanical process (99). A key function of inner hair cells is to release a chemical transmitter that diffuses across a synaptic cleft to activate specialized postsynaptic receptors and depolarize the afferent nerve fibers sufficiently to generate an action potential. There is general agreement that one chemical substance probably carries out this function. At other sites in the CNS where synaptic action is as rapid as in the cochlea the transmitter has been referred to as the transmitter of fast transmission although the chemical may not be the same at all fast transmission sites (52). This should in no way lead the reader to believe that only one chemical is released from hair cells during sound stimulation, for, in addition to the mediator of fast transmission, other chemicals are most probably released from hair cells, nerve endings, and even supporting cells, which then act on receptors located on the hair cells or afferents to alter responsiveness to the fast transmitter. These chemicals are called modulators to distinguish them from fast transmitters and have been found in the retina and other nervous structures (126).

In octavolateralis systems neither the identity of the hair cell transmitter(s), the nature of the afferent postsynaptic receptors, nor the molecular events associated with hair cell/afferent fiber interaction have been well established. Evidence largely from pharmacological studies has, however, provided considerable insight as to what the hair cell transmitter is not, although these substances may function as modulators. Thus, it is reasonably clear that the mediator of fast transmission is not acetylcholine (ACh), 5-hydroxytryptamine, norepinephrine, dopamine, glycine, taurine, or substance P (31,72,85). More recently, a number of substances, including excitatory amino acids (glutamate and aspartate), gamma-aminobutyric acid (GABA), a GABA-like compound, and the auditory nerve activating substance (ANAS), have been advanced as potential candidates. To date, the evidence best supports the hypothesis that the transmitter is an excitatory amino acid, possibly glutamate, or a structurally related compound. Before reviewing this evidence, a discussion of the criteria for transmitter identification is provided to serve as a framework for an evaluation of the merits of this hypothesis.

CRITERIA FOR NEUROTRANSMITTER/NEUROMODULATOR IDENTIFICATION

A number of criteria need to be satisfied in order to establish a chemical as the endogenous neurotransmitter at a specific synapse (130). The neuromodulator criteria are the same as for neurotransmitters except for the requirement that the chemical be excluded as acting like a neurotransmitter and instead be shown to modify the actions of the neurotransmitter (126). Among the transmitter criteria are the following:

1. Identical action: The transmitter candidate, when applied to the synapse, should elicit a postsynaptic response that mimics the response produced by natural stimulation of the presynaptic element.
2. Pharmacological identity: Substances that influence the natural postsynaptic response should also have the same influence on the response elicited by the transmitter candidate.
3. Stimulus-induced release: Stimulation of the presynaptic element should result in the release of the transmitter candidate, and this release should be dependent on extracellular calcium (Ca^{2+}).
4. Presynaptic location: The transmitter candidate must be shown to exist presynaptically associated with structures capable of its release.

5. Synthetic enzymes: Enzymes responsible for the biosynthesis of the transmitter candidate must be present in the presynaptic element of the synapse.
6. Inactivation mechanism: A mechanism must be demonstrated that can either remove the transmitter candidate from the synaptic cleft or inactivate its physiological influence on the postsynaptic receptors.

The inner ear offers a number of advantages for studies of these criteria for neurotransmitters and modulators. For example, in the cochlea, perilymph, which is in diffusional contact with the hair cells, is a convenient route for the administration of drugs in known concentrations and the collection of release samples for assay. In addition, a number of electrophysiological potentials can be recorded from the cochlea in the presence and absence of sound that reflect not only the functional integrity of the cochlea, but also various steps in the process of afferent neural excitation. Nevertheless, many theoretical and technological difficulties are encountered in the inner ear and other hair cell systems. For example, owing to the small size of the afferent terminals contacting hair cells in the cochlea, it is not yet technically feasible to test stringently the criteria of identical action and pharmacological identity with intracellular measurements of membrane potential and conductance changes. Pharmacological investigations of afferent transmission have therefore relied on less direct evidence obtained with extracellular measurements of afferent nerve activity. For this reason, many have viewed the stimulus-induced release criterion to be of critical importance in studies on the inner ear. The interpretation of release data is made difficult, however, by the small numbers of hair cells and the heterogeneity of the tissues involved. In the final analysis, one must be aware of and be willing to accept the many theoretical and technological difficulties associated with applying transmitter criteria to hair cell systems.

GLUTAMATE HYPOTHESIS IN HAIR CELL SYSTEMS

In comparison with the CNS, the evidence for excitatory amino acids as transmitters in the inner ear is rudimentary and has been the subject of much debate and controversy (33,44,76). There is also growing recognition that the hair cell transmitter may not be the same in all members of the octavolateralis system (98). For instance, the hypothesis that GABA may be a hair cell transmitter in the mammalian vestibular labyrinth (54,97) will be discussed in a later section. In this section, evidence pertaining to glutamate (Glu) in the mammalian cochlea and amphibian lateral line is surveyed. Some recent findings in other octavolateralis organs are also discussed. Much of the evidence presented is pharmacological in nature and has been obtained with drugs that have been used to distinguish multiple types of excitatory amino acid receptors in the CNS (128,129).

Identical Action

Some of the initial evidence for excitatory amino acids as the hair cell transmitter in the mammalian cochlea was provided by screening studies intended to establish the relative influence of various putative neurotransmitters on the sound-evoked whole nerve action potential (CAP) in guinea pigs (18,25) and cats (87). Of a number of putative transmitters perfused into the scala tympani (including GABA, L-alanine, β-alanine, taurine, histamine, serotonin, norepinephrine, epinephrine, octopamine, dopamine, and glycine) only Glu and aspartate (Asp) were found to reduce CAP amplitude markedly without influencing the cochlear microphonic (CM). It was hypothesized that the reductions induced by Glu and Asp were caused not by inhibition, but by an increase in discharge rate of the afferent nerve fibers, making them less responsive to sound. Bobbin (19,26) and Comis and Leng (38) confirmed this explanation, showing that both amino acids cause firing of individual auditory nerve fibers and reduce sound-evoked discharge rates.

Extending these observations, Bledsoe et al. (13) demonstrated that kainic acid (KA), a structural analog of Glu and selective agonist for one type of excitatory amino acid receptor (the kainate type), causes a dose-dependent reduction in the amplitude of CAP when introduced into the perilymph of the guinea pig cochlea. It does so by exciting afferent nerve fibers without affecting CM, the summating potential (SP), endocochlear potential (EP), or the crossed olivocochlear potential elicited by electrical stimulation of efferent fibers. These findings have since been confirmed by Kusakari et al. (88).

Jenison et al. (84) have also shown that quisqualic acid (QA), a selective agonist for a second type of excitatory amino acid receptor (the quisqualate type), reduces the amplitude of CAP without affecting CM in the guinea pig cochlea. Subsequently they found that QA increases and then decreases the firing of single afferent nerve fibers (82). They concluded that QA is approximately 100 times more potent than Glu and about five times more potent than KA. Thus, QA ranks as the most potent substance to affect selectively afferent nerve activity. In contrast, N-methyl-D-aspartate (NMDA), an agonist for yet a third type of receptor (the NMDA type), has been shown to have no detectable effect on guinea pig cochlear potentials or to have effects only at concentrations that are most possibly nonspecific and osmotic (28,84). Thus if NMDA receptors are present and functional in the cochlea, their role remains to be detected. The detection of NMDA receptor function in some other areas of the nervous system has required special techniques, which has led to the speculation that the receptor modulates fast synaptic transmission mediated by non-NMDA (e.g., KA and QA) receptors (39,90,94).

All these observations reveal that receptors for KA and QA are present and functional in the mammalian cochlea. Since the hair cell receptor potentials are largely unaffected, the site of action of these compounds is most probably postsynaptic. This contention, at least for KA, has received support from recent work by Pujol et al. (108) who have observed that KA in adult guinea pigs produces a selective swelling of afferent nerve terminals contacting inner hair cells. Neuronal swelling is indicative of the depolarizing and initial toxic actions of KA (105).

Although the mammalian cochlea is amenable to pharmacological study, much of our knowledge of the actions of Glu and its analogs comes from studies on simpler hair cell systems in which such experiments are technically easier to perform. A number of sensory organs have been studied, but pharmacological evidence in support of the Glu hypothesis has been obtained largely in the lateral line of the African clawed frog (*Xenopus laevis*). The lateral line in this amphibian is freestanding on the skin and consists of a number of sensory end-organs, termed stitches. They are distributed in rows over the animal's body and head, with each stitch containing a variable number of neuromasts in which are located the hair cells. The stitches are innervated by two myelinated afferent nerve fibers, which, in turn, innervate the neuromasts to make synaptic contact with the two populations of hair cells that are excited by water motion in opposite directions (112). The Xenopus lateral line has long been used as a model for understanding sensory transduction in the inner ear. The reasons for this include its relatively simple structure, the accessibility of the hair cells to experimental manipulations and controlled stimulation, and the viability of *in vitro* preparations for long periods of time. Moreover, hair cells in the lateral line are morphologically and mechanistically similar to inner hair cells of the cochlea.

Glu and Asp were among the first substances shown to induce an increase in the discharge rate of afferent fibers of the Xenopus lateral line (15,24,30,112,134). At high drug concentrations, responses are not sustained but are rapidly followed by postexcitatory suppression of spontaneous activity suggestive of a depolarization blockade. Similar biphasic responses have been reported to occur in CNS preparations (107). Bledsoe et al. (15) have demonstrated that the responses of the lateral line to QA and KA are comparable to the responses these agonists induce in the cochlea. Unlike the cochlea, however, the lateral line is quite responsive to NMDA, indicating that one distinction between the two octavolateralis organs is that the amino acid receptors within the lateral-line organ include those of the NMDA-preferring subtype. Whether NMDA receptors in the lateral line function in concert with non-NMDA receptors in a manner analogous to the dual receptor system proposed for the CNS remains to be determined (39,94).

With intracellular and extracellular measurements of nerve activity, Guth and associates (125) have studied the actions of Glu in the isolated semicircular canal of the frog (*Rana esculenta*). They reported that in the presence of a low-Ca^{2+}–high-Mg^{2+} solution (0.1 mM $CaCl_2$–10 mM $MgCl_2$), which blocks transmitter release, Glu failed to increase the discharge rate of afferent nerve fibers, but still produced a long-lasting postsynaptic depolarization. The conclusion was drawn that the increase in discharge rate produced by Glu in normal Ringer's solution is owing to a presynaptic action to induce release of the afferent transmitter from hair cells, whereas the nerve depolarization results from some nonspecific postsynaptic mechanism not linked to action potential generation. However, in marked contrast to Guth and associates, Annoni et al. (7) studied intracellular responses to Glu and other excitatory amino acids in the presence of low-Ca^{2+}–high-Mg^{2+} solutions in the semicircular canal of the frog (*Rana temporana*) and concluded the excitatory actions are mediated postsynaptically. A similar conclusion has been drawn by Akoev et al. (2) in the Lorenzinian ampullae of the skate, where Glu increased the spontaneous discharge rate of the afferent nerve in the presence of elevated Mg^{2+}. Also, in the lateral line of Xenopus, low-Ca^{2+}–high-Mg^{2+} solutions do not block excitatory responses to exogenously applied Glu, indicating a postsynaptic site of action (32). We have now extended these observations to include responses to KA and QA and conclude that these two subtypes of Glu receptors are located postsynaptically. Responses to NMDA are blocked by low-Ca^{2+}–high-Mg^{2+} solutions, but ion channels linked to NMDA receptors are known to be blocked by Mg^{2+} (8). Thus, no definite conclusion can yet be drawn about the pre- versus postsynaptic location of NMDA receptors.

Pharmacological Identity

Several compounds have been shown to antagonize the activation of excitatory amino acid receptors in various vertebrate CNS preparations (94,128). However, only three studies to date have examined the effects of amino acid antagonists in the mammalian cochlea. Fex and Martin (58) reported that the D,L-racemic mixture of aminoadipate, an NMDA receptor antagonist, had no effect on sound-evoked CAP or CM in the cat and concluded that the postsynaptic receptor of the hair cell transmitter on afferent nerve fibers is not the NMDA type. In a preliminary report Bobbin et al. (28) studied the actions of the D-isomer of aminoadipate and other NMDA-preferring antagonists, such as 2-amino-5-phosphonovalerate [2-amino-5-phosphonopentanate (APV or AP5)] and D-alpha-aminosuberate on guinea pig cochlear potentials and confirmed the findings of Fex and Martin (58). The lack of effect of aminoadipate in the mammalian cochlea is in marked contrast to its actions in the Xenopus lateral line and other hair cell systems (see later).

Bobbin et al. (28) studied the effects of non-NMDA antagonists at the relatively high concentration of 10 mM and reported that L(+)-2-amino-4-phosphonobutyrate (APB or AP4) was inactive, but glutamate diethyl ester (GDEE) abolished the CAP (86%) and reduced CM (60%). The broad spectrum excitatory amino acid antagonist *cis*-2-3-piperidine dicarboxylate (*cis*-2,3-PDA) caused a reduction in CAP (33%) and had no effect on the CM, whereas gamma-D-glutamylglycine (DGG) was less effective. They are termed broad spectrum antagonists because they block to a large extent all three receptor types (NMDA, QA, and KA). Bobbin and Ceasar (20) have recently extended the list of broad spectrum antagonists examined to kynurenic acid (KYN) and gamma-D-glutamylaminomethylsulfonic acid (GAMS). Although GAMS was not very powerful in antagonizing CAP, KYN reduced CAP magnitude at 0.6 mM, which was the lowest concentration tested. To date this is the first drug that is a glutamate antagonist that dramatically affects the CAP at a concentration lower than 10 mM. The drug was shown to be specific and selective for the CAP by its lack of effect on the CM, SP, and EP. In addition KYN had no effect on the efferent transmitter system (acetylcholine transmission) to the outer hair cells. This was demonstrated by the lack of effect of KYN on the slow potential evoked in the scala media by efferent stimulation. Strychnine applied after KYN readily blocked the slow potential demonstrating that drugs applied by the same route as KYN could readily affect the potential. Thus, Bobbin and Ceasar (20) concluded that KYN antagonized a non-NMDA receptor, possibly a KA or QA receptor, which mediates hair cell transmission in the cochlea. It appears that the cochlea is not unusual in its pharmacology of excitatory amino acids since other synaptic responses that are resistant to blockade by NMDA antagonists (such as APV) but that can be blocked by *cis*-2-3-PDA, DGG, GAMS, and KYN have now been described in a number of preparations, including spinal cord (41), olfactory cortex (120), hippocampus (40), striatum (77), cochlear nucleus (92), and retina (46).

In the Xenopus lateral line D-alpha-aminoadipate (DAA), but not L-alpha-aminoadipate, reversibly suppresses spontaneous activity and excitation induced by water motion at concentrations as low as 0.25 to 0.5 mM (11). The lack of an antagonist effect with the L-isomer, which had slight excitatory actions, indicates the actions of DAA are highly stereospecific. At these concentrations, DAA also selectively blocks responses to exogenously applied NMDA (1.0–2.0 mM), with less effect on responses to Glu and Asp (1.0–2.0 mM), and essentially no effect on KA-induced excitation (5–15 μM). Overall, these results strongly support the hypothesis that the afferent transmitter is an excitatory amino acid or structurally related compound and reveal that it acts, at least in part, on NMDA receptors.

Several additional compounds, including AP5, GDEE, *cis*-2,3-PDA, DGG, and KYN, have now been tested in the Xenopus lateral line (17). Of particular interest are the actions of *cis*-2,3-PDA, DGG, and KYN on spontaneous and stimulated activity. *Cis*-2,3-PDA and DGG are the most potent antagonists thus far tested, suppressing both spontaneous activity and water motion-induced excitation at concentrations as low as 50 to 100 μM. KYN is slightly less potent (125–250 μM). All three drugs act competitively at concentrations less than 500 μM. At 1 to 2 mM, they totally block motion-induced excitation at all magnitudes of stimulation (up to 30 dB above threshold), but do not completely abolish spontaneous activity (as much as 80% suppressed). *Trans*-2,3-PDA has virtually no effect on lateral-line activity at 1 to 2 mM, indicating that the actions of *cis*-2,3-PDA are structurally specific. Since *cis*-2,3-PDA, DGG, and KYN act on all three subtypes of receptors (NMDA, KA, and QA), these findings suggest that in addition to NMDA receptors, KA and possibly QA receptors are also involved in lateral-line afferent transmission. Evidence that non-NMDA receptors play a greater role in afferent synaptic transmission than previously envisioned has also been presented in the frog vestibular organ (7).

Under certain conditions, it appears that in the lateral line the antagonists dissociate spontaneous from stimulated activity. This is evident in the actions of *cis*-2,3-PDA, DGG, and KYN, with their ability to abolish stimulated responses without completely eliminating spontaneous activity. We have also found that AP5 at 125 to 250 μM selectively blocks NMDA responses and suppresses spontaneous activity, but not motion-induced excitation. At higher concentrations (0.5 to 1.0 mM), AP5 reduces motion-induced responses and suppresses excitation to KA and Glu. These findings suggest that different receptors may mediate spontaneous and stimulated activity in the lateral line. Although this contradicts classic views of neurotransmission, there is evidence in the CNS that ions, phospholipids, and guanyl nucleotides may regulate the activity and expression of excitatory amino acid receptors (67). Thus, it is conceivable that alterations of the physicochemical environment in the synapse during stimulation could alter the properties of receptors or unmask additional receptors. For instance, NMDA receptors may be utilized during spontaneous activity and at low levels of stimulation, whereas QA and KA receptors are activated by high intensity stimuli. Such speculation is compatible with the dual receptor system discussed earlier.

Aspirin has long been known to induce a reversible hearing loss in humans. This hearing loss is a special problem in patients with arthritis who must take 12 to 16 tablets of aspirin every day to reduce the arthritic inflammation. Therefore we tested the hypothesis that aspirin induces a hearing loss by antagonism of the hair cell transmitter and Glu. In preliminary results Glu and KA responses in the lateral line were antagonized by 0.3 to 1.25 mM salicylate (27). Spontaneous activity was antagonized at a lower concentration of salicylate than water motion-induced activity. These studies are being extended to mammals to test the hypothesis further.

In summary, the pharmacological data have revealed that in at least the mammalian cochlea, Xenopus lateral line, frog vestibular organ, and cat labyrinth (42), receptors for excitatory amino acids are present and functional. At least two of the receptor subtypes, those for KA and QA, are present in both organs and the available evidence suggests they are located postsynaptically on afferent nerve fibers. Moreover, there is compelling evidence that the endogenous afferent transmitter as well as exogenously applied Glu act on these excitatory amino acid receptors.

Stimulus-Induced Release

When attempting to identify a neurotransmitter a primary criterion of fundamental importance is to demonstrate that a substance is released from hair cells by stimulation of the end-organ (130). It is well established that the release of neurotransmitters requires Ca^{2+} and that the influx of Ca^{2+} into presynaptic elements after membrane depolarization is blocked by high concentrations of other divalent cations, such as Mg^{2+}. Although this concept is currently being challenged by several demonstrations of noncalcium-dependent release of chemicals known to be transmitters in other systems (126), it behooves the scientist to examine whether the release of a substance is dependent on extracellular Ca^{2+}.

In the cochlea several studies have examined the stimulus-induced release criterion by attempting to measure an increase in the concentration of substances in perilymph. Bledsoe et al. (12) perfused the cochlea with artificial perilymph and reported preliminary results of a small but significant increase in the concentration of Glu in the perfusate during periods of exposure to low-frequency sound. Others, using different techniques, have not observed this increase (45,95,96), but there are reports of other substances released by sound, including ANAS (118), a GABA-like substance (45), and methionine-enkephalin (45). Drescher and Drescher (44), however, observed at high levels of stimulation (115 dB sound pressure level) a release of Glu into perilymph above nonstimulated control levels. These conflicting results may reflect methodological difficulties inherent in studies of the mammalian ear. This seems especially evident in regard to GABA and enkephalin, which have been localized to efferent terminals in the cochlea (see later). It should be noted that none of these studies addressed the issue of whether any observed release was dependent on extracellular Ca^{2+}.

One interpretation for the lack of ability to detect a change in Glu levels with sound stimulation may be that not enough transmitter is released from the hair cells for detection, owing to efficient degradation or uptake into surrounding cells (see "Inactivation Mechanism"). Sound is, in fact, very difficult to shape so that both apical and basal regions of the cochlea are stimulated maximally. On the other hand, using depolarizing concentrations of potassium (K^+) to induce a synchronous release of transmitter from a large number of hair cells, Jenison et al. (83) have shown a K^+-stimulated, Ca^{2+}-dependent release of Glu and taurine into fluid bathing the hair cells of the guinea pig cochlea.

In the Xenopus lateral line, Bledsoe et al. (14) showed that vibrating water motion caused a greater release of Glu and Asp (but not glycine) from isolated skins containing the lateral line than from skins without it. Recently, utilizing a superfusion technique to enhance amino acid release and high levels of K^+ as a depolarizing stimulus, Bledsoe (10,16) demonstrated a K^+-induced, Ca^{2+}-dependent release of Glu, Asp, and two unidentified primary amines from the Xenopus lateral line. Based on retention time analysis of the HPLC assay one of these unknowns has since been tentatively identified as L-alpha-aminoadipate, which as we have previously shown has slight excitatory effects on lateral-line afferent nerve fibers (11).

Although a number of interpretations are possible, the results with K$^+$ stimulation are consistent with the hypothesis that the afferent transmitter released by hair cells in both the cochlea and lateral line is an excitatory amino acid. They further suggest a potential role for other substances in sensory transduction possibly as neuromodulators.

Presynaptic Location

Glu and Asp have been shown to be present in the organ of Corti (68). Owing to the involvement of these amino acids in a number of metabolic processes, their mere presence, however, is not sufficient evidence. In addition, they must be shown to exist presynaptically associated with structures (such as vesicles) capable of their release. Immunocytochemistry is a powerful tool for the discrete localization of substances in tissues. Most transmitters and neuroeffectors are small molecules that are generally not amenable to immunocytochemical procedures. Recently, however, techniques for producing antibodies to transmitter amino acids, including Glu, have been reported (106). Although this methodology has been used for other substances it has yet to be applied to hair cell systems to examine Glu localization. It certainly offers a potentially powerful approach for studies on sensory transduction.

Inactivation Mechanism

In the nervous system, the actions of amino acid transmitters are generally thought to be terminated by an active, Na$^+$-dependent uptake into neurons and glia (127). Uptake of Glu and other amino acids has been studied in the organ of Corti with conflicting results. Gulley et al. (71) and Schwartz and Ryan (117) demonstrated with radioautographic techniques that Glu preferentially labeled cochlear efferent fibers and terminals and questioned the role of Glu as the afferent transmitter. In contrast, Eybalin and Pujol (48) showed a preferential labeling of inner hair cells when incubations with radiolabeled Glu were followed by a postincubation without a tracer. It is widely accepted that in the CNS the metabolism of Glu and glutamine is compartmentalized. In an oversimplification, this is viewed in the following way. Glu released by nerve terminals is largely taken up by high-affinity, Na$^+$-dependent transport into glia where it is metabolized to glutamine by the enzyme glutamine synthetase. The glutamine is released back into the extracellular space and made available to nerve terminals where it is converted back to Glu by the enzyme glutaminase (GLNase). Eybalin and Pujol (48) postulated that a similar metabolic link between Glu and glutamine exists in the cochlea. The high levels of glutamine in the perilymph and the preferential labeling of hair cells with radiolabeled glutamine reported by Ryan and Schwartz (113) and Eybalin and Pujol (48) seems compatible with this hypothesis. Further studies of uptake and metabolism of Glu, glutamine, and related substances are needed to examine the role of Glu in sensory transduction.

Synthetic Enzymes

A number of enzymes, including GLNase, glutamine synthetase, ornithine aminotransferase, and aspartate aminotransferase (AAT) have been examined for their involvement in the metabolism of a transmitter pool of glutamate (65). Biochemical and cytochemical investigations of these enzymes have provided insight into Glu metabolism and potential glutamatergic pathways in the brain. Recent studies of cytoplasmic AAT have been of particular interest (6). However, owing to the extensive role of Glu in metabolism, no one metabolic pathway has been shown to be present only in glutamatergic neurons. For example, AAT, a ubiquitous enzyme, is present in glia (6) and has been localized by lead precipitation cytochemistry to inhibitory neurons in the cerebellum (93). Fex et al. (61) have demonstrated the presence of AAT-like immunoreactivity in the spiral ganglion cells and the medial system of efferent nerve fibers associated with outer hair cells of the guinea pig cochlea, but not within the hair cells. Recently, Fex et al. (62) demonstrated the presence of GLNase immunoreactivity in auditory nerve dendrites of inner hair cells and in the medial system of efferents, but again not within hair cells to any great extent. Since enzymes involved in transmitter metabolism would be expected to be present presynaptically, these findings could be construed as evidence against the Glu hypothesis. This should not be the case. Immunocytochemical techniques are especially sensitive to the amounts of antigenic substance present, with slight differences in level capable of producing either a positive or negative result. Thus, the lack of AAT- and GLNase-like immunoreactivity within hair cells may simply reflect the lower metabolic activity of these cells. It is of interest that AAT- and GLNase-like immunoreactivity is present in cochlear efferents, since there is no evidence that efferent terminals release excitatory amino acids as transmitters. This in itself questions the use of antibodies to AAT and GLNase as specific probes for transmitter-pool metabolism within the cochlea.

EFFERENT SYNAPTIC TRANSMISSION

Acetylcholine as an Efferent Transmitter

There is considerable evidence indicating that ACh is an efferent transmitter in the mammalian cochlea (31,74,85). The most persuasive pharmacological evidence is the demonstration that atropine (both tertiary and quaternary), D-tubocurarine, decamethonium, hexamethonium, other anticholinergic agents, and alpha-bungarotoxin, when applied intracochlearly, selectively block the effects of efferent stimulation without affecting any of the potentials associated with afferent transmission. Strychnine is a potent antagonist of efferent transmission, and this effect has been attributed to its anticholinergic properties rather than its antiglycinergic effects for which it is best known (74). The identical action criterion for ACh has also been examined by studying its influence on sound-evoked afferent activity. Intracochlear perfusions of ACh in combination with physostigmine [an acetylcholinesterase (AChE) inhibitor] produce an increase in the amplitude of CM evoked by low frequencies and a concurrent reduction in the amplitude of CAP (22). Both of these effects mimic the influence of efferent stimulation and both are blocked by curare

(23). Robertson and Johnstone (109) and Comis and Leng (38) demonstrated that the decrease in CAP reflects the suppression of the firing rates of afferent fibers. Recent evidence indicates that the efferents innervating the outer hair cells may induce a contraction of the outer hair cells and that ACh mimics this effect when applied to isolated outer hair cells (35). This was a preliminary study and the results need to be replicated. ACh is a quaternary nitrogen compound that can block potassium channels in high concentrations (132). Since potassium channels appear to play a prominent role in the hair cells, then ACh acting on these channels may account for the observed response rather than it being a receptor-mediated event. On the other hand, acetylcholine receptor stimulation has recently been shown to activate the synthesis of actin (70). This finding, together with the discovery of actin in the cells of the organ of Corti (101), suggests the possibility that the cholinergic efferents to the outer hair cells may exert a long-term modulation of basilar membrane motion by controlling the levels of actin in the outer hair cells. In addition, Schacht and Zenner (115) proposed that the motile responses of isolated outer hair cells may be linked to efferent stimulation of the phosphoinositide cascade, a transmembrane signaling system for neurotransmitters, modulators, and hormones that elevate intracellular Ca^{2+} levels.

One of the two key enzymes involved in the metabolism of ACh is AChE, which inactivates ACh by cleaving it into acetate and choline. Churchill et al. (37) and Schuknecht et al. (116) demonstrated that when the efferents of the olivocochlear bundle are sectioned and allowed to degenerate, AChE activity decreases to an undetectable level. This indicates that AChE is localized exclusively to efferent terminals and that enzymatic inactivation of ACh takes place presynaptically rather than postsynaptically on the surface of the hair cells or the afferent terminals. AChE drugs have also been shown to potentiate the actions of efferent stimulation (85), revealing that the enzyme is involved in terminating the action of the efferent transmitter.

Choline acetyltransferase (ChAT), the enzyme responsible for synthesizing ACh, has also been shown to be associated exclusively with efferent nerve terminals. Jasser and Guth (81) demonstrated that ChAT activity in the cochlea decreases below detectable levels after the efferents are sectioned and allowed to degenerate. Thus, other cochlear structures, including the hair cells, appear incapable of synthesizing ACh. This has been confirmed and extended by Altschuler et al. (5), who localized ChAT-like immunoreactivity to efferent terminals under both inner and outer hair cells using an immunofluorescence technique. Since the synthesis of ACh is thought to occur only in cholinergic neurons, these findings suggest that only cochlear efferent fibers use ACh as a transmitter.

The candidacy of ACh as the efferent transmitter has also been examined by analyzing perilymph for release of ACh with various stimulus conditions. Both Fex (55) and Norris and Guth (103) reported the detection of ACh-like activity in perilymph after electrical stimulation of the efferent system. Norris and Guth (103) demonstrated that ACh-like activity is not altered by exposing the cochlea to sound. Although these results are consistent with the premise that ACh is released by the efferent terminals, it remains to be determined whether the change in ACh-like activity is calcium dependent.

In addition to the mammalian cochlea, there is considerable evidence that ACh is the efferent transmitter in other hair cell systems. In the Xenopus lateral line,

Russell (111) showed that tetanic stimulation of efferents suppressed spontaneous activity of the afferent fibers. This effect was dependent on extracellular Ca^{2+} and blocked by high extracellular concentrations of Mg^{2+}. Thus, the suppression of afferent activity appears mediated by the release of a transmitter from efferent terminals induced by electrical stimulation. Russell also showed that curare and atropine both antagonize the effects of efferent stimulation. Cholinesterase activity has also been demonstrated in the lateral-line organ, as has the potentiation of efferent stimulation with the anticholinesterase, physostigmine (111). In addition, both ACh and ACh-like compounds have been shown to suppress spontaneous afferent activity, and this drug-induced suppression is blocked by prior treatment with curare or atropine (111).

In the Xenopus lateral line Winbery and Bobbin (131) reported that ACh and carbachol (a cholinergic agonist) increase spontaneous activity before producing suppression. This action of ACh contrasts with the reports (111) that the efferents suppress afferent activity in this system and to date the reason for these results remain unresolved. In later experiments designed to determine the mechanism of this response, the increase in activity owing to ACh and carbachol was compared with that caused by Glu (32). Atropine (1 μM) blocked the excitatory effects of ACh and carbachol while not affecting responses to Glu, indicating that ACh and Glu act on different receptors. Atropine (1 to 20 μM) had no effect on spontaneous or water motion-induced discharge rates. In addition, a low-Ca^{2+}–high-Mg^{2+} Ringer's solution blocked the excitatory response to ACh but not Glu. Therefore, it was postulated that ACh and carbachol act presynaptically to induce release of the afferent transmitter. Similar findings and conclusions were reported by Akoev et al. (1) in the Lorenzinian ampullae of the skate. In addition, Bernard et al. (9) reported that cholinergic agonists and electrical stimulation of efferents increase the spontaneous discharge rate of the afferent nerve in the *in vitro* frog semicircular canal. These excitatory responses were blocked by cholinergic antagonists and low-Ca^{2+}–high-Mg^{2+} Ringer's solution. In keeping with the previous two studies, these researchers concluded that the excitatory responses to ACh were mediated presynaptically and went on to speculate that the underlying mechanism was a hyperpolarized hair cell membrane potential generated by the experimental conditions. On the other hand, Guth et al. (75) stated that "In a manner analogous to efferent nerve stimulation, ACh produced both facilitatory and inhibitory changes in afferent firing rates." These authors concluded that ACh is the transmitter of the efferent vestibular nerve. Further studies on these excitatory actions of ACh must be carried out to clarify this situation.

In summary, the evidence for ACh as an efferent transmitter in hair cell systems is substantial. Nevertheless, there are gaps in our knowledge. For example, the release of ACh from efferent fibers in a Ca^{2+}-dependent manner has yet to be demonstrated. The pharmacological nature of the efferent receptors (muscarinic versus nicotinic) has also not been established conclusively. The introduction of isolated hair cell preparations to the armamentarium of auditory science may ultimately lead to a better understanding of the functional role of ACh as an efferent transmitter and its relationship to other potential efferent transmitters and modulators.

GABA—Afferent or Efferent Transmitter?

GABA, the alpha-decarboxylation product of Glu, is widely accepted as a major inhibitory neurotransmitter in the vertebrate nervous system (51). However, a transmitter function for GABA in hair cell systems is controversial and its overall role in synaptic processes in the inner ear and other octavolateralis organs remains unclear. This section surveys evidence indicating that, despite the situation in the cochlea, GABA may be an afferent transmitter in the vertebrate vestibular system. In addition, evidence suggesting that it may function in relationship to efferent innervation in the cochlea and the Xenopus lateral line is discussed.

Studying the synthesis of GABA from radioactive Glu in several hair cell preparations, Flock and Lam (64) were the first to suggest that GABA might be an afferent transmitter. These investigators did not, however, include the cochlea in their studies. Tachibana and Kuriyama (121), on the other hand, were unable to detect the presence of GABA in either inner or outer hair cells of the guinea pig cochlea. Others (59,68) also reported the levels of GABA as well as the activity of glutamic acid decarboxylase (GAD), the enzyme that synthesizes GABA from Glu, to be low in the cochlea. Furthermore, Desmedt and Monaco (43) and Bobbin and Guth (21) showed that thiosemicarbazide, an inhibitor of GAD, does not affect the sound-evoked CAP.

GABA applied both iontophoretically (123) and intracochlearly (21,25,86) does not affect sound-evoked cochlear potentials except at high concentrations that are probably nonspecific. Baclofen, an agonist for one class of presynaptic GABA receptor, also apparently has no influence on cochlear potentials (91). In addition, several investigators (21,43,86) showed that picrotoxin, a GABA antagonist, does not alter guinea pig afferent cochlear potentials. However, bicuculline methiodide, another GABA antagonist, does have a slight suppressive effect on the guinea pig CAP, but only at unusually high concentrations (25,86). Overall, these observations provide a strong argument against GABA as an afferent transmitter in the cochlea.

In contrast, Felix and Ehrenberger (53,54) demonstrated that GABA applied iontophoretically excites afferent nerve fibers in the saccule of the cat. The excitation is blocked by bicuculline, which also suppresses spontaneous activity of the afferent nerve fibers. Based on these findings the investigators suggested that GABA may be an afferent transmitter in the vestibular labyrinth. In support of this hypothesis, Flock and Lam (64) reported that the bullfrog basilar papilla, which has only afferent innervation, is capable of synthesizing GABA from radioactive Glu and that picrotoxin blocks spontaneous and evoked afferent activity in the semicircular canal of the skate. Systemically administered picrotoxin has also been shown to suppress vertigo in patients with peripheral vestibular disorders (47). Moreover, in a series of biochemical studies, Meza and associates (97) provided evidence that GABA may be an afferent transmitter in the crista ampullaris of the chick. Among their findings, they demonstrated the synthesis of GABA from radioactive Glu, a Na^+- and energy-dependent, high-affinity uptake system for [^3H]GABA, which may represent a transmitter inactivation mechanism, and the binding of [^3H]GABA to crude membrane preparations, which occurs in a manner analogous to an interaction with GABA receptors. Others have suggested that GABA immunoreactivity is present in the hair cells of the chick, whereas it is in the efferents of the squirrel monkey (124). However, it should be noted that both Guth and Norris (73) and Annoni et al. (7), studying the frog semicircular canal, reported no consistent excitation with GABA and its potent agonist muscimol. In those few instances when an excitatory response did occur, it was blocked by low-Ca^{2+}–high-Mg^{2+} solutions, indicating a presynaptic site of action. In addition, these investigators observed no effect of GABA antagonists (picrotoxin and bicuculline) on afferent spontaneous activity.

These results seem to suggest that in some, but not all, vestibular systems, GABA may play a role in sensory transduction, possibly as an afferent transmitter. On the other hand, some of the GABA may play a metabolic or modulator role.

There is some evidence to support a function of GABA in association with efferent innervation in the cochlea (3). Picrotoxin and bicuculline reduce the influence of efferent stimulation on the cochlea (86) and GABA uptake has been localized predominantly among the terminals of efferent fibers (71,117). Aminooxyacetic acid (AOAA) has rather complex effects on efferent stimulation (29) and as discussed previously AAT, an enzyme that AOAA inhibits, has been demonstrated in efferent nerve fibers (61). In addition, Drescher et al. (45) reported the presence of a GABA-like compound in natural guinea pig perilymph (possibly CSF since the cochlear aqueduct was patent) and showed that the amount of this substance increases during exposure to noise. The term GABA-like was used because the chromatographic analysis of this substance is indistinguishable from that of GABA. Fex and Altschuler (57) demonstrated the presence of GAD-like immunoreactivity and Fex et al. (60) and Eybalin and Pujol (49) demonstrated GABA itself in a small population of efferents in the guinea pig cochlea. The fact that only a small number of efferents is involved might explain why thiosemicarbazide, a GAD inhibitor, and GABA antagonists have been reported to have little, if any, ability to block the effects of efferent stimulation on sound-evoked afferent activity in the cochlea (21,43,86), and also why GABA, as discussed previously, does not mimic the effects of efferent stimulation on CAP and CM when applied intracochlearly except at unusually high concentrations. Thus, evidence does exist that suggests a role of GABA in the efferent system of the cochlea and raises the possibility that the pharmacology of the basal turn cells in the cochlea may be different from those in the more apical turns.

In the lateral line of Xenopus, GABA is a potent suppressor of spontaneous afferent nerve activity (15). Bicuculline blocks the inhibition produced by GABA in the lateral line and does so without affecting either the activity evoked by natural stimulation (water motion) or the increase in spontaneous activity induced by Glu or carbachol (32). Also, baclofen does not alter either spontaneous activity or the response evoked by natural stimulation. These results indicate that GABA acts on receptors separate from those activated by Glu, carbachol, or the endogenous afferent transmitter. Furthermore, it appears that these GABA receptors are of a subclass termed GABA-A receptors, which are blocked by bicuculline but insensitive to baclofen, rather than of the subclass termed GABA-B receptors, which are insensitive to bicuculline but sensitive to baclofen (34). These observations, in general, support the likelihood that GABA plays some role in efferent transmission. In view of the strong evidence that ACh is an efferent transmitter in both the inner ear and Xenopus lateral line, we have speculated that GABA's role is adjunct to that of ACh, possibly as a cotransmitter or as a transmitter for a second efferent system (15). A second GABAergic efferent system is compatible with the findings and suggestions of Fex and Altschuler (57) and Altschuler and Fex (3) in the cochlea.

In summary, there is no compelling evidence that GABA is an afferent transmitter in either the cochlea or lateral line. There is, however, evidence to support the role of GABA as an excitatory transmitter in the chick basal papilla and the vestibular labyrinth of mammals but not amphibians. In addition, there is evidence indicating that GABA may function in the efferent innervation of hair cells in both the cochlea and lateral line. It is clear that additional work is needed to elucidate the functional significance of GABA in synaptic processes of hair cell systems.

Modulator Chemicals

Fex and Altschuler (56) demonstrated an enkephalin-like immunoreactivity in the efferent olivocochlear neurons of the cochlea, but not in the spiral ganglion cells, the auditory nerve fibers, or the hair cells of the organ of Corti. Hoffman (79,80) identified two methionine-enkephalin fractions in cochleae from guinea pigs using HPLC separation and subsequent radioimmunoassay. Drescher et al. (45) detected a methionine-enkephalin-like component in perilymph and found it elevated in response to noise. These last investigators have suggested that the enkephalin may have been released from efferent terminals. Eybalin et al. (50) suggested that noise exposure lowers the cochlear levels of methionine-enkephalin. Fex and Altschuler (56) speculated that enkephalins may share a role with ACh in efferent transmission. In this regard, it is of interest that opiate peptides are known to suppress responses of brain neurons to microiontophoretic applications of Glu (133). Studying the effects of methionine-enkephalin on the specific binding of Glu to synaptic membranes, Kuznetsov and Godukhin (89) showed that methionine-enkephalin reduces the binding of Glu by decreasing the number of binding sites without affecting the binding affinity. They concluded that the suppressive effect of methionine-enkephalin is owing to an inhibitory influence of the peptide on Glu binding to its postsynaptic receptors. Whether opiates exert a similar modulating influence on Glu responses in hair cell systems remains to be established.

Other modulator substances have recently been suggested to be present in hair cell systems. Bryant and Guth (36) suggested that adenosine is a modulator of hair cell transmitter in the vestibular system of the frog. That ATP has an effect in the cochlea was demonstrated by Bobbin and Thompson (25). Calcitonin gene-related peptide has been demonstrated in the efferent fibers of the rat cochlea (122). Taurine has been demonstrated to be released from cells in the cochlea in a calcium-dependent manner (83). To date the action of taurine in the cochlea has not been detected (25), which suggests a possible modulator role. Release of Asp has been demonstrated (14,16,83) and its role may be as a modulator of Glu action. Altschuler et al. (4) demonstrated the enzyme for the synthesis of dopamine in the cochlea. Norris et al. (104) suggested that histamine may have activity in the frog vestibular labyrinth. Finally potassium, which appears to carry current in the cochlea, has been postulated as a modulator of synaptic transmission (126). It is clear that the list of potential modulators of synaptic processing in the inner ear is growing. Their functional role in sensory transduction remains to be established.

FUTURE DIRECTIONS

A major goal of studies on neurotransmitters and modulators in the inner ear is to provide information about the molecular mechanisms associated with sensory transduction. The identity of the chemicals and receptors involved and the chemical steps occurring after activation of those receptors are but a few of the chemical reactions occurring in the ear. It is readily apparent that many chemicals are probably released from every cell in the organ of Corti during sound exposure and so it is easy to accept the fact that many chemicals will be detected as released into a fluid bathing the cells. Certainly not all of them are transmitters or even modulators. The challenging questions are what is their function and what does their release tell us about the function of the various cells in the ear.

All the available evidence suggests that we must be willing to incorporate new and innovative lines of thinking into our research on neurotransmission and cellular communication in the ear. First, and perhaps foremost, is the possibility that the hair cell transmitter is not the same in all hair cell systems and also that neither is the transmitter of the efferent nerve fibers synapsing under the hair cells the same in all systems. Although Glu or a Glu-like compound remains the leading candidate in the mammalian cochlea and amphibian lateral line for the hair cell transmitter, this may not be the case in other organs, for example, ampullary electroreceptors of the catfish (98). The assertion that GABA is a hair cell excitatory transmitter in the mammalian vestibular labyrinth is a particularly intriguing postulate worthy of further study. As discussed by Annoni et al. (7), the possibility that GABA acts presynaptically to induce the release of the hair cell transmitter needs to be more closely examined. Likewise, although acetylcholine is the leading candidate for the transmitter of efferent fibers terminating under the hair cells, the existence of efferents that utilize GABA seems likely as is the probability that both may use polypeptides such as the enkephalins as cotransmitters or modulators. Second, as pointed out earlier, differential receptor activation may occur at different levels of sound exposure. Along similar lines is the likelihood that fast transmitters do not act alone but their actions are most probably modified by silent chemicals called modulators. In the final analysis, answers to these questions would be important not only in understanding vestibular versus cochlear physiology, but also for the development of selective drug therapies for vestibular versus cochlear disorders.

To date, much of the research on neurotransmitters and neuromodulators in the inner ear has been, by necessity, descriptive. We are now entering an era of new research in which many of the questions being posed concern functional aspects of synaptic mechanisms. It is anticipated that this trend will continue and progress to even more detailed analyses at the molecular level. In this regard, it is of interest that receptors for excitatory amino acids in the brain have been linked to the cyclic nucleotide system of transmembrane second messengers (such as cyclic AMP and cyclic GMP). ACh receptors (102) and, most recently, excitatory amino acid receptors (100) have also been linked to the newly described phosphoinositide cascade transmembrane signaling system (114). Biochemical second messengers have been implicated in the regulation of a number of synaptic processes including uncoupling of electrical synapses (110), neurotransmitter synthesis and release such as in the adrenal gland (66), ion channel regulation such as changes in potassium currents (78), and even of sensory transduction (69). Identifying the systems present and the functional role they may play in afferent and efferent synaptic processes will definitely prove to be an exciting avenue for future experimentation.

Studies on the molecular mechanisms of neurotransmission in the inner ear are entering an exciting new phase. The expectations are high that by providing a more complete understanding of synaptic processes we might explain various pathological states of the ear. In the brain, neurotransmission disorders may account for neuronal degenerative and other diseases; for example, Huntington's chorea and senile dementia may result from dysfunctions in excitatory amino acid mechanisms. KA, which has been widely used to produce excitotoxic models for degenerative diseases, has clear and selective excitatory actions on auditory nerve fibers. In this context, it is of interest that Spoendlin (119) reported in cases of Friedreich's ataxia selective degeneration of the VIIIth nerve with sparing of the organ of Corti. Clearly, once the transmitter systems of audition are identified, these and other disease manifestations may be better understood, explained, or treated.

ACKNOWLEDGMENTS

Portions of this chapter were published previously in *Seminars in Hearing*, 7:117–138, Thieme, Inc., New York, 1986, and are used here with permission.

The authors' research cited in this manuscript is supported by program project grants from the National Institutes of Health (NS-05785 to S.B., NS-16080 to R.P.B.), a grant from the University of Michigan Biomedical Research Council to S.B., a grant from NSF to R.P.B. (BNS-84-19241), and funds to Louisiana State University Medical School from the Kresge Foundation and the Louisiana Lions Eye Foundation.

REFERENCES

1. Akoev, G. N., Andrianov, G. N., and Sherman, N. O. (1983): Effects of acetylcholine and cholinolytics on the synaptic transmission in the ampullae of Lorenzini of the skate. *Comp. Biochem. Physiol. [C]*, 74:95–97.
2. Akoev, G. N., Andrianov, G. N., and Volpe, N. O. (1980): L-Glutamate as possible neurotransmitter in the ampullae of Lorenzini of the skate. *Neurosci. Lett.*, 20:307–312.
3. Altschuler, R. A., and Fex, J. (1986): Efferent neurotransmitters. In: *Neurobiology of Hearing: The Cochlea*, edited by R. A. Altschuler, R. P. Bobbin, and D. W. Hoffman, pp. 383–397. Raven Press, New York.
4. Altschuler, R. A., Jones, N., Reeks, K. A., and Fex, J. (1986): Tyrosine hydroxylase immunoreactivity marks a catecholaminergic system in the guinea pig organ of Corti. *Abstracts of the Ninth Midwinter Research Meeting of the Association for Research in Otolaryngology*, p. 91. Clearwater Beach, FL.
5. Altschuler, R. A., Kachar, B., Rubio, J. A., Parakkal, M. H., and Fex, J. (1985): Immunocytochemical localization of choline acetyltransferase-like immunoreactivity in the guinea pig cochlea. *Brain Res.*, 338:1–11.
6. Altschuler, R. A., Neises, G. R., Harmison, G. G., Wenthold, R. J., and Fex, J. (1981): Immunocytochemical localization of aspartate aminotransferase immunoreactivity in cochlear nucleus of the guinea pig. *Proc. Natl. Acad. Sci. USA*, 78:6553–6557.
7. Annoni, J.-M., Cochran, S. L., and Precht, W. (1984): Pharmacology of the vestibular hair cell-afferent fiber synapse in the frog. *J. Neurosci.*, 4:2106–2116.
8. Ascher, P., and Nowak, L. (1987): Electrophysiological studies of NMDA receptors. *Trends Neurosci.*, 10:284–287.
9. Bernard, C., Cochran, S. L., and Precht, W. (1985): Presynaptic actions of cholinergic agents upon the hair cell-afferent fiber synapse in the vestibular labyrinth of the frog. *Brain Res.*, 338:225–236.
10. Bledsoe, S. C., Jr. (1986): Pharmacology and neurotransmission of sensory transduction in the inner ear. In: *Seminars in Hearing*, edited by J. M. Miller, pp. 117–138. Thieme, New York.
11. Bledsoe, S. C., Jr., and Bobbin, R. P. (1982): Effects of D-alpha-aminodipate on excitation of afferent fibers in the lateral line of Xenopus laevis. *Neurosci. Lett.*, 32:315–320.
12. Bledsoe, S. C., Jr., Bobbin, R. P., and Chihal, D. M. (1981): Technique for studying sound-induced release of endogenous amino acids from the guinea pig cochlea. *Abstracts of the Association for Research in Otolaryngology*, p. 24. St. Petersburg, FL.
13. Bledsoe, S. C., Jr., Bobbin, R. P., and Chihal, D. M. (1981): Kainic acid: An evaluation of its action on cochlear potentials. *Hear. Res.*, 4:109–120.
14. Bledsoe, S. C., Jr., Bobbin, R. P., Thalmann, R., and Thalmann, I. (1980): Stimulus-induced release of endogenous amino acids from the Xenopus laevis lateral-line organ. *Exp. Brain Res.*, 40:97–101.
15. Bledsoe, S. C., Jr., Chihal, D. M., Bobbin, R. P., and Morgan, D. N. (1983): Comparative actions of glutamate and related substances on the lateral line of Xenopus laevis. *Comp. Biochem. Physiol. [C]*, 75:119–206.

16. Bledsoe, S. C., Jr., McLaren, J. D., and Meyer, J. R. (1986): Potassium-induced, calcium-dependent release of endogenous amino acids from the *Xenopus* lateral line. *Abstracts of the Ninth Midwinter Meeting of the Association for Research in Otolaryngology*, p. 89. Clearwater Beach, FL.

17. Bledsoe, S. C., Jr., Meyer, J. R., and Howland, M. M. (1985): Effects of excitatory amino acid receptor antagonists on synaptic excitation in the lateral line of Xenopus laevis. *Abstracts of the Association for Research in Otolaryngology*, p. 111. Clearwater Beach, FL.

18. Bobbin, R. P. (1976): Effects of putative transmitters on afferent cochlear transmission. *J. Acoust. Soc. Am.*, 60:S79.

19. Bobbin, R. P. (1979): Glutamate and aspartate mimic the afferent transmitter in the cochlea. *Exp. Brain Res.* 34:389–393.

20. Bobbin, R. P., and Ceasar, G. (1987): Kynurenic acid and gamma-D-glutamylaminomethylsulfonic acid suppresses the compound action potential of the auditory nerve. *Hear. Res.*, 25:77–81.

21. Bobbin, R. P., and Guth, P. S. (1970): Evidence that gamma-aminobutyric acid is not the inhibitory transmitter at the crossed olivocochlear nerve-hair cell junction. *Neuropharmacology*, 9:567–574.

22. Bobbin, R. P., and Konishi, T. (1971): Acetylcholine mimics crossed olivocochlear bundle stimulation. *Nature*, 231:222–223.

23. Bobbin, R. P., and Konishi, T. (1974): Action of cholinergic and anticholinergic drugs at the crossed olivocochlear bundle-hair cell junction. *Acta Otolaryngol. (Stockh.)*, 77:56–65.

24. Bobbin, R. P., and Morgan, D. N. (1980): Glutamate mimics the afferent transmitter in the Xenopus laevis lateral line. In: *Morphogenesis and Malformation of the Ear*, edited by R. J. Gorlin, pp. 107–109. Alan R. Liss, New York.

25. Bobbin, R. P., and Thompson, M. H. (1978): Effects of putative transmitters on afferent cochlear transmission. *Ann. Otol. Rhinol. Laryngol.*, 87:185–190.

26. Bobbin, R. P., and Thompson, M. H. (1978): Glutamate stimulates cochlear afferent nerve fibers. *Fed. Proc.*, 37:613.

27. Bobbin, R. P., Bledsoe, S. C., Jr., and Ceasar, G. (1985): Action of salicylate on the activity of afferent fibers in the *Xenopus laevis* lateral line. *Soc. Neurosci.*, 11:244.

28. Bobbin, R. P., Bledsoe, S. C., Jr., and Chihal, D. M. (1981): Effects of various excitatory amino acid antagonists on guinea pig cochlea potentials. *Abstracts of the Association for Research in Otolaryngology*, p. 27. St. Petersburg, FL.

29. Bobbin, R. P., Bledsoe, S. C., Jr., and Chihal, D. M. (1981): Effect of asphyxia and aminooxyacetic acid on the slow potential evoked by crossed olivocochlear bundle stimulation. *Hear. Res.*, 5:265–269.

30. Bobbin, R. P., Bledsoe, S. C., Jr., Chihal, D. M., and Morgan, D. N. (1981): Comparative actions of glutamate and related substances on the Xenopus laevis lateral line. *Comp. Biochem. Physiol.* [C], 69:146–147.

31. Bobbin, R. P., Bledsoe, S. C., Jr., and Jenison, G. L. (1984): Neurotransmitters of the cochlea and lateral line organ. In: *Recent Advances in Hearing Science*, edited by C. Berlin, pp. 159–180. College-Hill Press, San Diego.

32. Bobbin, R. P., Bledsoe, S. C., Jr., Winbery, S., Ceasar, G., and Jenison, G. L. (1985): Comparative actions of GABA and acetylcholine on the Xenopus laevis lateral line. *Comp. Biochem. Physiol.* [C], 80:313–318.

33. Bobbin, R. P., Bledsoe, S. C., Jr., Winbery, S. L., and Jenison, G. L. (1985): Actions of putative neurotransmitters and other relevant compounds on Xenopus laevis lateral line. In: *Auditory Biochemistry*, edited by D. G. Drescher, pp. 102–122. Charles C. Thomas, Springfield, IL.

34. Bowery, N. G., Hill, D. R., and Hudson, A. L. (1983): Characteristics of GABA receptor binding sites on rat whole brain synaptic membranes. *Br. J. Pharmacol.*, 78:191–206.

35. Brownell, W. E., Bader, C. E., Bertrand, D., and de Ribaupierre, Y. (1985): Evoked mechanical responses of isolated cochlear outer hair cells. *Science*, 227:194–196.

36. Bryant, G. M., and Guth, P. S. (1986): Adenosine has a neuromodulatory role in afferent transmission in the semicircular canal of the frog. *Abstracts of the Association for Research in Otolaryngology*, p. 120. Clearwater Beach, FL.

37. Churchill, J. A., Schuknecht, H. P., and Doran, R. (1956): Acetylcholinesterase activity in the cochlea. *Laryngoscope*, 66:1–15.

38. Comis, S. D., and Leng, G. (1979): Action of putative neurotransmitters in the guinea pig cochlea. *Exp. Brain Res.*, 36:119–128.

39. Cotman, C. W., and Iverson, L. L. (1987): Excitatory amino acids in the brain-focus on NMDA receptors. *Trends Neurosci.*, 10:263–265.

40. Crunelli, V., Forda, S., and Kelly, J. S. (1983): Blockade of amino acid-induced depolarizations and inhibition of excitatory postsynaptic potentials in rat dentate gyrus. *J. Physiol (Lond.)*, 341:627–640.

41. Davies, J., and Watkins, J. C. (1983): Role of excitatory amino acid receptors in mono- and polysynaptic excitation in the cat spinal cord. *Exp. Brain. Res.*, 49:280–290.

42. Dechesne, C., Raymond, J., and Sans, A. (1984): Action of glutamate in the cat labyrinth. *Ann. Otol. Rhinol. Laryngol.*, 93:163–165.
43. Desmedt, J. E., and Monaco, P. (1962): The pharmacology of a centrifugal inhibitory pathway in the cat's acoustic system. *Proc. First Intl. Pharmacol. Meet.*, 8:183–188.
44. Drescher, D. G., and Drescher, M. J. (1985): HPLC analysis of presumptive neurotransmitters in perilymph. In: *Auditory Biochemistry*, edited by D. G. Drescher, pp. 50–67. Charles C. Thomas, Springfield, IL.
45. Drescher, M. J., Drescher, D. G., and Medina, J. E. (1983): Effect of sound stimulation at several levels on concentrations of primary amines, including neurotransmitter candidates in perilymph of the guinea pig inner ear. *J. Neurochem.*, 41:309–320.
46. Dvorak, D. (1984): Off-pathway synaptic transmission in the outer retina of the axolotl is mediated by a kainic acid-preferring receptor. *Neurosci. Lett.*, 50:7–11.
47. Ehrenberger, K., Benkoe, E., and Felix, D. (1982): Suppressive action of picrotoxin, a GABA antagonist, on labyrinthine spontaneous nystagmus and vertigo in man. *Acta Otolaryngol. (Stockh.)*, 93:269–273.
48. Eybalin, M., and Pujol, R. (1983): A radioautographic study of [^{3}H]L-glutamate and [^{3}H]L-glutamine uptake in the guinea pig cochlea. *Neuroscience*, 9:863–871.
49. Eybalin, M., Parnaud, C., Geffard, M., and Pujol, R. (1988): Immunoelectron microscopy identifies several types of GABA-containing efferent synapses in the guinea pig organ of Corti. *Neuroscience (in press)*.
50. Eybalin, M., Rebillard, G., Jarry, T., and Cupo, A. (1987): Effect of noise level on the Met-enkephalin content of the guinea pig cochlea. *Brain Res.*, 418:189–192.
51. Fagg, G. E., and Foster, A. C. (1983): Amino acid neurotransmitters and their pathways in the mammalian central nervous system. *Neuroscience*, 9:701–719.
52. Fagg, G. E., Foster, A. C., and Ganong, A. H. (1986): Excitatory amino acid synaptic mechanisms and neurological function. *Trends Pharmacol. Sci.*, 85:357–363.
53. Felix, D., and Ehrenberger, K. (1982): The action of putative neurotransmitter substances in the cat labyrinth. *Acta Otolaryngol. (Stockh.)*, 93:101–105.
54. Felix, D., and Ehrenberger, K. (1985): The action of putative neurotransmitter substances in the mammalian labyrinth. In: *Auditory Biochemistry*, edited by D. G. Drescher, pp. 68–79. Charles C. Thomas, Springfield, IL.
55. Fex, J. (1968): Efferent inhibition in the cochlea by the olivocochlear bundle. In: *Ciba Foundation Symposium on Hearing Mechanisms in Vertebrates*, edited by A. V. S. de Reuck and J. Knight, pp. 169–181. Little, Brown, Boston.
56. Fex, J., and Altschuler, R. A. (1981): Enkephalin-like immunoreactivity of olivocochlear nerve fibers in cochlea of guinea pig and rat. *Proc. Natl. Acad. Sci. USA*, 78:1255–1259.
57. Fex, J., and Altschuler, R. A. (1984): Glutamic acid decarboxylase immunoreactivity of olivocochlear neurons in the organ of Corti of guinea pig and rat. *Hear. Res.*, 15:123–131.
58. Fex, J., and Martin, M. R. (1980): Lack of effect of DL-alpha-aminoadipate, an excitatory amino acid antagonist on cat auditory nerve responses to sound. *Neuropharmacology*, 19:809–811.
59. Fex, J., and Wenthold, R. (1976): Choline acetyltransferase, glutamate decarboxylase and tyrosine hydroxylase in the cochlea and cochlear nucleus of the guinea pig. *Brain Res.*, 109:575–585.
60. Fex, J., Altschuler, R. A., Kachar, B., Wenthold, R. J., and Zempel, J. M. (1986): GABA visualized by immunocytochemistry in the guinea pig cochlea in axons and endings of efferent neurons. *Brain Res.*, 366:106–117.
61. Fex, J., Altschuler, R. A., Wenthold, R. J., and Parakkal, M. H. (1982): Aspartate aminotransferase immunoreactivity in cochlea of guinea pig. *Hear. Res.*, 7:149–160.
62. Fex, J., Kachar, B., Rubio, J. A., Parakkal, M. H., and Altschuler, R. A. (1985): Glutaminase-like immunoreactivity in the organ of Corti of guinea pig. *Hear. Res.*, 17:101–113.
63. Flock, A. (1965): Electron microscopic and electrophysiological studies in the lateral-line canal organ. *Acta Otolaryngol. [Suppl.] (Stockh.)*, 199:1.
64. Flock, A., and Lam, D. M. K. (1974): Neurotransmitter synthesis in inner ear and lateral line sense organs. *Nature*, 249:142–144.
65. Fonnum, F. (1984): Glutamate: A neurotransmitter in mammalian brain. *J. Neurochem.* 42:1–11.
66. Forsberg, E. J., Rojas, E., and Pollard, H. B. (1986): Muscarinic receptor enhancement of nicotine-induced catecholamine secretion may be mediated by phosphoinositide metabolism in bovine adrenal chromaffin cells. *J. Biol. Chem.*, 261:4915–4919.
67. Foster, A., and Fagg, G. (1984): Acidic amino acid binding sites in mammalian neuronal membranes: Their characteristics and relationship to synaptic receptors. *Brain Res. Rev.*, 7:103–164.
68. Godfrey, D. A., Carter, J. A., Berger, S. J., and Matschinsky, F. M. (1976): Levels of putative transmitter amino acids in the guinea pig cochlea. *J. Histochem. Cytochem.*, 24:468–472.
69. Gold, G. H., and Nakamura, T. (1987): Cyclic nucleotide-gated conductances: A new class of ion channels mediates visual and olfactory transduction. *Trends Pharmacol. Sci.*, 8:312–316.

70. Greenberg, M. E., Ziff, E. B., and Greene, L. A. (1986): Stimulation of neuronal acetylcholine receptors induces rapid gene transcription. *Science*, 234:80–83.

71. Gulley, R. L., Fex, J., and Wenthold, R. J. (1979): Uptake of putative neurotransmitters in the organ of Corti. *Acta Otolaryngol. (Stockh.)*, 88:177–182.

72. Guth, P. S., and Melamed, B. (1982): Neurotransmission in the auditory system: A primer for pharmacologists. *Annu. Rev. Pharmacol. Toxicol.*, 22:383–412.

73. Guth, P. S., and Norris, C. H. (1984): Pharmacology of the isolated semicircular canal: Effect of GABA and picrotoxin. *Exp. Brain Res.*, 56:72–78.

74. Guth, P. S., Norris, C. H., and Bobbin, R. P. (1976): The pharmacology of transmission in the peripheral auditory system. *Pharmacol. Rev.*, 28:95–125.

75. Guth, P. S., Norris, C. H., Guth, S. L., Quine, D. B., and Williams, W. H. (1986): Cholinomimetics mimic efferent effects on semicircular canal afferent activity in the frog. *Acta Otolaryngol. (Stockh.)*, 102:194–203.

76. Guth, P. S., Norris, C. H., and Sewell, W. F. (1985): Primary afferent transmission in acoustico-lateralis organs. In: *Auditory Biochemistry*, edited by D. G. Drescher, pp. 41–49. Charles C. Thomas, Springfield, IL.

77. Herrling, P. L. (1985): Pharmacology of the corticocaudate excitatory postsynaptic potential in the cat: Evidence for its mediation by quisqualate- or kainate-receptors. *Neuroscience*, 14:417–426.

78. Higashida, H., and Brown, D. A. (1986): Two polyphosphatidylinositide metabolites control two K^+ currents in a neuronal cell. *Nature*, 323:333–335.

79. Hoffman, D. W. (1986): Opioid mechanisms in the inner ear. In: *Neurobiology of Hearing: The Cochlea*, edited by R. A. Altschuler, R. P. Bobbin, and D. W. Hoffman, pp. 371–382. Raven Press, New York.

80. Hoffman, D. W., Altschuler, R. A., and Fex, J. (1983): High-performance liquid chromatographic identification of enkephalin-like peptides in the cochlea. *Hear. Res.*, 9:71–78.

81. Jasser, A., and Guth, P. S. (1973): The synthesis of acetylcholine by the olivocochlear bundle. *J. Neurochem.*, 20:45–53.

82. Jenison, G. L., and Bobbin, R. P. (1985): Quisqualate excites spiral ganglion neurons of the guinea pig. *Hear. Res.*, 20:261–265.

83. Jenison, G. L., Bobbin, R. P., and Thalmann, R. (1985): Potassium-induced release of endogenous amino acids in the guinea pig cochlea. *J. Neurochem.*, 44:1845–1853.

84. Jenison, G. L., Winbery, S., and Bobbin, R. P. (1986): Comparative actions of quisqualate and N-methyl-D-aspartate, excitatory amino acid agonists, on guinea pig cochlear potentials. *Comp. Biochem. Physiol. [C]*, 84:385–389.

85. Klinke, R. (1981): Neurotransmitters in the cochlea and the cochlear nucleus. *Acta Otolaryngol. (Stockh.)*, 91:541–554.

86. Klinke, R., and Oertel, W. (1977): Evidence that GABA is not the afferent transmitter in the cochlea. *Exp. Brain Res.*, 28:311–331.

87. Klinke, R., and Oertel, W. (1977): Amino acids-putative afferent transmitter in the cochlea? *Exp. Brain Res.*, 30:145–148.

88. Kusakari, J., Arakawa, E., Ohyama, K., Rokugo, M., and Inamura, N. (1984): Effect of kainic acid upon N1 latency. *Laryngoscope*, 94:1365–1369.

89. Kuznetsov, V. I., and Godukhin, O. B. (1985): Mechanism of methionine-enkephalin modulation of glutamatergic transmission in the rat striatum. *Neurosci. Lett.*, 57:143–146.

90. MacDermott, A. B., and Dale, N. (1987): Receptors, ion channels and synaptic potentials underlying the integrative actions of excitatory amino acids. *Trends Neurosci.*, 10:280–284.

91. Martin, M. R. (1982): Baclofen and the brain stem auditory evoked potential. *Exp. Neurol.*, 76:675–680.

92. Martin, M. R. (1985): Excitatory amino acid pharmacology of the auditory nerve and nucleus magnocellularis of the chicken. *Hear. Res.*, 17:153–160.

93. Martinez-Rodriguez, R., Fernandez, B., Cevallos, C., and Gonzalez, M. (1974): Histochemical location of glutamic dehydrogenase and aspartate aminotransferase in chicken cerebellum. *Brain Res.*, 69:31–40.

94. Mayer, M. L., and Westbrook, G. L. (1987): The physiology of excitatory amino acids in the vertebrate central nervous system. *Prog. Neurobiol.*, 28:197–276.

95. Medina, J. E., and Drescher, D. G. (1981): The amino acid content of perilymph and cerebrospinal fluid from guinea pigs and the effect of noise on the amino acid composition of perilymph. *Neuroscience*, 6:505–509.

96. Melamed, B., Norris, C., Bryant, G., and Guth, P. (1982): Amino acid content of guinea pig perilymph collected under conditions of quiet or sound stimulation. *Hear. Res.*, 7:13–18.

97. Meza, G. (1985): Characterization of GABA-ergic and cholinergic neurotransmission in the chick inner ear. In: *Auditory Biochemistry*, edited by D. G. Drescher, pp. 80–101. Charles C. Thomas, Springfield, IL.

98. Nagai, R., Obara, S., and Kawaf, N. (1984): Differential blocking effects of a spider toxin on synaptic

and glutamate responses in the afferent synapse of the acousticolateralis receptors of Plotosus. *Brain Res.*, 300:183–187.

99. Neely, S. T., and Kim, D. O. (1986): A model for active elements in cochlear biomechanics. *J. Acoust. Soc. Am.*, 79:1472–1480.

100. Nicoletti, F., Iadarola, M. I., Wroblewski, J. T., and Costa, F. (1985): Excitatory amino acid receptors are coupled with inositol phospholipid metabolism in the rat central nervous system. *Soc. Neurosci. Abstr.*, 11:822.

101. Nielsen, D. W., and Slepecky, N. (1986): Stereocilia. In: *Neurobiology of Hearing: The Cochlea*, edited by R. A. Altschuler, R. P. Bobbin, and D. W. Hoffman, pp. 23–46. Raven Press, New York.

102. Nishizuka, Y. (1984): Turnover of inositol phospholipids and signal transduction. *Science*, 225:1365–1370.

103. Norris, C. H., and Guth, P. S. (1974): The release of acetylcholine (ACH) by the crossed olivocochlear bundle (COCB). *Acta Otolaryngol. (Stockh.)*, 77:318–326.

104. Norris, C. H., Guth, P. S., and Quine, D. B. (1987): The effects of histamine on the semicircular canal of the frog. *Abstracts of the Association for Research in Otolaryngology*, p. 107. Clearwater Beach, FL.

105. Olney, J. W., Fuller, T., and de Gubareff, T. (1979): Acute dendrotoxic changes in the hippocampus of kainate treated rats. *Brain Res.*, 176:91–100.

106. Ottersen, O. P., and Storm-Mathisen, J. (1984): Glutamate- and GABA-containing neurons in the mouse and rat brain, as demonstrated with a new immunocytochemical technique. *J. Comp. Neurol.*, 229:374–392.

107. Peet, M. J., Malik, R., and Curtis, D. R. (1983): Post excitatory depression of neuronal firing by acidic amino acids and acetylcholine in the cat spinal cord. *Brain Res.*, 263:162–166.

108. Pujol, R., Lenoir, M., Robertson, D., Eybalin, M., and Johnstone, B. M. (1985): Kainic acid selectively alters auditory dendrites connected with cochlear inner hair cells. *Hear. Res.*, 18:145–152.

109. Robertson, D., and Johnstone, B. M. (1978): Efferent transmitter substance in the mammalian cochlea: Single neuron support for acetylcholine. *Hear. Res.*, 1:31–34.

110. Rogawski, M. A. (1987): New directions in neurotransmitter action: Dopamine provides some important clues. *Trends Neurosci.*, 10:200–205.

111. Russell, I. J. (1971): The pharmacology of efferent synapses in the lateral line system of Xenopus laevis. *J. Exp. Biol.*, 54:643–658.

112. Russell, I. J. (1976): Amphibian lateral line receptors. In: *Frog Neurobiology: A Handbook*, edited by R. Llinas and W. Precht, pp. 513–549. Springer-Verlag, New York.

113. Ryan, A. F., and Schwartz, I. R. (1984): Preferential glutamine uptake by cochlear hair cells: Implications for the afferent cochlear transmitter. *Brain Res.*, 290:376–379.

114. Schacht, J. (1986): Biochemistry of cochlear function and pathology. In: *Seminars in Hearing*, edited by J. M. Miller, pp. 101–116. Thieme, New York.

115. Schacht, J., and Zenner, H. P. (1986): The phosphoinositide cascade in isolated outer hair cells: Possible role as second messenger for motile responses. *Hear. Res.*, 22:94.

116. Schuknecht, H. F., Churchill, J. A., and Doran, R. (1959): The localization of acetylcholinesterase in the cochlea. *Arch. Otolaryngol.* 69:549–559.

117. Schwartz, I. R., and Ryan, A. F. (1983): Differential labeling of sensory cell and neural populations in the organ of Corti following amino acid incubations. *Hear. Res.*, 9:185–200.

118. Sewell, W., Norris, C. H., Tachibana, M., and Guth, P. S. (1978): Detection of an auditory nerve-activating substance. *Science*, 202:910–912.

119. Spoendlin, H. (1974): Optic and cochleovestibular degenerations in hereditary ataxia: II. Temporal bone pathology in two cases of Friedreich's ataxia with vestibulo-cochlear disorders. *Brain*, 97:41–48.

120. Surtees, L., and Collins, G. G. S. (1985): Receptor types mediating the excitatory actions of exogenous L-aspartate and L-glutamate in rat olfactory cortex. *Brain Res.*, 334:287–295.

121. Tachibana, M., and Kuriyama, K. (1974): Gamma-aminobutyric acid in the lower auditory pathway of the guinea pig. *Brain Res.*, 69:370–374.

122. Takeda, N., Kitajiri, M., Girgis, S., Hillyard, C. J., MacIntyre, I., Emson, P. C. Shiosaka, S., Tohyama, M., and Matsunaga, T. (1986): The presence of a calcitonin gene-related peptide in the olivocochlear bundle in rat. *Exp. Brain Res.*, 61:575–578.

123. Tanaka, Y., and Katsuki, Y. (1966): Pharmacological investigations of cochlear responses and of olivocochlear inhibition. *J. Neurophysiol.*, 29:94–108.

124. Usami, S., Igarashi, M., and Thompson, G. C. (1987): GABA-like immunoreactivity in the squirrel monkey vestibular endorgans. *Brain Res.*, 417:367–370.

125. Valli, P., Zucca, G., Prigioni, I., Botta, L., Casella, C., and Guth, P. S. (1985): The effect of glutamate on the frog semicircular canal. *Brain. Res.*, 330:1–9.

126. Vizi, E. S. (1984): *Non-synaptic Interactions Between Neurons: Modulation of Neurochemical Transmission*, p. 260. John Wiley, New York.

127. Watkins, J. C., and Evans, R. H. (1981): Excitatory amino acid transmitters. In: *Annual Review of*

Pharmacology and Toxicology, 21, edited by R. George, R. Okum, and A. K. Cho, pp. 165–204. Annual Reviews, Palo Alto.

128. Watkins, J. C., and Olverman, H. J. (1987): Agonists and antagonists for excitatory amino acid receptors. *Trends Neurosci.*, 10:265–272.

129. Watkins, J. C., Evans, R. H., Mewett, K. N., Olverman, H. J., and Pook, P. (1986): Recent advances in the pharmacology of excitatory amino acids. In: *Excitatory Amino Acid Transmission*, edited by T. P. Hick, D. Lodge, and H. McLennan, pp. 19–26. Alan R. Liss, New York.

130. Werman, R. (1966): A review: Criteria for identification of a central nervous system transmitter. *Comp. Biochem. Physiol.*, 18:745–766.

131. Winbery, S. L., and Bobbin, R. P. (1983): Actions of acetylcholine and carbachol on the spontaneous activity of afferent fibers in the Xenopus laevis lateral line. *Abstracts of the Association for Research in Otolaryngology*, p. 47. St. Petersburg, FL.

132. Yarom, Y., Bracha, O., and Werman, R. (1985): Intracellular injection of acetylcholine blocks various potassium conductances in vagal motoneurons. *Neuroscience*, 16:739–752.

133. Zieglgansberger, W. (1980): Peptides in the regulation of neuronal function. In: *Peptides: Integrators of Cell and Tissue Function*, edited by F. E. Bloom, pp. 219–233. Raven Press, New York.

134. Zimmerman, D. McG. (1979): Onset of neural function in the lateral line. *Nature*, 282:82–84.

Physiology of the Ear,
edited by A. F. Jahn and J. Santos-Sacchi.
Raven Press, New York © 1988.

Introduction to Anatomy and Physiology of the Central Auditory Nervous System

D. P. Phillips

Department of Psychology, Dalhousie University, Halifax, Nova Scotia, Canada B3H 4J1

It is difficult to capture in a few pages the rapidly expanding wealth of information on the structural and functional organization of the central auditory nervous system. The account that follows is of necessity both highly selective and highly simplified in its treatment of the subject matter, and the reader is referred to other sources for detailed coverage of issues only lightly touched on here (4,8,16,21,30,68,75,94, 132,140). The organization of the material in the following pages is broadly hierarchical. It begins by sketching some of the dominant features of cochlear nerve fiber physiology and examining the physiological consequences of the various structural modes in which auditory nerve fiber input is disseminated in the cochlear nucleus. We turn then to examine the projections of the cochlear nucleus on the superior olivary nuclei and the inferior colliculus. Since the olivary nuclei receive input bilaterally from the cochlear nuclei, opportunity will be taken to examine both the form of the binaural interactions that emerge from that convergent input and the more general question of the neural basis of spatial hearing. We will then briefly examine the organization of the thalamocortical auditory system and conclude with an analysis of some of the peripheral and central auditory contributions to the neural correlates of noise masking and subjective loudness.

Although a knowledge of basic neurophysiology is assumed in this chapter, it will be of help to define some specific terms that are used throughout. The term *tuning curve* (or *frequency tuning curve* or *threshold tuning curve*) refers to the minimum tone intensity (expressed on dB sound pressure level, i.e., dB re 20 μPa) required to increase a neuron's spike discharge rate above spontaneous levels, plotted as a function of tone frequency (expressed in kHz). It is thus a curve that depicts the sensitivity of a neuron to tone frequency. The term *characteristic frequency* (CF) denotes the tone frequency to which a neuron is most sensitive, i.e., has the lowest absolute threshold for an excitatory response. The term *rate-level function* refers to a graph of spike discharge rate (expressed on spikes/sec or spikes/stimulus trial) plotted as a function of the sound pressure level of the stimulus used. This curve provides quantitative information on the threshold and intensity dynamic range of a neuron for the stimulus in question. Finally, the term *response area* refers to the total frequency-intensity domain within which a tonal stimulus is able to influence a neuron's spike discharge rate. Note that all of these terms can be applied as usefully to inhibitory responses as to excitatory ones.

One other preliminary issue merits consideration here. Much of the evidence on the stimulus–response functions of central auditory neurons has come from studies in anesthetized animals. The use of anesthesia is required since relatively invasive surgical procedures are needed. It raises the question, however, of the extent to which neuronal response properties, so visualized, accurately represent those of cells in the alert animal. This issue is far from resolved. Considering the auditory cortex, for example, it is abundantly clear that neuronal responses are significantly more vigorous and sustained in the alert animal than in the anesthetized one. The further, and possibly more important, question is whether the use of general anesthesia modifies the stimulus selectivity of cortical neurons. In this respect, where data are available to make the necessary comparisons, most or all of the physiological cell types seen in the anesthetized animal have also been described in the awake preparation. On the other hand, some cell types described for the cortex of awake animals have not been seen in the anesthetized animal. It is also often the case that the supragranular cortical layers are relatively unresponsive in the anesthetized animal, suggesting that general anesthesia depresses or silences some cells. It is therefore likely that studies of anesthetized animals may not reveal the full complement of afferent input to cortical (or other) auditory neurons. For further discussion of this issue, the reader is referred to a number of recent reports (4,31,105,112,146).

AUDITORY NERVE AND COCHLEAR NUCLEAR COMPLEX

The afferent auditory neurons of the VIIIth cranial nerve are bipolar cells with their perikarya located in the cochlear spiral ganglion. The dendrites of these neurons traverse the osseous spiral lamina to penetrate the organ of Corti and innervate, almost exclusively, the inner hair cells (127). Fibers innervating the pillar side of the inner hair cell base have systematically larger diameters than those innervating the modiolar side (63). The axons of spiral ganglion cells leave the cochlea, pass through the internal auditory meatus, and ramify within the cochlear nuclear complex. Since most electrophysiological studies of single elements in the VIIIth nerve have actually been based on axonal recordings, the identified elements have, by convention, been termed cochlear nerve fibers rather than spiral ganglion cells.

To the extent that each cochlear nerve fiber's input is functionally unitary (i.e., derived from a single inner hair cell), auditory nerve fibers form a relatively homogeneous physiological population. Each fiber has a clearly defined CF to which it is most sensitive, and spike discharge rates are sigmoidal (monotonic) functions of the level of a suprathreshold tonal or other stimulus. In response to a low-frequency tone of appropriate amplitude, most auditory nerve fibers group their spike discharges around integral multiples of the period of the stimulating sinusoid (57,89,114). If one examines the temporal disposition of spike response times within the period of the sine wave, then the spikes are typically found within a specifiable preferred half-period of the stimulus waveform. This phase-locked behavior follows from the functional polarization of hair cells, and therefore the sensitivity of hair cell depolarization to unidirectional elevations of the basilar membrane (19,33,89,106). Hair cell transmitter release is likely synchronized to the depolarization phase of the receptor potential; the AC component of the hair cell response, which dominates for low-stimulus frequencies, is thus able to synchronize transmitter release to the depolarizing half-period of the waveform. For high tone frequencies, where the DC component may dominate, there is little or no opportunity for any such synchronization (89). Phase locking of the spike discharges of cochlear nerve fibers is poor for tone frequencies above 3.5 kHz (89,114). At higher stimulus frequencies, the distribution of interspike intervals is continuous, with a mode often significantly less than 10 to 12 msec, and an exponentially declining tail (21).

Phase locking of the spike activity of cochlear nerve fibers extends to complex sounds that have significant low-frequency content (19). By means of long-term sampling of the discharges evoked by a complex periodic sound, it is possible to show that the probability of a spike discharge has a temporal distribution that follows the instantaneous amplitude of a partially rectified stimulus waveform (19). It is important to appreciate, however, that if the central nervous system uses a temporal code (i.e., distribution of interspike intervals) for the analysis of low-frequency stimuli, then it may do so as much by spatial sampling across cochlear nerve fibers as by temporal sampling within any single fiber.

Recent quantitative studies have distinguished two major groups of cochlear nerve fibers within this otherwise homogeneous population (27,62,119). The larger group (90%–95% of the total) has spontaneous discharge rates in excess of 18 spikes/sec, intensity dynamic ranges less than approximately 30 dB in breadth, clearly saturating rate-level functions, and the lowest absolute thresholds of fibers in any specified CF range. It is likely that these represent the large-diameter fibers. The smaller population has very low spontaneous rates, broader intensity dynamic ranges, less marked tendency to firing-rate saturation at high stimulus levels, and higher absolute thresholds. This physiological group probably represents the small-diameter fiber population (63).

The cochlear nuclear complex contains three major subdivisions, differentiated in both Nissl and Golgi material (14,21,88). These are the anteroventral (AVCN), posteroventral (PVCN), and dorsal (DCN) cochlear nuclei. Cochlear nerve fibers enter at the nerve root, which separates the AVCN from the PVCN and DCN. Within the nerve root, each primary afferent fiber bifurcates. The branching itself and the dissemination of axon terminals throughout the cochlear nuclei are highly orderly (65). The fibers penetrating the cochlear nucleus most deeply before branching have high CFs, whereas fibers deriving their input from more apical cochlear regions bifurcate ventrally, nearer the entry point of the nerve trunk. One axonal branch projects directly on AVCN neurons; the other gives off terminal branches in PVCN en route to DCN. The projection of the cochlear nerve on the cochlear nuclei is thus a divergent one. The terminal fields of the auditory nerve fibers within the cochlear nucleus subdivisions are, however, highly restricted. The result is that most of the postsynaptic neurons retain narrow excitatory response areas and well-defined CFs. Moreover, the recipient neurons are spatially arrayed according to the CFs conferred by their inputs. Each subdivision of the cochlear nucleus thus contains a relatively complete neural representation of cochlear place and hence the audible frequency range (30). This tonotopic organization is a cardinal feature of all the core nuclei of the central auditory pathway (4,68). Interestingly, the terminal axon arbors of the low spontaneous rate, saturation-resistant cochlear nerve fibers may have more branch points and be more ramifying than those of the high spontaneous rate group (32). By this means, some resistance to firing-rate saturation might be conferred on many central neurons.

Neuroanatomical specializations within the ventral and dorsal divisions of the cochlear nucleus impart quite different functional properties on AVCN, PVCN, and

DCN neurons (21,41,59,90). In the AVCN, some neurons (bushy cells in Golgi material) receive cochlear nerve input by way of synaptic endings termed end-bulbs of Held (13). These are large afferent endings with finger-like extensions that partially encapsulate the AVCN cell soma. They are most common among AVCN neurons of low CF (118), and only a very small number of such endings innervate any given AVCN cell. By means of these contacts, an afferent fiber may exert a dominant influence on the spike (action-potential) behavior of the postsynaptic AVCN neuron. It is in part for this reason that the response properties of these AVCN neurons in many respects resemble those of the low-CF afferent fibers by which they are innervated. Thus, the frequency tuning, response areas, driven and spontaneous interspike-interval distributions, and phase-locking behavior of many of these AVCN neurons may rather faithfully preserve that seen in the cochlear nerve (59,90,110).

The second major morphological population in the AVCN comprises the stellate neurons, which likely receive numerous button-like synaptic contacts from primary afferent fibers (13,14). These neurons display more varied and complex CF tone-evoked temporal patterns of spike discharges than do cochlear nerve fibers (109,110). Some of these neurons [the so-called chopper cells, cf. (90)] display distinct periodicities in the peristimulus-time histograms of their responses. These periodicities are unrelated to stimulus frequency. Quantitative studies of the fine temporal structure of these responses indicate that they are of a kind that may be shaped by a multiplicity of small-amplitude synaptic inputs (21,76,91). The interspike-interval distributions of the driven responses of these cells may have modes as short as 2 to 3 msec and be symmetrical, without the exponentially declining tail seen in the spike behavior of cochlear nerve fibers (110). In addition, many of these neurons may receive inhibitory inputs in the form of suppressive response areas flanking the excitatory one centered at CF (110,125).

An interesting recent finding is that the differences in the organization of synaptic input to bushy and stellate cells may be paralleled by differences in the electrical properties of the postsynaptic neuronal membranes (85,141). Bushy cells, in particular, exhibit bioelectrical specializations that may facilitate the faithful preservation of spike timing in the afferent input. These neurons display large but brief excitatory postsynaptic potentials. Intracellularly injected depolarizing current usually evokes a single-action potential in bushy cells. In addition, they possess a low-input resistance that requires a large synaptic current for postsynaptic depolarization, and it is likely that such currents are generated by the end-bulbs by which they are usually innervated. In contrast, stellate cells have a higher input resistance and respond to intracellularly injected current with trains of spike potentials. These postsynaptic properties may be viewed as complementary to the afferent innervation patterns of AVCN neurons in shaping the temporal organization of the spike discharges of those cells. The bushy cells are able to preserve the time structure of spike activity present in the afferent input. The stellate cells may not, but by virtue of their convergent input and bioelectric specializations, they are among the most vigorously discharging neurons in the auditory brainstem.

One of the major cell groups in the PVCN is the octopus cell (21). These neurons have long, paired dendrites oriented orthogonally to the incoming cochlear nerve fibers. There is evidence that these neurons may be more broadly tuned to tone frequency than are cochlear nerve fibers (110), which is perhaps to be expected given the spatial arrangement of their dendritic fields. These neurons also display strikingly transient discharge patterns to tonal stimuli and have been implicated in the coding of repetitive acoustic stimuli.

The DCN has a quite different neuronal circuitry. There are no end-bulbs of Held in the DCN: cochlear nerve axon terminals are more conventional in size and are found on a variety of morphological cell types. The output neurons of the DCN have been identified structurally and functionally using retrograde tracing (2,122) and antidromic activation (145) techniques, and are those neurons with fusiform peri-karya. Many of the smaller neurons in the DCN are intrinsic inhibitory neurons, and their connections onto the fusiform cells significantly shape both the temporal pat-terning of spike discharges and the effective response areas of those cells (31,41,42,111,112,125,146). Studied with tonal stimuli, a number of physiological cell types have been differentiated, most notably by the organization of their inhibitory inputs. The DCN output cells have small, circumscribed excitatory response areas, with strong inhibitory inputs from frequency–intensity domains on the low- and/or high-frequency sides and in high-intensity domains at CF. In some cases the dis-position of these inhibitory response areas corresponds well with the excitatory stimulus domains of smaller, neighboring cells. Where it has been possible to record pairs of such neurons simultaneously, and thereby correlate in time their spike dis-charges, activity in the presumed inhibitory interneurons is closely followed in time by suppression of discharges in the DCN output neuron (133).

One of the consequences of these inhibitory inputs is a marked selectivity of DCN output cells for stimulus amplitude (41,111,146). These neurons, because they are inhibited at high stimulus levels, have bell-shaped (nonmonotonic) rate-level func-tions for tones and may be excited by tones over exceedingly narrow frequency and intensity ranges. Sideband (lateral) inhibition in other DCN neurons imposes marked constraints on the spectral bandwidth of excitatory noise stimuli. This follows from the fact that broadband signals may invade both the excitatory and inhibitory re-sponse areas of DCN neurons, resulting in an effective cancellation of the excitatory afferent events.

SUPERIOR OLIVARY COMPLEX AND INFERIOR COLLICULUS

Bushy cells of the AVCN project directly on the ipsilateral and contralateral medial superior olivary nucleus (MSO) (26). Neurons in these pontine nuclei possess two densely tufted dendrites; those on the lateral side receive axon terminals from the ipsilateral AVCN, and those on the medial side derive their input from the contra-lateral AVCN (21,26,39,130). These axons reach their olivary destinations via the trapezoid body, which is a heavily myelinated fiber tract at the base of the brainstem containing fibers of a variety of sources and target nuclei. The axonal arbors of the ventral cochlear nucleus inputs to the MSO are tonotopically constrained. The MSO thereby contains a complete representation of the audible frequency range, although it may be somewhat biased in favor of low-CF neurons.

Cochlear nucleus neurons (likely modified bushy cells receiving a smaller variant of end-bulb contact from the VIIIth nerve) project directly on the ipsilateral lateral superior olivary nucleus (LSO) and indirectly on the contralateral LSO, by way of the medial nucleus of the trapezoid body (MNTB) of the target LSO side. Innervation of MNTB cells by cochlear nucleus axons is by means of specialized calyx-type endings partially encapsulating the MNTB cell soma (81). It is thought that the MNTB cells serve as inhibitory interneurons between the cochlear nucleus and the LSO. As in the case of the MSO, afferent input to the MNTB/LSO is tonotopically constrained. These factors serve to provide LSO cells with a net excitatory input from the ipsilateral ear, and a net inhibitory input of similar CF from the contralateral ear. In contrast to the MSO, the representation of the audible frequency range in the LSO may be somewhat biased in favor of high CF cells. The differing patterns of binaural convergence on MSO and LSO neurons have important consequences for the sensitivity of cells in those structures to interaural temporal and intensity disparities and, therefore, for mechanisms underlying binaural spatial hearing. With some exceptions (12,39,40), however, most of the detailed evidence on the physiology of superior olivary neurons has come from studies of cells in nuclei to which the olivary neurons project. We will therefore postpone discussion of that physiology until the efferent connections of the olivary nuclei have been described.

Surrounding the MSO and LSO are a number of cell groups deriving their ascending acoustic input bilaterally from the cochlear nuclei either by way of the trapezoid body or from the PVCN via the intermediate acoustic stria that leaves the cochlear nuclei and penetrates the olivary nuclei from their dorsal sides. Neurons in these satellite nuclei and in the LSO give rise to axons forming the olivocochlear bundles (64,113,134). Small cells within the LSO give rise to slender unmyelinated axons that descend through the ipsilateral cochlear nerve to terminate as small contacts located on the afferent terminals of cochlear nerve fibers innervating inner hair cells. These fibers make up the (uncrossed) olivocochlear bundle. Much larger neurons located outside the LSO, in the dorsomedial periolivary cell groups, give rise to large-diameter, myelinated axons that cross the midline to innervate outer hair cells in the contralateral cochlea. These fibers make up the crossed olivocochlear bundle (COCB). These descending connections, perhaps particularly those of the COCB, may serve to modulate cochlear sensitivity, possibly by influencing the contractile properties of the outer hair cells (cf. 15,34,36).

The ascending outputs of the olivary nuclei are directed to the inferior colliculi (IC), which are bilateral, mesencephalic relay nuclei for almost all ascending auditory projections. The MSO projections are almost exclusively ipsilateral, whereas those of the LSO are largely crossed (66,116). These fibers ascend via the lateral lemnisci, which are large myelinated fiber tracts lying close to the lateral surface of the brainstem. In addition, output fibers from the DCN form the dorsal acoustic stria, cross the midline, enter the lateral lemniscus, and ascend to the IC. A smaller direct ipsilateral projection from the ACVN also ascends via the lateral lemniscus to penetrate the IC. The lateral lemniscus itself contains two groups of cell bodies, the dorsal (DNLL) and ventral (VNLL) nuclei. Many neurons in the DNLL are binaurally influenced, and it is therefore likely that they derive a substantial input from the olivary nuclei (18). The VNLL, on the other hand, contains mostly neurons receiving a monaural contralateral input, likely derived from the contralateral cochlear nucleus (3). Both cell groups of the lateral lemniscus send axons to the IC. A net morphological result of these numerous axonal projection systems is that the outputs of each cochlea, which are disseminated throughout the numerous pontine auditory nuclei, regroup at the IC.

The structure and physiology of the IC have been described in detail. It contains three major subdivisions. The largest is the central nucleus (ICC), which, in Golgi material, has a distinctly laminar appearance. This derives in part from the spatial arrangement of its neurons' tufted dendritic processes: they provide the impression of curved laminae stacked in the dorsolateral-to-ventromedial direction. It is in the ICC that the vast majority of lateral lemniscus fibers terminate. On its dorsal and lateral margins, the ICC is bounded by the pericentral nucleus (ICP), which receives acoustic input, but whose function is largely unknown. On its caudal and ventral sides, the ICC is bounded by an external nucleus (ICX). The ICX likely derives at least part of its acoustic input from the ICC (7). Its descending outputs may be directed to brainstem nuclei involved in head, pinna, and/or eye movements to acoustic targets.

The ICC contains a single tonotopic organization, with dorsally located neurons tuned to low tone frequencies and ventrally located cells tuned to high frequencies (70,120). The axis of the tonotopic gradient is perpendicular to the morphological lamination, so that cells of any given CF are arrayed in curved planes or sheets. It is thus a remarkable feature of brainstem auditory system circuitry, as well as central nervous system ontogeny, that inputs from widely dispersed nuclei converge not only within a single mesencephalic nucleus, but within a single tonotopic framework. Within the ICC, inputs from various pontine auditory nuclei are not homogeneously distributed, even within iso-CF laminae. Thus, the DCN likely projects on neurons located ventrally and caudally in the ICC, despite the fact that the relevant iso-CF laminae may be more extensive. Neither, however, is the segregation of input to the ICC complete: in an elegant study, Semple and Aitkin (121) revealed that ICC neurons receiving short-latency, and presumably monosynaptic, input from the DCN often were also innervated by LSO neurons.

Relatively few authors have studied the physiology of superior olivary neurons directly, presumably for technical reasons (39). In contrast, the discharge characteristics of IC neurons, particularly those of the ICC, have been described in detail. At least in part, the response properties of ICC neurons must reflect those of the neurons from which the ICC cells receive their input. It is for these reasons that the properties of superior olivary neurons have, implicitly or explicitly, often been inferred from those of cells in the ICC (e.g., 61,115,142–144), the DNLL (18), or higher centers (5,20,103).

The physiology of neurons in the MSO and LSO is of special interest because the olivary nuclei are the structures in which information from the two ears first converges. This interest itself derives from the fact that many aspects of spatial hearing, particularly the ability to localize sound sources in space, are based on a comparison of the stimuli arriving at the two tympanic membranes. This fact in turn derives from physical acoustics. When a sound source is located in the mid-saggital plane, the stimuli impinging on the two tympanic membranes are closely matched in arrival time and intensity. For any sound source location outside the median plane, the additional path length to the farther ear and the sound shadowing effect of the head and pinnae impose interaural arrival time and intensity differences, respectively (95). The arrival time disparity, which may be as great as 400 μsec, generates an interaural phase difference, which, for low-frequency stimulus components, is within the temporal resolving power of central auditory neurons. The interaural intensity difference is most significant for signals with high-frequency content where the relevant stimulus wavelengths are smaller than the head diameter. These frequencies are those above 2 to 3 kHz and are therefore usually outside the range where sensitivity to interaural phase differences significantly shapes neuronal responses to binaural stimuli.

The neural mechanisms contributing to this comparison have been most thoroughly studied in the DNLL (18) and ICC (61,115,142–144). At those levels, it is apparent that the input from each ear has an excitatory response phase locked to a preferred half-cycle of the stimulus waveform. The remaining half-period may or may not be associated with an inhibitory response, in one or both monaural inputs. When the excitatory response phases arrive at the binaural neuron synchronously, that neuron responds vigorously. When the interaural phase disparity is varied from the optimal one, the excitatory response phase of one input partially or totally overlaps in arrival time with the inhibitory response phase from the opposite ear, resulting in a net cancellation of the excitatory input and a poor response. Because the low-frequency tones typically used to study these phenomena are themselves periodic (i.e., repeating sinusoids), increments in interaural phase delay result in a spike rate that is a periodic function of the delay; the period of the response cycle is equal to that of the stimulus waveform.

Low-CF neurons are often sensitive to tonal stimuli over relatively broad ranges of low stimulus frequencies. This has enabled study of sensitivity to interaural phase delay for different tone frequencies within a single neuron (115,143). Variations in interaural delay for each tone frequency produce a response rate that is a cyclical function of delay, the period of the response function reflecting that of the carrier tone. In many cases, the delay functions for the various tone frequencies coincide at a single point, referred to as the characteristic delay for that neuron. Where the point of coincidence occurs at a peak response rate, the time delay in the dichotic stimulus usually favors the contralateral ear (i.e., contralateral stimulus phase leads ipsilateral phase). When the delay functions have a common trough, that characteristic delay typically favors the ipsilateral ear (143). Two important consequences follow from these data. First, most neurons are maximally responsive to delays that favor the contralateral ear and therefore simulate contralateral sound source locations. Second, small changes in azimuth of a low-frequency sound source, and therefore in the interaural delay generated by that source, will have maximal effects on the identity and size of the discharging neuronal population when those changes occur over azimuthal ranges close to the midline.

Neurons in the LSO receive an excitatory input directly from the ipsilateral cochlear nucleus and an inhibitory input of comparable CF from the contralateral cochlear nucleus by way of the MNTB. Because the output of the LSO is largely crossed, this binaural input pattern is manifested as a contralateral-excitatory/ipsilateral-inhibitory one in neurons of the DNLL, ICC, and higher structures. The strengths of both the excitatory and inhibitory inputs are sensitive functions of stimulus level. Studied with binaural signals, the response rates of such neurons reflect the balance of excitatory and inhibitory events evoked by the stimuli at the two ears.

This sensitivity has been demonstrated by examining neuronal response rate for a constant contralateral (excitatory) tone level presented simultaneously with various ipsilateral (inhibitory) tone levels (5,18,20,103,115). These studies typically have revealed a sigmoidal function relating response rate to ipsilateral tone level, and therefore interaural intensity disparity. Generally, intensity differences favoring the contralateral ear (i.e., contralateral tone level exceeding the ipsilateral) evoke vigorous responses, whereas intensity disparities favoring the ipsilateral ear result in a profound, and often complete, suppression of the response that otherwise would result from stimulation of the contralateral ear alone. Over a restricted range of interaural intensity differences, response rate declines steeply with increasing ipsilateral intensity. This range of intensity disparities is centered close to zero. A further question is the stability of this sensitive range over variations in the absolute level of the binaural stimulus. In at least some instances, this range is invariant over wide ranges of absolute contralateral stimulus levels, suggesting that excitatory and inhibitory inputs may be, in those instances, closely matched in both threshold and intensity dependence.

In some rostral auditory nuclei, a second group of neurons sensitive to interaural intensity disparity has been described. These neurons discharge vigorously in response to simultaneous, equally intense CF tones at the two ears, but their spike discharge rates fall dramatically if either an interaural arrival time or intensity difference, favoring either ear, is introduced. These cells are unresponsive to monaural stimuli and have often been termed predominantly binaural (60,87,103,138). These neurons likely receive a sub-(spike)-threshold input from each ear. Summation of these inputs might reasonably be expected to occur in the event of their synchronous arrival at the binaural neuron. This synchrony of input would, however, be prevented by the presence of an arrival time disparity in the stimuli at the two ears or by an interaural intensity difference, in the latter case by means of the familiar latency–intensity relation.

NEURAL CODING OF ACOUSTIC SPATIAL INFORMATION AND THE QUESTION OF "EAR" REPRESENTATION IN THE CENTRAL AUDITORY SYSTEM

From the foregoing, it is apparent that there are some marked similarities in the sensitivities of the relevant central neurons to the interaural phase and intensity disparities that are cues for sound source azimuth. These similarities prompt a more general examination of neural sensitivity to sound source location, the cues in which that sensitivity has its genesis, and their behavioral consequences.

Neurons sensitive to interaural differences in the phase of low-frequency signals and those sensitive to interaural disparities in the intensity of high-frequency signals are maximally responsive to interaural disparities favoring the contralateral ear and are poorly responsive to, or actively inhibited by, disparities favoring the ipsilateral ear. These anisotropic distributions themselves have the consequence that small azimuthal shifts of a sound source may bring about the greatest changes in the identity and size of the responsive neural populations when those shifts are over azimuthal ranges close to the midline. It is important to recall, however, that the mechanisms shaping sensitivity to interaural phase and intensity differences are quite different: the former represents a cycle-by-cycle comparison of stimulus phase at the tympani and is achieved by means of a temporal interlacing of excitatory and inhibitory phase-locked events in the input from each ear; the latter reflects the net balance of excitatory input from one ear and inhibitory input from the other.

Recent measurements of the interaural time and intensity differences generated by the heads and pinnae of cats (79,117) have provided new evidence on the azimuthal dependence of interaural disparity magnitude that is of direct relevance here. Measured close to the tragus, interaural temporal and intensity disparities are negligible for stimuli located in the median plane and increase in magnitude with increasing sound source eccentricity. For both time and amplitude disparities, however, the relation between disparity magnitude and azimuth is often markedly nonlinear. The disparities increase steeply as source azimuths increase from 0° (midline) and tend toward plateau levels when source eccentricities exceed approximately 45°. For (tonal) stimuli then, the interaural disparity generated by a near-midline source may unambiguously specify source azimuth in the frontal (or caudal) sound field; such is less obviously the case at wide eccentricities. Central neurons have firing rates that are sensitive functions of interaural disparities over ranges close to zero. The central auditory nervous system may be seen, therefore, to be most sensitive to interaural time and intensity disparities where those disparities themselves most precisely specify sound source azimuth (95).

A further correspondence is relevant here. In humans studied with interaural phase and intensity differences, the ability of those cues to determine perceived source azimuth is greatest over cue ranges associated with perceived azimuths relatively close to the midline. Similarly, in human (74) and animal (55) free-field localization, the greatest acuity in localization is for sources close to the midline. Perhaps predictably then, behavioral sensitivity reflects neural sensitivity.

This discussion raises the question of the mechanisms used to localize sound sources at wider eccentricities where the interaural disparities are less precise in specifying source azimuth. Psychophysical evidence in humans (9,82,86) and physiological evidence in animals (25,35,73,96,123) suggests that sound pressure transformations incurred by the passive acoustical properties of the pinnae and external auditory meatuses may significantly enhance localization cues for sources at loci with nonzero azimuths and elevations. The pinna, at least in animals, has a distinct acoustical axis within the acoustic hemifield of the same side. This acoustical axis is manifested as a peak in the tympanic sound pressure level for sources located in the preferred direction; it reflects both amplification of signals on axis and attenuation of those sources whose locations are off axis (25,96). These properties have their basis in the joint effects of the resonance properties of the external auditory meatus and the diffraction of sound waves brought about by the pinna itself. As a result, the directional properties of the pinnae may significantly modify the interaural intensity disparities that would otherwise result from the sound shadowing effect of the head alone.

In free-field studies of the spatial selectivity of central auditory neurons, there has been agreement that neurons with restricted spatial receptive fields have those fields located almost exclusively in contralateral space (35,72,73,78,123). In most cases, these receptive fields are centered on the acoustical axis of the contralateral pinna. It is likely, however, that neural firing rates within the receptive field and the receptive field boundary itself may be shaped by both pinna directionality and binaural interactions (24,73,78,123,138). Thus, provided that information about pinna and/or head orientation is available, perhaps by efference copy or proprioception, pinna directionality might readily be utilized to enhance the dichotic localization cues and therefore sound-localization performance in the lateral auditory hemifields. It seems equally likely that if the locus of a sound source is known, then pinna directionality might be used, by active pinna/head movements, to improve the signal-to-noise ratio for that stimulus at the tympanum.

A second salient feature of the foregoing binaural interaction data is the contralateral bias in the effective interaural phase delays and intensity disparities for neurons rostral to the LSO. It has been argued that this contralateral bias extends to the range of time and intensity disparities encoded by the dynamic portions of the response rate–disparity functions and not simply disparities evoking maximal responses (95,103,143). These views are compatible with the evidence from the free-field studies, which indicates the near-exclusive contralateral location of acoustic spatial receptive fields of central neurons. Taken together, these data suggest that each side of the auditory nervous system (rostral to the LSO) processes spatial information only for the contralateral auditory hemifield and is independently capable of localizing sound sources in that acoustic hemifield.

This point takes on special significance from the fact that a widely expressed view of sound-localization mechanisms holds that it is a comparison of the outputs of the bilateral olivary nuclei that determines sound source laterality (10,11,44,135). The hypothesis outlined earlier suggests that such interhemispheric comparisons are unnecessary. It suggests that the relevant comparison is that of the stimuli at the two ears and that it is the process of this comparison in the superior olivary nuclei that confers a contralateral preference in the spatial properties of higher neurons. Two independent lines of evidence support this view. First, transections of the commissural fiber tracts of the auditory system, with the obvious exception of the trapezoid body mediating the binaural comparison, are without effect on the free-field sound-localization performance of animals (77). Second, unilateral ablation of central auditory nuclei rostral to the olivary nuclei results in profound deficits in the performance of sound localization tasks, but only for responses to sources in the sound field contralateral to the lesion (55,56,58,66,95). The contralaterality of acoustic spatial deficits following from unilateral brain damage may extend to humans (46,98). It seems unlikely that hypotheses postulating interhemispheric comparisons as necessary for normal lateralization or localization performance can sustain these data.

Interestingly, animals with bilateral lesions of the primary auditory cortex are unable to localize sound sources within either hemifield, although they retain the ability to distinguish sound source laterality, i.e., left from right (58). This ability is equally preserved in animals with unilateral lesions (55). These data suggest that the neural mechanisms subserving localization within an auditory hemifield may be quite different from those underlying discriminations between the acoustic hemifields.

One further ramification of these data merits consideration. The binaural interactions developed in the brainstem auditory neurons are conferred onto higher neurons, including those of the cortex. Thus, the vast majority of cortical cells are binaurally influenced and show the now familiar contralateral bias in their spatial properties (10,20,22,73,103). It is important to recognize that this contralateral bias in spatial selectivity does not derive from the relative effectiveness of stimuli at the two ears in influencing those cells: the spatial selectivity is generated by binaural computations and would be minimal without them. These and other considerations have raised the question of in what sense the contralateral ear should be thought of as dominant in each cerebral hemisphere as is usually held to be the case (29,98). It is noteworthy in this respect that many of the assessment techniques revealing contralateral ear deficits after unilateral brain damage have inherent in them the feature of compromising or eliminating some of the normal contributions of the ipsilateral ear inputs (e.g., dichotic listening tasks). It seems plausible that the ipsilateral and contralateral acoustic inputs to the cerebral hemispheres have only partially overlapping functional roles and that it is the contralateral projections that are relatively selectively accessed by those tests. It may thus be more parsimonious to think of the apparent contralaterality of ear deficits after unilateral cerebral lesions as special cases of a more general contralateral spatial representation in the auditory nervous system. To some extent, these conclusions parallel those in the visual system: visual cortex neurons are largely binocular but process spatial information only for the contralateral visual field. The difference between spatial representation in the visual and auditory systems derives from the fact that in vision the contralaterality is a direct consequence of the decussating projection of the peripheral receptor sheets, whereas in audition the contralaterality may be necessarily computational in origin.

Jenkins and Merzenich (56) provided a new insight into the nature of spatial information coding in the central auditory system. They unilaterally ablated focal regions of the cat's primary auditory cortex that represented a single, narrow range of tone frequencies and then tested the animals in a free-field sound localization task using tonal stimuli. These animals showed poor performance only for sources in the sound field contralateral to the lesion and for stimulus frequencies deprived of cortical representation. This suggests that the coding of sound localization cues is accomplished over frequency-specific pathways, a conclusion that is entirely consistent with the tonotopic framework within which convergence of information from the two ears occurs (see above).

MEDIAL GENICULATE BODY AND AUDITORY CORTEX

Neurons in the laminated ICC direct their ascending axons largely to the laminated, ventral division of the medial geniculate body (MGv) (80,137), which is the major thalamic relay nucleus of the auditory system. The projection is bilateral, but the ipsilateral projection is the more dense. In principle, this projection may be thought of as a sheet-to-sheet one, since both the ICC (70,120) and MGv (5,50) are tonotopically organized and the ascending projection is thus tonotopically constrained. The MGv is bordered by a number of related nuclear groups. Some of these nuclei receive a highly intra- and/or intermodal convergent input, whereas others may be purely auditory and perhaps tonotopically organized (51,101). Insofar as the acoustic input to these cell groups is concerned, ascending input is likely derived variously from the ICC, ICX, and ICP, whereas some descending input may be derived from cortical fields (7,23,42).

Thalamocortical connectivity in the auditory system is complex but organized according to understandable principles. The connections are strictly ipsilateral and largely reciprocal. The auditory sensory cortex in cats and primates contains a number of subfields that are distinguishable on physiological and cytoarchitectonic grounds (16,17,54,67,107). Many of these fields are tonotopically organized, and the boundaries between them are usually marked by reversals in tonotopic neural CF sequences at the fields' mutual borders. Cortical fields so distinguished usually have different patterns of thalamic connections. A primary field (AI) is defined cytoarchitectonically as koniocortex and by the strength and topography of its connections with the MGv (16). Other tonotopic cortical fields may also receive input from MGv but with significant input also from nuclei surrounding the MGv. In the cat, which has been studied most thoroughly, identified nontonotopic fields, which are thought to contain neurons broadly tuned to tone frequency, may derive their ascending input exclusively from thalamic cell groups other than the MGv.

Thalamic afferent fibers to the cortex terminate most densely in layer IV and the deeper parts of layer III. By means of numerous vertical connections at any given cortical locus, thalamic input to layer IV is indirectly disseminated among neurons in different cortical strata at that locus. It is likely for this reason that neurons studied at any given site in AI have similar CFs regardless of their depth beneath the pial surface (69,102). In this sense, the auditory cortex may be thought of as a two-dimensional structure. The tonotopic organization of a cortical field is expressed in the form of iso-CF strips—roughly linear spatial arrays of neurons with similar CFs, oriented orthogonal to the tonotopic axis (17,68). The projection of the MGv onto AI (or other tonotopic fields) is thus a convergent, sheet-to-strip one (6,49,68).

The presence of these iso-CF strips has raised the question of whether some other stimulus parameter is represented along the cortical dimension orthogonal to CF. Imig and Adrian (47) provided evidence that cortical neurons of similar CF but different binaural interaction patterns might be segregated from each other within the iso-CF strips. This general notion has been confirmed by a number of more recent studies (71,108). These studies have led to the view that AI should be thought of as a tonotopic array on which are superimposed patches or territories of binaural response-specific neurons. The binaural patches are variable in shape, sometimes being strip-like and oriented orthogonally to isofrequency lines but often appearing smaller and less obviously organized in their topography. There has been some disagreement over what should be considered the relevant binaural classifications used to characterize these territories and whether the patches should be considered functional columns spanning all cortical strata or more simply a manifestation of segregated thalamic input to layer IV, where most recordings are made.

Imig and his colleagues (48,52,53) have provided detailed evidence on cortico-cortical connections within the auditory cortex, with special reference to the extent to which patterns of connectivity are related to the functional properties of neurons contributing to those connections. The cortical territories within AI that contain neurons demonstrating summative binaural interactions (i.e., binaural responses stronger than either monaural response at the same stimulus level) have reciprocal connections with tonotopically homotypic, binaurally similar patches in the contra-lateral hemisphere. In contrast, cortical territories in AI containing cells demon-strating suppressive binaural interactions (i.e, binaural responses weaker than the stronger monaural response at the same stimulus level) have more sparse callosal connectivities but may participate more strongly in ipsilateral corticocortical con-nections. Corticocortical connections may thus be constrained not only by CF but also by binaural interaction pattern.

Most of the quantitative evidence on the response properties of auditory cortex neurons has come from studies of the primary field, AI. It is a major task confronting central auditory neurophysiology to establish the specific functional roles of the cortical fields outside AI (cf. 104,132,147). Within AI, as may be inferred from the preceding paragraphs, the CFs, narrow frequency tuning, and binaural interactions of brainstem neurons are preserved in cortical cells (20,22,102,103). Recent studies indicate that some of the more complex cell types characterized by mixed excitatory-inhibitory response areas, originally described for the dorsal cochlear nucleus, are also found in AI (97,105). These cell types may also be segregated in AI, in patches that do not respect the boundaries of territories defined by binaural properties. If this finding is confirmed, then it will suggest that superimposed on AI's frequency organization are multiple, incompletely overlapping topographies representing other facets of stimulus processing. Equally interesting is the fact that the presence of patches, or modules, of different cell types itself indicates that the convergence of input onto AI is incomplete. These observations provide a testimony to the specificity of the convergence of input in the ascending auditory system.

There has been a long-standing interest in the sensitivity of cortical neurons to temporally and spectrally complex sounds, including frequency- and amplitude-modulated tones and species-specific vocalizations (84,136,139). There is little doubt that some cortical neurons may display marked selectivity for particular complex stimuli. Primate cortical neurons, whose responsiveness is restricted to single elements of extensive vocalization repertoires, and cat cortical cells showing profound sensitivity to direction of frequency change have been described. The extent to which such selectivity is predictable from the other properties of those neurons, notably the overlap between the stimulus spectra and the neurons' excitatory/inhibitory response areas, and the dynamic properties of central neural responses (see below), is only beginning to be investigated systematically (38,83,93,100,126,131,132).

Three features of the responses of cortical neurons to complex, temporally varying stimuli are, however, becoming increasingly clear. The first is that cortical neuron responsiveness to a given complex sound probably depends less on the global, non-acoustic properties of the stimulus (meaning or behavioral relevance) than on the acoustic nature of the elements of which the signal is composed (38,83). Thus, the effectiveness of a species-specific vocalization in exciting primate cortical cells is largely unaffected by reversing the vocalization (38), which presumably eliminates its behavioral significance. In such cases, the temporal organization of spike discharges may tend to follow the component acoustic structures of the vocalization and its reversed analog.

Second, it is likely that the net excitatory or inhibitory effect exerted by a complex sound on the responses of a cortical neuron is at least partially understandable in terms of the spectral overlap between the stimulus and the excitatory and inhibitory tone response areas of the neuron (100,126,136). A recent study of the responses of cat cortical cells to linear amplitude modulations of CF tones pointed to this overlap as a prominent factor determining neural tuning to the rate of amplitude change (100). Thus, the relative effectiveness of low- or high-speed modulations of a continuous CF tone may be shaped by the splatter of stimulus energy into a neuron's inhibitory stimulus domains; this spectral splatter is a necessary consequence of linear amplitude change, and it is likely that the increasingly wide-spectrum nature of the stimulus at high modulation speeds contributes to the band-pass tuning of cortical cells to modulation velocity.

Third, the response of a cortical neuron to a given element of a temporally varying signal may be significantly conditioned or influenced by the response to the immediately preceding stimulus events. This effect has been noted in a diverse range of studies. Thus, the response of primate cortical cells to a human vowel sound is significantly modified by the (acoustic) identity of the preceding consonant (128); the response of a cortical neuron to isolated vocalization fragments is commonly greater than that to the whole vocalization from which the fragments are drawn (83); finally, sensitivity to a tone pulse is dramatically modified by the nature of the response evoked by a preceding tone (1,124,131) or noise pulse (89). These data suggest that the neural response(s) evoked by a stimulus event may outlast that triggering stimulus and, in so doing, modify the response to a subsequent stimulus component in a complex sound.

To date, two mechanisms have been proposed as contributing to such effects. One is the time course of the excitatory or inhibitory response evoked by the relevant stimulus element (124,131). The other is a rapid, short-term adaptation of the neuron's sensitivity to the effective level of the stimulus element (93,99,100). Both of these mechanisms are of a kind that might reasonably be expected to confer neural sensitivity to the temporal sequence of components within a temporally complex stimulus. Interestingly, the finding that sensitivity to such a stimulus might be shaped by the responses to successive individual components is entirely compatible with a recent account of human speech perception (129). This requires neural sensitivity not to the linguistic (global) identity of a speech sound, but to individual acoustic elements and their sequencing. A further question is whether such properties are unique to cortical neurons or are also properties of the thalamic inputs. There is some evidence that the former might be the case in some instances (28,128).

NEURAL CORRELATES OF NOISE MASKING: OBSERVATIONS THAT MAY BE RELEVANT TO THE NEURAL BASIS OF PERCEIVED LOUDNESS

Cochlear nerve fibers and auditory cortex neurons have both been studied quantitatively for the effects of continuous wide-spectrum noise masking on their sensitivity to tonal stimulation. An examination of these studies is instructive here for two reasons. First, they have provided evidence on the neural correlates of tone (or other signal) sensitivity shifts seen in normal listeners under conditions of noise masking. Second, they have provided evidence that may be relevant to understanding the increased rate of loudness growth (recruitment) with elevations in stimulus level that is seen in both normal listeners under conditions of masking and patients with cochlear disease.

All cochlear nerve fibers are excited by wide-band noise of appropriate level. As with their responses to tones, their spike rates for noise are a monotonic function of noise level and show only modest adaptation over the duration of the stimulus. A continuous noise background therefore sets a base rate of spike discharges on which the response to a simultaneously presented CF tone must be superimposed. The further effects of continuous noise backgrounds on the responses to tone pulses have been described in detail (27,37). In the presence of noise levels that raise the base rate of spike discharges, the range of spike rates available for encoding tone level is truncated. This follows from the fact that cochlear nerve fibers have limited maximal firing rates. In addition, the part of the tone rate-level function that survives the baseline elevation is displaced toward higher tone intensities. This shift likely has its basis in basilar membrane nonlinearities in which the tone-evoked vibration of the locus innervated by the fiber is constrained by the more widespread mechanical response to the noise. If the background noise level is elevated, there is a higher base rate of response, further foreshortening of the spike rate range available to encode the tone intensity, and an increase in the tone sensitivity shift that roughly matches the increase in noise level. There is no increase in the slope of that part of the tone function that survives the baseline elevation brought about by the noise.

Now recall that cortical neurons receive a highly convergent but tonotopically constrained afferent input. It is for this reason that the majority of AI neurons have retained their tuning to a CF while acquiring a wealth of other properties (binaural input, sideband inhibition in their response areas, nonmonotonic rate-level functions) that arise initially in spatially separate brainstem nuclei. It is thus very likely that the threshold tuning curve of a cortical neuron actually represents the envelope of the best sensitivities of a large number of inputs with similar CFs but varying thresholds and other properties (99). In addition, cortical neuron responses, particularly in the anesthetized animal, are strongly transient and locked in time to the onset of a stimulus event whether that event is the occurrence of a tone pulse or a modulation of an otherwise invariant signal (100). There is evidence that the transient nature of these responses, whether excitatory or inhibitory, is owing in part to short-term adaptation (93). Two important consequences follow from this. First, continuous background noise has little effect on the base discharge rate of cortical cells, so that the full range of a cortical neuron's spike rates is available for the encoding of tone presented against that background. Second, the neuron's threshold for tonal (or other) stimulation is elevated to the effective level of that background, so that the whole tone rate-level function is displaced toward higher tone intensities. This sensitivity shift may be shaped by the same stimulus and transduction factors that produce the sensitivity shifts in cochlear nerve fibers (94). Once the background noise level is above threshold for inducing this sensitivity shift, then, as in the case of cochlear nerve fibers, further increments in noise level are roughly matched by increases in the tone sensitivity loss (97,99).

Further, a least some cortical neurons show a significant steepening of their rate-level functions for masked tones (93,99). This is perhaps to be expected: if cortical cells receive multiple inputs at the test tone frequency and those inputs have different absolute thresholds, then only those inputs whose thresholds are exceeded by the noise level will have their sensitivities shifted toward higher tone levels. This will, in the masked state, bring into closer register the otherwise dispersed thresholds of inputs at the stimulating frequency. A supra-(masked)-threshold tone may therefore simultaneously activate more inputs to the neuron than an unmasked tone of the same suprathreshold level. Since the spike output of a cortical neuron likely reflects the sum of its inputs, a steepened rate-level function for masked tones results. Note that mask-induced steepening of this kind is probably not possible in an auditory nerve fiber: it receives a unitary input from the single inner hair cell it contacts. It is the convergent nature of input onto cortical cells and the dynamic character of those inputs (or of the cortical responses to them) that may shape cortical sensitivity to masked signals.

These observations have a number of implications (94,99). The tone-sensitivity shifts brought about by continuous noise in both cochlear nerve fibers and auditory cortex neurons parallel in form those seen psychophysically in normal listeners under conditions of noise masking. In both cases the sensitivity loss is linearly related to noise amplitude, with a slope close to unity (94). Second, it is tempting to speculate that the steepened tone rate-level functions seen in cortical cells might represent a neural correlate of the loudness recruitment seen in normal listeners for loudness judgments of masked tones. In this respect, cochlear damage also produces behavioral threshold elevations and loudness recruitment, and there is evidence that the rate-level functions of cochlear nerve fibers innervating damaged organs of Corti are displaced toward higher stimulus levels and are steeper than usual (45,94). As mentioned, this steepening does not occur in cochlear nerve fiber responses to masked tones. This suggests that if the slope of rate-level functions contributes to the rate of perceived loudness growth, then the processes responsible for recruitment in cochlear pathology are expressed at the level of cochlear output, whereas those underlying recruitment in noise masking are predominantly or totally central in origin.

The question of how different stimulus amplitudes might be represented in the pattern of spike activity across the neural populations making up any specified auditory nucleus is now addressed. We have seen that acoustic signals of a given frequency excite neurons tuned to that frequency and that central neurons are spatially arrayed in tonotopic fashion. There is abundant evidence that some features of the spatial location of a sound source may be encoded in the activity of neurons sensitive to variously small ranges of interaural disparities specifying source azimuth. Whether the mammalian auditory system contains a map of acoustic space, perhaps in the form of neurons arrayed in an orderly fashion according to their restricted spatial sensitivities, is currently a contentious issue (72,73,95,123,138).

Central auditory neurons manifest their sensitivity to stimulus level in either of two forms of rate-level function. Some neurons, after the fashion of all cochlear nerve fibers, have monotonic rate-level functions so that their spike discharge rates tend toward saturation at high stimulus amplitudes. Any such neuron whose excitatory threshold is exceeded by the test-tone level will respond to that tone, and for increasingly intense signals, the population of discharging neurons will expand to include those elements whose sensitivities are exceeded by the increased stimulus level. Other neurons have nonmonotonic rate-level functions and these cells are excited relatively selectively by signals whose levels are close to those cells' own optimal stimulus levels. For cells of similar CF, there appear to be nonmonotonic elements with diverse preferred sound pressure levels (22,104). For these neuronal populations, stimulus intensity may be signaled as much in the identity of the discharging neurons as in the absolute size of the discharging population. In bats (132), the auditory cortex contains a subfield consisting almost exclusively of nonmonotonic cells that are spatially arrayed according to their preferred stimulus amplitudes. High concentrations of these cells have also been found in the cortex of cats (104) and primates (22,92), but no map of stimulus level has yet been described. An intriguing implication of the noise-masking studies is that neither the threshold nor the optimal stimulus levels of central neurons should be considered static: they each may be a sensitive function of the level of background stimulation. This would make for a very dynamic map indeed, or perhaps a map not of absolute stimulus level but of signal-to-noise ratio.

ACKNOWLEDGMENTS

Some of the research described in this chapter was supported by NSERC grant U0442 to the author. Special thanks are due to colleagues whose influences guided the development of some of this research: J. F. Brugge, M. S. Cynader, S. E. Hall, and D. R. F. Irvine.

REFERENCES

1. Abeles, M., and Goldstein, M. H., Jr. (1972): Responses of single units in the primary auditory cortex of the cat to tones and to tone pairs. *Brain Res.*, 42:337–352.
2. Adams, J. C. (1979): Ascending projections to the inferior colliculus. *J. Comp. Neurol.*, 183:519–538.
3. Aitkin, L. M., Anderson, D. J., and Brugge, J. F. (1970): Tonotopic organization and discharge characteristics of single neurons in nuclei of the lateral lemniscus in the cat. *J. Neurophysiol.*, 33:421–440.
4. Aitkin, L. M., Irvine, D. R. F., and Webster, W. R. (1984): Central neural mechanisms of hearing. In: *Handbook of Physiology. Section 1, Volume 3, Part 2*, edited by I. Darian-Smith, pp. 675–737. American Physiology Society, Bethesda, MD.
5. Aitkin, L. M., and Webster, W. R. (1972): Medial geniculate body of the cat: Organization and responses to tonal stimuli of neurons in ventral division. *J. Neurophysiol.*, 35:365–380.
6. Andersen, R. A., Knight, P. L., and Merzenich, M. M. (1980): The thalamocortical connections of AI, AII and the anterior auditory field (AAF) in the cat: Evidence for two largely segregated systems of connections. *J. Comp. Neurol.*, 194:663–701.
7. Andersen, R. A., Roth, G. L., Aitkin, L. M., and Merzenich, M. M. (1980): The efferent projections of the central nucleus and the pericentral nucleus of the inferior colliculus in the cat. *J. Comp. Neurol.*, 194:649–662.
8. Aslin, R. N. editor (1986): *Advances in Neural and Behavioral Development. Vol. 2*. Ablex, Norwood, NJ.
9. Batteau, D. W. (1967): The role of the pinna in human localization. *Proc. R. Soc. Lond. [Biol.]*, 168:158–180.
10. Benson, D. A., and Teas, D. C. (1976): Single unit study of binaural interaction in the auditory cortex of the chinchilla. *Brain Res.*, 103:313–338.
11. Bergeijk, W. A. van (1962): Variation on a theme of Békésy: A model of binaural interaction. *J. Acoust. Soc. Am.*, 34:1431–1437.
12. Boudreau, J. C., and Tsuchitani, C. (1968): Binaural interaction in the cat superior olive S segment. *J. Neurophysiol.*, 31:442–454.
13. Brawer, J. R., and Morest, D. K. (1975): Relations between auditory nerve endings and cell types in the cat's anteroventral cochlear nucleus seen with the Golgi method and Nomarski optics. *J. Comp. Neurol.*, 160:491–506.
14. Brawer, J. R., Morest, D. K., and Kane, E. C. (1974): The neuronal architecture of the cochlear nucleus of the cat. *J. Comp. Neurol.*, 155:251–299.
15. Brownell, W. E., Bader, C. R., Bertrand, D., and de Ribaupierre, Y. (1985): Evoked mechanical responses of isolated cochlear outer hair cells. *Science*, 227:194–196.
16. Brugge, J. F. (1975): Progress in neuroanatomy and neurophysiology of auditory cortex. In: *The Nervous System. Vol. 3: Human Communication and Its Disorders*, edited by E. L. Eagles, pp. 97–111. Raven Press, New York.
17. Brugge, J. F. (1982): Auditory cortical areas in primates. In: *Cortical Sensory Organization. Vol. 3. Multiple Auditory Areas*, edited by C. N. Woolsey, pp. 59–70. Humana Press, Clifton, NJ.
18. Brugge, J. F., Anderson, D. J., and Aitkin, L. M. (1970): Responses of neurons in the dorsal nucleus of the lateral lemniscus of cat to binaural tonal stimulation. *J. Neurophysiol.*, 33:441–458.
19. Brugge, J. F., Anderson, D. J., Hind, J. E., and Rose, J. E. (1969): Time structure of discharges in single auditory nerve fibers of the squirrel monkey in response to complex periodic sounds. *J. Neurophysiol.*, 32:386–401.
20. Brugge, J. F., Dubrovsky, N. A., Aitkin, L. M., and Anderson, D. J. (1969): Sensitivity of single neurons in auditory cortex of cat to binaural tonal stimulation; effects of varying interaural time and intensity. *J. Neurophysiol.*, 32:1005–1024.
21. Brugge, J. F., and Geisler, C. D. (1978): Auditory mechanisms of the lower brainstem. *Annu. Rev. Neurosci.*, 1:363–394.
22. Brugge, J. F., and Merzenich, M. M. (1973): Responses of neurons in auditory cortex of the macaque monkey to monaural and binaural stimulation. *J. Neurophysiol.*, 36:1138–1158.
23. Calford, M. B., and Aitkin, L. M. (1983): Ascending projections to the medial geniculate body of the cat: Evidence for multiple, parallel auditory pathways through the thalamus. *J. Neurosci.*, 3:2365–2380.

24. Calford, M. B., Moore, D. R., and Hutchings, M. E. (1986): Central and peripheral contributions to coding of acoustic space by neurons in inferior colliculus of cat. *J. Neurophysiol.*, 55:587–603.
25. Calford, M. B., and Pettigrew, J. D. (1984): Frequency dependence of directional amplification of the cat's pinna. *Hear. Res.*, 14:13–19.
26. Cant, N. B., and Casseday, J. H. (1986): Projections from the anteroventral cochlear nucleus to the lateral and medial olivary nuclei. *J. Comp. Neurol.*, 247:457–476.
27. Costalupes, J. A., Young, E. D., and Gibson, D. J. (1984): Effects of continuous noise backgrounds on rate response of auditory nerve fibers in cat. *J. Neurophysiol.*, 51:1326–1344.
28. Creutzfeldt, O., Hellweg, F.-C., and Schreiner, C. (1980): Thalamocortical transformation of responses to complex auditory stimuli. *Exp. Brain Res.*, 39:87–104.
29. Efron, R. (1985): The central auditory system and issues related to hemispheric specialization. In: *Assessment of Central Auditory Dysfunction. Foundations and Clinical Correlates*, edited by M. L. Pinheiro and F. E. Musiek, pp. 143–154. Williams and Wilkins, Baltimore.
30. Evans, E. F. (1975): The cochlear nerve and cochlear nucleus. In: *Handbook of Sensory Physiology. Vol. 5, Pt. 2*, edited by W. D. Keidel and W. D. Neff, pp. 1–108. Springer-Verlag, Heidelberg.
31. Evans, E. F., and Nelson, P. G. (1973): The responses of single neurons in the cochlear nucleus of the cat as a function of their location and anesthetic state. *Exp. Brain Res.*, 17:402–427.
32. Fekete, D. M., Rouiller, E. M., Liberman, M. C., and Ryugo, D. K. (1984): The central projections of intracellularly labelled auditory nerve fibers in cats. *J. Comp. Neurol.*, 229:432–450.
33. Flock, A. (1971): Sensory transduction in hair cells. In: *Handbook of Sensory Physiology. Vol. 1*, edited by W. Lowenstein, pp. 396–441, Springer, Berlin.
34. Flock, A. (1985): Motility in outer hair cells and its structural substrate. *Assn. Res. Otolaryngol. Abstr.*, 8:175–176.
35. Fuzessery, Z. M., and Pollak, G. D. (1985): Determinants of sound location selectivity in bat inferior colliculus: A combined dichotic and free-field study. *J. Neurophysiol.*, 54:757–781.
36. Geisler, C. D. (1986): A model of the effect of outer hair cell motility on cochlear vibrations. *Hear. Res.*, 24:125–131.
37. Gibson, J. D., Young, E. D., and Costalupes J. A. (1985): Similarity of dynamic range adjustment in auditory nerve and cochlear nuclei. *J. Neurophysiol.*, 53:940–958.
38. Glass, I., and Wollberg, Z. (1983): Responses of cells in the auditory cortex of awake squirrel monkeys to normal and reversed species-specific vocalizations. *Hear. Res.*, 9:27–33.
39. Goldberg, J. M., and Brown, P. B. (1968): Functional organization of the dog superior olivary complex: An anatomical and electrophysiological study. *J. Neurophysiol.*, 31:639–656.
40. Goldberg, J. M., and Brown, P. B. (1969): Response of binaural neurons of dog superior olivary complex to dichotic tonal stimulation: Some physiological mechanisms of sound localization. *J. Neurophysiol.*, 32:613–636.
41. Goldberg, J. M., and Brownell, W. E. (1973): Discharge characteristics of neurons in anteroventral and dorsal cochlear nuclei of cat. *Brain Res.*, 64:35–54.
42. Graybiel, A. M. (1972): Some fiber pathways related to the posterior thalamic region in the cat. *Brain Behav. Evol.*, 6:363–393.
43. Greenwood, D. D., and Goldberg, J. M. (1970): Response of neurons in the cochlear nucleus to variations in noise bandwidth and to tone-noise combinations. *J. Acoust. Soc. Am.*, 47:1022–1040.
44. Hall, J. L. (1965): Binaural interaction in the accessory superior-olivary nucleus of the cat. *J. Acoust. Soc. Am.*, 37:814–823.
45. Harrison, R. V. (1985): The physiology of the normal and pathological cochlear neurones—some recent advances. *J. Otolaryngol.*, 14:345–356.
46. Hochster, M. E., and Kelly, J. B. (1981): The precedence effect and sound localization by children with temporal lobe epilepsy. *Neuropsychologia*, 19:46–55.
47. Imig, T. J., and Adrian, H. O. (1977): Binaural columns in the primary field (AI) of cat auditory cortex. *Brain Res.*, 138:241–257.
48. Imig, T. J., and Brugge, J. F. (1978): Sources and terminations of callosal axons related to binaural and frequency maps in primary auditory cortex of the cat. *J. Comp. Neurol.*, 182:637–660.
49. Imig, T. J., and Morel, A. (1984): Topographic and cytoarchitectonic organization of thalamic neurons related to their targets in low-, middle-, and high-frequency representations in cat auditory cortex. *J. Comp. Neurol.*, 227:511–539.
50. Imig, T. J., and Morel, A. (1985): Tonotopic organization in ventral nucleus of medial geniculate body in the cat. *J. Neurophysiol.*, 53:309–340.
51. Imig, T. J., and Morel, A. (1985): Tonotopic organization in lateral part of posterior group of thalamic nuclei in the cat. *J. Neurophysiol.*, 53:836–851.
52. Imig, T. J., and Reale, R. A. (1980): Patterns of cortico-cortical connections related to tonotopic maps in cat auditory cortex. *J. Comp. Neurol.*, 192:293–332.
53. Imig, T. J., and Reale R. A. (1981): Ipsilateral corticocortical projections related to binaural columns in cat primary auditory cortex. *J. Comp. Neurol.*, 203:1–14.

54. Imig, T. J., Ruggero, M. A., Kitzes, L. M., Javel, E., and Brugge, J. F. (1977): Organization of auditory cortex in the owl monkey (Aotus trivirgatus). *J. Comp. Neurol.*, 171:111–128.
55. Jenkins, W. M., and Masterton, R. B. (1982): Sound localization: effects of unilateral lesions in central auditory pathways. *J. Neurophysiol.*, 47:987–1016.
56. Jenkins, W. M., and Merzenich, M. M. (1984): Role of cat primary auditory cortex for sound localization behavior. *J. Neurophysiol.*, 52:819–847.
57. Johnson, D. (1980): The relationship between spike rate and synchrony in response of auditory nerve fibers to single tones. *J. Acoust. Soc. Am.*, 68:1115–1122.
58. Kavanagh, G. L., and Kelly, J. B. (1987): Contribution of auditory cortex to sound localization by the ferret (Mustela putorius). *J. Neurophysiol.*, 57:1746–1766.
59. Kiang, N. Y-S., Pfeiffer, R. R., Warr, W. B., and Backus, A. S. N. (1965): Stimulus coding in the cochlear nucleus. *Ann. Otol. Rhinol. Laryngol.*, 74:463–485.
60. Kitzes, L. M., Wrege, K. S., and Cassady, J. M. (1980): Patterns of responses of cortical cells to binaural stimulation. *J. Comp. Neurol.*, 192:455–472.
61. Kuwada, S., and Yin, T. C. T. (1983): Binaural interaction in low frequency neurons in the inferior colliculus of the cat. I. Effects of long interaural delays, intensity, and repetition rate on the interaural delay function. *J. Neurophysiol.*, 50:981–999.
62. Liberman, M. C. (1978): Auditory nerve responses from cats raised in a low-noise chamber. *J. Acoust. Soc. Am.*, 63:442–455.
63. Liberman, M. C. (1982): Single-neuron labelling in the cat auditory nerve. *Science*, 216:1239–1241.
64. Liberman, M. C., and Brown, M. C. (1986): Physiology and anatomy of single olivocochlear neurons in the cat. *Hear. Res.*, 24:17–36.
65. Lorente de No, R. (1979): Central representation of the eighth nerve. In: *Ear Diseases, Deafness and Dizziness*, edited by V. Goodhill, pp. 64–83. Harper and Row, New York.
66. Masterton, R. B., and Imig, T. J. (1984): Neural mechanisms for sound localization. *Annu. Rev. Physiol.*, 46:275–287.
67. Merzenich, M. M., and Brugge, J. F. (1973): Representation of the cochlear partition on the superior temporal plane of the macaque monkey. *Brain Res.*, 50:275–296.
68. Merzenich, M. M., and Kaas, J. H. (1980): Principles of organization of sensory-perceptual systems in mammals. In: *Progress in Psychobiology and Physiological Psychology. Vol. 9*, edited by J. M. Sprague and A. N. Epstein, pp. 1–42. Academic Press, New York.
69. Merzenich, M. M., Knight, P. L., and Roth, G. L. (1975): Representation of cochlea within primary auditory cortex in the cat. *J. Neurophysiol.*, 38:231–249.
70. Merzenich, M. M., and Reid, M. D. (1974): Representation of the cochlea within the inferior colliculus of the cat. *Brain Res.*, 77:397–415.
71. Middlebrooks, J. C., Dykes, R. W., and Merzenich, M. M. (1980): Binaural response-specific bands in primary auditory cortex (AI) of the cat: Topographical organization orthogonal to isofrequency contours. *Brain Res.*, 181:31–48.
72. Middlebrooks, J. C., and Knudsen, E. I. (1984): A neural code for auditory space in the cat's superior colliculus. *J. Neurosci.*, 4:2621–2634.
73. Middlebrooks, J. C., and Pettigrew, J. D. (1981): Functional classes of neurons in primary auditory cortex of the cat distinguished by sensitivity to sound location. *J. Neurosci.*, 1:107–120.
74. Mills, A. W. (1958): On the minimum audible angle. *J. Acoust. Soc. Am.*, 30:237–246.
75. Møller, A. R. (1983): *Auditory Physiology*. Academic Press, New York.
76. Molnar, C. E., and Pfeiffer, R. R. (1968): Interpretation of spontaneous spike discharge patterns of neurons in the cochlear nucleus. *Proc. IEEE*, 56:993–1004.
77. Moore, C. N., Casseday, J. H., and Neff, W. D. (1974): Sound localization: The role of the commissural pathways of the auditory system of the cat. *Brain Res.*, 82:13–26.
78. Moore, D. R., Hutchings, M. E., Addison, P. D., Semple, M. N., and Aitkin, L. M. (1984): Properties of spatial receptive fields in the central nucleus of the cat inferior colliculus. II. Stimulus intensity effects. *Hear. Res.*, 13:175–188.
79. Moore, D. R., and Irvine, D. R. F. (1979): A developmental study of the sound pressure transformation by the head of the cat. *Acta Otolaryngol. (Stockh.)*, 87:434–440.
80. Morest, D. K. (1965): The laminar structure of the medial geniculate body of the cat. *J. Anat.*, 99:143–160.
81. Morest, D. K. (1973): Auditory neurons of the brain stem. *Adv. Otorhinolaryngol.*, 20:337–356.
82. Musicant, A. D., and Butler, R. A. (1984): The influence of pinnae-based cues on sound localization. *J. Acoust. Soc. Am.*, 75:1195–1200.
83. Newman, J. D., and Symmes, D. (1979): Feature detection by single units in squirrel monkey auditory cortex. *Exp. Brain Res.* (suppl. 2):140–145.
84. Newman, J. D., and Wollberg, Z. (1973): Multiple coding of species-specific vocalizations in the auditory cortex of squirrel monkeys. *Brain Res.*, 54:287–304.
85. Oertel, D. (1983): Synaptic responses and electrical properties of cells in brain slices of the mouse anteroventral cochlear nucleus. *J. Neurophysiol.*, 3:2043–2053.

86. Oldfield, S. R., and Parker, S. P. A. (1984): Acuity of sound localisation: A topography of auditory space. II. Pinna cues absent. *Perception*, 13:601–617.
87. Orman, S. S., and Phillips, D. P. (1984): Binaural interactions of single neurons in posterior field of cat auditory cortex. *J. Neurophysiol.*, 51:1028–1039.
88. Osen, K. K. (1969): Cytoarchitecture of the cochlear nuclei in the cat. *J. Comp. Neurol.*, 136:453–484.
89. Palmer, A. R., and Russell, I. J. (1986): Phase-locking in the cochlear nerve of the guinea-pig and its relation to the receptor potential of inner hair cells. *Hear. Res.*, 24:1–15.
90. Pfeiffer, R. R. (1966): Classification of response patterns of spike discharges for units in the cochlear nucleus: tone-burst stimulation. *Exp. Brain Res.*, 1:220–235.
91. Pfeiffer, R. R., and Kiang, N. Y-S. (1965): Spike discharge patterns of spontaneous and continuously stimulated activity in the cochlear nucleus of anesthetized cats. *Biophys. J.*, 5:301–316.
92. Pfingst, B. E., and O'Connor, T. A. (1981): Characteristics of neurons in auditory cortex of monkeys performing a simple auditory task. *J. Neurophysiol.*, 45:16–34.
93. Phillips, D. P. (1985): Temporal response features of cat auditory cortex neurons contributing to sensitivity to tones delivered in the presence of continuous noise. *Hear. Res.*, 19:253–268.
94. Phillips, D. P. (1987): Stimulus intensity and loudness recruitment: Neural correlates. *J. Acoust. Soc. Am.*, 82:1–12.
95. Phillips, D. P., and Brugge, J. F. (1985): Progress in neurophysiology of sound localization. *Annu. Rev. Psychol.*, 36:245–274.
96. Phillips, D. P., Calford, M. B., Pettigrew, J. D., Aitkin, L. M., and Semple, M. N. (1982): Directionality of sound pressure transformation at the cat's pinna. *Hear. Res.*, 8:13–28.
97. Phillips, D. P., and Cynader, M. S. (1985): Some neural mechanisms in the cat's auditory cortex underlying sensitivity to combined tone and wide-spectrum noise stimuli. *Hear. Res.*, 18:87–102.
98. Phillips, D. P., and Gates, G. R. (1982): Representation of the two ears in the auditory cortex: A re-examination. *Int. J. Neurosci.*, 16:41–46.
99. Phillips, D. P., and Hall, S. E. (1986): Spike-rate-intensity functions of cat cortical neurons studied with combined tone-noise stimuli. *J. Acoust. Soc. Am.*, 80:177–187.
100. Phillips, D. P., and Hall, S. E. (1987): Responses of single neurons in cat auditory cortex to time-varying stimuli. II. Linear amplitude modulations. *Exp. Brain Res.*, 67:479–492.
101. Phillips, D. P., and Irvine, D. R. F. (1979): Acoustic input to single neurons in pulvinar-posterior complex of cat thalamus. *J. Neurophysiol.*, 42:123–136.
102. Phillips, D. P., and Irvine, D. R. F. (1981): Responses of single neurons in physiologically defined primary auditory cortex (AI) of the cat: Frequency tuning and responses to intensity. *J. Neurophysiol.*, 45:48–58.
103. Phillips, D. P., and Irvine, D. R. F. (1981): Responses of neurons in physiologically defined area AI of cat cerebral cortex: Sensitivity to interaural intensity differences. *Hear. Res.*, 4:299–307.
104. Phillips, D. P., and Orman, S. S. (1984): Responses of single neurons in posterior field of cat auditory cortex to tonal stimulation. *J. Neurophysiol.*, 51:147–163.
105. Phillips, D. P., Orman, S. S., Musicant, A. D., and Wilson, G. F. (1985): Neurons in the cat's primary auditory cortex distinguished by their responses to tone and wide-spectrum noise. *Hear. Res.*, 18:73–86.
106. Pickles, J. O. (1985): Recent advances in cochlear physiology. *Prog. Neurobiol.*, 24:1–42.
107. Reale, R. A., and Imig, T. J. (1980): Tonotopic organization in auditory cortex of the cat. *J. Comp. Neurol.*, 192:265–291.
108. Reale, R. A., and Kettner, R. E. (1986): Topography of binaural organization in primary auditory cortex of the cat: Effects of changing interaural intensity. *J. Neurophysiol.*, 56:663–682.
109. Rhode, W. S., Oertel, D., and Smith, P. H. (1983): Physiological response properties of cells labelled intracellularly with horseradish peroxidase in cat ventral cochlear nucleus. *J. Comp. Neurol.*, 213:448–463.
110. Rhode, W. S., and Smith, P. H. (1986): Encoding timing and intensity in the ventral cochlear nucleus of the cat. *J. Neurophysiol.*, 56:261–286.
111. Rhode, W. S., and Smith, P. H. (1986): Physiological studies on neurons in the dorsal cochlear nucleus of cat. *J. Neurophysiol.*, 56:287–307.
112. Rhode, W. S., Smith, P. H., and Oertel, D. (1983): Physiological response properties of cells labelled intracellularly with horseradish peroxidase in cat dorsal cochlear nucleus. *J. Comp. Neurol.*, 213:426–447.
113. Robertson, D. (1985): Brainstem location of efferent neurones projecting to the guinea pig cochlea. *Hear. Res.*, 20:79–84.
114. Rose, J. E., Brugge, J. F., Anderson, D. J., and Hind, J. E. (1967): Phase-locked response to low-frequency tones in single and auditory nerve fibers of the squirrel monkey. *J. Neurophysiol.*, 30:769–793.
115. Rose, J. E., Gross, N. B., Geisler, C. D., and Hind, J. E. (1966): Some neural mechanisms in the

inferior colliculus of the cat which may be relevant to localization of a sound source. *J. Neurophysiol.*, 29:288–314.

116. Roth, G. L., Aitkin, L. M., Andersen, R. A., and Merzenich, M. M. (1978): Some features of the spatial organization of the central nucleus of the inferior colliculus of the cat. *J. Comp. Neurol.*, 182:661–680.

117. Roth, G. L., Kochhar, R. K., and Hind, J. E. (1980): Interaural time differences: Implications regarding the neurophysiology of sound localization. *J. Acoust. Soc. Am.*, 68:1643–1651.

118. Rouiller, E. M., Cronin-Schreiber, R., Fekete, D. M., and Ryugo, D. K. (1986): The central projections of intracellularly labeled auditory nerve fibers in cats: an analysis of terminal morphology. *J. Comp. Neurol.*, 249:261–278.

119. Sachs, M. B., and Abbas, P. J. (1974): Rate versus level functions for auditory-nerve fibers in cats: Tone burst stimuli. *J. Acoust. Soc. Am.*, 56:1835–1847.

120. Semple, M. N., and Aitkin, L. M. (1979): Representation of sound frequency and laterality by units in central nucleus of cat inferior colliculus. *J. Neurophysiol.*, 42:1626–1639.

121. Semple, M. N., and Aitkin, L. M. (1980): Physiology of pathway from dorsal cochlear nucleus to inferior colliculus revealed by electrical and auditory stimulation. *Exp. Brain Res.*, 41:19–28.

122. Semple, M. N., and Aitkin, L. M. (1981): Integration and segregation of input to the cat inferior colliculus. In: *Neuronal Mechanisms of Hearing*, edited by J. Syka and L. M. Aitkin, pp. 155–161. Plenum Press, New York.

123. Semple, M. N., Aitkin, L. M., Calford, M. B., Pettigrew, J. D., and Phillips, D. P. (1983): Spatial receptive fields in cat inferior colliculus. *Hear. Res.*, 10:203–215.

124. Shamma, S. A., and Symmes, D. (1985): Patterns of inhibition in auditory cortical cells in awake squirrel monkeys. *Hear. Res.*, 19:1–13.

125. Shofner, W. P., and Young, E. D. (1985): Excitatory/inhibitory response types in the cochlear nucleus: Relationship to discharge patterns and responses to electrical stimulation of the auditory nerve. *J. Neurophysiol.*, 54:917–940.

126. Sovijarvi, A. R. A. (1975): Detection of natural complex sounds by cells in the primary auditory cortex of the cat. *Acta Physiol. Scand.*, 93:318–335.

127. Spoendlin, H. (1967): The innervation of the organ of Corti. *J. Laryngol.*, 81:717–738.

128. Steinschneider, M., Arezzo, J., and Vaughan, H. G. (1982): Speech evoked activity in the auditory radiations and cortex of the awake monkey. *Brain Res.*, 252:353–365.

129. Stevens, K. N. (1980): Acoustic correlates of some phonetic categories. *J. Acoust. Soc. Am.*, 68:836–842.

130. Stotler, W. A. (1953): An experimental study of the cells and connections of the superior olivary complex of the cat. *J. Comp. Neurol.*, 98:401–432.

131. Suga, N. (1965): Analysis of frequency-modulated sounds by auditory neurones of echo-locating bats. *J. Physiol. (Lond.)*, 179:26–53.

132. Suga, N. (1982): Functional organization of the auditory cortex: representation beyond tonotopy in the bat. In: *Cortical Sensory Organization. Vol. 3. Multiple Auditory Areas*, edited by C. N. Woolsey, pp. 157–218. Humana, Clifton, NJ.

133. Voigt, H. F., and Young, E. D. (1980): Evidence of inhibitory interactions between neurons in dorsal cochlear nucleus. *J. Neurophysiol.*, 44:76–96.

134. Warr, W. B. (1975): Olivocochlear and vestibular efferent neurons of the feline brain stem: Their location, morphology and number determined by retrograde axonal transport and acetylcholinesterase histochemistry. *J. Comp. Neurol.*, 161:159–182.

135. Whitfield, I. C. (1971): Mechanisms of sound localization. *Nature*, 233:95–97.

136. Whitfield, I. C., and Evans, E. F. (1965): Responses of auditory cortical neurones to stimuli of changing frequency. *J. Neurophysiol.*, 28:655–672.

137. Winer, J. A. (1985): The medial geniculate body of the cat. *Adv. Anat. Embryol. Cell Biol.*, 86:1–98.

138. Wise, L. Z., and Irvine, D. R. F. (1985): Topographic organization of interaural intensity difference sensitivity in deep layers of cat superior colliculus: Implications for auditory spatial representation. *J. Neurophysiol.*, 54:185–211.

139. Wollberg, Z., and Newman, J. D. (1972): Auditory cortex of squirrel monkey: Response patterns of single cells to species-specific vocalizations. *Science*, 175:212–214.

140. Woolsey, C. N. editor (1982): *Cortical Sensory Organization. Vol. 3. Multiple Auditory Areas*. Humana Press, Clifton, NJ.

141. Wu, S. H., and Oertel, D. (1984): Intracellular injection with horseradish peroxidase of physiologically characterized stellate and bushy cells in slices of mouse anteroventral cochlear nucleus. *J. Neurophysiol.*, 4:1577–1588.

142. Yin, T. C. T., Chan, J. C. K., and Irvine, D. R. F. (1986): Effects of interaural time delays of noise stimuli on low-frequency cells in the cat's inferior colliculus. I. Responses to wideband noise. *J. Neurophysiol.*, 55:280–300.

143. Yin, T. C. T., and Kuwada, S. (1983): Binaural interaction in low-frequency neurons in inferior colliculus of the cat. III. Effects of changing frequency. *J. Neurophysiol.*, 50:1020–1042.
144. Yin, T. C. T., Kuwada, S., and Sujaku, Y. (1984): Interaural time sensitivity of high-frequency neurons in the inferior colliculus. *J. Acoust. Soc. Am.*, 76:1401–1410.
145. Young, E. D. (1980): Identification of response properties of ascending axons from dorsal cochlear nucleus. *Brain Res.*, 200:23–37.
146. Young, E. D., and Brownell, W. E. (1976): Response to tones and noise of single cells in dorsal cochlear nucleus of unanesthetized cats. *J. Neurophysiol.*, 39:282–300.
147. Zeki, S. M. (1978): Functional specialization in the visual cortex of the rhesus monkey. *Nature*, 274:423–428.

Physiology of the Ear,
edited by A. F. Jahn and J. Santos-Sacchi.
Raven Press, New York © 1988.

The Development of Stimulus Coding in the Auditory System

*Dan H. Sanes and **Edwin W Rubel

*Departments of Otolaryngology, and Physiology and Biophysics, New York University
Medical Center, New York, New York 10016; and **Department of Otolaryngology,
University of Washington, Seattle, Washington 98195*

Studies of auditory system maturation typically present a system that becomes progressively more competent at responding to the full range of sound stimuli. Toward this end, an impressive array of functional parameters has now been developmentally characterized in a variety of species. The underlying rationale for describing each parameter is that it has perceptual relevance to the animal. For example, the dramatic improvement in sensitivity of the cochlea and auditory nervous system during the initial period of hearing must certainly be responsible for concomitant behavioral improvements. Such clarity in the relationship between function and perception is, however, often missing. It is quite unclear how an animal's ability to discriminate relative sound levels is represented in the central nervous system, although there are numerous reports documenting the maturation of intensity coding by cochlear and neural elements. In all likelihood these functional properties will eventually be causally related to sensory perception; however, our current state of knowledge argues for a careful appraisal of relevance when considering differences between early and adult function. Therefore, a primary aim of this chapter is to distinguish between those functional properties that appear to underlie perceptual tasks and those that are at present of unknown importance.

A second goal is to determine the locus of functional changes. This is a most important task if we are to pursue the cellular mechanisms underlying functional ontogeny. One may then be in a position to compare auditory system development with that of other sensory systems. From a clinical perspective, this approach will also facilitate our understanding of otological disease etiology and suggest favorable animal models for their elucidation.

Finally, we will explore the importance of auditory activity prior to the mature transduction of airborne sound. This sustained or spontaneous electrical activity of developing neurons has been linked to maturational events in two ways. First, activity may have a trophic influence, and second, it may be informative during the period when nerve cells form specific connections: hence the long-standing interest of psychologists and physiologists in the possibility that humans and other animals hear *in utero* (5). This issue has long been a focus of research in the visual pathway and deserves evaluation in the auditory system.

This review is not intended as an archival survey. Instead we focus on several important issues and the experimental findings that allow greatest insight. It is our hope that this approach will provide a framework for evaluating additional data as they are generated or encountered. The reader is referred to other reviews for comprehensive summaries of the developmental literature (81,84,87).

FREQUENCY RESPONSE

Precise frequency detection is necessary for all species. If hair cells (the first element to transform pressure waves into an electrical signal) responded unselectively to all frequencies, the poor signal-to-noise ratios would severely compromise the detection of species-specific vocalizations (e.g., speech sounds) and localization cues. Regardless of its evolutionary *raison d'être*, frequency selectivity has come to influence a wide range of sensory percepts; therefore its ontogeny is of primary interest. Four important topics will be considered within this context: the extent to which change is homogeneous across the cochlea's frequency axis, the cellular processes underlying the generation of frequency selectivity, the possibility that frequency selectivity is a distinct maturational event in the central auditory system, and the development of cochlear tonotopy.

Until now there has been no direct functional assay of frequency tuning at the level of the cochlea during development. The most pertinent data come from tone-on-tone masking procedures and single auditory nerve fiber recordings. The first assay (22) relies on a poorly understood interaction between neighboring regions of the cochlea during which activation of one region suppresses activity in a second region. The general procedure consists of recording the whole nerve action potential at the round window (N_1 response) to a pure-tone probe. A second tonal stimulus, the masker, is increased in intensity until the evoked-response amplitude is reduced by an arbitrary amount. A plot of masker frequency versus the intensity at which it must be presented to decrease the evoked response by a fixed amount is known as a compound action potential tuning curve (APTC). The shape of APTCs is comparable to that of single-fiber threshold tuning curves, where the lowest intensity to elicit a response is plotted against stimulus frequency (24,41).

The sharpening of N_1 APTCs occurs very rapidly in the chick (73), within 5 to 7 days of the first evoked activity (97). Similarly, the maturation of N_1 APTCs in rodents occurs during a period of 3 to 5 days following the onset of hearing (15,103). Frequency selectivity in the kitten exhibits a more extended maturational time course, whether it is assayed by APTCs (15) or with single-fiber data (81).

Maturation Across the Frequency Axis

Given that cochlear frequency selectivity does improve with age, there are data to suggest that this process should first occur for high-frequency regions. Foremost among these is the consistent observation that the cochlea first achieves morphological maturity at basal locations (3,35,44,51,62,70,76,114). There is also reason to believe that basal loci are the first to function (89), although they respond to lower frequencies in young animals (discussed later). Auditory nerve fibers in the kitten with characteristic frequencies of 1, 3, and 7 kHz appear to have different rates of maturation such that the 7-kHz fibers are the first to reach an adult state (Fig. 1) (81). Woolf and Ryan (120) noted that only high-frequency neurons (i.e., charac-

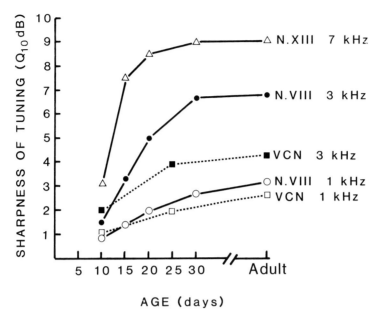

FIG. 1. Development of frequency selectivity in the auditory nerve and cochlear nucleus of the kitten. The measure of frequency selectivity, the Q_{10} value, is computed by dividing best frequency by the effective bandwidth at 10 dB above threshold. The Q_{10} value is large for sharply tuned neurons. Auditory nerve fibers reach functional maturity between postnatal days 20 and 30, with the higher frequency neurons doing so first. Although values from cochlear nucleus neurons were binned across a larger age range, they appear to mature with roughly the same time course. (Adapted from refs. 12 and 80.)

teristic frequencies greater than 4 kHz) in the gerbil cochlear nucleus have adult-like tuning at the youngest ages examined. It was also found that in 6-month-old infants, frequency discrimination is better for high than low frequencies, in relation to adults (65). However, there are four sets of data that do not support this trend. The development of frequency selectivity in APTCs of both the chick (73) and mouse (98) show equivalent rates of maturation across frequency. In addition, a single-unit analysis of tuning in the lateral superior olivary nucleus of the gerbil failed to demonstrate a faster rate of maturation for high-frequency neurons (95). Finally, Olsho et al. (67) recently showed that in 3-month-old human infants, frequency discrimination is poorer at high frequencies (i.e., >4 kHz) than at lower frequencies (i.e., <4 kHz).

Cellular Considerations

An interpretation of these physiological results must finally rely on the elucidation of the cellular bases of frequency selectivity. From a developmental perspective there are no compelling results in support of any particular mechanism. It has been proposed that the outer hair cells and/or their efferent innervation are responsible for the enhancement of tuning. The first suggestion rests on the experimental finding that selective destruction of the outer hair cells results in broader (i.e., immature-like) cochlear tuning properties (23,33,50). The second suggestion is based on the

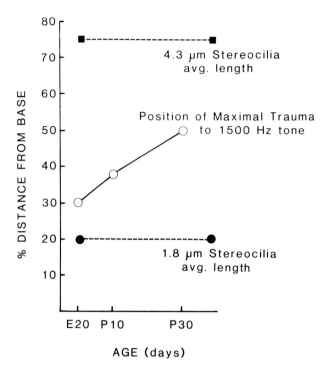

FIG. 2. Ontogeny of the tonotopic map and stereocilia length in the chick basilar papilla. The position of maximal damage produced by a 1,500-Hz tone is found at progressively more apical locations with increasing age. However, the stereocilia length remains constant at these loci during the same period. (Adapted from refs. 88 and 110.)

temporal correlation of enhanced tuning with the significant increase in efferent terminals at the base of outer hair cells (14,72).

More recently, a comprehensive morphogenetic description of the chick basilar papilla (i.e., cochlea) has allowed us to entertain the possibility that modification of stereocilia length, a parameter that is correlated with the frequency axis in adult animals (109), may underlie the ontogeny of frequency tuning (110). A comparison of stereocilia width and length with the maturation of cochlear physiology (73,97) suggests a number of incongruities (Fig. 2). For example, stereocilia length has attained adult proportions over 70% of the cochlea's extent by embryonic day 21 (110). However, these same cochlear regions encode progressively higher frequencies during the next 10 to 30 days (59,60,86,88). If stereocilia length exclusively determined the frequency selectivity of a hair cell in the chick cochlea, then one would have expected the tonotopic map to be stable by embryonic day 21. Similarly, the width of stereocilia reaches an adult proportion by embryonic day 17, well before functional stability.

Studies on the emergence of frequency tuning in newly generated electroreceptors (i.e., a hair cell derivative) have indicated that biophysical changes within each sensory cell, independent of mechanical transduction, may contribute to the generation of mature coding properties (123). This process is likely to involve ontogenetic change in the number, type, and localization of ion channels within the sensory cell's membrane.

Although the ideas presented above are at present among the viable alternatives, it should be emphasized that developmental approaches to cochlear morphology, biochemistry, pharmacology, and metabolism remain largely unexplored. As these data become available, it is worth considering their relationship to the following certainties. The basilar membrane, whose deflection activates the hair cells, is tuned as sharply as the sensory elements that transform mechanical energy to electrical (50,78,100). Furthermore, the sensitivity of this mechanism is energy dependent and hence prone to trauma (18,34,77). The extent to which each cell type in the cochlea contributes to basilar membrane vigor may provide a clue as to its developmental contribution during the maturation of frequency selectivity.

A Consideration of Central Processes

We have primarily focused on the generation of tuning at the cochlear level in the preceding discussion. Since the central auditory pathway preserves both the tonotopic axis of the cochlea and its level of frequency tuning, it seems reasonable to inquire whether there are central mechanisms to ensure that fidelity is maintained. The most direct way to ascertain whether central auditory neurons are broadly tuned (at a time when the periphery has reached an adult state) is to compare the tuning of single auditory nerve fibers with that of central neurons in the same animal, thus controlling for biological and experimental variability. This very difficult experiment has never been attempted. Unfortunately, there is also an absence of quantitative between-subject data; where quantitative data do exist, there are inevitable differences in stimulus presentation, tuning criteria, and data reduction methodologies.

At present, the most suitable comparison of frequency selectivity at two loci can be made for eighth nerve fibers (81) and anteroventral cochlear nucleus (AVCN) neurons in the cat (12). Although neurons at both loci respond to a more limited range of frequencies with increasing age, there does not appear to be a difference in the time course of this sharpening (Fig. 1). These data support the proposition that there are no central mechanisms contributing to the maturation of frequency tuning; AVCN neurons simply mirror the ontogenetic state of the cochlea (12). A second system for which this comparison can be made is the mouse cochlea and cochlear nucleus. In this case the measure of selectivity is APTCs, originally used to assay the ability of one tone to suppress the response evoked by a second tone at the level of the cochlea. However, it is conceivable that APTCs obtained with the evoked response from central structures may reflect neural integration as well. APTCs obtained from the eighth nerve have become maturely tuned by postnatal day 16 (103), whereas the APTCs obtained in the cochlear nucleus do not obtain a mature state until postnatal days 18 to 24, depending on frequency (98).

A recent developmental study of neuronal function in the lateral superior olivary nucleus (LSO) of the gerbil (95) contained two pieces of evidence indicating that central processes may be involved in the maturation of frequency selectivity. Since the broad tuning of neurons in young animals can be attributed to cochlear immaturity, comparisons were made of neurons characterized within the same neonatal animal. If one of the neurons exhibited adult-like properties, then the cochlea would obviously be capable of endowing central neurons with mature frequency selectivity; unusually broad tuning is postulated as having a neural basis in this case. It was found that dramatic disparities in tuning were possible within animals of postnatal ages 13 to 16 days. Figure 3A shows a plot of best frequency versus tuning for several unit pairs in 15- to 16-day-old gerbils. A second line of evidence for inherent central maturation derived from the observation that some neurons responded to an unusual range of frequencies in 13- to 16-day-old animals. A common characteristic of their response areas was the presence of a second discrete range of frequencies capable of eliciting a response from the neuron, a phenomenon not generally seen in adults. Figure 3B depicts one such response area. It seems unlikely that such a response type would be attributable to an immature cochlea.

Development of the Place Code

An event that underlies and undoubtedly influences the maturation of frequency selectivity is the progressive appearance of a high-frequency response. That is, the cochlea originally transduces only low frequencies along the length of the cochlea, even though the basal (i.e., high frequency) region appears structurally well advanced. The appearance of an adult frequency range and the shift in tonotopy along the cochlea's length have been reviewed in detail elsewhere (61,87). We will only briefly consider this ontogenetic event.

There are now several independent lines of evidence to indicate that basal regions of the cochlea encode successively higher frequencies as an animal ages. This was first demonstrated in the chick, where it was found that the same high-intensity tonal stimulus traumatized progressively more apical positions along the basilar papilla (i.e., cochlea) in older animals (Fig. 2) (86,88). In addition, neurons at distinct loci within central auditory nuclei respond to successively higher frequencies with age (59,60). If the afferent connections to these neurons are not shifting, then their changing frequency response must be attributed to a change in the spatial encoding of frequency along the basilar membrane. Both cochlear (42,121) and central (94) measurements of this process have also been made in the gerbil, indicating a shift of 1 to 2 octaves in the frequency map during the first 3 to 4 postnatal weeks. Finally, a behavioral analysis has indicated that rat pups, conditioned to respond to an 8-kHz tone at postnatal day 15, respond optimally to a 12-kHz tone when tested 3 days later (47). The most parsimonious explanation for all of these results is an alteration of the cochlea's frequency map during development.

In summary, a trend toward better frequency selectivity is apparent from the onset of hearing. The locus of greatest functional change is most likely the cochlea. In addition, the limited evidence available suggests that the central auditory system may contribute to the sharpened tuning. Even with such obvious physiological correlates of frequency selectivity, the bothersome question remains: Are we quantifying the appropriate parameters? For example, cochlear hair cells and single neurons encode broader frequency ranges as stimulus intensity is raised. In apparent opposition to this is the psychophysical observation that frequency discrimination (i.e., the smallest detectable change in frequency) is enhanced as intensity is raised (104). Perhaps the challenge of future developmental studies lies in the characterization of response to novel stimulus paradigms or analysis of ensemble activity patterns.

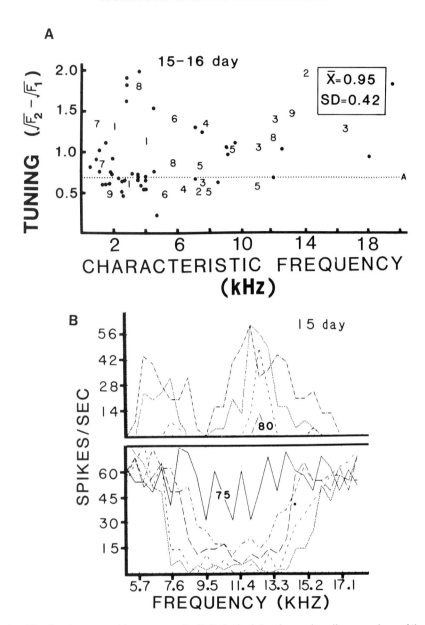

FIG. 3. The development of frequency selectivity in the lateral superior olivary nucleus of the gerbil. **A:** The frequency tuning of neurons recorded in 15- to 16-day-old animals. The measure of tuning, $\sqrt{F_2} - \sqrt{F_1}$, is computed by subtracting the square root of the lower limit of effective stimulus frequencies from the upper limit at 15 dB above threshold. In this case, larger values denote more broadly tuned neurons. For each number, corresponding to neurons recorded in the same animal, one of the cells responded with adult selectivity, whereas the other was outside of the adult range. The dotted line is the mean value for all adult neurons. **B:** Bigeminal response area. The range of frequencies eliciting (**top**) or inhibiting (**bottom**) a response from a neuron in the LSO of a 15-day-old animal. Each line depicts the response at a particular intensity. The intensity of the sound stimulus at threshold is indicated in dB SPL. Note that two discrete frequency ranges excite the cell, whereas its inhibitory response area is merely broad.

INTENSITY RESPONSE

Intensity discrimination is a perceptual quality whose functional basis is still poorly understood (40). We may only characterize the maturation of sensory properties that are likely to bear some relationship to the eventual correlates. Nearly all studies have chosen to examine the response amplitude (e.g., cochlear microphonic) or response rate (e.g., neuronal action potentials per second) as a function of sound level. Within the constraints of these data, maturation of the following coding properties will be discussed: the detection threshold, dynamic range, and interaural intensity differences.

Threshold

A maturational increase in sensitivity of the auditory system to sound stimuli is well documented at both the behavioral and electrophysiological levels (30). As with frequency selectivity, a primary question concerns locus. Although the ontogenetic increase in middle ear admittance does not appear to restrict the frequency range of the cochlea, it may limit sensitivity in hamsters (74,75,99). However, it is unclear whether middle ear properties limit the development of sensitivity in the chick, since admittance increases for approximately 70 days after thresholds have reached adult levels (97,99).

The gerbil auditory system has recently been proposed as a model in which to evaluate the ontogenesis of cochlear sensitivity, since the morphology of the external meatus and middle ear appears relatively mature before the onset of hearing (36). The development of cochlear nucleus neuron thresholds follows the chronology observed for the cochlear microphonic (119,120). A functional analysis of the gerbil middle ear is still needed to verify that the cochlea is the limiting factor in this system. Beyond the level of the cochlea there is no apparent lag in the maturation of threshold in mice (29,98,102,103) or cats (1,11,31).

The cellular correlates of threshold improvement at the level of the cochlea remain unexplored. The candidates include the opening of the inner spiral sulcus (3,71,79), the latent maturation of outer hair cells (21), changes in basilar membrane dimensions (56), and the generation of an endolymphatic ionic concentration (by the stria vascularis) necessary to drive hair cell receptor potentials (57). Wada (114) and Rubel (84,85) stressed the developmental synchrony of these and other factors that may be involved in threshold improvement. An intriguing challenge for future research is to discover the process(es) that may underlie this synchrony.

Dynamic Range

The appearance of a mature dynamic range is difficult to study because individual elements in the adult auditory pathway encode a much smaller range of intensities than the system as a whole is capable of encoding. That is, neurons are typically able to modulate their discharge rate over a 20 to 50-dB range of intensities, whereas humans are known to perceive a 100 to 120-dB range. There are two commonly advanced explanations. The first, based on variation in absolute threshold (58), suggests that different neurons encode portions of the entire dynamic range beginning

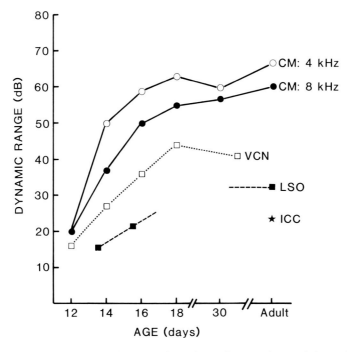

FIG. 4. The development of dynamic range along the auditory pathway of the gerbil. A response increment occurs over a larger range of intensities as maturation progresses for the cochlear microphonic (CM) and discharge rate in the cochlear nucleus (VCN) and lateral superior olive (LSO). The dynamic range for a population of neurons in the inferior colliculus (ICC) of the adult gerbil is shown for comparison. The time course for increasing dynamic range is similar for all three loci examined. (Adapted from refs. 95,101,119,120.)

at threshold. The second is based on the consideration that more intense stimuli recruit progressively greater numbers of neurons (2). Neither of these possibilities has been explored from a developmental perspective.

Quantitative descriptions of dynamic range in the cochlea, ventral cochlear nucleus, and lateral superior olivary nucleus of the gerbil allow for ontogenetic comparison. The cochlear dynamic range improves by approximately 30 to 40 dB during the first several days of hearing (119). These data are qualitatively similar to those obtained at the level of the cochlear nucleus (120) and the lateral superior olivary nucleus (95). The developmental enhancement of dynamic range for these three regions, shown in Fig. 4, illustrates two points. First, the gerbil auditory system encodes less than half the adult range at the onset of hearing. Second, the rate of maturation is equivalent at these three loci despite the apparent diminution of dynamic range in the central nuclei. This correspondence of rate becomes more apparent if the ranges are presented as a percentage of adult values (not shown). We may also compare a measure of the resolution with which these two central nuclei encode intensity: the change in discharge rate obtained for a 1-dB change in intensity. Neurons in the ventral cochlear nucleus have values of 4.8 discharges/sec/dB at 14 days, increasing to 8 in the adult [calculated from data presented in Woolf and Ryan (120)]. The values obtained in the lateral superior olive are remarkably similar, going from 4.7 discharges/sec/dB at 13 to 14 days to 9.2 in the adult (95). At the present time, then, there is no indication that the maturation of intensity coding consists of other than a dynamic periphery.

Interaural Intensity Differences

The development of intensity discrimination is, in turn, consequential for the binaural localization of sound. Psychophysical studies have implicated interaural intensity differences (IID) as a major azimuthal cue, especially for high-frequency sounds (90,108). The lateral superior olivary nucleus (LSO), a structure receiving binaural auditory input in the ventral brainstem, contains neurons whose discharge rate is proportional to the IID (i.e., azimuthal sound source location). Neurons in LSO are excited by acoustic stimuli at the ipsilateral ear and inhibited by stimuli at the contralateral ear (8,9,37). Therefore, a sound source emanating from the ipsilateral field would be expected to evoke a greater response from the excitatory system owing to the decrement in sound level across the head.

The IID response properties of neurons in the gerbil LSO were examined near hearing onset and in the adult (95). The shape of normal adult IID functions (Fig. 5A), negatively sloped curves that are linear over most of their course, describe the decrement in discharge rate as the contralateral sound level becomes relatively greater than the ipsilateral level. The IID functions in animals 13 to 16 days of age are somewhat less uniform in shape (Fig. 5B and C) than those of adults. They also encode a significantly smaller range of IID values (e.g., 18 dB in 13–14 day animals and 28 dB in adults) and have a poorer resolution, much as the monaural rate-intensity functions do. Qualitatively similar results have been obtained in the inferior colliculi of the cat and bat (10,64).

Figure 6 emphasizes the reduced ability of LSO neurons in 13- to 16-day-old gerbils to encode absolute IIDs compared with adults. Furthermore, these neurons are better able to encode intensity differences corresponding to contralateral loci (e.g., contralateral intensity greater than ipsilateral intensity) as maturation progresses. The threshold for inhibition is also significantly lower than for excitation early in development. An interesting pharmacological correlate of this result has recently been described (93,96). The development of the presumptive receptor molecule-mediating inhibition in the LSO, the glycine receptor, was found to have a relatively greater concentration in neonatal than adult gerbils (although this may be limited to one portion of the nucleus).

TEMPORAL RESPONSE

Of the five common sensory pathways, the auditory system is most sensitive to temporal discrimination. Perhaps this is best intuited by considering the predominant form that our art takes: although visual art may be complex within a defined space (e.g., over the span of a canvas) but invariant over time, the world of music relies on great temporal complexity. At a much simpler level, we will consider the ontogeny of coding properties that may be related to the time of detection (i.e., latency), integration of stimuli over time (i.e., adaptation), and frequency discrimination (i.e., phase locking).

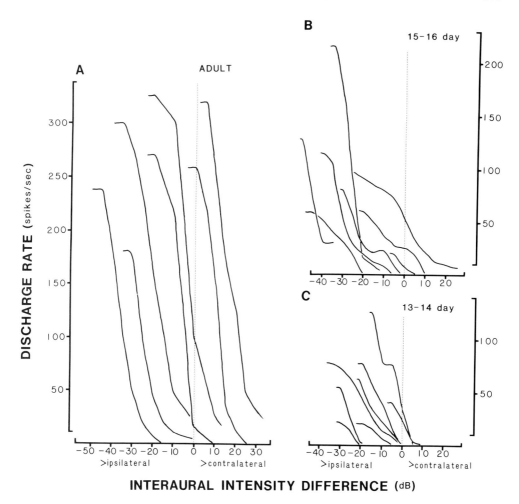

FIG. 5. The development of interaural intensity difference functions in the gerbil LSO. Each curve shows the decrement in a neuron's discharge rate (ordinate) as the stimulus level (abscissa) becomes relatively greater at the contralateral (i.e., inhibitory) ear. The vertical dotted line in each graph indicates equivalent sound level at each ear. **A:** The response of neurons in adult animals. **B:** The response of neurons in 15- to 16-day-old animals. **C:** The response of neurons in 13- to 14-day-old animals. Note the irregular shape of the curves in the younger animals.

Latency

The developmental decrease in response latency, as assayed with evoked potentials, has been well documented for the cochlea (79) and central locations (32,43,82). The most complete examination of latency considers its maturation at several levels of the auditory system and over a broad age range in the unanesthetized kitten (69,115). The strategy used was to monitor the electrical discharges generated by populations of auditory neurons with electrodes located within (69) or outside of (115) the skull. Since the amplitude of the response can be quite small under these conditions, a large number of evoked potentials were averaged for every stimulus parameter. An example is shown in Fig. 7A in which the waves denoted by larger

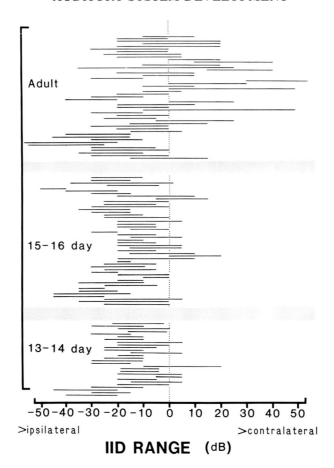

FIG. 6. The range of interaural intensity differences encoded during maturation. The linear portion of each IID function is positioned over the intensity differences to which the neuron altered its discharge rate. The IID values are given as contralateral sound level relative to ipsilateral sound level. Negative values (>ipsilateral) are comparable to a sound source located in the hemifield ipsilateral to the LSO neuron. A value of zero is equivalent to a sound source at the midline. Positive values (>contralateral) are comparable to a sound source located in the contralateral hemifield. It can be seen that the population of LSO neurons in adult gerbils encode a greater range of interaural intensities (i.e., azimuthal locations) than those in 15- to 16- or 13- to 14-day-old animals.

Roman numerals are presumed to be determined by signals from progressively more rostral auditory centers.

The evoked potential data not only document the chronology of latency decrease but illustrate three additional points (Fig. 7B). First, it is apparent that there are two phases of latency decline, a rapid linear process followed by a slower exponential decline. Second, the total magnitude of decline is greater for later occurring waves (i.e., more rostral auditory areas). Finally, the duration over which the latency decline is observed is prolonged for later occurring waves. Clearly, both cochlear and central mechanisms must operate to account for the differential magnitude and rate of development. For wave I, Walsh et al. (115) argued that the source of delay is predominantly owing to cochlear travel time and synaptic immaturity during the phase of linear decline. After this point they favor an improvement in conduction

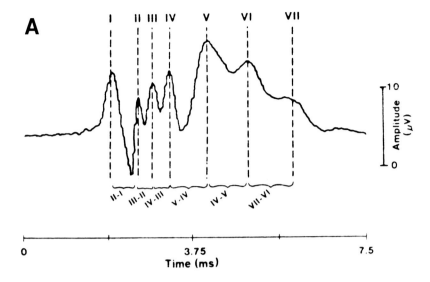

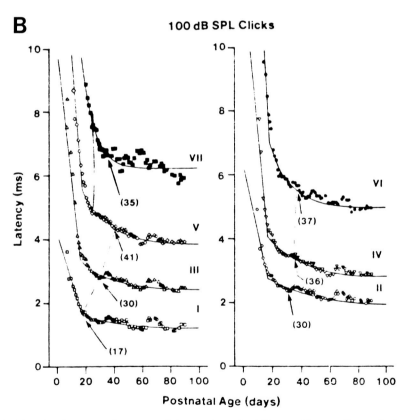

FIG. 7. The development of response latency along the kitten auditory pathway. **A:** An example of the evoked potentials from which latencies were determined. Each identifiable voltage peak is labeled with a Roman numeral. The later occurring waves are thought to arise from more rostral auditory centers. **B:** The decrement in response latency with increasing age is shown for the voltage peaks identified in A. A very rapid improvement occurs before day 20 and gradually decreases thereafter. The postnatal days at which latency reaches adult levels are shown in parentheses for each peak. (From ref. 115.)

velocity along the axon, presumably caused by increasing fiber diameter and myelination. As noted by Eggermont (27), the evoked potentials emanate from a large population of neurons and, hence, the measured latency reflects the degree to which neurons discharge synchronously. Precise timing of discharge is considered in more detail in the next section.

Adaptation

There are certain auditory processes that are more sensitive to increasing stimulus duration. That is, the auditory system appears to integrate information over time. To the extent that the pathway fatigues to repeated or continuous stimulation, the underlying percepts should be negatively affected. Temporal integration may affect threshold values (25,28,38,46,68), the perceived loudness of a sound (6,107), and localization of stimuli (52,111).

Sensory or neural elements of the auditory pathway are especially prone to adaptation or habituation during early development (16,32). Two studies have examined this phenomenon parametrically with qualitatively similar results. A comparison of evoked potentials from the mouse cochlear nerve and inferior colliculus indicates different ontogenetic rates with respect to their ability to respond continuously to stimuli (92). The click-evoked potentials from these two structures were monitored as stimulus rate and duration were increased, with a decrease in response amplitude indicating fatigue. Figure 8 illustrates the following response to increasing stimulus rates for three age groups. At the higher repetition rates the cochlear response (i.e., N_1) has reached adult levels by day 18, whereas the inferior colliculus continues to mature. Saunders et al. (97) demonstrated a similar differential development of following response between the receptor potential (i.e., cochlear microphonic) and brainstem response in the chick. There are at present no data concerning the cellular basis of this initial adaptation or habituation along the auditory pathway, although synaptic fatigue is common following synaptogenesis. Given a delayed maturation of temporal integration for more rostral central auditory nuclei, it will be interesting to compare behavioral studies that examine the effect of stimulus rate and duration on detection thresholds. One related measure of temporal coding that has been investigated in young infants is the ability to detect gaps in a continuous noise. Olsho and Halpin (66) recently showed that the duration of a gap must be as much as 10 times as long for detection by 3-month-old infants than for adults.

Phase Locking

So far we have principally considered functional assays of maturation that rely on the mere presence or magnitude of an electrical response. This is somewhat misleading because the temporal pattern of neural activity may be the informative code in certain situations. Auditory nerve fibers are particularly accurate in encoding low-frequency sounds by discharging at only a single phase of the stimulus waveform (83). A tone of 200 Hz should, therefore, lead to periodic discharges at 5-msec intervals, although some of these intervals may be missed. A measure of the degree to which action potentials are locked to the stimulus cycle, the vector strength, is 0 if there is a random relationship and 1.0 if there is perfect phase synchrony (39).

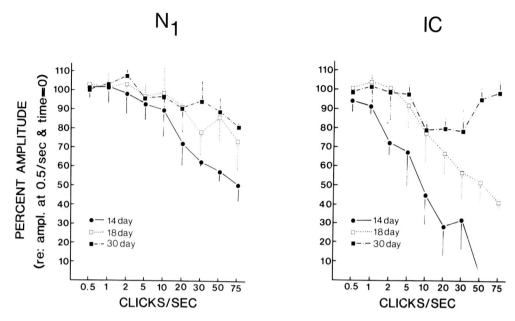

FIG. 8. The maturation of stimulus following in the auditory nerve (N_1) and midbrain (IC) of the mouse. A decrease in evoked-potential amplitude (ordinate) with increasing click repetition rates (abscissa) indicates that fewer neurons are synchronously driven by the click stimuli. The following response at 14 days postnatal is significantly poorer than at 30 days for both the N_1 and IC responses. It should be noted that the N_1 following response is essentially mature by day 18, whereas the IC response is not, especially for greater click repetition rates. (From ref. 92)

An evaluation of phase locking has recently been obtained at the level of the auditory nerve (49) and anteroventral cochlear nucleus (11) of the kitten. At the level of the auditory nerve, phase locking approaches adult levels during the first 3 postnatal weeks, especially for stimulus frequencies above 600 Hz (Fig. 9). For cochlear nucleus neurons, whose vector strength is equivalent to that of auditory nerve fibers (11), maturation appears to continue even after 8 weeks. Therefore, as with response latency and adaptation, the ability of neurons to phase lock relies, at least partially, on central ontogenetic mechanisms. It will be of great interest and importance to elucidate the underlying biophysical and anatomical bases of this process. The synapse is an obvious locus at which to begin the search, although the number of parameters ensures complexity. Finally, the effects of immature temporal properties on the neural coding of interaural time differences and the localization of low-frequency sounds provide fertile ground for future advances.

ELECTRICAL ACTIVITY AND DEVELOPMENT

Does the amount or pattern of neural activity influence the maturation of auditory response properties? This question has perhaps derived more from our respect of such ordered complexity than from a wealth of observations. The original motivation comes from studies on the kitten visual cortex showing that alterations in the amount and pattern of retinal activity lead to functional changes in cortical neurons (45,118).

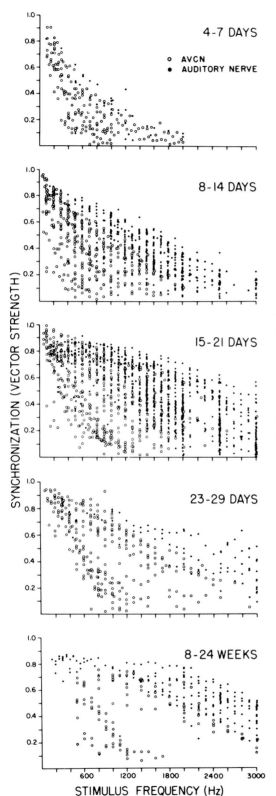

FIG. 9. The maturation of phase locking for neurons in the auditory nerve and anteroventral cochlear nucleus (AVCN) of the kitten. A vector strength of 1.0 indicates that a neuron's response was strongly associated with a particular phase of the stimulus waveform. The most sensitive AVCN neurons lag behind those in the auditory nerve in each age range. It should be noted that AVCN neurons appear to sort into two populations during development, one phase sensitive and the other not. (From ref. 49.)

There is no better introduction to the topic than a brief discussion of these results. In kittens that had been monocularly deprived beginning by postnatal days 6 to 18, Wiesel and Hubel (117) found a drastic reduction in the fraction of cortical neurons that could be driven by the deprived eye. This result led them to predict that binocularly deprived animals would have cortical neurons that did not respond to stimulation of either eye. However, a normal percentage of the visually excitable cells was found to be binocular (118). This result prompted them to consider not only afferent activity levels, but also the "interrelationships between the various sets of afferents."

Hubel and Wiesel (45) offered a second line of evidence for the effect of activity in a study on strabismic cats. In this case the timing of afferent activity from the two eyes to binocular neurons was quite disparate because their receptive fields were misaligned. The visual cortices of experimental animals were depleted of binocularly driven cells. Hubel and Wiesel (45) concluded that absence of temporal synchrony, in conjunction with the activation of at least one afferent pathway, may lead to functional elimination of a second set of afferents. During the past 20 years the intricacies and addenda of activity effects have been well documented in the visual system. One caution applies to the majority of reports in this field: they generally consider the induction of abnormal response properties in a previously normal population rather than directly examining the mechanisms that act during ontogeny. Since the influence of activity is still a nascent issue among auditory physiologists, we may obtain both instruction and caution from the visual system literature.

The amount of afferent activity has been implicated in maintaining postsynaptic neuron morphology because of the deleterious effects attendant to sound attenuation and inner ear insult during early development (7,19,20,106,112,116). Since the focus of this chapter is on functional attributes, this discussion is limited to influences of activity on their maturation. We will first consider two studies that address frequency coding, one concerned with response latency, and then turn our attention to those that concentrate on binaural interactions. Unfortunately, in selective rearing studies, an effort is seldom made to determine the neural discharge rate or pattern imposed by the manipulation (92,113).

Monaural Properties

The frequency tuning of single neurons in the mouse inferior colliculus was quantified for both normal animals and those reared in an acoustic environment that imposed distinct firing patterns on these neurons (91). The environment consisted of repetitive clicks at 20/sec, a stimulus pattern that continuously entrains a large proportion of primary afferents (Fig. 8) (92) from the onset of hearing (i.e., postnatal days 12–13) until a time when tuning curves should be adult-like (i.e., postnatal days 19–24). Click-reared animals had significantly broader tuning curves than did normally reared mice, particularly for units with best frequencies in the 10 to 15 kHz range (Fig. 10). The lack of a robust effect beyond these bounds may be owing to the rearing stimulus (e.g., the clicks had little energy above 15 kHz) and the characteristics of inferior colliculus neurons (e.g., low-frequency neurons have high thresholds and habituate more rapidly). Broadened tuning curves were not observed when a second stimulus regimen was employed, consisting of repetitive pulses of

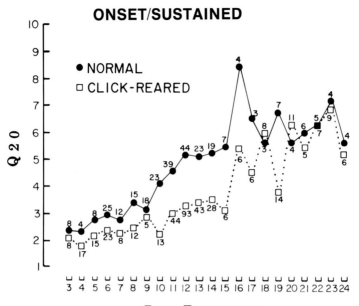

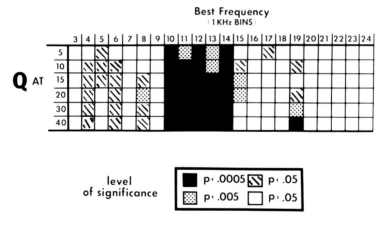

FIG. 10. The difference in frequency selectivity between neurons from normal and click-reared mice. The measure of tuning, Q_{20} values, is obtained by dividing best frequency by effective bandwidth at 20 dB above threshold. In this case, larger values indicate sharper tuning. Each point in the graph (**top**) is the mean Q_{20} value obtained from units in 1 kHz best frequency groups. The number of units comprising each mean is indicated. The mean values from click-reared animals are noticeably lower than those of normals, indicating that frequency selectivity was affected by the environmental manipulation. A summary of significant differences between normal and click-reared animals (**bottom**) is given for Q values obtained at 5, 10, 15, 20, 30, and 40 dB above threshold. Reading across the "Q at 20" line on the summary table would detail where significant differences exist for the plot of Q_{20} versus best frequency. (From ref. 92.)

two added frequencies. There was no evidence of cochlear damage (i.e., both N_1 and single-unit thresholds were normal in click-reared animals) nor were changes in latency or spontaneous activity apparent. The results suggest that mature frequency tuning is influenced by the pattern of electrical activity in the periphery. The precise locus of change is still unknown and may be located in the cochlea or the central nervous system.

A second approach to frequency coding has used behavioral analysis to determine the effects of acoustic environment during development in the chick (48). Animals were reared with earplugs *in ovo* such that there was a fairly uniform 40-dB attenuation of sound across a 0.125- to 4-kHz range. On post-hatch days 3 to 4, the animals were first habituated to an 800-Hz tone (i.e., failure to elicit peep suppression and an orienting response) and then probed with five frequencies to construct a frequency generalization gradient. The chick would be expected to show the same behavioral response, habituation, to tones other than 800 Hz if they were perceptually equivalent. Acoustic attenuation resulted in broader behavioral generalization gradients: experimental animals responded in the same manner to 800 to 900 Hz, whereas control animals treated 850 and 900 Hz as novel stimuli. The result could not easily be attributed to a damaged cochlea as thresholds were normal following earplug removal. Recent observations from this laboratory (113) revealed that manipulations that attenuate sound by an equivalent amount (e.g., middle ear bone removal) do not affect the normally high spontaneous activity levels within the primary brainstem nuclei. Therefore, the behavioral results may be attributable to alterations in the pattern of evoked activity. As with the previous study, the locus of change is unknown.

An effect of sound attenuation on response latency has been demonstrated in rats reared with unilateral ligature of the external auditory meatus (17). This experimental atresia produced an attenuation of 25 dB or greater. After 3 to 5 months the ear canal was reopened and the latency of single neurons in the inferior colliculus to click stimuli was determined. Those neurons recorded in experimental animals having a best frequency above 10 kHz had significantly increased response latencies, although a few were within the normal adult range. This alteration of temporal coding was attributed to events central to the eighth nerve since the N_1 latency was equivalent in normal and experimental animals.

Binaural Properties

The consequences of unilateral sound attenuation on interaural intensity difference functions or behavioral localization are quite discordant in the studies to date. Essentially the same manipulation, unilateral meatal ligature, has been performed once on rats (105) and twice on kittens (13,63), leading to three different conclusions. Normal animals show a balance between excitatory and inhibitory inputs, emanating from the contralateral and ipsilateral ears, respectively. In rats reared with monaural attenuation, the efficacy of the inhibitory input is altered (105). The nonligated ear shows an enhanced suppressive influence in the ipsilateral colliculus, whereas the deprived ear is significantly poorer at suppressing activity in its ipsilateral colliculus. The excitatory inputs from normal and manipulated ears are similar in facilitating a neural response. It should be noted that both of these neural changes would tend to shift IID coding further from the norm than the shift expected from a ligature alone. One would predict that neurons no longer modulate their firing rate to the available range of free-field intensity differences, and the animal is, therefore, poorer at localizing sound, whether the earplugs remain in place or are removed.

When cats are reared under similar conditions, but pure tonal stimuli instead of clicks are used to evoke a response, apparently opposite results are obtained (63). Inhibitory inputs from the nonligated ear are less effective at suppressing neural activity in the inferior colliculus. A compensation of this sort could allow neurons to modulate their discharge rate to the original range of IID values (when the ligature remained in place). However, the lack of normal IID function shape at extreme intensity differences indicate that these neural alterations would also lead to degenerate perceptual abilities. Neither the experiment on the rat nor the one on the kitten is completely explicable in terms of peripheral threshold shifts attendant to the original ligation.

A second group has repeated the experiment on kitten but assayed functional state at the cortical level (13). In this case there was no effect of ligation that could not be attributed to the substantial cochlear threshold shifts found in experimental animals. With ligature in place, then, these neurons would not be expected to alter their firing rate over a physiological range of intensity differences. Clearly, such a broad range of outcomes is disturbing. The lack of resolution requires a parametric study that carefully documents the level of attenuation and its affect on activity levels, intra-animal alterations in cochlear versus central threshold, and the effects on inhibitory versus excitatory processes.

Monaural attenuation has a profound effect on auditory localization in the barn owl. If animals are reared with one ear plugged, they gradually compensate for the imposed interaural intensity and time differences (53,54) and are able to localize sound accurately. Immediately following removal of the plug the owls were unable to localize sounds correctly, but young animals (less than 40 weeks) gradually readjusted to normal responsiveness (55). Perhaps the most disconcerting problem posed by these results is that none of the binaural response properties found in the rat or cat central auditory system after unilateral attenuation is consistent with behavioral compensation. Both sets of physiological data would predict an impairment of localization ability. It is possible that novel binaural discharge properties (with ear plugs in place) are capable of eliciting the appropriate behavioral response. Alternatively, auditory neurons in the barn owl may compensate for the peripheral deficit by altering the strength of certain synaptic inputs such that the original change in discharge corresponds to the original interaural stimulus differences. The complexity of attenuation effects across the owl's frequency range, coupled with our rudimentary knowledge of neural correlates to localization, make this an interesting but daunting experimental system.

SUMMARY AND CONCLUSIONS

Our present understanding of functional ontogeny is predominantly composed of descriptive work contrasting the neonatal and adult states. The apparent differences are, for the most part, not currently explicable in terms of morphological, biophysical, or molecular changes. However, we may expect this deficiency to be short-lived (4,26,122). At the other extreme, the studies reviewed in this chapter indicate a need for behavioral models such that physiologically examined properties may be judged as nontrivial. We may also begin the search for neural correlates to other perceptual properties, including masking level differences and the precedence effect. The ontogeny of these processes may highlight central mechanisms that have heretofore gone unexplored. Finally, the effects of acoustic environment on auditory development are far from clear. It is only through the careful documentation of sensory maturation, the discharge pattern of neurons from the earliest time points, and the neural transform of environmental sound that such an evaluation will be made.

REFERENCES

1. Aitkin, L. M., and Moore, D. R. (1975): Inferior colliculus. II. Development of tuning characteristics and tonotopic organization in central nucleus of the neonatal cat. *J. Neurophysiol.*, 38:1208–1216.
2. Allanson, J. T., and Whitfield, I. C. (1965): The cochlear nucleus and its relation to theories of hearing. In: *Third London Symposium on Information Theory*, pp. 269–284. Butterworth, London.
3. Anggard, L. (1965): An electrophysiological study of the development of cochlear function in the rabbit. *Acta Otolaryngol. [Suppl.] (Stockh.)*, 203:1–64.
4. Anniko, M. (1985): Histochemical, microchemical (microprobe), and organ culture approaches for the study of auditory development. *Acta Otolaryngol. [Suppl.] (Stockh.)*, 421:10–18.
5. Birnholz, J. C., and Benacerraf, B. R. (1983): The development of human fetal hearing. *Science*, 222:516–518.
6. Boone, M. M. (1973): Loudness measurements on pure tone and broad band impulsive sounds. *Acustica*, 29:198–204.
7. Born, D. B., and Rubel, E. W. (1988): Afferent influences on brain stem auditory nuclei of the chicken: Presynaptic action potentials regulate protein synthesis in n. magnocellularis neurons. *J. Neurosci.*, 8:901–919.
8. Boudreau, J. C., and Tsuchitani, C. (1968): Binaural interaction in the cat superior olive s-segment. *J. Neurophysiol.*, 31:442–454.
9. Boudreau, J. C., and Tsuchitani, C. (1970): Cat superior olive s-segment cell discharge to tonal stimulation. In: *Contributions to Sensory Physiology, Vol. 4*, edited by W. D. Neff, pp. 143–213. Academic, New York.
10. Brown, P. E., Grinnell, A. D., and Harrison, J. B. (1978): The development of hearing in the pallid bat, *Antrozous pallidus*. *J. Comp. Physiol.*, 126:169–182.
11. Brugge, J. F., Javel, E., and Kitzes, L. M. (1978): Signs of functional maturation of peripheral auditory system in discharge patterns of neurons in anteroventral cochlear nucleus of kitten. *J. Neurophysiol.*, 41:1557–1579.
12. Brugge, J. F., Kitzes, L. M., and Javel, E. (1981): Postnatal development of frequency and intensity sensitivity of neurons in the anteroventral cochlear nucleus of kittens. *Hear. Res.*, 5:217–229.
13. Brugge, J. F., Orman, S. S., Coleman, J. R., Chan, J. C. K., and Phillips, D. P. (1985): Binaural interactions in cortical area AI of cats reared with unilateral atresia of the external ear canal. *Hear. Res.*, 20:275–287.
14. Carlier, E., and Pujol, R. (1978): Role of inner and outer hair cells in coding sound intensity: An ontogenetic approach. *Brain Res.*, 147:174–176.
15. Carlier, E., Lenoir, M., and Pujol, R. (1979): Development of cochlear frequency selectivity tested by compound action potential tuning curves. *Hear. Res.*, 1:197–201.
16. Chaloupka, Z., and Myslivecek, J. (1960): A contribution to the ontogenetical development of the auditory analyzer. *Cesk. Fysiol.*, 9:423–424.
17. Clopton, B. M., and Silverman, M. S. (1978): Changes in latency and duration of neural responding following developmental auditory deprivation. *Exp. Brain Res.*, 32:39–47.
18. Cody, A. R., and Johnstone, B. M. (1980): Single auditory neuron response during acute acoustic trauma. *Hear. Res.*, 3:3–16.
19. Coleman, J. R., and O'Connor, P. (1979): Effects of monaural and binaural sound deprivation on cell development in the anteroventral cochlear nucleus of rats. *Exp. Neurol.*, 64:553–566.
20. Conlee, J. W., and Parks, T. N. (1981): Age- and position-dependent effects of monaural acoustic deprivation in nucleus magnocellularis of the chicken. *J. Comp. Neurol.*, 202:373–384.
21. Dallos, P., Billone, M. C., Durrant, J. D., Wang, C.-Y., and Raynor, S. (1972): Cochlear inner and outer hair cells: Functional differences. *Science*, 177:356–358.

22. Dallos, P., and Cheatham, M. A. (1976): Compound action potential (AP) tuning curves. *J. Acoust. Soc. Am.*, 59:591–597.
23. Dallos, P., and Harris, D. (1978): Properties of auditory nerve responses in absence of outer hair cells. *Neurophysiol.*, 41:365–383.
24. Dolan, T. G., Mills, J. H., and Schmiedt, R. A. (1985): A comparison of brainstem, whole-nerve AP and single-fiber tuning curves in the gerbil: Normative data. *Hear. Res.*, 17:259–266.
25. Dooling, R. J. (1979): Temporal summation of pure tones in birds. *J. Acoust. Soc. Am.*, 65:1058–1060.
26. Drescher, D. G. editor (1985): *Auditory Biochemistry*. Charles C. Thomas, Springfield, IL.
27. Eggermont, J. J. (1985): Evoked potentials as indicators of auditory maturation. *Acta Otolaryngol.* [*Suppl.*] (*Stockh.*), 421:41–47.
28. Ehret, G. (1976): Temporal auditory summation for pure tones and white noise in the house mouse (*Mus musculus*). *J. Acoust. Soc. Am.*, 59:1421–1427.
29. Ehret, G. (1976): Development of absolute auditory thresholds in the house mouse (*Mus musculus*). *J. Am. Audiol. Soc.*, 1:179–184.
30. Ehret, G. (1985): Behavioral studies on auditory development in mammals in relation to higher nervous system functioning. *Acta Otolaryngol.* [*Suppl.*] (*Stockh.*), 421:31–40.
31. Ehret, G., and Romand, R. (1981): Postnatal development of absolute auditory thresholds in kittens. *J. Comp. Physiol. Psychol.*, 95:304–311.
32. Ellingson, R. J., and Wilcott, R. C. (1960): Development of evoked responses in visual and auditory cortices of kittens. *J. Neurophysiol.*, 23:363–375.
33. Evans, E. F. (1975): The sharpening of cochlear frequency selectivity in the normal and abnormal cochlea. *Audiology*, 14:419–442.
34. Evans, E. F., and Klinke, R. (1974): Reversible effects of cyanide and furosemide on the tuning of single cochlear nerve fibers. *J. Physiol.* (*Lond.*), 242:129–131.
35. Fermin, C. D., and Cohen, G. M. (1984): Developmental gradients in the embryonic chick's basillar papilla. *Acta Otolaryngol.* (*Stockh.*), 97:39–51.
36. Finck, A., Schneck, C. D., and Hartman, A. F. (1972): Development of cochlear function in the neonate mongolian gerbil (*Meriones unguiculatus*). *J. Comp. Physiol. Psychol.*, 78:375–380.
37. Galambos, R., Schwartzkopf, J., and Rupert, A. (1959): Microelectrode study of superior olivary nuclei. *Am. J. Physiol.*, 197:527–536.
38. Garner, W. F., and Miller, G. A. (1947): The masked threshold of pure tones as a function of duration. *J. Exp. Psychol.*, 37:293–303.
39. Goldberg, J. M., and Brown, P. B. (1969): Response of binaural neurons of dog superior olivary complex to dichotic tonal stimuli: Some physiological mechanisms of sound localization. *J. Neurophysiol.*, 32:613–636.
40. Green, D. M. (1976): *An Introduction to Hearing*. Lawrence Erlbaum, Hillsdale, NJ.
41. Harris, D. M. (1979): Action potential suppression, tuning curves, and thresholds: Comparison with single fiber data. *Hear. Res.*, 1:133–154.
42. Harris, D. M., and Dallos, P. (1984): Ontogenetic changes in frequency mapping of a mammalian ear. *Science*, 225:741–743.
43. Hecox, K., and Galambos, R. (1974): Brainstem auditory evoked responses in human infants and adults. *Arch. Otolaryngol.*, 99:30–33.
44. Hirokawa, N. (1978): The ultrastructure of the basillar papilla of the chick. *J. Comp. Neurol.*, 181:361–374.
45. Hubel, D. H., and Wiesel, T. N. (1965): Binocular interaction in striate cortex of kittens reared with artificial squint. *J. Neurophysiol.*, 28:1041–1059.
46. Hughes, J. W. (1946): The threshold of audition for short periods of stimulation. *Proc. R. Soc. Lond.* [*Biol.*], 133:486–490.
47. Hyson, R. L., and Rudy, J. W. (1987): Ontogenetic change in the analysis of sound frequency in the infant rat. *Dev. Psychobiol.*, 20:189–208.
48. Kerr, L. M., Ostapoff, E. M., and Rubel E. W. (1979): Influence of acoustic experience on the ontogeny of frequency generalization gradients in the chicken. *J. Exp. Psychol.*, 5:97–115.
49. Kettner, R. E., Feng, J.-Z., and Brugge, J. F. (1985): Postnatal development of the phase-locked response to low frequency tones of auditory nerve fibers in the cat. *J. Neurosci.*, 5:275–283.
50. Khanna, S. M., and Leonard, D. G. B. (1986): Relationship between basilar membrane tuning and hair cell condition. *Hear. Res.*, 23:55–70.
51. Kikuchi, K., and Hilding, D. (1965): The development of the organ of Corti in the mouse. *Acta Otolaryngol.* (*Stockh.*), 60:207–222.
52. Knudsen, E. I., and Konishi, M. (1979): Mechanisms of sound localization by the barn owl (*Tybo alba*). *J. Comp. Physiol.*, 133:13–21.
53. Knudsen, E. I., Knudsen, P. F., and Esterly, S. D. (1982): Early auditory experience modifies sound localization in barn owls. *Nature*, 295:238–240.

54. Knudsen, E. I., Esterly, S. D., and Knudsen, P. F. (1984): Monaural occlusion alters sound localization during a sensitive period in the barn owl. *J. Neurosci.*, 4:1001–1011.
55. Knudsen, E. I., Knudsen, P. F., and Esterly, S. D. (1984): A critical period for the recovery of sound localization accuracy following monaural occlusion in the barn owl. *J. Neurosci.*, 4:1012–1020.
56. Kraus, H.-J., and Aulbach-Kraus, K. (1981): Morphological changes in the cochlea of the mouse after the onset of hearing. *Hear. Res.*, 4:89–102.
57. Kuipers, W. (1974): Na-K-ATPase activity in the cochlea of the rat during development. *Acta Otolaryngol. (Stockh.)*, 78:341–344.
58. Liberman, M. C. (1978): Auditory-nerve response from cats raised in a low-noise chamber. *J. Acoust. Soc. Am.*, 63:442–455.
59. Lippe, W. R., and Rubel, E. W. (1983): Development of the place principle: Tonotopic organization. *Science*, 219:514–516.
60. Lippe, W. R., and Rubel, E. W. (1985): Ontogeny of tonotopic organization of brainstem auditory nuclei in the chicken: Implications for development of the place principle. *J. Comp. Neurol.*, 237:273–289.
61. Lippe, W. R., Ryals, B. M., and Rubel E. W. (1986): Development of the place principle. In: *Advances in Neural and Behavioral Development Volume 2*, edited by R. Aslan, pp. 155–203. Ablex, Norwood.
62. Mikaelian, D., and Ruben, R. J. (1965): Development of hearing in the normal CBA-J mouse. *Acta Otolaryngol. (Stockh.)*, 59:451–461.
63. Moore, D. R., and Irvine, D. R. F. (1981): Plasticity of binaural interaction in the cat inferior colliculus. *Brain Res.*, 208:198–202.
64. Moore, D. R., and Irvine, D. R. F. (1981): Development of responses to acoustic interaural intensity differences in the cat inferior colliculus. *Exp. Brain Res.*, 41:301–309.
65. Olsho, L. W. (1984): Infant frequency discrimination. *Infant Behav. Dev.*, 7:27–35.
66. Olsho, L. W., and Halpin, C. F. (1987): Gap detection thresholds of 3-, 6-, and 12-month-old human infants. *Assoc. Res. Otolaryngol. Abst.*
67. Olsho, L. W., Koch, E. G., and Halpin, C. F. (1987): Level and age effects in infant frequency discrimination. *J. Acoust. Soc. Am.*, 82:454–464.
68. Plomp, R., and Bouman, M. A. (1959): Relation between hearing threshold and duration for tone pulses. *J. Acoust. Soc. Am.*, 31:749–758.
69. Pujol, R. (1972): Development of tone burst responses along the auditory pathway in the cat. *Acta Otolaryngol. (Stockh.)*, 74:383–391.
70. Pujol, R., and Marty, R. (1970): Postnatal maturation in the cochlea of the cat. *J. Comp. Neurol.*, 139:115–126.
71. Pujol, R., and Hilding, D. (1973): Anatomy and physiology of the onset of auditory function. *Acta Otolaryngol. (Stockh.)*, 76:1–10.
72. Pujol, R., Carlier, E., and Lenoir, M. (1980): The sensory hair cell. Ontogenetic approach to inner and outer hair cell function. *Hear. Res.*, 2:423–430.
73. Rebillard, G., and Rubel, E. W. (1981): Electrophysiological study of the maturation of auditory responses from the inner ear of the chick. *Brain Res.*, 229:15–23.
74. Relkin, E. M., Saunders, J. C., and Konkle, D. F. (1979): Development of middle-ear admittance in the hamster. *J. Acoust. Soc. Am.*, 126:133–139.
75. Relkin, E. M., and Saunders, J. C. (1980): Displacement of the malleus in neonatal golden hamsters. *Acta Otolaryngol. (Stockh.)*, 90:6–15.
76. Retzius, G. (1884): *Das Gehorogan der Wirbeltiere. II. Das Gehororgan der Reptilien, der Vogel, und der Saugetiere*. Samson and Wallin, Stockholm.
77. Robertson, D., and Manley, G. A. (1974): Manipulation of frequency analysis in the cochlear ganglion of the guinea pig. *J. Comp. Physiol.*, 91:363–375.
78. Robles, L., Ruggero, M. A., and Rich, N. C. (1986): Basilar membrane mechanics at the base of the chinchilla cochlea. I. Input-output functions, tuning curves, and response phases. *J. Acoust. Soc. Am.*, 80:1364–1374.
79. Romand, R. (1971): Maturation des potentiels cochleaires dans la periode perinatale chez le chat et chez le cobaye. *J. Physiol. (Paris)*, 63:763–782.
80. Romand, R. editor (1983): *Development of Auditory and Vestibular Systems*. Academic Press, New York.
81. Romand, R. (1983): Development in the frequency selectivity of auditory nerve fibers in the kitten. *Neurosci. Lett.*, 35:271–276.
82. Rose, J. E., Adrian, H., and Santibanez, G. (1957): Electrical signs of maturation in the auditory system of the kitten. *Acta Neurol. Latinoam.*, 3:133–143.
83. Rose, J. E., Brugge, J. F., Anderson, D. J., and Hind, J. E. (1967): Phase-locked response to low-frequency tones in single auditory nerve fibers of the squirrel monkey. *J. Neurophysiol.*, 30:769–793.

84. Rubel, E. W. (1978): Ontogeny of structure and function in the vertebrate auditory system. In: *Handbook of Sensory Physiology Vol. IX*, edited by M. Jacobson, pp. 135–237. Springer-Verlag, New York.
85. Rubel, E. W. (1985): Strategies and problems for future studies of auditory development. *Acta Otolaryngol. [Suppl.] (Stockh.)*, 421:114–128.
86. Rubel, E. W., and Ryals, B. M. (1983): Development of the place principle: Acoustic trauma. *Science*, 219:512–514.
87. Rubel, E. W., Born, D. E., Deitch, J. S., and Durham, D. (1984): Recent advances toward understanding auditory system development. In: *Hearing Sciences: Recent Advances*, edited by C. Berlin, pp. 109–157. College-Hill Press, San Diego.
88. Ryals, B. M., and Rubel, E. W. (1985): Ontogenetic changes in the position of hair cell loss after acoustic overstimulation in avian basillar papilla. *Hear. Res.*, 19:135–142.
89. Ryan, A. F., Woolf, N. K., and Sharp, F. R. (1982): Functional ontogeny in the central auditory pathway of the mongolian gerbil. *Exp. Brain Res.*, 47:428–436.
90. Sandel, T. T., Teas, D. C., Fedderson, W. E., and Jeffress, L. A. (1955): Localization of sound from single and paired sources. *J. Acoust. Soc. Am.*, 68:858–875.
91. Sanes, D. H., and Constantine-Paton, M. (1985): The sharpening of frequency tuning curves requires patterned activity during development in the mouse, *Mus musculus. J. Neurosci.*, 5:1152–1166.
92. Sanes, D. H., and Constantine-Paton, M. (1985): The development of stimulus following in the cochlear nerve and inferior colliculus of the mouse. *Dev. Brain Res.*, 22:255–267.
93. Sanes, D. H., Geary, W., Wooten, G. F., and Rubel, E. W. (1987): The quantitative distribution of the glycine receptor in the auditory brain stem of the gerbil. *J. Neurosci.*, 7:3793–3802.
94. Sanes, D. H., Merickel, M., and Rubel, E. W. (1987): Development of the tonotopic map in the lateral superior olivary nucleus of the gerbil. *J. Comp. Neurol. (in press)*.
95. Sanes, D. H., and Rubel, E. W. (1988): The functional ontogeny of inhibition and excitation in the gerbil auditory brain stem. *J. Neurosci.*, 8:682–700.
96. Sanes, D. H., and Wooten, G. F. (1987): The development of glycine receptor distribution in the lateral superior olivary nucleus of the gerbil. *J. Neurosci.*, 7:3803–3811.
97. Saunders, J. C., Coles, R. B., and Gates, G. R. (1973): The development of auditory evoked responses in the cochlea and cochlear nuclei of the chick. *Brain Res.*, 63:59–74.
98. Saunders, J. C., Dolgin, K. G., and Lowry, L. D. (1980): The maturation of frequency selectivity in C57BL/6J mice studied with auditory evoked response tuning curves. *Brain Res.*, 187:69–79.
99. Saunders, J. C., Kaltenbach, J. A., and Relkin, E. M. (1983): The structural and functional development of the outer and middle ear. In: *Development of Auditory and Vestibular Systems*, edited by R. Romand, pp. 3–25. Academic Press, New York.
100. Sellick, P. M., Patuzzi, R., and Johnstone, B. M. (1982): Measurement of basilar membrane motion in the guinea pig using the Mossbauer technique. *J. Acoust. Soc. Am.*, 72:131–141.
101. Semple, M. N., and Kitzes, L. M. (1985): Single unit responses in the inferior colliculus: Different consequences of contralateral and ipsilateral stimulation. *J. Neurophysiol.*, 53:1483–1498.
102. Shnerson, A., and Willott, J. F. (1979): Development of inferior colliculus response properties in C57BL/6J mouse pups. *Exp. Brain Res.*, 37:373–385.
103. Shnerson, A., and Pujol, R. (1982): Age-related changes in the C57BL/6J mouse cochlea. I. Physiological findings. *Dev. Brain Res.*, 2:65–75.
104. Shower, E. G., and Biddulph, R. (1931): Differential pitch sensitivity of the ear. *J. Acoust. Soc. Am.*, 2:275–287.
105. Silverman, M. S., and Clopton, B. M. (1977): Plasticity of binaural interaction. I. Effects of early auditory deprivation. *J. Neurophysiol.*, 40:1266–1274.
106. Smith, Z. D. J., Gray, L., and Rubel, E. W. (1983): Afferent influences on brainstem and auditory nuclei of the chicken: N. laminaris dendritic length following monaural conductive hearing loss. *J. Comp. Neurol.*, 220:199–205.
107. Stephens, S. D. G. (1974): Methodological factors influencing loudness of short duration sounds. *J. Sound Vib.*, 37:235–246.
108. Stevens, S. S., and Newman, E. B. (1936): The localization of actual sources of sound. *Am. J. Psychol.*, 48:297–306.
109. Tilney, L. G., and Saunders, J. C. (1983): Actin filaments, stereocilia, and hair cells of the birds cochlea. I. Length, number, width, and distribution of stereocilia of each hair cell are related to the position of the hair cell on the cochlea. *J. Cell. Biol.*, 96:807–821.
110. Tilney, L. G., Tilney, M. S., Saunders, J. C., and DeRosier, D. J. (1986): Actin filaments, stereocilia, and hair cells of the bird cochlea. III. The development and differentiation of hair cells and stereocilia. *Dev. Biol.*, 116:100–118.
111. Tobias, J. V., and Zerlin, S. (1959): Lateralization threshold as a function of stimulus duration. *J. Acoust. Soc. Am.*, 31:1591–1594.
112. Tucci, D. L., and Rubel, E. W. (1985): Afferent influences on brain stem auditory nuclei of the

chicken: Effects of conductive and sensorineural hearing loss in N. magnocellularis. *J. Comp. Neurol.*, 238:371–381.

113. Tucci, D. L., Born, D. E., and Rubel, E. W. (1987): Changes in spontaneous activity and CNS morphology associated with conductive and sensorineural loss in chickens. *Ann. Otol. Rhinol. Laryngol.*, 96:343–350.

114. Wada, T. (1923): Anatomical and physiological studies on the growth of the inner ear of the albino rat. *Am. Anat. Mem.*, 10:1–74.

115. Walsh, E. J., McGee, J., and Javel, E. (1986): Development of auditory evoked potentials in the cat. II. Wave latencies. *J. Acoust. Soc. Am.*, 79:725–744.

116. Webster, D. B., and Webster, M. (1979): Effects of neonatal conductive hearing loss on brain stem auditory nuclei. *Ann. Otol. Rhinol. Laryngol.*, 88:684–688.

117. Wiesel, T. N., and Hubel, D. H. (1963): Single cell responses in striate cortex of kittens deprived of vision in one eye. *J. Neurophysiol.*, 26:1003–1017.

118. Wiesel, T. N., and Hubel, D. H. (1965): Comparison of monocular deprivation and binocular deprivation in cortex of cats. *J. Neurophysiol.*, 28:1029–1040.

119. Woolf, N. K., and Ryan, A. F. (1984): The development of auditory function in the cochlea of the mongolian gerbil. *Hear. Res.*, 13:277–283.

120. Woolf, N. K., and Ryan, A. F. (1985): Ontogeny of neural discharge patterns in the ventral cochlear nucleus of the mongolian gerbil. *Dev. Brain Res.*, 17:131–147.

121. Yancy, C., and Dallos, P. (1985): Ontogenic changes in cochlear characteristic frequency at a basal turn location as reflected in the summating potential. *Hear. Res.*, 18:189–195.

122. Young, S., and Rubel, E. W. (1986): Embryogenesis of arborization pattern and topography of individual axons in n. laminaris of the chicken brain stem. *J. Comp. Neurol.*, 254:425–459.

123. Zakon, H. H. (1986): The emergence of tuning in newly generated tuberous electroreceptors. *J. Neurosci.*, 6:3297–3308.

Physiology of the Ear,
edited by A. F. Jahn and J. Santos-Sacchi.
Raven Press, New York © 1988.

Functional Morphology of the Vestibular System

Matti Anniko

Department of Oto-Rhino-Laryngology and Head and Neck Surgery, and Otologic Research Laboratories, Umeå University Hospital, S-901 85 Umeå, Sweden

ANATOMICAL OVERVIEW

The organs for maintenance of equilibrium are located in the vestibular part of the inner ear. The inner ear is divided into a pars superior (vestibular labyrinth), a pars inferior (cochlea), and an endolymphatic system. The membranous labyrinth of the inner ear consists of three membranous semicircular canals located within their corresponding bony canals; the utricle and saccule, with the bony vestibule; the ductus cochlearis (scala media) in the bony cochlea; and the endolymphatic duct and sac in the bony aqueduct of the vestibule. There are six neuroepithelial areas in each labyrinth: one in each macula, the macula utriculi and the macula sacculi; one in each ampulla, the crista ampullaris; and one in the cochlear duct, the organ of Corti. The last area is the only one concerned with the hearing; all the others have to do with the equilibrium.

The vestibular labyrinth is comprised of two statoconial organs, the utricle and the saccule, and three cristae ampullares located in an enlargement (ampulla) of the semicircular duct (Figs. 1 and 2). The maculae and cristae ampullares are special regions of the vestibular labyrinth that contain the receptor cells that mediate the sense of equilibrium. The two maculae are stimulated by linear acceleration and the effect of gravity, whereas the three cristae ampullares register angular acceleration (rotation) in the same plane as the semicircular duct that is irritated.

The membranous labyrinth is enclosed by a similarly shaped but wider osseous labyrinth, filled with endolymph, and connected to the osseous labyrinth through fine fibrous strands. The space between the membranous labyrinth and the osseous labyrinth is filled with perilymph (perilymphatic space) (Fig. 3).

The utricle is an elliptical sac lying in the upper posterior part of the vestibule from which the membranous semicircular canals originate. The semicircular ducts all comprise slightly more than half a circle. The three semicircular ducts open into the utricle through five apertures in its posterior wall. The anterior and posterior semicircular ducts merge into a common duct (crus commune) immediately before they open into the utricle. The anterior (superior) semicircular canal is orientated perpendicular to the long axis of the temporal bone. The posterior semicircular canal is orientated at a right angle into the axis of the anterior semicircular canal. In this way the two semicircular canals form an angle of approximately 45° with the median plane. The lateral semicircular canal is positioned in a plane perpendicular to the

457

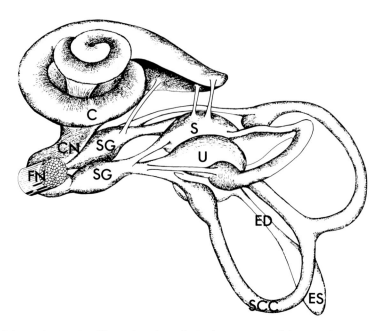

FIG. 1. Schematic drawing illustrating the principal structures of the membranous labyrinth. C, cochlea; CN, cochlear nerve; SG, Scarpa's ganglion; U, utricle; S, saccule; FN, facial nerve, ES, endolymphatic sac; ED, endolymphatic duct; SCC, semicircular canal.

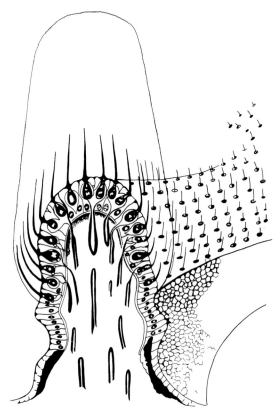

FIG. 2. Schematic drawing of the crista ampullaris in the guinea pig labyrinth illustrating the sensory cells and their relation to the innervating nerve fibers. The sensory hair bundles from the hair cells protude into channels of the cupula resting on the top of the crista surface. (From ref. 70.)

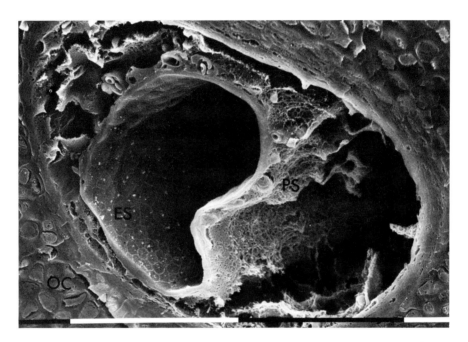

FIG. 3. Scanning electron micrograph of a cross section of a semicircular canal of 1-day-old CBA/CBA mouse. The epithelial lining of the endolymphatic space (ES) comprises flattened epithelial cells of the squamous cell type. The perilymphatic space (PS) contains fibrous strands from the membranous semicircular canal to the walls of the adjacent bony labyrinth. OC, otic capsule. Bar = 0.1 mm.

anterior and posterior semicircular canals forming an anteriorly open angle of approximately 30° with the horizontal plane.

The smaller spherical saccule is located anterior to the utricle. A short and narrow canal, the ductus reuniens, emanates from the lower part of the saccule and connects it with the membranous cochlea (i.e., the cochlear duct). The utricle and the saccule are connected by the utriculosaccular duct. The two organs are thus connected and continue backward through the vestibular aqueduct as the slender endolymphatic duct. This duct terminates in a blind enlargement, the endolymphatic sac, under the dura of the posterior surface of the temporal bone.

The epithelium in the two maculae and the three cristae ampullares is made up of hair cells, specialized receptor cells for the sense of equilibrium, and supporting cells. Two types of hair cells are distinguished, types I and II (Fig. 4). The two hair cell types differ primarily in their different patterns of innervation, whereas their cytological differences are few. The two types of sensory cells are common to the saccule, the utricle, and the three cristae ampullares.

THE HAIR CELL

Hair cells are mechanoreceptors in the sensory organs for hearing and equilibrium in vertebrates, and in the lateral-line organs of fish and in aquatic amphibians. The mechanosensitive cell of the acousticolateralis system is characterized by a bundle

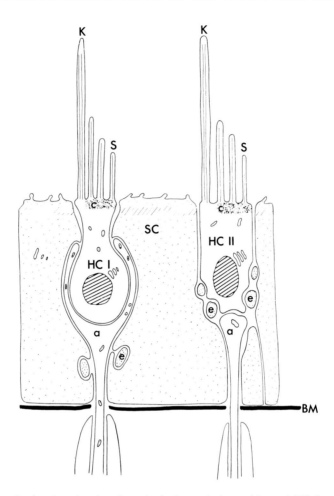

FIG. 4. Schematic drawing showing the principal morphology of types I (HC I) and II (HC II) hair cells. a, afferent nerve; e, efferent nerve; c, cuticle; K, kinocilium; S, stereocilium; BM, basal membrane; and SC, supporting cell.

of hairs at its apex. These hairs, one kinocilium and many stereocilia, are regularly arranged in rows that differ systematically in length (Fig. 4). Each vestibular hair cell possesses a morphological polarization determined by the relative position of the kinocilium and the stereocilia (70). The morphological polarization of the hair cell reflects also its functional polarization (49). The adult kinocilium is always located in the periphery of the sensory hair bundle. In the crista ampullaris of the horizontal ampulla, the kinocilium is found on the side of the bundle toward the utricle, whereas the kinocilium is located on the canal side of the crista in the two vertical semicircular canals. The location of the kinocilium thus coincides with the direction of excitation of the hair cell. Because of the curved form of the macula utriculi, it exhibits a more complicated pattern of hair cell orientation (Fig. 5A). Emanating from a point in the medial part of the macula, the striolar region, the kinocilia are pointing in gradually altering directions from anterior passing lateral to posterior covering approximately a semicircle (18). In a zone along the anterior,

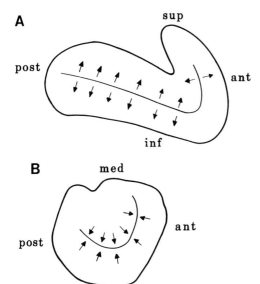

FIG. 5. Schematic drawings showing the morphological polarization of sensory hairs in the mammalian utricle (**A**) and saccule (**B**). The orientation of the sensory epithelia has a characteristic pattern determined by the location of the kinocilium of the hair bundle, indicated by arrows.

lateral, and posterior margins of the macula, the hair cells are oriented with their kinocilia pointing in opposite directions. In the macula of the saccule a similar pattern of hair cell polarization may be seen (Fig. 5B).

Type I Hair Cell

This sensory cell is flask shaped and its cell body is surrounded to slightly below its upper surface by a calyx formed from the terminal end of an afferent nerve fiber (Figs. 4 and 6). In general, only one afferent nerve ending encloses one hair cell. The upper surface of the hair cell contains between 40 and 100 stereocilia and 1 kinocilium. The stereocilia are continuous with the surface membrane and may be considered as enlarged, specialized microvilli. The stereocilia are arranged in a step-like, "organ pipe" fashion, with the longest stereocilium positioned adjacent to the kinocilium. The kinocilium is always longer than the longest stereocilia. Immediately below the hair cell surface, a cuticle is located that is composed of actin filaments. A large rounded nucleus is located in the central part of the bulbous area of the cell. The cytoplasm contains the usual organelles of vertebrate cells (mitochondria, endoplasmic reticulum, Golgi complexes). Efferent nerve endings regularly synapse with the afferent calyx, mostly at its base.

Type II Hair Cell

These cells are considered to be phylogenetically older than type I hair cells. Type II sensory cells have a cylindrical shape and can vary considerably in length (Fig. 4). The arrangement of stereocilia and the kinocilium is the same as on type I hair cells. However, both afferent and efferent nerve endings synapse with type II cells, generally in the lower one-third of the cell body.

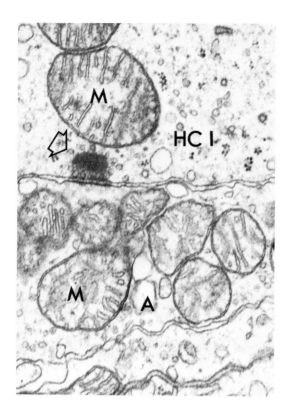

FIG. 6. Transmission electron micrograph showing an afferent synapse of a type I hair cell (HC I). The synaptic body is indicated with an arrow. A, afferent nerve calyx; M, mitochondrion. ×25,500.

Surface Morphology of the Hair Cells

In the adult vestibular epithelium, types I and II sensory cells are distinguished by the surface morphology of their stereocilia (35,41,42,47). Although there are differences in all vestibular organs between their central and peripheral zones in the height of the hair cell type I stereocilia, these are generally thicker and taller than the stereocilia of the neighboring type II hair cells. Individual stereocilia of type I cells resemble inverted baseball bats with thicker club-like tops and tapered, thinner shafts. During recent years, interconnections between stereocilia have been demonstrated (53). The micromechanics of sensory hairs have so far been analyzed mainly in cochlear sensory cells. Interconnections between sensory hairs are, however, present also in the vestibular hair cells. Stereocilia are coupled not only with each other but also to the kinocilium (22,26,34). During stimulation of a hair cell all sensory hairs thus become stimulated. In the cochlea of birds and mammals, the length of the stereocilia and the number of sensory hairs per cell are related to frequency selectivity (30,44,67,71). Also the tonotopic organization of the saccular maculae of reptiles, amphibians, and fish is reflected in hair bundle size (56). Considerably less is known about mammalian vestibular hair cells.

Cytoskeletal Organization of the Hair Cell

The skeletal framework of the mammalian cell is a very complex structure responsible for cell morphology and internal organization. The cytoskeleton is composed of the major filament systems (microfilaments, intermediate filaments, and microtubules) and many interconnecting structural elements. In hair cells, each stereocilium is comprised of extensively cross-linked bundles of actin filaments (19,20,67). At the point of contact between the stereocilium and the apical portion of the hair cell, there is a network of actin filaments in the cuticular plate. The central filaments in the stereocilia enter the cuticular plate as a rootlet. Using the quick-freeze, deep-etch technique, Hirokawa (29) showed that many actin filaments from each stereocilium enter the cuticular plate and are connected to the apical cell membrane by tiny branched connecting units. Actin filaments in the cuticular plate are also connected to each other by fine filaments, 3 nm in thickness and 74 ± 14 nm in length. These 3-nm filaments interconnect actin filaments not only of the same polarity but of also opposite polarity. In the cuticular region, adjacent actin filaments often show opposite polarities. At the apical lateral margins of the hair cell two populations of actin filaments occur, one just below the tight junction as a network and the other as a ring at the level of the intermediate junction. Because of the alternating polarities of actin filaments, this ring may be contractile. Mircotubules are also found in the apical part of the hair cell. Most microtubules run parallel to the long axis of the cell so that they insert with one end into the cuticular plate. The microtubules are cross-linked with actin filaments in the cuticular plate. Immunocytochemical analyses have shown that alpha-actinin and myosin are localized in the cuticular plate region (16) and fimbrin exists in the stereocilia (21). Since myosin is present in the apical part of the hair cell, the ring of actin could potentially be contractile. Hirokawa (29) suggested that the function of this ring in hair cells is to maintain the stiffness of the apical cell surface and squeeze the surface of the cell and push stereocilia upwards.

The functional organization of actin filaments in hair cells has recently been reviewed by Tilney et al. (67,68). Although motile responses owing to contractility of the hair cell cytoskeleton have been shown in outer hair cells of the cochlea (75), considerably less is known about the vestibular hair cells. Anniko and Thornell (7) showed in human vestibular organs that a particularly strong fluorescence for filamentous (F-) actin occurred at the apical surfaces of both the supporting cells and sensory cells in all vestibular organs but not outside the hair cell-containing regions (Fig. 7). The high amounts of F-actin in vestibular organs give them an extreme stiffness in relation to surrounding structures.

The distribution of intermediate filament proteins has recently been analyzed in human vestibular organs (66). Vestibular hair cells have a weak positivity for vimentin, whereas supporting cells in all vestibular organs show strong positivity, except the epithelial lining in the endolymphatic space outside the vestibular organs. Considerable variations occur in positivity for different subgroups of cytokeratins in the epithelial lining of the endolymphatic space. Differences in cytokeratin composition occur also in epithelia where morphological differences in cell configuration between adjacent cells are not distinguished. The characterization of intermediate filament proteins shows that the cells of the inner ear have an extremely high degree of complexity of their cytoskeleton.

Hair Cell Junctions

The presence of junctional complexes in the inner ear sensory epithelium has been documented in several animal species as well as in the human (2,37). Intercellular

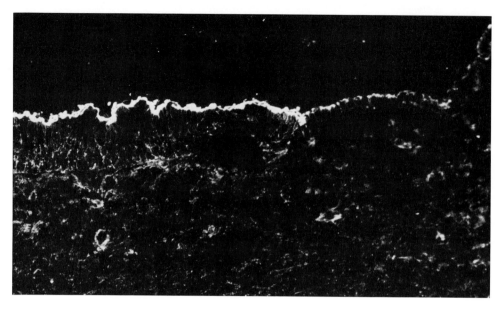

FIG. 7. The distribution of filamentous (F-) actin in the macula utriculi of the 14-week-old human fetus is shown with the immunofluorescence technique. A strong fluorescence is found at the apical surfaces of both sensory and supporting cells, whereas only a weak staining occurs in adjacent epithelia outside the macula. ×135.

junctions play an important role in the maintenance of the highly specific inner ear environment (endolymph) and hair cell function. The tight junction is located in the apical portion (closest to the lumen) of epithelial cells (Fig. 8). Below this, the zonulae adherentes and punctate maculae adherentes, or desmosomes, are present. The tight junction always lines the entire lumen surface of an epithelial cell and acts as a permeability barrier to fluids and ions. The zonulae adherentes and the desmosomes act as mechanical couplers between epithelial cells. The gap junction is found on the lateral surface of an epithelial cell below the level of the tight junction and acts as an electronic coupler allowing ions and/or electrical currents to pass from one cell to another (9).

During embryonic differentiation, an uncoupling occurs of the gap junctions of those epithelial cells that differentiate into innervated vestibular hair cells (8,23). The uncoupling ensures that the individual hair cell functions electrotonically independent of the adjacent hair cells and the adjacent supporting cells.

Function of the Hair Cell

The basic electrophysiological principle in the hair cell is the biphasic directional response of stereocilia to stimuli approaching from opposite directions. Displacement of sensory hairs toward the kinocilium is accompanied by a depolarization of the hair cell and an increased discharge rate in adjacent afferent nerve fibers, whereas displacement in the opposite direction is accompanied by a hyperpolarization and a decreased discharge frequency. The functional polarization in directional selec-

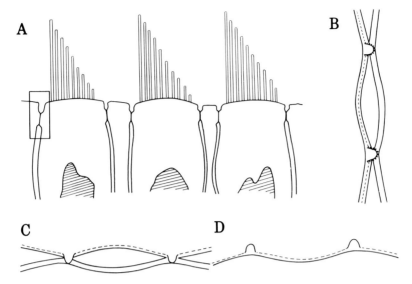

FIG. 8. Schematic representation of tight junctional complexes in apical portion of cells of vestibular sensory epithelia. **A**: Plasma membranes of adjacent sensory and supporting cells are closely apposed near their endolymphatic surfaces. **B**: Enlarged view of area bounded by rectangle in A. Trilaminar structure of plasma membrane of both supporting cell (**left**) and hair cell (**right**) is shown. Freeze-fracture plane (*dotted line*) passes through supporting cell membrane and reveals two surfaces shown in C and D. **C**: E-face or hexoplasmic monolayer facing cell's exterior shows series of troughs. **D**: P-face or protoplasmic monolayer adjacent to cell's interior shows series of ridges corresponding to troughs on E-face.

tivity of individual hair cells, originally described by Loewenstein and Wersäll (49) in the ray (raya clavata), has now been extended to a wide variety of species ranging from cyclostomes (50) to mammals (24,25). The principles for stereociliary function are applicable also to otolith (17,48) and lateral line organs (18). Most studies have so far been performed on cochlear hair cells, but the basic principles are similar in vestibular hair cells.

The mechanoelectrical transduction of the hair cell takes place at or near the distal end of stereocilia (33). A displacement of the stereocilia toward the kinocilium causes an increase in membrane conductance (and a decrease in the membrane potential). When the stereocilia are displaced in the opposite direction, the conductance is decreased (and the cells become hyperpolarized) (31,32). A change in the resistance caused by mechanical stimulation modulates a steady current flow across the hair cell membrane and is driven by the electrical potential differences across this membrane (14). The resulting changes of the membrane potentials are the receptor potentials that modulate the spontaneous release of neurochemical transmitters at the afferent synapse of the hair cell. However, the ionic selectivity of the transduction channels is nonspecific (12). Calcium seems essential to the transduction process in the lateral-line organ and may carry a major part of the receptor current across the transducer membrane of the hair cell (59). However, calcium may also control the ionic permeability of the transducer membrane.

Electron probe microanalysis offers a sophisticated and specialized approach for localizing calcium in different cell types (52,72). By use of the energy dispersive X-ray microanalysis technique, Anniko et al. (4) showed that elemental calcium could be detected both in the stereocilia and in the supranuclear cytoplasm of both types of vestibular hair cells. Flock et al. (21) demonstrated that the stereocilia are composed of actin filaments and that their rootlets contain tubulin. This finding suggests that the stiffness of the stereocilia can be regulated by the contractile protein by means of calcium. Anniko et al. (5) have previously been able to localize calcium in stereocilia and in the upper part of cytoplasm of both outer and inner hair cells in the cochlea. Thus, the results from microprobe analysis are in accordance with physiological and cytochemical evidence that calcium is involved in the mechano-transduction of sensory cells.

FUNCTIONAL ORGANIZATION OF THE SEMICIRCULAR CANALS

Head movements in the horizontal plane around the vertical axis produce angular accelerations resulting in displacement of endolymph in the membranous horizontal semicircular duct of the inner ear. The magnitude of the fluid displacement is greatest when the plane of the head movement coincides with the plane of the semicircular duct and decreases in a cosine function as the angle between these planes increases (13). The cupula, a highly specialized gelatinous extracellular substance overlying the crista ampullaris, has an elastic restoring force so that at the end of the angular acceleration it returns to its normal resting position. The sequences of the cupular bending and return have been described as a mechanical operation of the semicircular canal. For a given head movement of angular acceleration a number of anatomical and mechanical factors influence the extent to which the cupula will be bent and the time course of this bending: the radius of curvature of the entire semicircular duct, the radius of the duct, the viscosity and density of endolymph, and the stiffness of the cupula (54,55). The dynamic range of average human cupular motion is between 520 Å and 10 μm. In response to the head rotation, horizontal canal neurons increase their rate of firing during angular acceleration to the ipsilateral side and decrease during angular acceleration to the contralateral side. The afferent innervation exhibits a bidirectional response. The directions of excitatory and inhibitory accelerations are identical for all afferents innervating a single semicircular canal ampulla and consistent with Ewald's first law. Traditionally, the response dynamics of peripheral neurons were thought to mirror dynamics of the cupula–endolymph system. However, it has now been established that adaptation occurs in the response of both peripheral and central vestibular neurons.

Suzuki and co-workers (64) and Suzuki and Harada (65) analyzed the physiological significance of the mode of cupular movement. The swing-door deflection seems physiologically most effective in producing the optimum increase in response rate as well as maintaining the time course of the tonic response. Perception of rotatory movements can be elicited primarily by swing-door deflection, since these provoke both phasic and tonic responses that can eventually reflect both length and magnitude of angular velocity. The physiology of the maculae is only partially known, but they represent organs for linear acceleration and gravity. Their morphological polarization is also represented by a functional polarization.

THE VESTIBULAR GANGLION

The afferent neurons innervating the vestibular organs are bipolar cells with their neuronal cell bodies within the internal auditory canal. The vestibular ganglion (or

Scarpa's ganglion) consists of two parts corresponding to the superior vestibular nerve and the inferior vestibular nerve (74). In most vertebrate species, except humans, the cell bodies are enclosed by a myelin sheath. Until recently, only one type of vestibular ganglion cell was recognized using light microscopy or electron microscopy. Using immunomorphological techniques, however, Thornell et al. (66) showed that the human vestibular ganglions contain two distinct subpopulations of cell bodies: those staining for neurofilament proteins and those lacking this immunoreactivity. Similar observations on neurofilament staining were made by Anniko et al. (6) for vestibular ganglion cells in the newborn mouse. Furthermore, Spassova (63) claimed that in the cat two populations can be distinguished by routine morphology. Sans et al. (60) documented that vestibular ganglion cells in the cat express two types of immunocytochemical reaction for vitamin D-dependent calcium-binding proteins. Type II hair cells stained intensely for this protein, whereas the immunoreactivity of type I was very weak, if present at all. It is tempting to speculate that the different populations of vestibular ganglion cells could be correlated with the different populations of vestibular hair cells.

In the human, the intensely neurofilamentous immunoreactive ganglion cells were irregularly scattered within the vestibular ganglia (66) in contrast to the findings in the newborn mouse (6) where the subpopulations of neurofilament expressing ganglion cells were close together. Further analysis is necessary to determine if such an aggregation of vestibular ganglion cells represents a vestibulotopic organization in a similar way as the tonotopic organization in the cochlea along the basilar membrane. Further evidence for a subpopulation of the vestibular ganglion cells was documented by Ylikoski et al. (73) showing strong substance P-like reactivity in 30% to 40% of the cells in the vestibular ganglia and neural elements in the vestibular sensory epithelia, notably in the afferent nerve calyces of type I hair cells.

THE CUPULA

Above the epithelium of the crista ampullaris a mass of extracellular, highly specialized material (the cupula) is located, extending from the epithelial cell surface to the roof of the ampulla (Fig. 9). A fibrillar network occurs in the cupula. These filaments are between 30 Å and 100 Å in diameter (36,70). The chemical composition of the cupula is only partially known. Histochemical studies indicate the presence of acid mucopolysaccharides (15,38). X-ray diffraction of cupular material shows two bands between 4.57 Å and 4.81 Å and between 10 Å and 14 Å. Thus, the cupula consists to a large extent of protein, which is in accordance with the morphological features of extrusion of cytoplasmic material during cupular development. In spite of their superficial similarity, elemental analysis of the tectorial membrane and the cupula reveals considerable qualitative differences (1). Distinct elemental peaks have been identified for sodium, phosphorus, sulfur, chlorine, potassium, and calcium in the tectorial membrane, whereas only minor peaks for chlorine and potassium are obtained for the cupula. However, this technique does not allow analysis of elements with an atomic weight below that of sodium, which must influence the interpretation of the results obtained from a structure composed mainly of organic material.

The cupula forms a tight diaphragm across the ampulla, which is most easily displaced at the center. In light microscopy of the crista there is always a translucent

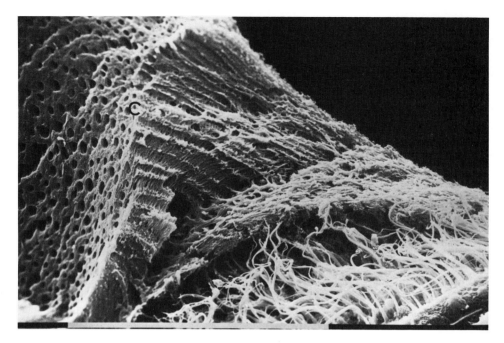

FIG. 9. Scanning electron micrograph showing the apical portion of the mouse crista ampullaris with overlying cupula (C). Sensory hairs protrude above the hair cell surfaces. Cupular canals are identified. Bar = 0.1 mm.

area of varying width between the surface of the hair cells and the cupula. The same finding is seen in otolithic membranes. This area has been named the subcupular space and constitutes a slit through which the hairs pass into the organized canal-like structures of the cupula (Fig. 9). The presence of the cupular canals have been observed in the human (40), guinea pig (70), bullfrog (27), mouse (46), and other species. In general, the canals are larger in the central part and smaller at the periphery of the cupula. The diameter of the individual canal is larger at the base and smaller toward the apex. The relationship between the cupula and the underlying sensory cilia bundles is of great interest for understanding the micromechanics involved in mechanosensory transduction. The tall ciliary bundles are inserted into cupular canals, in the guinea pig, human, and mouse, but short stereociliary bundles are in general free-standing.

Electrophysiological studies using single-unit nerve responses of vestibular sensory organs show the presence of regular (or static) and irregular (dynamic) units (13,17,24,25,51). Type I hair cells, located mainly in the central (striolar) zone and innervated mostly by thick fibers, are static receptors with a regular discharge pattern; type II hair cells, found mainly in the peripheral zone and innervated by small fibers, are dynamic receptors with an irregular discharge pattern. Goldberg and Fernández (25) suggested that regular units may be considered as static receptors, the response of which is related to the displacement of the cupula or otolithic membrane. Irregular units are considered as dynamic receptors, which show adaptation and are sensitive to both the degree of mechanical displacement (static) and the velocity of the displacement (dynamic). Variations in the response dynamics may reflect differences in the physiology of the two types of hair cells and the afferent terminals, in the modal coupling of the sensory hairs to the gelatinous membrane, or in both. In mammals, type I hair cell ciliary bundles are more loosely coupled to the overlying membrane than the type II hair cell bundles (43,46).

The physiology and motion patterns of the cupula have not been fully documented, and even the mechanisms of normal cupular motion still remain controversial. Dohlman (15) described swing-door movement of the entire cupula, but Hillman and McLaren (28) claimed that a movement occurs that is based on a diaphragmatic displacement of the midportion of the cupula. Suzuki and Harada (65) assumed that the cupula can be easily bent in the axis parallel to the crista but not in the vertical axis.

OTOCONIA

The initial event in vestibular hair cell transduction is the moving of the sensory cilia by displacement of overlying structures (cupula or otoconial/statoconial membrane). The statoconial layer (or membrane) is made up of a gelatinous layer, a subcupular meshwork, and otoconia. The utricular and saccular maculae have an overlying mineral layer or otoconial mass (Fig. 10), whereas the tectorial membrane of the organ of Corti and the cupula of the cristae ampullares are normally devoid of any mineral layer. Otoconia are not inert structures but are subject to changes during their life span (58,69). In humans, some of the otoconia grow throughout childhood and many otoconia disappear with advancing age. In mammals, otoconia consist of calcium carbonate in the form of calcite; in amphibia, in the form of aragonite; and in lamprey, in the form of calcium phosphate (10,11). In general, an

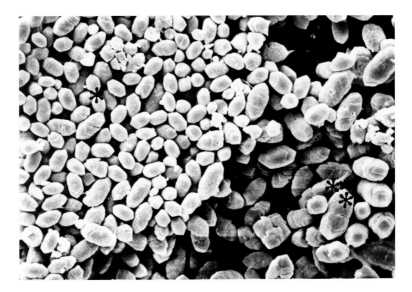

FIG. 10. Scanning electron micrograph of utricular otoconia from Shaker-2 mouse. Small otoconia (*) are located in the striolar region whereas larger otoconia are found immediately outside the striola (**). ×1,600.

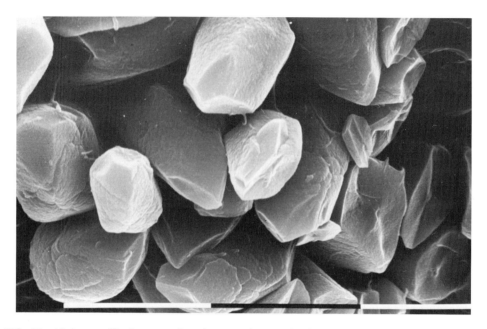

FIG. 11. High magnification scanning electron micrograph of utricular otoconia of the CBA/CBA mouse. The otoconia have rounded bodies with pointed tips that have three planar (rhombohedron) surfaces. Bar = 10 μm.

organic nucleus is found in otoconia. Some otoconia are partially embedded in the gelatinous layer, and the rest are held together by the gelatinous substance. The gelatinous layer and the subcupular meshwork are formed of acid mucopolysaccharides and glycoproteins. Considerable species differences occur in the shape, size, chemical composition, and mode of formation of otoconia.

The length of otoconia ranges from 0.1 μm to 25 μm in the guinea pig and as much as 30 μm in the human. In some species, such as the rat, the saccular otoconia are much larger than those in the utricle. Small otoconia are located mainly on the surface, the outer margin of the statoconial layer, and in the striolar zone (Fig. 10). Neither the mechanisms responsible for the peculiar anatomical distribution of otoconia of different sizes nor the corresponding functional significance are known. The majority of mammalian calcite otoconia have rounded bodies with pointed tips that have three planar (rhombohedron) surfaces (Fig. 11). The ultrastructure of mineralized (and partly mineralized) otoconia shows an internal organization of fine, spindle-shaped calcite crystals and fibrillar organic substance. The arrangement of calcite crystals closely mimics the fibrillar arrangement of the organic substance. In the central core (the nucleus), the spindles, when present, are arranged almost parallel with the long axis of the otoconium or they appear amorphous (45).

There are distinct differences in the composition of the organic material (and calcite) in different locations (such as the nucleus, terminal faces and body) within the otoconia. Mature otoconia have a very limited calcium turnover that occurs at their outer surfaces (57,58). In the gerbil, the incorporation of calcium represented a fraction rate of 0.1% with a half-life of approximately 11 days.

In humans, otoconia change their elemental content with aging before morphological changes are observed, indicating a phosphatization of aging otoconia with transformation from calcite into apatite through reaction with phosphate ions (3).

THE EPITHELIAL LINING OF NONSENSORY AREAS OF THE MEMBRANOUS LABYRINTH

The wall of the membranous labyrinth is composed of an epithelial layer and a connective tissue layer. The epithelium in nonsensory areas is single layered. In most areas of the labyrinth, including the semicircular canals, some areas of the utricle, the roof of the ampulla, and the saccule, the epithelium is undifferentiated and of the squamous cell type. In other areas, the epithelium is differentiated into a secretory epithelium with several types of cells (dark cells and light cells).

The dark cells are found on either side of the vestibular organs. In principle, the localization of the dark-cell epithelium is rather similar among a number of mammalian species including the human. Although a particular species-dependent variation in the pattern of the distribution occurs, the dark cells are found in the walls of all ampullae. Dark cells participate in the fluid homeostasis for preservation of the unique high-potassium and low-sodium content of endolymph. On the utricular side of the crista ampullaris, the dark-cell epithelium forms a continuous layer around the opening to the utricle from the roof of the ampulla to its floor. The entire posterior endolymphatic wall of the utricle is lined with dark cells. On the anterior wall of the utricle, dark cells are not found in the immediate periphery of the macula, but this area is lined with well-defined cuboidal cells. Dark-cell epithelium also occurs on the lateral wall of the common crus. Dark cells are not found in the wall of the saccule. The dark-cell epithelium consists of cells with multiple pinocytotic vesicles close to their luminal surface, suggesting fluid passage through the cells. A large number of infoldings occurs at the basal end of the dark cell toward the basal membrane. These infoldings contain numerous mitochondria. The nucleus of the dark cell is displaced toward the surface, which is covered with microvilli of varying lengths (39,62). The dark cells are structurally similar to ion-transporting epithelia in renal tubules, ciliary plexus, choroid plexus, and the like. The dark cells with basal infoldings represent a transport mechanism from tissue fluid to endolymph, whereas the transport in or between the cells with lateral infoldings should be from the endolymph to the tissue fluid (62).

The planum semilunatum consists of columnar cells in the area between the sensory cell region and that of the dark-cell epithelium. The functional significance of cells in the planum semilunatum has still to be analyzed.

The supporting cells between the sensory cells in the vestibular organs are in general columnar, but their structure varies from species to species. Small microvilli are found on the surface of supporting cells. In higher animals and birds, a membrana reticularis is found at the upper surface of the supporting cell. The membrana reticularis represents a ring of dense substance close to the cell membrane. The distance between two supporting cells is rather constant whereas the distance between supporting cells and hair cells can vary widely, being approximately 80 Å to 175 Å (61).

Recent immunomorphological investigations (66) have shown that a considerable similarity in cytoskeletal composition occurs between all secretory/reabsorptive epithelia in the inner ear. The intermediate filament protein composition, as analyzed with monoclonal antibodies against a number of cytokeratins, showed a similar positivity in the stria vascularis, the dark-cell epithelium around vestibular organs, and in cells lining the endolymphatic duct and sac.

CONCLUDING REMARKS

The peripheral vestibular organs have a very complex pattern for registration of orientation in space. The hair cell is the receptor cell of the auditory, vestibular, and related sensory systems. The hair cell renders sensory inputs into electrical signals and performs this task by use of a variety of mechanical, hydrodynamic, and electrical strategies to measure stimulation with extreme sensitivity. A mechanical tuning (frequency selectivity) occurs at the hair cell level, suggesting that variations in hair bundle morphology are of functional significance. The different physiological functions of stereocilia and kinocilia may be associated with different properties of their cytoskeletal components, the cell membrane, and the structures linking the actin core of stereocilia and cuticular plate and the hair cell membrane. The specialized hair cell surface, as represented by stereocilia and kinocilia, makes contact with auxiliary structures (cupula or otolithic membrane). Both the hair cells and overlying structures are needed for the finely graded mechanisms of mechanoelectric transduction. The rapid expansion of immunomorphological knowledge, using monoclonal antibodies against well-defined cytoskeletal proteins at both the light microscopic and electron microscopic levels, makes it possible to further analyze the extremely high complexity of the inner ear and also make new correlations between structure and function.

ACKNOWLEDGMENTS

This work was supported by grants from the Swedish Medical Research Council (12X-7305), the Ragnar Söderberg and Torsten Söderberg Foundation, the Foundation Tysta Skolan, and the University of Umeå. The skilled technical assistance of Andrea Lotz, Ann-Louise Grehn, and Monika Andersson is gratefully acknowledged.

REFERENCES

1. Anniko, M., and Wróblewski, R. (1980): Elemental composition of the mature inner ear. *Acta Otolaryngol. (Stockh.)*, 90:25–32.
2. Anniko, M., and Wróblewski, R. (1984): The freeze fracture technique in inner ear research. *Scan. Electron Microsc.*, IV:2067–2075.
3. Anniko, M., Ylikoski, J., and Wróblewski, R. (1984): Microprobe analysis of human otoconia. *Acta Otolaryngol. (Stockh.)*, 97:283–289.
4. Anniko, M., Lim, D., and Wróblewski, R. (1985): Energy dispersive X-ray microanalysis of individual vestibular hair cells. *Arch. Otorhinolaryngol.*, 242:161–166.
5. Anniko, M., Lim, D., and Wróblewski, R. (1985): Elemental composition of individual cells and tissues in the cochlea. *Acta Otolaryngol. (Stockh.)*, 98:439–453.
6. Anniko, M., Thornell, L.-E., Gustafsson, H., and Virtanen, I. (1986): Intermediate filaments in the newborn inner ear of the mouse. *Adv. Otorhinolaryngol.*, 48:98–106.

7. Anniko, M., and Thornell, L.-E. (1987): Cytoskeletal organization of the human inner ear. IV. Expression of actin in vestibular organs. *Acta Otolaryngol. [Suppl.] (Stockh.)*, 437:65–76.
8. Bagger-Sjöbäck, D., and Anniko, M. (1984): Development of intercellular junctions in the vestibular end organ. A freeze fracture study in the mouse. *Ann. Otol. Rhinol. Laryngol.*, 93:89–95.
9. Bennett, M. V. L., Makajima, Y., and Pappas, C. D. (1967): Physiology and ultrastructure of electronic junctions. I. Supramedullary neurons. *J. Neurophysiol.*, 30:161–179.
10. Carlström, D., and Engström, H. (1955): The ultrastructure of statoconia. *Acta Otolaryngol. (Stockh.)*, 45:14–18.
11. Carlström, D. (1963): A crystallographic study of vertebrate otoliths. *Biol. Bull.*, 125:441–463.
12. Corey, D. P., and Hudspeth, A. J. (1979): Ionic basis of the receptor potential in a vertebrate hair cell. *Nature*, 281:675–677.
13. Curthoys, I. S. (1983): The development of function of primary vestibular neurons. In: *Development of Auditory and Vestibular Systems*, edited by R. Romand, pp. 425–461. Academic Press, New York.
14. Davies, H. (1965): A model for transducer action in the cochlea. *Cold Spring Harbor Symp. Quant. Biol.*, 30:181–190.
15. Dohlman, G. F. (1971): The attachment of the cupulae, otolith and tectorial membranes to the sensory cell areas. *Acta Otolaryngol. (Stockh.)*, 71:89–105.
16. Drenckhahn, D., Kellner, J., Mannherz, H. G., Groschel-Stewart, U., Kendrick-Jones, J., and Scholey, J. (1982): Absence of myosin-like immunoreactivity in stereocilia of cochlear hair cells. *Nature*, 300:531–532.
17. Fernández, C., Goldberg, J. M., and Abend, W. K. (1972): Response to static tilts of peripheral neurons innervating otolith organs of the squirrel monkey. *J. Neurophysiol.*, 35:978–997.
18. Flock, Å. (1965): Electron microscopic and electrophysiological studies on the lateral line canal organ. *Acta Otolaryngol., [Suppl.] (Stockh.)*, 199:1–90.
19. Flock, Å, and Cheung, H. (1977): Actin filaments in sensory hairs of the inner ear receptor cells. *J. Cell Biol.*, 75:339–343.
20. Flock, Å, Cheung, H., and Utter, G. (1981): Three sets of actin filaments in sensory cells of the inner ear. Identification and functional orientation determined by gel electrophoresis, immunofluorescence and electron miscroscopy. *J. Neurocytol.*, 10:133–147.
21. Flock, Å, Bretscher, A., and Weber, K. (1982): Immunohistochemical localization of several cytoskeletal proteins in inner ear sensory and supporting cells. *Hear. Res.*, 6:75–89.
22. Flock, Å., and Strelioff, D. (1984): Studies on hair cells in isolated coils from guinea pig cochlea. *Hear. Res.*, 15:11–18.
23. Ginsberg, R. D., and Gilula, N. B. (1979): Modulation of cell junctions during differentiation of the chicken otocyst sensory epithelium. *Dev. Biol.*, 68:110–129.
24. Goldberg, J. M., and Fernández, C. (1971): Physiology of peripheral neurons innervating semicircular canals of the squirrel monkey. I. Resting discharge and response to constant angular accelerations. *J. Neurophysiol.*, 34:635–660.
25. Goldberg, J. M., and Fernández, C. (1975): Vestibular mechanisms. *Annu. Rev. Physiol.*, 37:129–162.
26. Hillman, D. E. (1969): New ultrastructural findings regarding a vestibular ciliary apparatus and its possible functional significance. *Brain. Res.*, 13:407–412.
27. Hillman, D. E. (1974): Cupular structure and its receptor relationship. *Brain Behav. Evol.*, 10:52–68.
28. Hillman, D. E., and McLaren, J. W. (1979): Displacement configuration of semicircular canal cupulae. *Neuroscience*, 4:1989–2000.
29. Hirokawa, N. (1986): Cytoskeletal architecture of the chicken hair cells revealed with the quick-freeze, deep-etch technique. *Hear. Res.*, 22:41–54.
30. Holton, T., and Hudspeth, A. J. (1983): A micromechanical contribution to cochlear tuning and tonotopic organization. *Science*, 222:508–510.
31. Hudspeth, A. J., and Corey, D. P. (1977): Sensitivity, polarity, and conductance change in the response of vertebrate hair cells to controlled mechanical stimuli. *Proc. Natl. Acad. Sci. USA*, 76:2407–2411.
32. Hudspeth, A. J., and Jacobs, R. (1979): Stereocilia mediate transduction in vertebrate hair cells. *Proc. Natl. Acad. Sci. USA*, 76:1506–1509.
33. Hudspeth, A. J. (1982): Extracellular current flow and the site of transduction by vertebrate hair cells. *J. Neurosci.*, 2:1–10.
34. Hudspeth, A. J. (1983): Mechanoelectrical transduction by hair cells in the acousticolateralis sensory system. *Annu. Rev. Neurosci.*, 6:187–215.
35. Hunter-Duvar, J. M., and Hinojosa, R. (1984): Vestibule: Sensory epithelia. In: *Ultrastructural Atlas of the Inner Ear*, edited by J. Friedmann and J. Ballantyne, pp. 211–244. Butterworths, London.
36. Iurato, S., and De Petris, S. (1967): Otolithic membranes and cupulae. In: *Submicroscopic Structure of the Inner Ear*, edited by S. Iurato, pp. 216–218. Pergamon, New York.

37. Jahnke, K. (1975): The fine structure of freeze-fractured intercellular junctions in the guinea pig inner ear. *Acta Otolaryngol. [Suppl.] (Stockh.),* 336:1–40.
38. Jensen, C. E., and Vilstrup, P. (1960): On the chemistry of human cupulae. *Acta Otolaryngol. (Stockh.),* 52:383.
39. Kimura, R., Lundquist, P.-G., and Wersäll, J. (1963): Secretory epithelial linings in the ampullae of the guinea pig labyrinth. *Acta Otolaryngol. (Stockh.),* 57:517–530.
40. Kolmer, W. (1926): Ueber das Verhalten der Dachmembranen zum Sinnesepithel. *Arch. Ohrenheilk,* 116:10–26.
41. Lim, D. J. (1976): Morphological and physiological correlates in cochlear and vestibular sensory epithelia. *Scan. Electron Microsc.,* V:269–276.
42. Lim, D. J. (1977): Fine morphology of the tectorial membrane: Fresh and developmental. *INSERM Symp.,* 68:47–60.
43. Lim, D. J. (1977): Ultra anatomy of sensory end-organs in the labyrinth and their functional implications. In: *Proceedings of the Shambaugh 5th International Workshop on Middle Ear Microsurgery and Fluctuant Hearing Loss,* edited by G. E. Shambaugh, Jr. and J. J. Shea, pp. 16–27. Strode Publishers, Huntsville, AL.
44. Lim, D. J. (1980): Cochlear anatomy related to cochlear micromechanics. A review. *J. Acoust. Soc. Am.,* 67:1686–1695.
45. Lim, D. J. (1984): The development and structure of the otoconia. In: *Ultrastructural Atlas of the Inner Ear,* edited by I. Friedmann and J. Ballantyne, pp. 245–267. Butterworths, London.
46. Lim, D. J., and Anniko, M. (1985): Developmental morphology of the mouse inner ear. A scanning electron microscopic observation. *Acta Otolaryngol. [Suppl.] (Stockh.),* 422:1–69.
47. Lindeman, H. H., Ades, H., and West, R. W. (1973): Scanning electron microscopy of the vestibular end organs. In: *Proceedings 5th Symposium on the Vestibular Organs in Space Exploration,* pp. 145–156. NASA, Washington, DC.
48. Loe, P. K., Tomko, D. L., and Nerner, G. (1973): The neural signal of angular head position in primary afferent vestibular nerve axons. *J. Physiol. (Lond.),* 230:29–30.
49. Loewenstein, O., and Wersäll, J. (1959): A functional interpretation of the electron microscopic structure of the sensory hairs in the cristae of elasmobranch Raja clavata in terms of directional sensitivity. *Nature,* 184:1807–1808.
50. Loewenstein, O. (1970): The electrophysiological study of the responses of the isolated labyrinth of the lamprey (Lampetra fluviatilis) to angular acceleration, tilting and mechanical vibration. *Proc. R. Soc. Lond. [Biol.],* 174:419–434.
51. Loewenstein, O. E. (1974): Comparative morphology and physiology. In: *Handbook of Sensory Physiology, Vol. VI/1. Vestibular System, Part 1: Basic Mechanisms,* edited by H. H. Kornhuber, pp. 75–120. Springer-Verlag, Berlin.
52. McGraw, C. F., Somlyo, A. V., and Blaustein, M. P. (1980): Probing for calcium at presynaptic nerve terminals. *Fed. Proc.,* 39:2796–2799.
53. Neugebauer, D.-Ch., and Thurm, U. (1985): Interconnections between the stereovilli of the fish inner ear. *Cell Tissue Res.,* 240:449–453.
54. Oman, C. M. (1981): The influence of duct and utricular morphology on semicircular canal response. In: *Vestibular Function and Morphology,* edited by E. Gualitieroth, pp. 251–274. Springer-Verlag, New York.
55. Oman, C. M., Marcus, E. N., and Curthoys, I. S. (1987): The influence of semicircular canal morphology on endolymph flow dynamics. *Acta Otolaryngol. (Stockh.),* 103:1–13.
56. Platt, C., and Popper, A. N. (1984): Variation in lengths of ciliary bundles on hair cells along the macula of the sacculus in two species of teleost fishes. *Scan. Electron Microsc.,* IV:1915–1924.
57. Preston, R. L., Johnsson, L.-G., Hill, H. J., and Schacht, J. (1975): Incorporation of radioactive calcium into otolithic membranes and middle ear ossicles of the gerbil. *Acta Otolaryngol. (Stockh.),* 80:269–273.
58. Ross, M. D. (1979): Calcium ion uptake and exchange in otoconia. *Adv. Otorhinolaryngol.,* 25:26–33.
59. Sand, O. (1975): Effects of ionic environments on the mechanosensitivity of lateral line organs in the mudpuppy. *J. Comp. Physiol.,* 102:27–42.
60. Sans, A., Etchecopar, B., Brehier, A., and Thomasset, M. (1986): Immunocytochemical detection of vitamin D dependent calcium binding protein (CaBP-28K) in vestibular sensory hair cells and vestibular ganglion neurones of the cat. *Brain Res.,* 364:190–194.
61. Smith, C. A. (1967): Utricle and saccule. In: *Submicroscopic Structure of the Inner Ear,* edited by S. Iurato, pp. 175–195. Pergamon Press, Oxford, London.
62. Smith, C. A. (1970): The extra-sensory cells of the vestibule. In: *Biochemical Mechanisms in Hearing and Deafness,* edited by M. M. Paparella, pp. 171–185. Charles C. Thomas, Springfield, IL.
63. Spassova, I. (1982): Fine structure of the neurones and synapsis of the vestibular ganglion of the cat. *J. Hirnforsch.,* 23:652–669.
64. Suzuki, M., Harada, Y., and Sugatan, Y. (1984): An experimental study on a function of the cupula.

Effect of cupula removal on the ampullary nerve action potential. *Arch. Otorhinolaryngol.*, 241:75–81.

65. Suzuki, M., and Harada, Y. (1985): An experimental study on the physiological significance of the mode of cupular movement. *Arch. Otorhinolaryngol.*, 242:57–62.

66. Thornell, L.-E., Anniko, M., and Virtanen, I. (1987): Cytoskeletal organization of the human inner ear. I. Expression of intermediate filaments in vestibular organs. *Acta Otolaryngol.* [*Suppl.*] (*Stockh.*), 437:5–28.

67. Tilney, L. G., and Saunders, J. C. (1983): Actin filaments, stereocilia and hair cells of the bird cochlea. I. Length, number, width, and distribution of stereocilia of each hair cell are related to the position of hair cell on the cochlea. *J. Cell Biol.*, 96:807–821.

68. Tilney, L. G., Egelman, E. H., De Rosier, D. J., and Saunders, J. C. (1983): Actin filaments, stereocilia and hair cells of the bird cochlea. II. Packing of actin filaments in the stereocilia and in the cuticular plate and what happens to the organization when the stereocilia are bent. *J. Cell Biol.*, 96:822–834.

69. Veenhof, V. B. (1969): *The Development of Statoconia in Mice.* North-Holland, Amsterdam.

70. Wersäll, J. (1956): Studies on the structure and innervation of the sensory epithelium of the cristae ampullares in the guinea pig. *Acta Otolaryngol.* [*Suppl.*] (*Stockh.*), 126:1–85.

71. Wright, A. (1984): Dimensions of the cochlear stereocilia in man and the guinea pig. *Hear. Res.*, 13:89–98.

72. Wróblewski, R., Anniko, M., and Sakai, T. (1984): A unique striated muscle: Further morphological and X-ray microanalytical investigations of the stapedius muscle in the guinea pig by using thin and thick cryosections. *J. Submicrosc. Cytol.*, 16:479–485.

73. Ylikoski, J., Eränkö, L., and Päiviranta, H. (1984): Substance P-like immunoreactivity in the rabbit inner ear. *J. Laryngol. Otol.*, 98:759–765.

74. Ylikoski, J., and Galey, F. R. (1984): The vestibular ganglion. In: *Ultrastructural Atlas of the Inner Ear*, edited by I. Friedmann and J. Ballantyne, pp. 290–305. Butterworths, London.

75. Zenner, H. P. (1986): Motile responses in outer hair cells. *Hear. Res.*, 22:83–90.

Physiology of the Ear,
edited by A. F. Jahn and J. Santos-Sacchi.
Raven Press, New York © 1988.

Injury and Repair in the Eighth Cranial Nerve

D. Marbey

Laboratory of Otolaryngology, New Jersey Medical School, University of Medicine and Dentistry of New Jersey, Newark, New Jersey 07103-2757

The structure and topography of the eighth cranial nerve are responsible for its susceptibility to injury (22,23). It has a long central glial segment and a short peripheral segment (22); the latter is too short to accommodate any elongation without tearing. Middle cranial fossa fractures (23) may disrupt the cochlear nerve in its course from the internal auditory meatus to the cochlear nuclei in the brainstem. Even blunt head trauma that does not result in skull fracture can harm the auditory nerve (22,23). Damage to the eighth nerve as a complication of bacterial meningitis or encephalitis (64) may be attributed to the absence of perineurium in the cochlear bony foramina and the glial dome structure. Because the eighth nerve is enclosed within bony structures for a significant part of its course, even relatively small space-occupying lesions can have extremely damaging effects.

Cochlear implants may be used to replace the function of the damaged organ of Corti (27) and generate electrical activity in the acoustic nerve in the damaged auditory system. However, restoration of hearing based on direct electrical stimulation of the eighth nerve has limited use (27,79,84,85); an unknown but minimal amount of intact auditory fibers is needed.

The response of neural injury has been studied in mammals, submammalian vertebrates, and invertebrates. Recovery of audition following eighth nerve injury depends on recovery or regeneration of the damaged structure. Whereas eighth nerve regeneration following injury has been observed in certain lower forms of life (e.g., the turtle and frog), regeneration of the adult mammalian cochlear nerve (69,71,73) has not been observed, indicating that in mammals the return of audition after neural injury is limited to injuries that leave the nerve relatively intact. This chapter examines mechanisms of nerve injury, repair, and regeneration both in general and in specific relation to the auditory nerve.

REVIEW OF THE CONSEQUENCES OF NERVE INJURY IN MAMMALS

Axotomy produces characteristic responses in neuronal soma and in the nerve fiber proximal and distal to the lesion (3,17,34,36). The proximal axon segment shows degeneration in the myelin sheath and microtubules. Wallerian degeneration in the distal fragment begins with the disruption of microtubules and microfilaments. The myelin sheath becomes segmented and disintegrates.

Response of neuronal cell bodies to axotomy is important in axonal repair. Axons depend on their somata for growth and maintenance. Somatal chromatolytic reaction

(24,37,55,83) to nerve transection results in the production of components (axoplasm, microtubules, neurofibrils, etc.) necessary for the reformation of an axonal fiber. These components are produced in the parental soma and transported via axonal transport to the axonal tip (38,45). The tip enlarges to form a growth cone, a cytoplasmic mobile structure (14,86) that subsequently elongates as a regenerating axon. Axonal regeneration (34) is the replacement of damaged cytoplasmic processes by parental somata. Complete regeneration (45) requires that axon fibers regrow from the point of injury and reform their original patterns.

Some mammalian peripheral nerves are able to regenerate successfully after transection. Degenerating axons and myelin of distal portions of transected nerves are removed by Schwann cells. Replacement fibers (nerves) grow for centimeters and penetrate the distal nerve stump of Schwann cell remnants and their basal laminae (1,2,34,45,65). Schwann cells multiply within basal laminae to form longitudinal columns (15,29,78). Regenerating nerve fibers grow through spaces between the basal laminae and the plasma membranes of Schwann cells (15,29). Basal laminae "scaffolds" (29) provide an effective route for regeneration of axons to appropriate synaptic sites.

Successful regeneration in the adult mammalian central nervous system (CNS) is limited (3,34,36,58). After transecting adult CNS axons, degenerating myelin and axonal remnants are cleared at a slower rate than after peripheral axotomy (1,2). In the CNS, wallerian degeneration involves astrocytes and microglia (1,2,68). Oligodendrocytes, the myelinating cells of the CNS, do not form well-aligned columns as do Schwann cells in the peripheral nervous system. Instead, an intertwining dense network of collagen (6) and glial processes (1,2,88) is found at the site of injury. The dense astroglial scar may act as a physical barrier to regenerating axons in the mammalian CNS and contribute to the failure of effective regeneration (6,16,17,56,90). Even when axonal branches from proximal segments elongate they fail to regenerate to their targets (1,2,59).

Minimizing glial scar formation caused by injury to central nervous tissue has been attempted (6,34); experimental laboratory mammals have been treated with piromen (6,34), triiodothyronine (6,34), L-thyroxine (6,34), and the enzymes hyaluronidase, trypsin, and elastase (6,34). Conflicting observations of the effects of those substances on regeneration provide little evidence for successful reduction of glial scar formation.

THE MAMMALIAN EIGHTH NERVE

The mammalian auditory nerve is of CNS origin for most of its extent (13,22,57,64). The glial dome, the transition point between central and peripheral portions of a nerve (7,75), is located at the base of the modiolus (22,64) in the rat. Lesions within the internal auditory meatus and along the course of the acoustic nerve to the cochlear nuclei in the brainstem disrupt CNS tissue. Regeneration within the adult mammalian CNS has not been observed.

Experimentally transected auditory nerves of adult mammals do not regenerate successfully (66,67,69,70,82). Studies have shown that intentionally disrupted central or peripheral processes of bipolar ganglion neurons result in anterograde or wallerian degeneration (69,70,74); distal segments separated from neuronal soma disintegrate.

Somata of spiral ganglia are similarly affected and appear swollen after damage to their neural processes (73,74). The swollen adult mammalian spiral ganglion neurons are not able to regenerate eighth nerve processes. Although many spiral ganglion neurons in the cat (73,74) form reactive peripheral sprouts to the basal aspect of inner hair cells after axotomy, 90% to 95% of these cells and their processes degenerate. The remaining 5% to 10% of spiral ganglion cells have processes that innervate mostly outer hair cells and few inner hair cells (69,70,72–74); numerous unmyelinated fibers with unknown targets (74) or "giant" fibers (73,74) innervate inner hair cells in long-term surviving animals. Efferent auditory nerves (74) may start regenerating in long-term survivors but not reach their targets.

Exposure of experimental laboratory mammals to ototoxic drugs and acoustic trauma leads to hair cell and neuronal degeneration. It is unclear whether neural degeneration is secondary to hair cell damage (32,35,42,43,71) or if spiral ganglion neurons are directly involved (33,43,81). Studies have shown that perikarya of spiral ganglia form reactive sprouts following acoustic trauma (89) or administration of ototoxic drugs (31,43,76,77,81). Reactive collateral sprouts eventually die and neuronal degeneration ensues.

EIGHTH NERVE TRANSECTION IN SUBMAMMALIAN VERTEBRATES

Adult CNS tissue of some submammalian vertebrates (fish, amphibians, reptiles) reacts differently to injury than that of mammals. Neural structures of central origin regenerate successfully (16,17,34,58). The phenomenon of eighth nerve regeneration has been observed in several species.

In one group of studies (92–95), eighth cranial nerve fibers were transected in the frog, an anamniote. Results showed that auditory fibers regenerate into the ipsilateral primary brainstem auditory nuclei 35 to 42 days post-transection and there form functional connections (92–95).

It is not surprising to find regeneration within the frog auditory nervous system. Studies have shown that amphibian astrocytes (11,61,62,90) do not block optic nerve outgrowth following optic nerve injury. Neurites are able to elongate through neuroglial scars at transection sites; gliosis is thought to enhance fiber elongation (11,62,90). The phenomenon has been compared with vertebrate peripheral nerve regeneration. Astrocytes in transected amphibian optic nerve (11,61,62,90) are thought to extend glial cytoplasmic processes; these processes surround, organize, and guide growing optic nerve fibers. Perhaps regenerating eighth nerve fibers are led to postsynaptic sites, the cochlear nuclei, in a similar manner.

Although the regenerative properties of nervous system tissue in anamniotes are well established, regenerative phenomena of various nervous tissues in the amniotic reptile are largely uninvestigated. Amniotes evolved 120 million years after anamniotes (63) and conceivably may react differently to neural injury than earlier evolved species. In response to axotomy, auditory nerve fibers and ganglion cells of the amniote, the red-eared turtle, show pathological changes similar to those in the mammal (50–53,69,70,73,74). In contrast to the mammal, however, turtle auditory ganglion cells can regenerate axons into the appropriate area of the cochlear nucleus 45 to 50 days following transection (Figs. 1 and 2). To date, the turtle is the only amniote in which eighth nerve afferent regeneration has been reproducibly demonstrated.

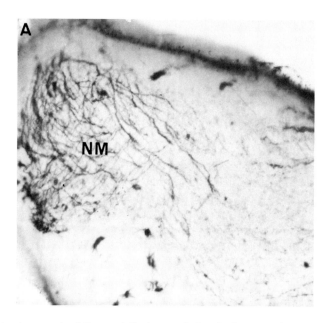

FIG. 1. A photomicrograph of the medulla (coronal plane) of a control (unoperated) turtle; the eighth nerve has not been sectioned. Horseradish peroxidase (HRP) reaction product is present in the nucleus magnocellularis following an injection of HRP into the ipsilateral cochlear duct. Horseradish peroxidase is also transported anterogradely to the nucleus angularis (not shown) after a cochlear duct injection of HRP. Dorsal is toward the top, medial is to the left. Neutral red, ×150.

With regard to the turtle eighth cranial nerve, the interaction between elongating axons and their microenvironment at the site of injury is important (3,34,45,90); the location of the injury will dictate the ensuing events. That is, if the turtle eighth cranial nerve were axotomized in its CNS extent, regenerating axons would have extended through a microenvironment of astrocytes as occurs with amphibia (11,61,62). However, if the nerve were sectioned in its peripheral nervous system domain, regenerating fibers would have been led initially by Schwann cells and their

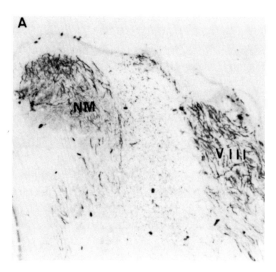

FIG. 2. A photomicrograph of the nucleus magnocellularis (coronal plane) of a turtle surviving 67 days after transection of the eighth nerve. Following an injection of HRP into the cochlear duct, eighth nerve fibers are filled with reaction product through the nucleus. HRP is also transported anterogradely to the nucleus angularis (not shown) after cochlear duct injection of HRP. Dorsal is toward the top, medial is to the left. Neutral red, ×75.

basal laminae, as in other systems (1,2,15,29,45), to the glial dome. Once there, regenerating axons would have projected through the transition zone to enter the CNS.

Using immunocytochemically labeled astrocytes as markers for the CNS, the location of the turtle eighth nerve transection site in those previous studies (50–53) was determined to be peripheral (54). Since the nerve was axotomized peripherally, regenerating eighth nerve axons of the turtle were presumably guided initially by Schwann cells and their basal laminae to the glial dome. Once regenerating axons projected through the glial dome, axons continued to extend to the cochlear nuclei in a microenvironment of astrocytes. If turtle astrocytes are similar to those of amphibia, regenerating eighth nerve axons may have been guided to their postsynaptic sites as previously described (11,61,62,90).

The examination of regenerative phenomena of the eighth cranial nerve in earlier evolved species provides insight into problems associated with mammalian auditory nerve regeneration. Mammalian spiral ganglion cells may not be able to regenerate eighth nerve fibers; if any auditory axons are formed, they may be blocked by astroglial scarring and unable to reach CNS cochlear nuclei.

EXPERIMENTAL ATTEMPTS TO ENHANCE NERVE REGENERATION

Methods to circumvent proposed obstacles of mammalian CNS regeneration are being explored. Transplants of embryonic and immature nervous system tissue have been used to induce neural growth (9,10,39–41). Fetal and early postnatal brain tissue from specific brain regions of rodents (10,21) have been transplanted into the same area of adult hosts. Cells of the graft complete their development within the host (10,21). In fact, fibers from transplants project to and form connections in the adult host similar to those of normal animals.

Transplanting adult nervous system tissue (1,2,5,18) has also been used to reconstitute damaged mammalian CNS tissue. Adult mammalian peripheral nerves have been transplanted into adult mammalian CNS (and vice versa) (1,2,5,18,19). Axons from injured spinal cord, brainstem, thalamus, and cerebral cortex are able to grow along peripheral nervous system grafts up to but not into CNS tissue. Central nervous system neurons are able to extend axons following injury in peripheral nervous system microenvironment.

Similar transplantation techniques might be applied experimentally to the mammalian auditory system. An autologous peripheral nerve graft could be interposed between severed ends of the eighth nerve to provide a milieu in which spiral ganglion neurons can generate and project axons to cochlear nuclei. Clinical application is limited; compromising normal innervation to obtain a suitable nerve for transplantation may not be practical.

An interesting variation to peripheral nerve grafting has been shown with the auditory and facial nerves of cats (79,84,85). The severed distal end of a facial nerve was approximated to the severed proximal end of the eighth nerve in a cat, and growth into the auditory brainstem was demonstrated by 9 to 18 months. Perhaps the motor component of the facial nerve was guided by degenerative debris of the severed eighth nerve, as occurs in others systems (44). However, the facial nerve's axons did not appear to make synaptic contact with cochlear neurons.

Alternative techniques for neural repair that involve manipulations of the nerve's microenvironment are in developmental stages. Transected ends of peripheral nerves regenerate when placed into artificial nerve guides constructed with various synthetic materials, including amicon acrylic copolymer (80), silicone (30,46,47), gortex (91), and bioresorbable materials (48,49). Optic nerve regeneration has been reported with guides composed of bioresorbable materials (48,49). The application of polyethylene glycol has been used to functionally reconnect severed crayfish giant axons *in vitro* (8); however, similar results have not been obtained with severed rat sciatic nerve. Also, fibrin matrix has been used to stimulate peripheral nerve regeneration with some success (87).

Interestingly, electrical stimulation may enhance neuronal regeneration. For example, accelerated frog neurite outgrowth (26) and lamprey spinal cord regeneration (12) occur under the influence of extracellular electric fields. Indeed, Frank (20) has reported human peripheral nerve regeneration can be stimulated in this manner.

CONCLUSION

The eighth cranial nerve may be injured by tumors (70,73), trauma (25,43,70,73,89), bacterial infections (13,64,70,73), and ototoxic drugs (28,43,60,70,73). Because of its liability to injury, studies of its repair are important and promise clinical applicability. These studies are in preliminary stages. Although eighth nerve regeneration has been demonstrated in frogs and turtles, and patterns of eighth nerve degeneration and regeneration following injury are similar to that observed in mammalian peripheral nerves and other central nerves of fish and amphibia, at present mammalian eighth nerves cannot be induced to regenerate. Continued research must identify critical factors that permit complete functional mammalian eighth nerve regeneration, which can eventually be applied in the clinical setting.

ACKNOWLEDGMENT

The author thanks Dr. R. Browner for reading initial drafts of this manuscript.

REFERENCES

1. Aguayo, A. J., David, S., Richardson, P., and Bray, G. (1982): Axonal elongation in peripheral and central nervous system transplants. In: *Cellular Neurobiology, Volume 3*, edited by S. Federoff and L. Hurtz, pp. 215–234. Academic Press, New York.
2. Aguayo, A. J., Richardson, P., David, S., and Benfey, M. (1982): Transplantation of neurons and sheath cells—a tool for the study of regeneration. In: *Repair and Regeneration of the Nervous System*, edited by J. G. Nicholls, pp. 91–108. Springer-Verlag, New York.
3. Anderson, H. J., Rapporteur, T., Aguayo, A. J., et al. (1982): Early responses to neural injury. In: *Repair and Regeneration of the Nervous System*, edited by J. G. Nicholls, pp. 315–339. Springer-Verlag, New York.
4. Barrett, C. P., Donati, E., and Guth, L. (1984): Differences between adult and neonatal rats in their astroglial responses to spinal injury. *Exp. Neurol.*, 84:374–385.
5. Benfey, M., and Aguayo, A. J. (1982): Extensive elongation of axons from rat brain into peripheral nerve grafts. *Nature*, 296:150–152.
6. Berry, M. (1979): Regeneration in the central nervous system. In: *Recent Advances in Neuropathology*, edited by Smith and Cavanagh, pp. 67–111. Churchill Livingston, New York.
7. Berthold, C., and Carlstedt, T. (1977): II. General organization of the transitional area in S1 dorsal

rootlets. Observations on the morphology at the transition between peripheral and central nervous system in the cat. *Acta Physiol. Scand.* [*Suppl.*], 46:23–42.

8. Bittner, G. D., Ballinger, M. L., and Raymond, M. A. (1986): Reconnection of severed nerve axons with polyethylene glycol. *Brain Res.*, 367:351–355.
9. Bjorklund, A., Bjerre, G., and Steveni, U. (1974): Has nerve growth factor a role in the regeneration of central and peripheral catcholamine neurons? In: *Dynamics of Degeneration and Growth in Neurons*, edited by K. Fuxe, L. Olson, and Y. Zotterman, pp. 389–409. Pergamon Press, New York.
10. Bjorklund, A., and Steveni, U. (1977): Reformation of the severed septohippocampal cholinergic pathway in the adult rat by transplanted septal neurons. *Cell Tissue Res.*, 185:289–302.
11. Bohn, R., Reier, P. J., and Sourbeer, E. (1982): Axonal interactions with connective tissue and glial substrata during optic nerve regeneration in Xenopus larvae and adults. *Am. J. Anat.*, 165:397–419.
12. Borgens, R. B., Roederer, E., and Cohen, M. J. (1981): Enhanced spinal cord regeneration in lamprey by electrical fields. *Science*, 213:611–617.
13. Brodeal, A. (1981): The auditory system. In: *Neurological Anatomy in Relation to Clinical Medicine*, edited by A. Brodeal, pp. 602–639. Oxford University Press, New York.
14. Bunge, M. B., Johnson, M. I., and Argiro, V. J. (1983): Studies of regenerating nerve fibers and growth cones. In: *Spinal Cord Reconstruction*, edited by C. C. Kao, R. P. Bunge, and P. J. Reier, pp. 99–120. Raven Press, New York.
15. Bunge, R. P. (1981): Contribution of tissue culture studies to our understanding of the basic processes in peripheral nerve regeneration. In: *Posttraumatic Peripheral Nerve Regeneration, Experimental Basis, and Clinical Implications*, edited by A. Gorio, H. Millesi, and S. Mingrino, pp. 105–113. Raven Press, New York.
16. Clemente, C. D. (1955): Structural regeneration in the mammalian central nervous system and the role of neuroglia and connective tissue. In: *Regeneration in the Central Nervous System*, edited by W. F. Windle, pp. 147–161, Charles C. Thomas, Springfield, IL.
17. Clemente, C. D. (1964): Regeneration in the vertebrate central nervous system. *Int. Rev. Biol.*, 6:257–301.
18. David, S., and Aguayo, A. (1982): Axonal elongation into peripheral nervous system "bridges" after central nervous system injury in adult rats. *Science*, 214:931–933.
19. Duncan, I., Aguayo, A. J., Bunge, R., and Wood, P. (1981): Transplantation of rat Schwann cells grown in tissue culture into mouse spinal cord. *J. Comp. Neurol. Sci.*, 49:241–252.
20. Frank, E. (1982): Adaptive and maladaptive regeneration in the spinal cord. In: *Repair and Regeneration of the Nervous System*, edited by J. G. Nicholls, pp. 243–254. Springer-Verlag, New York.
21. Freed, W., Pelow, M., Karoum, F., et al. (1980): Restoration of dopaminergic function by grafting fetal substantia nigra to the caudate nucleus long-term behavioral, biochemical, and histochemical studies. *Ann. Neurol.*, 8:510–519.
22. Gamble, H. J. (1976): Spinal and cranial nerve roots. In: *The Peripheral Nerve*, edited by D. N. Landon, pp. 330–354. John Wiley, New York.
23. Gray, H. (1974): The nervous system. In: *Gray's Anatomy*, edited by T. Pickering Pick and R. Howden, pp. 639–810. Running Press, Philadelphia.
24. Harkonen, M., and Kaufman, F. (1973): Metabolic alterations in the axotomized superior cervical ganglion of the cat. I. Energy metabolism. *Brain Res.*, 65:127–139.
25. Hawkins, J. E. (1973): Comparative otopathology: Aging, noise, and ototoxic drugs. *Adv. Otorhinolaryngol.*, 20:125–141.
26. Hinkle, L., McCraig, C. D., and Robinson, K. R. (1981): The direction of growth differentiating neurons and myoblasts from frog embryo in an applied electric field. *J. Physiol.*, 314:121–136.
27. Hochmair-Desoyer, I. J., Hochmair, E. S., Burian, K., and Fischer, R. E. (1981): Four years of experience with cochlear prostheses. *Med. Prog. Technol.*, 8:107–119.
28. Hunter-Duvar, I. M., and Mount, R. J. (1978): The organ of Corti following ototoxic antibiotic treatment. *Scan. Electron Microsc.*, 11:423–430.
29. Ide, C., Tohyama, K., Yokota, R., Nitatori, T., and Onoduro, S. (1983): Schwann cell basal lamina and nerve regeneration. *Brain Res.*, 288:61–75.
30. Jenq, C. B., and Coggeshall, R. E. (1986): Regeneration of transected rat sciatic nerves after using isolated nerve fragments as distal inserts in silicone tubes. *Exp. Neurol.*, 91:154–162.
31. Johnsson, L. G. (1972): Symposium on basic ear research. II. Strial atrophy in clinical and experimental deafness. *Laryngoscope*, 82:1105–1125.
32. Johnsson, L. G. (1974): Sequence of degeneration of Corti's organ and its first-order neurons. *Ann. Otol.*, 83:294–303.
33. Kellerhals, B. (1967): Die morphologie des ganglion spirale cochleae. *Acta Otolaryngol.* (*Stockh.*), Suppl. 226.
34. Kiernan, J. A. (1979): An explanation of axonal regeneration in the mammalian nervous system. *Biol. Dev.*, 54:155–197.
35. Kohhonen, A. (1965): Effect of some ototoxic drugs on the pattern and innervation of cochlear sensory cells in the guinea pig. *Acta Otolaryngol.* [*Suppl.*] (*Stockh.*), 208:10–70.

36. Kreutzberg, G. W. (1982): Acute neural reaction to injury. In: *Repair and Regeneration of the Nervous System*, edited by J. G. Nicholls, pp. 57–69. Springer-Verlag, New York.
37. Kreutzberg, G. W., and Emmert, H. (1980): Glucose utilization of motor nuclei during regeneration: A 14C 2-deoxyglucose study. *Exp. Neurol.*, 70:712–716.
38. Kreutzberg, G. W., and Schubert, P. (1971): Changes in axonal flow during regeneration of mammalian motor nerves. *Acta Neuropathol. [Suppl.] (Berl.)*, 5:70–75.
39. Kromer, L., Bjorklund, A., and Steveni, U. (1980): Innervation of embryonic hippocampal implants by regenerating axons of cholinergic septal neurons in the adult rat. *Brain Res.*, 210:153–171.
40. Kromer, L., Bjorklund, A., and Steveni, U. (1981): Regeneration of the septohippocampal pathways in adult rats is promoted by utilizing embryonic implants as bridges. *Brain Res.*, 210:173–200.
41. LeGros Clark, W. (1940): Neuronal differentiation in implanted fetal cortical tissue. *J. Neurol. Psychol.*, 3:263–272.
42. Liberman, M. C., and Kiang, N. Y. S. (1978): Acoustic trauma in cats. Cochlear pathology and auditory-nerve activity. *Acta Otolaryngol. [Suppl.] (Stockh.)*, 358:7–63.
43. Lim, D. J. (1976): Ultrastructural cochlear changes following acoustic hyperstimulation and otoxicity. *Ann. Otol.*, 85:740–751.
44. Lo, R., and Levine, R. (1981): Anatomical evidence for the influence of degenerating pathways on regenerating optic fibers following surgical manipulations in the visual system of the goldfish. *Brain Res.*, 210:61–68.
45. Lund, R. D. (1978): *Development and Plasticity of the Brain. An Introduction.* Oxford University Press, New York.
46. Lundborg, G., Dahlin, L. B., Danielsen, N., et al. (1982): Nerve regeneration in silicone chambers: Influence of gap length and of distal stump components. *Exp. Neurol.*, 76:361–375.
47. Lundborg, G., Gelberman, R. H., Longo, F. M., Powell, H. C., and Varon, S. (1982): *In vivo* regeneration of cut nerves encased in silicone tubes. Growth across a six-millimeter gap. *J. Neuropathol. Exp. Neurol.*, 41:412–422.
48. Madison, R., DaSilva, C. F., Dikkes, P., Chiu, T. T., and Sidman, R. L. (1985): Increased rate of peripheral nerve regeneration using bioresorbable nerve guides and a laminin-containing gel. *Exp. Neurol.*, 88:767–772.
49. Madison, R., Sidman, R. L., Chiu, T. H., and Nyilas, E. (1983): Bioresorbable nerve guides bridge transected optic nerve. *Neurosci. Abstr.*, 9:770.
50. Marbey, D., and Browner, R. (1984): Reconnection of the eighth nerve fibers after transection in the red-eared turtle. *Neurosci. Abstr.*, 10:1024.
51. Marbey, D., and Browner, R. (1984): The reconnection of auditory posterior root fibers in the red-eared turtle, *Chrysemys scripta elegans. Hear. Res.*, 15:88–94.
52. Marbey, D., and Browner, R. (1986): Regeneration of the eighth nerve fibers after transection in the red-eared turtle, *Chrysemys scripta elegans.* Abstr. IXth Midwinter Res. Meet. ARO, p. 24.
53. Marbey, D., and Browner, R. (1987): Regeneration of the eighth nerve fibers after transection in the red-eared turtle, *Chrysemys scripta elegans. J. Morphol.*, 193:197–216.
54. Marbey, D., and Santos-Sacchi, J. (1986): Immunocytochemical demonstration of astrocytes in the eighth cranial nerve of the red-eared turtle. *Exp. Neurol.*, 94:141–148.
55. Murray, M., and Grafstein, B. (1969): Changes in the morphology and amino acid incorporation of regenerating goldfish optic neurons. *Exp. Neurol.*, 23:544–568.
56. Nathaniel, E., and Nathaniel, D. (1981): The reactive astrocyte. *Adv. Cell. Neurobiol.*, 2:249–301.
57. Nemecek, S., Parizek, J., Spacek, J., and Nemeckova, J. (1969): Histological, histochemical, and ultrastructural appearance of the transitional zone of the cranial and spinal nerve roots. *Folia Morphol.*, V.X.VII:171–181.
58. Nicholls, J. G. (1982): Introduction. In: *Repair and Regeneration of the Central Nervous System*, edited by J. G. Nicholls, pp. 1–5. Springer-Verlag, New York.
59. Ramon y Cajal, S. (1928): *Degeneration and Regeneration of the Nervous System* (translated by R. M. May). Oxford University Press, New York.
60. Reddy, J. B., and Igarashi, M. (1962): Changes produced by kanamycin. Early histologic manifestations in the inner ears of cats. *Arch. Otolaryngol.*, 76:146–150.
61. Reier, P. J. (1961): Penetration of grafted astrocytic scars by regenerating optic nerve axons in *Xenopus tadpoles. Brain Res.*, 154:61–68.
62. Reier, P. J., Stensaas, L. J., and Guth, L. (1983): The astrocytic scars as an impediment to regeneration in the central nervous system. In: *Spinal Cord Reconstruction*, edited by C. C. Kao, R. P. Bunge, and P. J. Reier, pp. 163–195. Raven Press, New York.
63. Romer, A. S. (1970): *The Vertebrate Body.* W. B. Saunders, Philadelphia.
64. Ross, M. D., and Burkel, W. (1971): Electron microscopic observations of the nucleus, glial dome, and meninges of the rat acoustic nerve. *Am. J. Anat.*, 130:73–92.
65. Sanes, J. R. (1982): Regeneration of synapses. In: *Repair and Regeneration of the Nervous System*, edited by J. G. Nicholls, pp. 127–154. Springer-Verlag, New York.

66. Schuknecht, H. F. (1953): Lesions of the organ of Corti. *Trans. Am. Acad. Ophthalmol. Otolaryngol.*, 57:366–382.
67. Schuknecht, H. F., and Woeller, W. C. (1955): An experimental and clinical study of deafness from lesions of the cochlear nerve. *J. Laryngol.*, 69:75–77.
68. Skoff, R. P. (1975): The fine structure of pulse labeled (^{3}H-thymidine cells) in degenerating rat optic nerve. *J. Comp. Neurol.*, 161:595–611.
69. Spoendlin, H. (1971): Degeneration behavior of the cochlear nerve. *Arch. Klin. Exp. Ohr. Nas. U. Kehlk. Heilk.*, 200:275–291.
70. Spoendlin, H. (1975): Retrograde degeneration of the cochlear nerve. *Acta Otolaryngol. (Stockh.)*, 79:266–275.
71. Spoendlin, H. (1976): Anatomical changes following various noise exposures. In: *Effects of Noise on Hearing*, edited by D. Henderson. Raven Press, New York.
72. Spoendlin, H. (1981): Afferent innervation of cochlear hair cells. Abstr. IVth Midwinter Res. Meet. ARO, pp. 97–99.
73. Spoendlin, H. (1984): Factors inducing retrograde degeneration of the cochlear nerve. *Ann. Otol. Rhinol. Laryngol.*, 93:76–81.
74. Spoendlin, H., and Suter, R. (1976): Regeneration in the VIII nerve. *Acta Otolaryngol. (Stockh.)*, 81:228–236.
75. Tarlov, M. (1937): Structure of the nerve root. I. Nature of the junction between the central and the peripheral nervous system. *Arch. Neurol. Psychiatr.*, 37:1338–1355.
76. Terayama, Y., Kaneko, Y., Kawamoto, K., and Saki, N. (1977): Ultrastructural changes of the nerve elements following disruption of the organ of Corti. *Acta Otolaryngol. (Stockh.)*, 83:291–302.
77. Terayama, Y., Kaneko, Y., Tanaka, K., and Kawamoto, K. (1979): Ultrastructural changes of the nerve elements following disruption of the organ of Corti. *Acta Otolaryngol. (Stockh.)*, 88:27–36.
78. Thomas, P. K. (1974): Nerve injury. In: *Essays on the Nervous System*, edited by R. Bellairs and E. G. Gray, pp. 44–70. Oxford University Press, New York.
79. Thumfart, W., Finkenzeller, P., and Wigand, M. E. (1979): Grafting and electrical stimulation of the auditory nerve in cats. *Arch. Otorhinolaryngol.*, 224:79–83.
80. Uzman, B. G., and Villegas, G. M. (1983): Mouse sciatic nerve regeneration through semipermeable tubes: A quantitative model. *J. Neurosci. Res.*, 9:325–338.
81. Webster, M., and Webster, D. B. (1981): Spiral ganglion neuron loss following organ of Corti loss: A quantitative study. *Brain Res.*, 212:17–30.
82. Wever, E. G., and Neff, W. D. (1947): A further study of the effects of partial section of the auditory nerve. *J. Comp. Physiol. Psychol.*, 40:217–226.
83. Whitnall, M., and Grafstein, B. (1983): Changes in perikaryal organelles during axonal regeneration in goldfish retinal ganglion cells: An analysis of protein synthesis and routing. *Brain Res.*, 272:49–56.
84. Wigand, M. E. (1979): Experimental grafting of the auditory nerve. *Rev. Laryngol.*, 100:115–118.
85. Wigand, M. E., Thumfart, W., Berg, M., and Schmidt, H. (1978): Experimental grafting of the auditory nerve. *Arch. Otolaryngol.*, 104:325–328.
86. Willard, M., and Skene, J. H. P. (1982): Molecular events in axonal regeneration. In: *Repair and Regeneration of the Nervous System*, edited by J. G. Nicholls, pp. 71–90. Springer-Verlag, New York.
87. Williams, L. R., and Varon, S. (1986): Experimental manipulations of the microenvironment within a nerve regeneration chamber. Abstr. IXth Midwinter Res. Meet. ARO, p. 204.
88. Windle, W. F. (1956): Regeneration of axons in the vertebrate central nervous system. *Physiol. Rev.*, 36:426–440.
89. Wright, C. G. (1976): Neural damage in the guinea pig after noise exposure. A light microscopic study. *Acta Otolaryngol. (Stockh.)*, 82:82–94.
90. Wujek, J., and Reier, R. (1984): Astrocytic membrane morphology: Differences between mammalian and amphibian astrocytes after axotomy. *J. Comp. Neurol.*, 222:607–619.
91. Young, B. L., Begovac, P., Stuart, D. G., and Goslow, G. E. (1984): An effective sleeving technique in nerve repair. *J. Neurosci. Meth.*, 10:51–58.
92. Zakon, H. H. (1983): Reorganization of connectivity in amphibian central auditory system following VIIIth nerve regeneration: Time course. *J. Neurophysiol.*, 49:1410–1427.
93. Zakon, H. H. (1986): Regeneration and recovery of function in the amphibian auditory system. Abstr. IXth Midwinter Res. Meet. ARO, pp. 205–206.
94. Zakon, H. H., and Capranica, R. R. (1981): Reformation of organized connections in the auditory system after regeneration of the eighth nerve. *Science*, 213:242–244.
95. Zakon, H. H., and Capranica, R. R. (1981): An anatomical and physiological study of regeneration of the eighth nerve in the leopard frog. *Brain Res.*, 209:325–338.

Physiology of the Ear,
edited by A. F. Jahn and J. Santos-Sacchi.
Raven Press, New York © 1988.

Patch Clamp Recording from Hair Cells

*James P. Dilger and **Joseph Santos-Sacchi

*Departments of Anesthesiology, and Physiology and Biophysics, State University of New York at Stony Brook, Stony Brook, New York 11794-8480; and **Laboratory of Otolaryngology, New Jersey Medical School, University of Medicine and Dentistry of New Jersey, Newark, New Jersey 07103-2757

All cells, including hair cells, utilize the cell membrane to create and maintain an intracellular ionic composition that differs from that of the extracellular fluid. A variety of cellular functions are then driven by the resulting concentration and electrical potential gradients. Many of these functions rely on specialized integral membrane proteins that function as gatable transmembrane pores or channels. The probability that the gate of a particular channel is open or closed depends on various external and/or internal influences, including changes in transmembrane potential, the binding of chemical transmitters to receptors, intracellular messengers, or mechanical stimuli. Upon opening, a channel permits the passage of ions, and the magnitude of ion flux through the open channel depends on the electrochemical forces—ion concentrations and driving voltage—acting on the particular ion. Channels are usually classified according to the physiologically important ion that permeates them (e.g., K^+, Na^+, Ca^{2+}, or Cl^-).

Since the gating of many ion channels is voltage dependent, the ideal way to investigate the properties of these channels is to experimentally set (or clamp) the cell membrane potential to a given value and measure the resulting current. The conventional two-electrode voltage clamp (10) has been used on relatively large cells with great success. The technique involves inserting two electrodes into a cell, one for measuring voltage and one for injecting current into the cell. When the voltage is clamped to the cell's resting potential, the net current flowing across the membrane is zero (the cell is in electrochemical equilibrium) and the voltage clamp circuit does not pass any current. To change the membrane potential to a new level, current is injected into the cell. Intrinsic membrane currents will flow in response to the voltage step and these currents will tend to cause the membrane potential to deviate from the clamped value. The voltage electrode senses this tendency and a feedback loop in the voltage clamp circuit compensates for it by injecting more or less current into the cell. A good voltage clamp will quickly set the membrane potential at the desired level and keep it there. The amount of injected current needed to maintain the potential is equal in magnitude to the intrinsic currents flowing through ion channels. Thus, the current output of the voltage clamp circuit provides us with a measure of the cell's ionic currents.

Electrophysiologists have used conventional voltage clamp recording techniques since the 1950s to identify and characterize ionic currents in cells arising from the concerted activity of the many thousands of ion channels in the cell membrane.

Because of the large number of channels involved in producing these currents, information about the underlying, unitary channel events is obscured and only indirect estimates of the size and duration of these events could be made. In 1976, however, Neher and Sakmann (13) developed a method for making low-resolution current recordings from single acetylcholine receptor channels in muscle cells. During the next few years, they and their colleagues dramatically improved the resolving power of the technique (9) so that currents as small as 1 pA (10^{-12} A) lasting only tens of microseconds could be reliably measured. Since 1981, single-channel currents of many species of ionic channels from a wide variety of cells have been recorded using the patch clamp technique. These measurements provide previously unavailable, direct information about the gating and permeability properties of channels. In addition, a variation of the patch clamp technique, whole cell recording, allows voltage clamp measurements to be made on very small cells (such as mammalian neurons) for which conventional techniques are unreliable.

In this chapter we present a brief description of single-channel recording and analysis techniques (see references 9 and 17 for more detailed information), examine some of the results that have been reported thus far from experiments on hair cells, and indicate the ways in which the technique may contribute to our understanding of auditory processes.

PATCH CLAMP RECORDING TECHNIQUES

In patch clamp recording, a small patch of membrane (several square micrometers in area), containing only one or a few ion channels, is electrically isolated from the rest of the cell membrane (Fig. 1). Formation of a patch is achieved by slowly lowering the tip of a patch pipette onto the surface of the cell. Gentle suction is then applied to the inside of the pipette and, under ideal conditions, a high resistance seal of 10 to 100 gigaohms (1 gigaohm = 10^9 ohms) is obtained between the cell membrane and the pipette. Using a feedback amplifier and current-voltage converter, the investigator can clamp the voltage across this patch and measure any current that flows through it. If the patch contains one or more ion channels and the appropriate stimulus for channel opening is present, the current recording may reveal the step-like transitions of channels alternating between open (conducting) and closed (nonconducting) configurations (Fig. 1B).

There are four patch configurations in which single-channel recordings can be made (Fig. 1A). The one described previously, the cell-attached patch, is always the initial step toward producing the others. There are two excised patch configurations: inside-out patches, in which the intracellular side of the membrane patch is exposed to the saline bathing solution (and the extracellular side of the patch is exposed to the solution in the pipette) and outside-out patches, which have the opposite orientation. Recording from excised patches has the advantage that the solution bathing one side of the patch can be readily exchanged during the experiment, but has the possible disadvantage that essential intracellular factors may be lost upon excision from the cell. Finally, single-channel recording can sometimes be performed during whole-cell voltage clamp after disruption of the cell-attached patch. If the resistance of the entire cell membrane is sufficiently high, the background current and noise may be low enough to allow single-channel events to be distinguished (15).

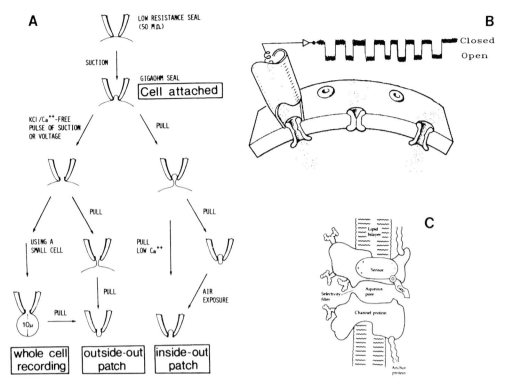

FIG. 1. **A:** Schematic of gigaohm seal formation and the four types of patch clamp recording configurations. (From ref. 17.) The glass pipette has a heat-polished tip with a diameter of 1 to 2 μm. It is filled with a saline solution and connected to the amplifier circuit with a silver chloride wire. The cells are placed in a saline bathing solution that is electrically grounded. For successful patch clamp recording, the surface of the cell membrane must be clean, that is, free of connective tissue and debris. All saline solutions used in the experiment are strained through a 0.2-μm filter to avoid plugging the tip of the pipette. There are two sources of suitable cells: cells grown in tissue culture and cells dissociated directly from animal tissue, sometimes with the aid of enzymes. **B:** High magnification schematic showing a patch electrode sealed around a single-membrane channel. The amplified single-channel currents reveal step-like transitions that correspond to the opening and closing of the channel. (Redrawn from ref. 7.) **C:** Detailed schematic of a hypothetical single channel. The channel protein spans the lipid bilayer providing an aqueous pore for charged ions to pass through. The particular type of ion that permeates the channel is determined by the channel's selectivity filter. The channel gate is controlled by a sensor moiety of the channel protein. The type of sensor determines which stimulus will open the gate. (From ref. 10.)

DATA ANALYSIS AND INTERPRETATION

Conventional and whole-cell voltage clamp (macroscopic current) techniques are usually the first electrophysiological methods used to identify and enumerate the various ionic currents present in a cell (Fig. 2). It is only when the study goes beyond this classification stage that the power of patch clamp recording is realized. The magnitude of the measured macroscopic current (I) is equal to the product of three parameters: (a) the number (N) of channels present in the cell, (b) the current (i) passed by each individual channel, and (c) the probability (p) that channels are open.

$$I = Nip$$

It is usually not possible to determine the value of these parameters separately using

A   HC53B

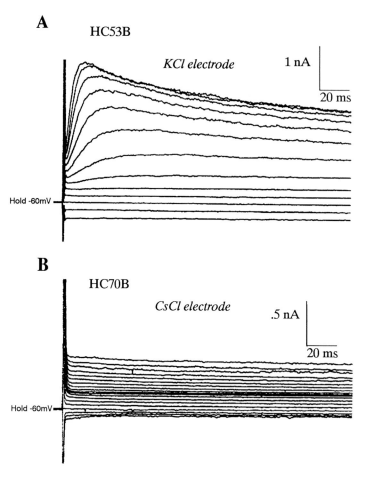

FIG. 2. Whole cell recordings from an isolated outer hair cell. **A:** Recording made with electrode solution containing 140 mM KCl. The membrane potential was either depolarized (upward traces) or hyperpolarized (downward traces) in increments of 10 mV for 200 msec from a holding potential of −60 mV. The I–V relation for outer hair cells is nonlinear since depolarization above about −40 mV elicits a voltage- and time-dependent outward current. **B:** Recording made with electrode solution containing 140 mM CsCl. In this case the I–V relation is more linear because intracellular cesium ions block the voltage- and time-dependent outward current. The blockage observed here on replacement of K^+ and Cs^+ indicates that the outward current is normally carried by potassium ions. This illustrates how whole-cell voltage clamp can be used to identify individual components of the whole-cell current.

macroscopic recording techniques. The basic advantage of single-channel recording is that it allows one to evaluate each of the three parameters: the single-channel current is the amplitude of the channel events, the open-channel probability is the fraction of time that channels spend in the open state, and the number of channels in the cell can be calculated by dividing the whole-cell current by the other two parameters or, in some instances, by various counting procedures.

In its simplest application, patch clamp recording can be used as an assay to test for the presence or absence of a certain type of channel activity in a given cell membrane. Although this can also be accomplished with other voltage clamp techniques (and often more simply), an additional feature of patch recording is that the distribution of channels over the surface of the cell membrane can readily be studied.

The open-channel properties of channels, conductance (permeability) and ion selectivity, can help the investigator associate what is seen on the macroscopic current scale with the single-channel events. As noted previously, channels are usually identified by the physiologically important ion that permeates them. Further classification is made by specifying the conductance of the channel (which will, of course, depend on the concentration of permeant ions used in the experiment) and by noting the type of stimulus that activates the channel. For example, in some cell membranes there are voltage-gated Na^+ channels, 200 pS (siemens are the reciprocal of ohms; 1 pS = 10^{-12} S), Ca^{2+}-activated K^+ channels, and mechanically activated nonselective cation channels. Ions that do not permeate but rather block the channel are also useful agents for identification purposes. Occasionally, the open-channel properties are studied for the sake of understanding permeability mechanisms themselves—the patch clamp technique has greatly assisted these studies.

The kinetic properties of channels reveal information about the various conformational states of the channel protein and how the gating parameter (e.g., voltage, mechanical stimulus) induces a change in state. To determine the number of these states and the transition rates between states, one must consider the distribution of open and closed durations of single channels. In practice, the investigator, aided by a computer program, determines the occurrence of channel openings and closings in digitized records of channel activity by observing when the current trace crosses some threshold value (usually, one-half the amplitude of the single-channel current). The durations of closed and open intervals are then accumulated into separate histograms. If it is assumed that there are two discrete conductance states of a channel, one closed and one open, and that the opening and closing transition rates are constant in time, stochastic analysis (4) predicts that both the open- and closed-duration histograms will exhibit a single exponential distribution. The mean open time (or the time constant of the exponential distribution of open times) is then simply the reciprocal of the rate constant for channel closing. (A parallel relationship holds for the mean closed time and the rate constant for channel opening.) Frequently, however, several exponentials are necessary to accurately fit duration histograms. A general rule is that the number of exponential components in the open (closed) duration histogram is equal to the minimum number of open (closed) states needed in a kinetic model that fully accounts for the data. Numerical values for transition-rate constants can also be obtained from these multi-exponential distributions.

Although the value of stochastic analysis of single-channel data to those who model channel activation processes is obvious, such analyses can also be used to address issues concerning cell physiology. One may want to know if a particular channel can respond to a stimulus on a time scale appropriate for the supposed physiological function of the channel. If a channel is thought to play an important role in sound transduction, for example, we would expect that the channel should be able to respond to sound stimuli with a very short latency. The manifestation of this property on the single-channel level is a component in the closed-duration histogram with a correspondingly short time constant. However, the converse of this (brief closed duration components imply short activation latencies) is not necessarily true, and there has been some confusion about this issue in the literature. The presence of a brief closed time component may reflect only the final step in the activation of the channel whereas the entire activation process may last considerably longer. Only when a full kinetic description of channel activation is presented can one assess whether a channel is fast enough to be involved in sound transduction. Alternatively, single-channel experiments can be designed to measure directly the latency of channel opening.

RESULTS OF PATCH CLAMP RECORDING FROM HAIR CELLS

The application of electrophysiological recording techniques to the study of hair cells is still at a stage where whole-cell and single-channel currents are being identified and characterized. Moreover, the correlations between these currents and physiological phenomena are generally unknown. Here, we will summarize some of the findings that have been reported on single-channel recordings from three isolated hair cell preparations: guinea pig outer hair cells, chick vestibular hair cells, and turtle hair cells.

Three groups of investigators identified K^+ channels in guinea pig outer hair cells (2,8,18). One of these groups also reported on 22-pS and 40-pS Cl^- channels in these cells (8). There appear to be at least three different conductance species of K^+ channels; two of them may be Ca^{2+}-activated (i.e., internal Ca^{2+} is the ligand that opens the channel) and one of these Ca^{2+}-activated K^+ channels has a very high conductance, about 200 pS (Fig. 3). High conductance Ca^{2+}-activated K^+ channels are seen in many types of cells, although the physiological role of these channels is usually unknown. One group suggested that a Ca^{2+}-activated K^+ channel is responsible for the resting membrane potential of outer hair cells (3). Presumably, this would require the presence of functional Ca^{2+} channels in the membranes of outer hair cells. In fact, depolarization-induced inward currents have been observed in outer hair cells in the presence of high extracellular concentrations of barium (19), suggesting the existence of Ca^{2+} channels in these cells (Ba^{2+} is often used as a Ca^{2+} substitute in studies of Ca^{2+} channels; Ca^{2+} channels are actually more permeable to Ba^{2+} than to Ca^{2+}).

In his studies on chick vestibular hair cells, Ohmori (14) identified two classes of inward rectifier K^+ channels (a type of voltage-gated potassium channel that, unlike most other voltage-gated channels, opens on hyperpolarization from the resting membrane potential). It is likely that these channels function to restore the resting potential of the cell after some hyperpolarizing stimulus, but this remains to be demonstrated. Vestibular hair cells also exhibit a Ca^{2+} current under whole-cell voltage clamp, but the channel events underlying this current have not be detected.

While making single-channel measurements during whole-cell voltage clamp, Ohmori (15,16) discovered a channel that is activated by the mechanical deflection of the hair cell bundle at the apical end of the cell (Fig. 4). There is now good evidence that these channels are the mechanical transducers of the cell. These channels have a conductance of about 50 pS and are selective for cations over anions, but are not very selective between Na^+ and K^+. Ca^{2+} ions are required for the channel's activity.

For some time, it has been known that the aminoglycoside antibiotics are ototoxic;

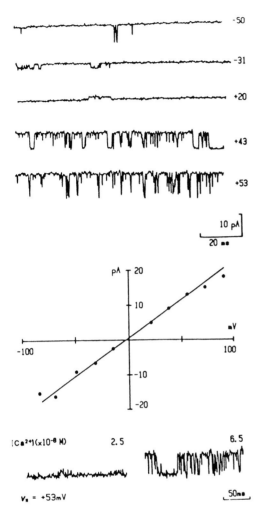

FIG. 3. The top portion of the figure shows single-channel currents at various holding potentials obtained from an inside-out patch of the basolateral membrane of an outer hair cell. Below, the current magnitude versus holding potential is plotted, and the slope of the fitted line indicates a conductance of 220 pS for this channel. The channel was determined to be K^+ selective and is gated by intracellular Ca^{2+}. These channels are activated by Ca^{2+} concentrations greater than 2.5×10^{-8} M. The bottom portion of the figure shows single-channel currents under conditions below and above Ca^{2+} activation levels. (From ref. 2.)

indeed, using conventional electrophysiological techniques, it has been shown that application of these drugs on the apical surfaces of hair cells interferes with hair cell transduction (5,11). Ohmori (15) extended these observations by investigating the effect of streptomycin and neomycin on mechanosensitive currents in chick vestibular hair cells. These drugs were found to block the mechanosensitive current. Close examination of the reported data suggests that both the single-channel current and the open-channel probability were reduced by neomycin. Although further experiments would be necessary to justify this speculation (the intent of the author of this study was to use a pharmacological assay to identify the channel rather than to investigate the mechanism of channel block per se), it should be apparent that single-channel studies are more powerful than macroscopic voltage clamp techniques for determining the mechanisms of action of drugs at a molecular level.

In 1981, Crawford and Fettiplace (6) demonstrated that hair cells of the turtle cochlea respond with damped oscillations of the membrane potential on the injection

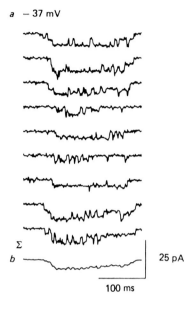

a − 37 mV

Σ
b

100 ms

25 pA

FIG. 4. Single-channel currents recorded in whole-cell configuration during mechanical displacement of vestibular hair cell stereociliar bundle. **a:** Several current records at a holding potential of −37 mV during 148-msec step displacements of the hair bundle. Note the step-like transitions of inward (downward) current, characteristic of single-channel currents. **b:** The ensemble average of the individual records in a. (From ref. 15.)

of small extrinsic DC currents (Fig. 5) This phenomenon has been demonstrated in other hair cell systems but not in the mammal. The frequency of the oscillation is dependent on the location of the cell along the sensory epithelium and correlates well with the tone frequency to which the cell responds maximally. Using the whole-cell voltage clamp technique on isolated hair cells, Lewis and Hudspeth (12) determined that two membrane currents active near the resting potential, an inward Ca^{2+} current and an outward Ca^{2+}-activated K^+ current, are most likely responsible for the observed phenomenon, since blocking these currents reduced or abolished the oscillations.

Art and Fettiplace (1) recorded single K^+ channels from turtle cochlear hair cells in an attempt to analyze further the oscillatory behavior of these cells. The K^+ channels have a conductance of about 100 pS and are activated by depolarizing voltage pulses. Interestingly, the activation time constant of these channels varied between 2 and 20 ms from cell to cell; those cells that demonstrate higher frequency oscillations have shorter time constants. The authors speculated that the kinetic behavior of these channels may underlie the specific tuning characteristics of hair cells along the sensory epithelium. This exciting result gives some insight into how an interplay between Ca^{2+} and K^+ channels in the hair cell may contribute to the resonant frequency tuning of these cells.

The application of the patch clamp technique to the study of hair cells is a recent development. However, within the last few years many important findings have added to our understanding of the complex physiology of hair cells. The examples discussed in this chapter are proof of this. Continued exploitation of this technique by auditory physiologists will contribute not only to an understanding of normal hair cell transduction and synaptic mechanisms, but also to a more basic understanding of pathologies that affect the peripheral auditory system.

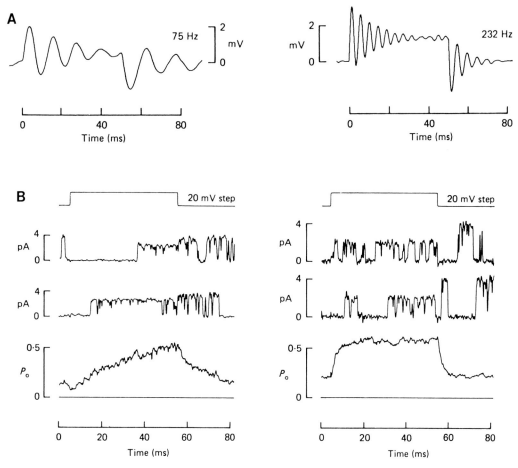

FIG. 5. **A:** Damped oscillations of the membrane potential in isolated turtle cochlear hair cells from the low (**left**) and high (**right**) frequency portion of the sensory epithelium in response to a 50-msec depolarizing current pulse. The frequency of membrane resonance is correlated with the initial tonotopic location of the cell along the epithelium. **B:** Single K^+ channel currents from a low-frequency cell (**left**) and a high-frequency cell (**right**) in response to a 20-mV voltage pulse. Two current traces from each cell are shown. Below the current traces, the ensemble probability (obtained from a large number of current traces) that a channel is open throughout the stimulus demonstrates a dramatic difference between the two cells. The open probability increases exponentially after the onset of the voltage pulse, but the associated time constant for the low-frequency cell is much longer than that of the high-frequency cell. The time constants are consistent with the range of resonant frequencies observed in low- and high-frequency cells. Thus the kinetics of these channels may underlie the macroscopic electrical phenomenon found in these cells. (From ref. 1.)

ACKNOWLEDGMENT

This work has been supported by NIH grant R23 NS21581 (J.P.D.) and NS21380 (J.S.S.) and a Research Career Development Award to J.S.S.

REFERENCES

1. Art, J. J., and Fettiplace, R. (1987): Variation of membrane properties in hair cells isolated from the turtle cochlea. *J. Physiol. (Lond.)*, 385:207–242.
2. Ashmore, J. F., and Meech, R. W. (1986): Three distinct potassium channels in outer hair cells isolated from the guinea-pig cochlea. *J. Physiol. (Lond.)*, 371:29P.
3. Ashmore, J. F., and Meech, R. W. (1986): Ionic basis of the resting potential in outer hair cells isolated from the guinea pig cochlea. *Nature*, 322:368–371.
4. Colquhoun, D., and Hawkes, A. G. (1983): The principles of the stochastic interpretation of ion-channel mechanisms. In: *Single Channel Recording*, edited by B. Sakmann and E. Neher, pp. 135–174. Plenum Press, New York.
5. Corey, D. P., and Hudspeth, A. J. (1979): Response latency of vertebrate hair cells. *Biophys. J.*, 26:499–506.
6. Crawford, A. C., and Fettiplace, R. (1981): An electrical tuning mechanism in turtle cochlear hair cells. *J. Physiol. (Lond.)*, 312:377–412.
7. Evans, P., and Levitan, I. editors (1986): Ion channels and receptors. *J. Exp. Biol.*, 124.
8. Gitter, A. H., Zenner, H. P., and Fromter, E. (1986): Membrane potential and ion channels in isolated outer hair cells of guinea pig cochlea. *ORL J.*, 48:68–75.
9. Hamill, O. P., Marty, E., Neher, E., Sakmann, B., and Sigworth, F. J. (1981): Improved patch-clamp techniques for high-resolution current recording from cells and cell-free membrane patches. *Pflugers Arch.*, 391:85–100.
10. Hille, B. (1984): *Ionic Channels of Excitable Membranes*. Sinauer Associates, Sunderland, MA.
11. Hudspeth, A. J., and Corey, D. P. (1977): Sensitivity, polarity and conductance change in the response of vertebrate hair cells to controlled mechanical stimuli. *Proc. Natl. Acad. Sci. USA*, 74:2407–2411.
12. Lewis, R. S., and Hudspeth, A. J. (1983): Voltage and ion dependent conductances in solitary vertebrate hair cells. *Nature*, 304:538–541.
13. Neher, E., and Sakmann, B. (1976): Single channel currents recorded from membrane of denervated frog muscle fibres. *Nature*, 260:799–802.
14. Ohmori, H. (1984): Studies of ionic currents in the isolated vestibular hair cell of the chick. *J. Physiol. (Lond.)*, 350:561–581.
15. Ohmori, H. (1985): Mechano-electrical transduction currents in isolated vestibular hair cells of the chick. *J. Physiol. (Lond.)*, 359:189–218.
16. Ohmori, H. (1984): Mechanoelectrical transducer has discrete conductances in the chick vestibular hair cell. *Proc. Natl. Acad. Sci. USA*, 81:1888–1891.
17. Sakmann, B., and Neher, E. editors (1983): *Single-Channel Recording*. Plenum Press, New York.
18. Santos-Sacchi, J., and Dilger, J. P. (1986): Patch clamp studies on isolated outer hair cells. *Advances in Auditory Neuroscience: The IUPS Satellite Symposium on Hearing*. Lone Mountain Conference Center, San Francisco, California.
19. Santos-Sacchi, J., and Dilger, J. P. (1987): Whole cell currents and mechanical responses of isolated outer hair cells (*submitted*).

Physiology of the Ear,
edited by A. F. Jahn and J. Santos-Sacchi.
Raven Press, New York © 1988.

Auditory Evoked Magnetic Fields

Samuel J. Williamson and Lloyd Kaufman

Neuromagnetism Laboratory, Departments of Physics and Psychology, New York University, New York, New York 10003

Electrical activity in the human brain produces a magnetic field in the space surrounding the head, as well as a distribution of electric potential across the scalp (24). Magnetic measurements during the past decade have shown that studies of this field can often locate the position of neural activity with a resolution of a few millimeters. For this reason *neuromagnetism*, as the study of these fields is called, is playing an increasingly important role in psychophysiology and clinical research. As we shall show, studies of the *magnetoencephalogram* (MEG) complement the conventional studies of the scalp electrical potential, or *electroencephalogram* (EEG), in identifying active neural sources. One major difference between the MEG and EEG is that the brain and surrounding tissues are transparent to magnetic fields of interest, so that they emerge from the head without distortion. If we imagine the head as a conductor with concentric shells of differing resistivity, then measurements of the field outside the scalp can be directly interpreted in terms of the underlying currents, without regard to the actual values of resistivity (9). By contrast, the EEG is very much affected by intervening layers of tissue, especially the skull, which imposes a barrier of high resistivity.

Biomagnetic fields have been observed from many organs of the body since 1963, when Baule and McFee (2) first revealed the magnetic field of the heart. Neuromagnetic fields are much weaker because their current sources are weaker than those of the heart. The typical field measured next to the scalp is about 100 femtotesla (100×10^{-15} tesla) in magnitude. In contrast the earth's magnetic field is typically 70 microtesla (70×10^{-6} tesla), roughly a billion times stronger. It is the weakness of neuromagnetic fields that has made their measurement a technical challenge. Advent of the superconducting interference device (SQUID) to biomagnetic studies enabled Cohen (6,7) to determine the first map of an alpha rhythm field. The first reports of sensory evoked responses came 3 years later from studies of the visual system (4,21), followed shortly by a method to locate neural activity (5).

PRINCIPLES OF MAGNETIC MEASUREMENTS

The conventional sensor for recording neuromagnetic fields is illustrated in Fig. 1. The high sensitivity of this instrument is made possible by the phenomenon of superconductivity, and at its heart is the SQUID. The superconducting components are mounted within a bath of liquid helium (at a temperature of $-269°C$) to sustain the superconducting state. A vacuum-insulated vessel known as a *dewar* minimizes

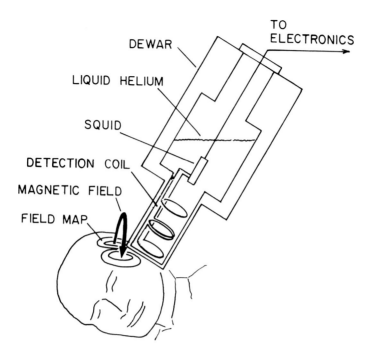

FIG. 1. Arrangement for monitoring the magnetic field of the brain, with a system based on the SQUID detector.

the helium evaporation rate and supports the SQUID. A key element of the system is the *detection coil*, a coil of superconducting wire mounted at the bottom of the dewar close to the head. Detection coils come in many forms to suit specific purposes, the example in Fig. 1 being called a *second-order gradiometer*. It consists of three individual coils wound in series, the center one being wound in the opposite direction with twice as many turns as each of the end coils. Whenever a magnetic field is applied to the detection coil, say by an active region of the brain, an induced current of superconducting electrons flows through the coil and along its leads to a second superconducting coil in series with the first, placed close to the SQUID. This current, which is proportional to the applied field, imposes a magnetic field on the SQUID, and the latter's response is monitored by a set of electronic circuits at room temperature. Thus the output voltage of the SQUID electronics is strictly proportional to the field originally applied to the detection coil. The details of the SQUID are not relevant to our discussion, the essential point being that the sensor's response is linear and extends over the bandwidth from DC to well over 5 kHz.

The principal challenge in field measurements is presented by environmental magnetic noise (15). AC magnetic fields from motors, elevators, and subways are many orders of magnitude greater than neuromagnetic fields, and consequently much emphasis has been directed toward avoiding this noise. The construction of an elaborate magnetically shielded room enabled Cohen to make many pioneering discoveries of a wide variety of biomagnetic effects, but an effective enclosure is expensive (12). An alternative way to reduce noise is with a detection coil having the form of a second-order gradiometer. This geometry makes the detection coil less sensitive to

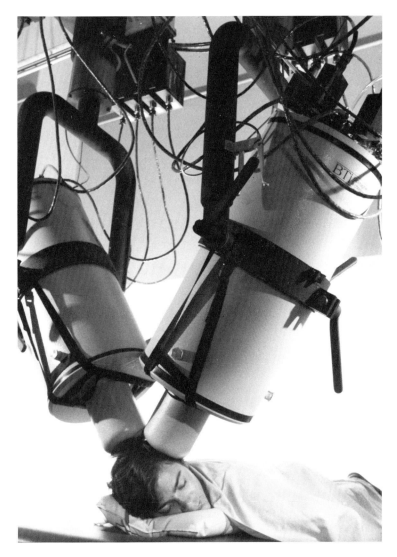

FIG. 2. Neuromagnetic installation with two dewars supported over the subject, each containing seven SQUID sensors. (Courtesy Biomagnetic Technologies, Inc., San Diego.)

the comparatively uniform magnetic fields from distant sources, while the coil remains sensitive to a nearby source, such as that in the brain, because the field is much stronger at the closest coils.

Traditionally, determining a field map was a laborious procedure because it involves sequential measurements at a large number of positions, typically 30 or more for reasonable resolution. However, within the past 2 years systems with multiple sensors have been developed that greatly enhance speed and accuracy (11,18,25). Figure 2 shows two dewars, each containing seven sensors in operation at the New York University Medical Center. Each dewar also has four sensors monitoring the magnetic noise, so that their outputs can be used to reduce the noise in the data of

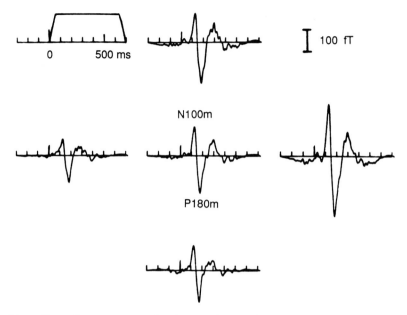

FIG. 3. Magnetic auditory responses simultaneously recorded by a five-sensor system, whose four outer detection coils are separated by 2 cm from the center one. The diagram at the upper left, which depicts the horizontal time scale, shows the amplitude of a tone as it is linearly increased, maintained for approximately 700 msec, and decreased. (From ref. 25.)

interest. The present emphasis in technical development is toward increasing the number of sensors that can simultaneously measure the field at various positions over the scalp. It is reasonable to expect that within 5 years a system will be available for measurements at, say 100 positions, so that measurements can be completed within a matter of minutes.

One important illustration of the capability of multiple-sensor measurements is shown by the five traces in Fig. 3, obtained simultaneously over the right hemisphere near the anterior end of the sylvian fissure. They show averaged responses evoked by 700-msec tone bursts. The first pronounced positive field component has a latency of approximately 100 msec, and so, by analogy with evoked potential notation, it is called N100m. The ''m'' is added because its source may well differ from that of the N100 component of the potential. The subsequent negative component is called P180m, and the last upward deflection, which would continue for a longer time if it were not attenuated by the bandpass filter used to reduce noise, is known as the steady field. These components had been observed by Elberling et al. (8) and by Hari et al. (10) shortly after Reite et al. (14) reported the first observation of auditory evoked magnetic activity.

One important feature in Fig. 3 is that the ratio of N100m amplitude to the P180m amplitude varies with position over the scalp. This indicates that these components do not arise from precisely the same source in the brain: one source is shifted in position, and perhaps rotated with respect to the other. The fact that the two sources differ in position by as much as 1 cm was demonstrated by Pelizzone et al. (13) from detailed mapping of the field patterns over the side of the head. As we shall now illustrate, this ability of magnetic studies to show subtle differences in the locations of neural activity is an important step toward establishing a functional map of the auditory sensory area.

SOURCES OF FIELD

As illustrated in Fig. 1, a localized source in the head produces a magnetic field pattern where the field emerges from the head (positive field) in one region of the scalp and enters the head at another. Since field lines are continuous, without beginning or end, the field must curve around inside the head to close the loop. We call the position of strongest field in each region an *extremum*. The source of such a field pattern is well represented by a short segment of current, called a *current dipole*, positioned under the center of the pattern and oriented parallel to the scalp at right angles to the line between the extrema. The depth of the current dipole is determined by the distance between these extrema (23).

The opposite field directions at the two extrema are illustrated in Fig. 4 for auditory responses. These measurements were taken at approximately the posterior and anterior ends of the sylvian fissure. Detailed mapping shows that the corresponding current dipole sources of all four components (P45m, N100m, P180m, and SF) lie in or near auditory cortex, and their orientations lie closely perpendicular to the fissure (1,10). Such sources may be explained by intracellular currents associated with populations of pyramidal cells, which lie in the cortex and have a preferential alignment that is perpendicular to the surface of the cortex. The pyramidal cells, and perhaps other cells with preferred alignment, are believed to give rise to many features seen in the electroencephalogram as well.

Cellular Currents

It is helpful to consider the cellular basis for a current dipole model to appreciate which aspects of a current pattern give rise to the magnetic field. Consider for the sake of illustration a pyramidal cell, which has tree-like extensions (*dendrites*) projecting from the cell body toward the outer layers of the cortex, and an axon projecting inward. When an adjacent cell excites a portion of a dendrite at a synapse, the resulting change in permeability of the cell membrane allows an influx of positive ions into the cell, which diffuse along the dendrite toward the cell body. This *intracellular current* produces a positive charge at the head of the flow, while leaving a negative charge near the synapse. The charge distribution causes a reverse flow of current in the surrounding medium, and this *extracellular current* is as large as the intracellular current.

According to the law of Biot and Savart (3), the field at any position can be computed by summing the contributions from each small region of the current pattern, suitably weighted according to distance and orientation. In fact, summing contributions from each volume of space, it is easy to show that the most significant contribution comes from the intracellular current. By contrast the transmembrane current gives a negligible contribution because the volume of the membrane is so small. Moreover the extracellular current gives no contribution whatsoever in a medium of uniform electrical conductivity, because contributions from symmetrically arranged portions of the dipolar flow pattern cancel exactly. This was shown

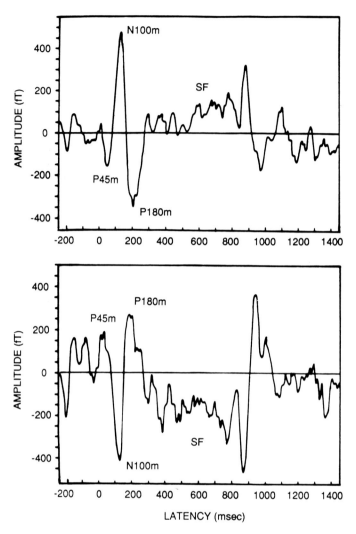

FIG. 4. Transient auditory responses over the right hemisphere for a 250-Hz tone of 800-msec duration, averaged over 100 epochs. Recorded over the posterior end (**upper panel**) and anterior end (**bottom panel**) of the sylvian fissure. (Adapted from ref. 1.)

mathematically by Swinney and Wikswo (20), who carried out numerical calculations for a realistic neural model that predicts the strengths of the fields from intracellular, transmembrane, and extracellular currents. Measurements on an isolated axon of the crayfish verify the theory (19).

The field from a single cell, or neuron, is too weak to detect outside the scalp by present sensors (22). Indeed, the typical neuromagnetic field strength outside the scalp requires that approximately 10^4 neurons contribute simultaneously. Although this may seem a large number, we should keep in mind that approximately 10^5 neurons lie under each square millimeter of cortex, so the total area of active cortex may be relatively small. As yet little is known of the exact distribution of active neurons that gives rise to neuromagnetic fields, so this estimate must be considered as very tentative.

NEURAL LOCALIZATION

Now we turn to examples of how neuromagnetic techniques have been applied with the notion that through source localization it is possible to reveal significant aspects of brain function, either normal or abnormal.

One example of such a functional map was provided by Romani et al. (17) who addressed the question as to whether humans have a tone map across the auditory cortex, that is, whether tones of different frequency evoked activity at different locations. They presented a tone whose amplitude was smoothly turned on and off at a rate of approximately 32 Hz and searched for a magnetic field that varied at this same rate. The resulting field patterns shown in Fig. 5 for four tones indicate that the distance separating the field extrema increases with increasing tone frequency. This shows directly that the source lies deeper within the sylvian fissure for tones of higher frequency. Indeed, there is a regular mathematical relationship between the distance separating one source from its neighbors: the distance across the cortex from one source to another increases as the logarithm of the frequency. This kind of tone map shows that each octave (factor of 2 in frequency) of the

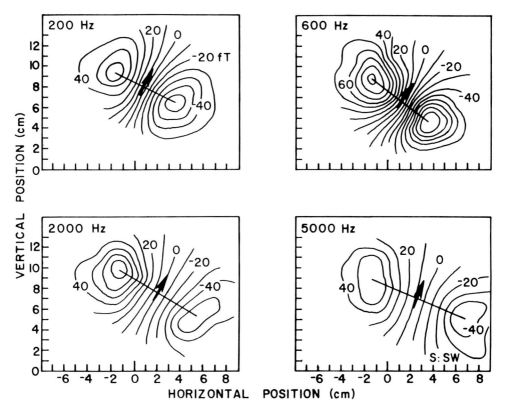

FIG. 5. Field patterns over the right hemisphere evoked by tones of the indicated frequencies. The origin of the coordinate system (0,0) is the ear canal, with the horizontal axis pointing toward the corner of the eye at (9,0) and vertical axis directed toward the top of the head. Values for the contours of constant field are indicated in femtotesla. Arrows denote the locations of the underlying sources, with the direction of each arrow showing the current direction. (From ref. 16.)

frequency scale spans an equal distance across the cortex, much like the arrangement of keys on a piano keyboard. One implication is that the human auditory cortex devotes the same number of neurons to each octave in frequency. This kind of study is just the first step toward a better understanding of how neural circuits are organized to provide our perception of sound.

OVERVIEW

In this brief survey of neuromagnetic recording we have emphasized source localization and resolution. Many observations support the theoretical notion that magnetic field patterns are generally more sharply confined over the active portion of the brain than are electric potential patterns. This implies that the task of identifying individual sources is made easier in cases where several sources are active in various regions of the brain. Indeed, all the evidence to date points to the source of the magnetic field as being the intracellular current in active neurons. In this sense the magnetic technique provides a direct measure of brain activity. The three-dimensional localization of a particular source is thus independent of the nature of intervening tissue, at least to a first approximation.

Finally, we should remark that both the magnetic and electrical techniques have limitations that may be largely overcome by using both techniques together. A limitation of the MEG is that it is insensitive to currents oriented perpendicular to the scalp; and a limitation of the EEG is the problem of separating patterns from different simultaneously active sources. One promising avenue to overcoming these difficulties is the four-step procedure in which the MEG is first analyzed to determine the underlying sources tangential to the scalp. The second step is to compute the scalp distribution of electric potential from these sources using a suitable head model. The third step is to subtract these predictions from the measured pattern of the EEG. And the fourth step is to identify the underlying sources of this pattern, which represents the effect of sources perpendicular to the scalp. Wood et al. (26) carried out such a four-step procedure with some success to analyze early activity in the primary somatosensory cortex evoked by electrical stimulation of the wrist.

In this brief presentation we have outlined the methods by which neuromagnetic studies can be used to determine the location in three dimensions of active regions of the auditory cortex. It is clear that the magnetic technique will play an increasingly important role in auditory research as a result of this localizing ability.

ACKNOWLEDGMENT

Supported in part by Air Force Office of Scientific Research grant F49620-85-K-0004.

REFERENCES

1. Arthur, D. L., Flynn, E. R., and Williamson, S. J. (1987): Source localization of long latency auditory evoked magnetic fields in human temporal cortex. *Electroencephalogr. Clin. Neurophysiol.*, Suppl. 40:429–439.

2. Baule, G. M., and McFee, R. (1963): Detection of the magnetic field of the heart. *Am. Heart J.*, 66:95–96.

3. Bleaney, B. I., and Bleaney, B. (1976): *Electricity and Magnetism*, 3rd ed. Oxford University Press, Oxford.

4. Brenner, D. Williamson, S. J., and Kaufman, L. (1975): Visually evoked magnetic fields of the human brain. *Science*, 190:480–482.

5. Brenner, D., Lipton, J., Kaufman, L., and Williamson, S. J. (1978): Somatically evoked magnetic fields of the human brain. *Science*, 199:81–83.

6. Cohen, D. (1968): Magnetoencephalography: Evidence of magnetic fields produced by alpha rhythm currents. *Science*, 161:784–786.

7. Cohen, D. (1972): Magnetoencephalography: Detection of the brain's electrical activity with a superconducting magnetometer. *Science*, 175:664–666.

8. Elberling, C., Bak, C., Kofoed, B., Lebech, J., and Saermark, K. (1981): Magnetic auditory responses from the human brain. *Scand. Audiol.*, 10:203–207.

9. Grynszpan, F., and Geselowitz, D. B. (1973): Model studies of the magnetocardiogram. *Biophys. J.*, 13:911–925.

10. Hari, R., Aittoniemi, K., Jarvinen, M.-L., Katila, T., and Varpula, T. (1980): Auditory evoked transient and sustained magnetic fields of the human brain. *Exp. Brain Res.*, 40:237–240.

11. Ilmoniemi, R., Hari, R., and Reinikainen, K. (1984): A four-channel SQUID magnetometer for brain research. *Electroencephalogr. Clin. Neurophysiol.*, 58:467–473.

12. Kelhä, V. O., Pukki, J. M., Peltonen, R. S., Penttinen, A., Ilmoniemi, R. J., and Heino, J. J. (1981): Design, construction, and performance of a large-volume magnetic shield. *IEEE Trans. Magn.*, MAG-18:260–270.

13. Pelizzone, M., Williamson, S. J., and Kaufman, L. (1985): Evidence for multiple areas in the human auditory cortex. In: *Biomagnetism: Applications and Theory*, edited by H. Weinberg, G. Stroink, and T. Katila, pp. 326–330. Pergamon Press, New York.

14. Reite, M., Eldrich, J., Zimmerman, J. T., and Zimmerman, J. E. (1979): Human magnetic auditory evoked fields. *Electroencephalogr. Clin. Neurophysiol.*, 45:114–117.

15. Romani, G. L., Williamson, S. J., and Kaufman, L. (1982): Biomagnetic instrumentation. *Rev. Sci. Instrum.*, 53:1815–1845.

16. Romani, G. L., Williamson, S. J., and Kaufman, L. (1982): Tonotopic organization of the human auditory cortex. *Science*, 216:1339–1340.

17. Romani, G. L., Williamson, S. J., Kaufman, L., and Brenner, D. (1982): Characterization of the human auditory cortex by the neuromagnetic method. *Exp. Brain Res.*, 47:381–393.

18. Romani, G. L., Leoni, R., and Salustri, C. (1985): Multichannel instrumentation for biomagnetism. In: *SQUID '85: Superconducting Quantum Interference Devices*, edited by H. D. Hahlbohm and H. Lübbig, pp. 919–932. Walter de Gruyter, Berlin.

19. Roth, R. J., and Wikswo, J. P., Jr. (1985): The magnetic field of a single axon. *Biophys. J.*, 48:93–109.

20. Swinney, K. R., and Wikswo, J. P., Jr. (1980): A calculation of the magnetic field of a nerve action potential. *Biophys. J.*, 32:719–731.

21. Teyler, T. J., Cuffin, B. N., and Cohen, D. (1975): The visual evoked magnetoencephalogram. *Life Sci.*, 17:683–692.

22. Tripp, J. H. (1981): Biomagnetic fields and current flow. In: *Biomagnetism*, edited by S. N. Erné, H. D. Hahlbohm, and H. Lübbig, pp. 207–215. Walter de Gruyter, Berlin.

23. Williamson, S. J., and Kaufman, L. (1981): Evoked cortical magnetic fields. In: *Biomagnetism*, edited by S. N. Erné, H. D. Hahlbohm, and H. Lübbig, pp. 353–402. Walter de Gruyter, Berlin.

24. Williamson, S. J., Romani, G. L., Kaufman, L., and Modena, I. (1983): *Biomagnetism: An Interdisciplinary Approach*. Plenum Press, New York.

25. Williamson, S. J., Pelizzone, M., Okada, Y., Kaufman, L., Crum, D. B., and Marsden, J. R. (1984): Magnetoencephalography with an array of SQUID sensors. In: *Proceedings of the Tenth Cryogenic Engineering Conference*, edited by H. Collan, P. Berglund, and M. Krusius, pp. 339–348. Butterworth, Guildford.

26. Wood, C. C., Cohen, D., Cuffin, B. N., Yarita, M., and Allison, T. (1985): Electrical sources in human somatosensory cortex: Identification by combined magnetic and potential recordings. *Science*, 227:1051–1053.

Physiology of the Ear,
edited by A. F. Jahn and J. Santos-Sacchi.
Raven Press, New York © 1988.

Auditory Brain Mapping

Frank H. Duffy

*Department of Neurology, Children's Hospital and Harvard Medical School,
Boston, Massachusetts 02115*

Dawson's 1950 report (15,32) of a human scalp-recorded response to peripheral nerve stimulation opened the era of the evoked potential (EP). Soon attention turned to the slow cortical responses evoked by acoustic stimuli as reviewed by Davis in 1965 (14). Nonetheless by 1969, according to Callaway (9), it was widely thought that such long latency EPs were only of limited clinical value, primarily for audiometry in neonates. The demonstration of the human far-field brainstem auditory EP (BAER, ABR) by Jewett and Williston in 1971 (40) focused attention on this short latency phenomenon. As is well known, the 5- to 10-msec ABR has proven a reliable clinical indicator of auditory and brainstem function and is now a test offered by most audiometry and clinical neurophysiology laboratories (10,13). The term far field arose because the recording electrodes placed on the scalp vertex and ear are far from the brainstem source of the electric field. With the advent of the ABR, attention shifted away from the long latency EP, especially the long latency auditory EP. Moreover, as summarized by Chiappa (10),

> long latency potentials often have poor waveform consistency among normal subjects and are easily altered by changes in many psychological variables, such as inattention and drowsiness. . . . changes thus induced in shape, amplitude and latency of the waveforms make it difficult to obtain consistent and reproducible results . . .

To a large extent the long latency AER became the focus of psychophysics laboratories whose interests were in the investigation of such effects and was dropped from clinical practice.

BRAIN ELECTRICAL ACTIVITY MAPPING

Topographic Mapping

Based in part on the critical observation of Jeffreys and Axford (39) that evoked potential components should be defined by their topographic distribution over the scalp as well as by their latency and polarity, we began our study of brain electrical activity mapping (BEAM) (19,21). We hypothesized that a major factor limiting extraction of clinically useful information from EEG and EP data was the inability of the human eye to discriminate the massive amounts of information contained within the apparently simple EP or EEG tracings. From the perspective of EP analysis,

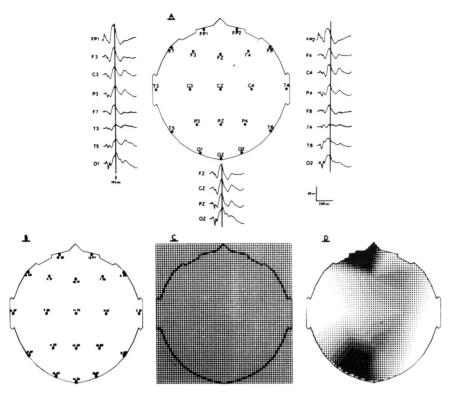

FIG. 1. Construction of topographic images from evoked potential data by the BEAM methodology. Example of the construction of a topographic map for EP data. Mean EPs are formed from each of 20 recording sites. Each EP is divided into 128 4-msec intervals, and the mean voltage value for each interval is calculated. In (**A**) the individual EPs are shown for the electrode locations indicated on the head diagram. In (**B**) the mean voltage values at these locations are shown for the interval beginning 192 msec after the stimulus (the vertical line in A indicates this time on the EPs). Next the head region is treated as a 64 × 64 matrix; the resulting 4,096 spatial domains are illustrated in (**C**). Each domain is assigned a voltage value by linear interpolation from the three nearest known points. Finally, for display, the raw voltage values are fitted to a discrete-level, equal-interval intensity scale as shown in (**D**). Although a VER is used to illustrate the mapping process, the same procedure is used for mapping other data including the AER.

the limiting factor appeared to be the mental gymnastics necessary to spatially map complex and interactive data from multiple electrode placements. The need to simultaneously integrate information from multiple channels in space and time constitutes a mental *tour de force*. A common solution for EP data has been to limit analyses to only one or at most a few electrodes. A consequence of this, of course, is the loss of spatial information.

Our goal, therefore, was to develop a method for topographic mapping and then devise a method for resynthesizing spatial and temporal aspects of the continuous data. As can be seen in Fig. 1, meaningful visualization of information from 20 scalp electrodes is greatly enhanced when represented as a topographic image. Then, to integrate the temporal aspects of the EP, serial topographic images are created and viewed by the cinematographic technique known as cartooning. In general, 128 images are utilized, each representing data summarizing 4 msec of the usual 512-msec poststimulus period. Any sampling schedule can, of course, be used. By means of such spatiotemporal representations, it is possible to see relationships that are otherwise invisible to the neurophysiologist.

Significance Probability Mapping

As we began to use BEAM to evaluate normal subjects and clinical patients, we became aware that it was often difficult to define normality and detect clinical abnormality by simple inspection of topographic images. For example, it was not altogether clear from visual inspection when an asymmetry was within normal limits and when it passed out of bounds. To solve this analytic deficiency, in 1981 we developed the technique of significance probability mapping (SPM) (20). This procedure, illustrated in Fig. 2, directly images statistical information and provides maps of where a subject differs from a normative data base (Z transform), where one group differs from another (t statistic), and where difference exists among three or more groups (F statistic). Virtually any statistic, e.g., Mahalanobis distance, principal components, Wilk's lambda, can be so mapped (12). In any case the goal is to image deviancy from some standard—usually data of a control group. SPM provides the clinician and researcher with an objective tool in the quest for detection of abnormality.

DATA GATHERING AND MANAGEMENT

All subjects are studied in a typical neurophysiology laboratory where both EEG and EP tests are performed. Twenty Grass gold cup scalp electrodes are applied with collodion in the standard 10–20 format as used for EEG (38). An additional four electrodes are applied to the face to permit monitoring and analyses of artifact (e.g., eye blink, eye movement, muscle activity, body movement, EKG). Data gathered for all clinical and most research studies include both EEG and EP states. Details of EEG data gathering, spectral analyses, visual EP, and associated topographic imaging techniques are covered elsewhere (21). The long latency AER is elicited by a minimum of 100 to a maximum of 500 tone pips delivered from earphones or loudspeakers placed on either side of the subject. Each pip consists of 50 msec of a 1,000-kHz sine wave with a 10-msec rise and fall time at intensity 92 db SPL. Resulting wave-shape amplitude and morphology of the long latency AER are relatively insensitive to tone pip parameters but are very sensitive to issues such as selective attention, level of consciousness, medication, and time-locked artifact (muscle spike or blink). Accordingly the EEG paper tracing is continued throughout tone pip presentation so as to ensure alertness, awakeness, and freedom from artifact. Stimulus presentation is often interrupted by the technologist to assure alertness. If the subject appears drowsy s/he is allowed to sleep for 15 to 30 minutes after which s/he is briskly walked down the corridor and given tea or coffee to drink before the study is continued. The study is performed with eyes closed to diminish random and/or time-locked eye blink.

On occasion we use a more complex stimulus to evoke the AER. The two words "tyke" and "tight," which differ only by one phoneme, were processed by computer to be alike in amplitude and duration. These words, randomly alternated, are used as stimuli. A task is superimposed in which we ask the subject to count the number

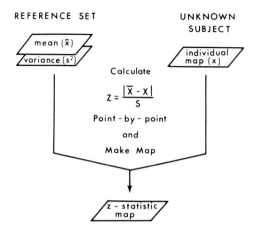

REFERENCE SET

mean ($\bar{x}$)
variance (s^2)

UNKNOWN SUBJECT

individual map (x)

Calculate

$$Z = \frac{|\bar{x} - x|}{S}$$

Point – by – point

and

Make Map

z – statistic map

A UNKNOWN vs REFERENCE

SET 1

map 1
+
map 2
+
.
.
.
+
map n

Sum

Individual

Maps

Point – by – point

SET 2

map 1
+
map 2
+
.
.
.
+
map n

Calculate Mean

and Variance

and

Make Maps

set 1 mean
variance

set 2 mean
variance

Calculate t – Statistic

and

Make Map

t – statistic map

B SET 1 vs SET 2

FIG. 2. Topographic imaging of abnormality: SPM. **A** demonstrates the formation of a Z-statistic SPM. The Z transform represents the number of SDs by which an individual's observations differs from the mean of a reference set. For BEAM, the Z statistic is calculated individually for each of the 20 to 32 scalp electrodes between the data of a subject and those of a normative control population. The resulting 20 to 32 Z values are then interpolated according to the procedure shown in Fig. 1 to produce the Z-SPM. The product is a display of a subject's deviation from normal in units of standard deviation in such a way that the spatial relations of the original BEAM image are retained. Z-SPM are ordinarily used in clinical practice to define abnormality in individual subjects. **B** demonstrates the formation of a t-statistic SPM. Student's t statistic quantifies the separation between two sets of measures, taking into account not only the difference between the mean value of each group but also the variability within each group. Thus the t value is lower for the same difference in group mean when the variance in either or both groups increases. For BEAM, the t statistic is calculated individually for each of the 20 to 32 scalp electrodes between the data from one group of subjects and those from another group. The resulting 20 to 32 t values are then mapped as per Fig. 1 to produce the t-SPM. The product is a topographic display of where the brain electrical activity of one group differs from that of another. Ordinarily t-SPM are used in research to delineate where a pathologic population differs from a control population.

of "tykes" for the first half of the session and "tights" for the second half. All responses are averaged to form the resulting tight-tyke auditory evoked response (TTAER).

During the study, the voltage level is adjusted to reject segments containing high-voltage artifact (usually blink, movement, or muscle). It is particularly important to situate the subject to minimize, or preferably eliminate, muscle tension artifact. Bickford and colleagues (4–6,11,37) clearly showed that, when high-intensity click stimuli are given during periods of increased neck muscle tension, time-locked myogenic potentials (part of a microreflex system) may contaminate the early portions of the long latency AER.

A minimum of five separate averages of just more than 100 responses each are superimposed and visually inspected. If there is reasonable wave-shape coincidence, they are averaged together to form single EPs from each electrode.

RESEARCH EXAMPLES

The short latency ABR serves two functions. It is used as a specific probe of the auditory system from peripheral receptor to thalamus. It also serves as a less specific but nonetheless clinically important probe of brainstem function. Indeed there is clinically useful correspondence among ABR components I-V and brainstem nuclear gray matter. The ABR is a primary neurophysiologic probe of subthalamic function (10).

The long latency AER complements the value of the ABR in that it appears to be derived from hemispheric generators above the level of the thalamus. As such, the AER is considered a probe of cortical function. Unfortunately the hemispheric generators of the human AER remain undetermined and no doubt complex. Arezzo et al. (1) reported that in the primate even the earliest AER components appear to be derived from multiple complex generators. Thus the AER does not share with the ABR established relationships to specific underlying brain anatomical structures. At best, the AER can be modeled as being derived from four dipole sources, one anterior and one posterior in each temporal lobe (51).

Despite uncertainty as to its specific origins, the long latency AER has seen considerable use in research where it functions as general probe of cortical auditory function. We will show examples in dyslexia and schizophrenia research in which the AER has been used productively in conjunction with topographic mapping.

Dyslexia

Our first application was to the area of developmental reading disability. We undertook an evaluation of children with developmental dyslexia, an entity not known to have fixed lesions demonstrable by CT scan. To assess the potential of our technique, we attempted to look at a very restricted question: Would it be possible for us to determine meaningful regional topographic differences in brain electrical activity between control subjects and a very restricted group of dyslexic persons? To eliminate extraneous variables, we limited our study to boys aged 10 to 12 years, most of whom were right-handed and all of whom suffered only from dyslexia. All selected children were more than 1.5 years retarded in age-expected reading ability but were free of attentional deficit disorder or other forms of learning disability, "hard" neurologic findings, psychiatric disturbance, or epilepsy. We analyzed these children by means of both EEG and EP paradigms ranging, in each condition, from the simple passive state to the highly activated state where cognitive or language tasks were demanded of the subject while under observation. To accomplish data analysis, we used the SPM technique. The task was to compare two groups, normal boys and dyslexic boys. The appropriate statistical measure of between-group difference was Student's *t*-test; thus controls and dyslexics were compared for a given condition by means of a topographic display of the t statistic, known as the t-SPM. The function of the t-SPM was to delineate graphically regions of between-group difference (20,22).

Given the strong association of dyslexia with other disorders of language and communication, it was pleasing that regional differences were demonstrated in response to auditory stimulation. Differences occurred predominantly overlying the left posterior lateral hemisphere regions most often associated with language function. Between-group difference was also found in the central parietal mid- and posterior temporal areas, extending back almost to the occipital region on the left, regions known to produce aphasia when lesioned.

Using blood flow mapping techniques, Larsen and Lassen and colleagues (42,43) demonstrated cerebral activation in normal subjects when reading silently or aloud that coincided almost exactly with the regional differences found in our study of dyslexic boys by AER and other means. We concluded from these results that dyslexia appears to represent dysfunction in the entire area normally involved in language function and that this system was more widely distributed than commonly appreciated. Figure 3 shows regional difference between our normal and dyslexic boys for the click AER and a more complex TTAER.

Schizophrenia

There is a growing literature on specifically lateralized or localized abnormalities in schizophrenia. This research has utilized such techniques as cerebral blood flow measurements (27,33–35), positron emission tomography (PET) (8,24,58), and CT scans (57) to elucidate abnormalities of brain structure and function. The CT scan is an excellent tool for studying brain anatomy but is not capable of revealing brain function. PET scans and cerebral blood flow studies suffer from the disadvantage of being invasive and of requiring the subject to maintain a particular state for relatively long periods of time. These latter disadvantages are particularly problematic when dealing with schizophrenic patients. Thus investigators have turned to neurophysiology, which has the advantages of measuring brain function and being noninvasive and relatively inexpensive. Although most studies, including our own, have emphasized EEG (25,26,29,36,45,47) others have found interesting changes with EP data (7,50,52) again including our own studies (45,46).

In our study, where both medicated and unmedicated schizophrenics were compared with age-matched normative controls, EEG and visually evoked response (VER) data demonstrated frontal and left hemispheric differences by t-SPM (45). These findings were in accord with the frontal lobe changes in metabolic activity reported by Ingvar and Franzen (34) and supported the notion of hypofrontality.

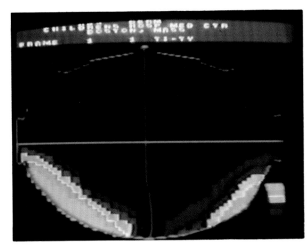

FIG. 3. Electrophysiologic difference in dyslexia-pure: a summary t-SPM. This t-SPM summarizes the results of our original study of boys with dyslexia pure (see text). Data are shown within a schematic map of the head in vertex view with nose above, occiput below, left ear to left and right ear to right. Only those regions achieving a two-tailed t value corresponding to the $P < 0.02$ level are shown. These regions demonstrate where dyslexic boys, as a group, differ from nondyslexic boys. Note the prominent involvement of the left temporal-parietal regions and to a much lesser degree the right. These regions were demonstrated by the click and "tight-tyke" AER. In our initial study the left anterior and medial frontal differences were delineated by EEG data. In subsequent work we found AER differences in these regions as well.

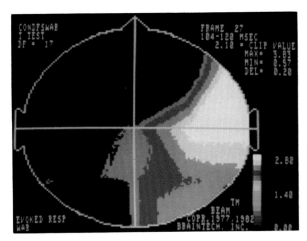

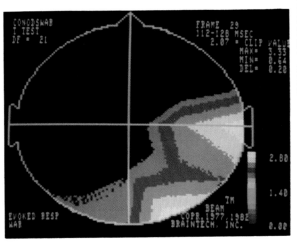

FIG. 4. Right hemispheric group difference by topographic AER in schizophrenia. Both images are t-SPM that delineate difference between a group of schizophrenic patients and age-matched control subjects. **A** illustrates group difference between drug-free schizophrenics during the 104- to 124-msec latency epoch of the long latency AER ($t_{max} = 3.83$). **B** illustrates a similar difference between medicated schizophrenics and controls for 112 to 132 msec of the AER ($t_{max} = 3.33$). The AER was uniquely useful in detecting right hemispheric differences in schizophrenia (see text).

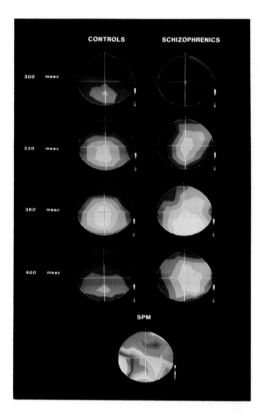

FIG. 5. Left hemispheric group difference in schizophrenia by the click-elicited P300. The topographic distribution of P300 activity at 300, 320, 360, and 400 msec after stimulus for both the control and medicated schizophrenic population. Scaling of colors was adjusted to allow topography in lower amplitude schizophrenic group to be clearly visible; color scale ranges from −5 to +5 uV in controls and −2 to +2 uV in schizophrenics. Lowest (negative) values are represented by blues; larger (positive) values, by reds, yellows, and white, in that order. Compared with controls, P300 development in schizophrenics shows maxima that are displaced anteriorly and to the right and deficiency of activity in left temporal region. At the bottom, the significance probability map (see text) shows regions of maximal separation between schizophrenic and control groups. Lowest t values are shown by blues, with larger values indicated by yellows, reds, and white, in that order. White codes regions containing t values greater than 2.10. Maximal separation occurred at left middle and posterior temporal electrode sites.

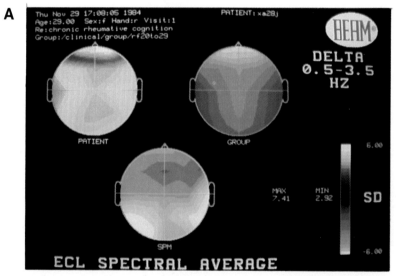

FIG. 6. Left posterior temporal abnormality in a patient with temporal lobe epilepsy personality syndrome. Three Z-statistic SPM are shown for a 29-year-old woman with the presenting complaint of "chronic ruminative condition" and the final diagnosis of temporal lobe epilepsy personality syndrome. Three sets of three BEAM images are shown. Within each set the patient data are shown at the upper left, the control data at the upper right, and the corresponding Z-SPM below. **A** shows globally augmented 0.5 to 3.5 Hz delta maximal in both posterior temporal regions (left > right) reaching a maximum Z value of 7.41 SD. *(Fig. 6 continues on page 514A.)*

Left parietal-posterior temporal differences supported Sherwin's findings (53) from a study of behaviorally disturbed temporal lobe epileptics that psychosis has its origins in the left hemisphere.

Surprisingly, the AER in our study (45) highlighted right hemispheric difference, as shown in Fig. 4.

It is of interest that a topographically extensive difference was found between schizophrenics (medicated and unmedicated) and normal controls in the right central temporal region only during the auditory EP. The physiologic significance of this finding is not clear. Neuropsychologic studies are now being performed to search for meaningful correlates of these unexpected right hemispheric findings. Although the meaning of the finding is not yet clarified, the value of the long latency AER combined with mapping in elucidating neurophysiologic data is clearly demonstrated.

In another study (46) we examined the P300 in schizophrenics. The P300 is a late component of the human EP that is elicited by stimuli, in any modality, that are both relevant to the subject and surprising (16). It is positive in amplitude and usually has a latency in the range of 250 to 450 msec. Investigators agree that this P300 provides some index or correlate of the brain's response to changes in attended stimuli. Study of this wave, therefore, is of great importance in schizophrenia, a disease in which the fundamental disorder may be the brain's inability to focus on relevant stimuli. The P300 latency has been correlated with stimulus evaluation time (16), and its amplitude with the probability of occurrence and the task relevance of a stimulus, as well as the motivation of the subject (17,23,55).

Several related cognitive models of the P300 have been proposed. Donchin (18) suggested that the P300 is a manifestation of the process whereby an unexpected event leads to a subject's revising his or her hypothesis about what is expected in the environment. Posner (49) postulated that the P300 correlates with the activity of a limited-capacity system and is intimately related to the degree of conscious effort expended in processing a signal. In fact, there is probably a family of late positive waves, some of which may be related to an orienting response and others to more selective attentional and cognitive processes (56).

The paradigm used in our research for evoking and defining the P300 component was based on that of Goodin et al. (30). This paradigm has the advantage of taking into account any effects of the unattended "oddball" stimulus and subtracting out all components and any time-locked artifacts common to the attended and unattended conditions. We recorded auditory EPs after infrequent high-pitched (1,070 Hz) and frequent low-pitched (960 Hz) tone pips.

The major finding, shown in Fig. 5, is that the wave form in the schizophrenics had a persistent deficiency of activity in the left middle and posterior temporal regions throughout its development (46). The amplitude of the schizophrenic P300 over the left temporal lobe was reduced. To our knowledge, these findings provide the first evidence for asymmetric topographic development of the P300 in schizophrenia. Many studies have pointed to a left hemispheric abnormality in schizophrenics, and these P300 findings support that hypothesis (48).

Depth recordings in epileptics have indicated that the P300 appears to be generated from subcortical structures (59) and in particular the hippocampus and amygdala (31), findings that are supported by brain electromagnetic studies (41).

Our P300 findings, therefore, point to a disturbance in the function of the limbic system of the left hemisphere in schizophrenia. This is consistent with neurochemical evidence (44,54) that limbic system disturbances are important in the etiology of schizophrenia.

These data emphasize the important role that the AER and its relative the P300 may play in electrophysiologic investigations of brain function that employ topographic mapping.

CLINICAL EXAMPLES

For the past 4 years BEAM has been offered by our laboratory as a clinical test. We have performed approximately 1,500 clinical studies and are currently performing 500 per year, limited only by the availability of technical help and equipment. Each study produces an extensive EEG polygraphic record that is classically analyzed. In addition, data recorded during the "eyes open alert" and "eyes closed alert" states are spectrally analyzed (after artifact removal), topographically mapped, and compared with an age appropriate normative data base (Z-SPM) to delineate abnormalities. The long latency flash VER and click AER are similarly generated, mapped, and compared with normative data. In our experience this combination of traditional EEG reading and modern quantitative topographic analysis has greatly enhanced the clinical value of neurophysiologic data.

As one might anticipate, patients are referred largely by neurologists and psychiatrists. We do not employ our technique to diagnose patients. Instead BEAM studies provide critical pieces of information to assist in the formation of a diagnosis by the referring clinician. BEAM does not diagnose dyslexia or schizophrenia. Moreover, such specific questions are seldom put to BEAM. Rather most studies are searches for unexpected neurophysiologic abnormality of a sort that might alter clinical thoughts about diagnosis. For example, most classic schizophrenics have near-normal brain electrical activity. If a patient referred with the diagnosis of schizophrenia were to show unusual and abnormal brain activity, this might suggest an unexpected organic etiology.

To illustrate the clinical use(s) of BEAM (especially the contribution of the long latency AER), several case examples are presented.

Temporal Lobe Epilepsy Personality

A 29-year-old woman was referred because of "chronic ruminative syndrome." She was being seen by a psychiatrist for refractory, chronic depression. Her standard EEG was read as probably normal; however, her spectral analysis topography revealed increased bilateral posterior temporal slowing, left more than right (Fig. 6A). The long latency VER strongly implicated the left parietal and left posterior temporal regions (Fig. 6B). The long latency AER also demonstrated a major left posterior temporal abnormality (Fig. 6C).

As such focal findings should not be seen in simple depression, she was referred for neurologic consultation to rule out organic pathology. Her subsequent CT scan was normal. Detailed historical review revealed, for the first time, three spells suggestive of partial complex epilepsy. Although the classic neurologic examination was normal, she was very serious, loquacious, and completely preoccupied with moral issues. Historically she admitted to keeping a detailed diary, and although she

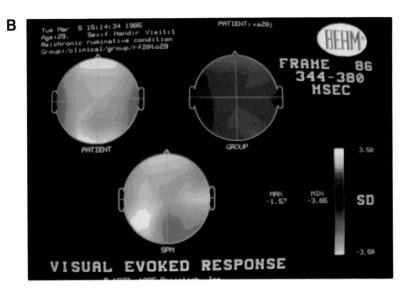

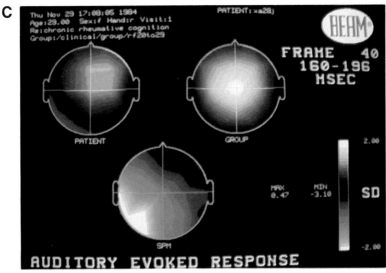

FIG. 6. (*continued*) **B** shows augmented negative activity of the VER from 344 to 380 msec by 3.65 SD in the left posterior temporal/parietal region. **C** shows augmented left posterior temporal/parietal activity of the AER from 160 to 196 msec. These three spatially congruent abnormalities lead to the recognition of an electrophysiologic abnormality and eventually the collection of complex historical data to synthesize the clinically important diagnosis (see text).

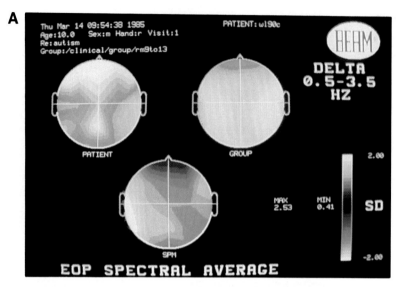

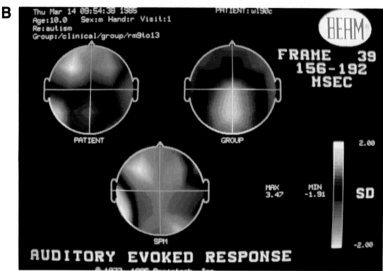

FIG. 7. Left temporal abnormality in an autistic with language difficulty. Two sets of three BEAM images according to the convention of Fig. 6 are shown. Data are shown for a 10-year-old boy with autism. Note in **A** the increased left temporal 0.5- to 3.5-Hz delta activity by 2.53 SD. In **B** there is regionally aberrant AER positive activity in the 156- to 192-msec epoch by 3.47 SD. Such regional abnormalities are often seen in autism (see text).

denied a religious conversion, she admitted dwelling on religious issues. Her sexual behavior swung between periods of complete inactivity to intensive overactivity. In short she demonstrated all the features of the "personality of temporal lobe epilepsy syndrome" as described by Bear (2,3), e.g., hyperlexia, hypergraphia, religious preoccupation, absence of a sense of humor associated with extreme seriousness and hypo/hypersexuality. Bear suggested that the syndrome resulted from temporal lobe (limbic system) overactivity produced by subclinical epileptic activity.

The repetitive BEAM abnormalities in the same location served to draw attention to the left posterior temporal region (Fig. 6). Had it not been for these convincing electrophysiologic abnormalities, it is unlikely that her syndrome would have been recognized. The AER findings were crucial in that they provided confirmation of regional abnormality also shown by the spectral EEG and VER data. She has responded well to anticonvulsant therapy.

Autism

The 10-year-old son of a successful businessman was referred for evaluation of autism. Since childhood he had demonstrated classic manifestations of autism, including diminished eye contact, preference for objects over people, repetitive movements including circular rotation, and pronoun reversal (28). He had been placed in intensive behavioral therapy with excellent results. Eye contact was excellent and his interactive skills had improved. Nonetheless he continued to show expressive and receptive language difficulties. He was referred for a BEAM study, the results of which are summarized in Fig. 7. Note the augmented (abnormal) left temporal delta (Fig. 7A) and abnormal left posterior temporal AER activity (Fig. 7B). In our experience (*unpublished data*), left temporal abnormalities are common in autism and may explain the language difficulties that are often uncovered in these children as they mature and become more interactive.

In autism the AER has proven to be one of the more important delineators of regional electrophysiologic abnormality.

Dyslexia in the Adult

A 41-year-old male was referred by a behavioral neurologist for confirmation of a history of childhood dyslexia. Current neurologic examination revealed little to support the past history of apparent reading disability, as the patient had eventually acquired slightly above average reading skills.

The BEAM examination revealed normal classic EEG, spectral EEG, and VER analysis. The AER, however, was abnormal in the left parietal and posterior temporal regions over two 40-msec epochs (Fig. 8A and B). Such left posterior findings, limited to the AER, are consistent with the clinical history of dyslexia (22). Here the AER served as a unique indicator of a minor but persisting neurophysiologic abnormality.

SUMMARY AND CONCLUSIONS

Topographic mapping of brain electrical activity has proven a useful adjunct to electrophysiologic studies from both the research and clinical perspectives. As we have illustrated, its use in research is to delineate topographically specific between- or among-groups differences to enhance an understanding of regional brain difference. The AER serves as a probe of hemispheric function. In several studies auditory stimulation has produced results not seen by analyses of EEG or VER data.

From the clinical perspective, studies of individual patients yield data useful in establishing a clinical diagnosis. As illustrated, the technique is not intended to replace the clinician by performing stand-alone automated diagnosis. Indeed the three dissimilar case histories all indicated left posterior AER abnormalities. As demonstrated, BEAM data are of maximum value when evaluated in the light of full historical information and need to be interpreted by skilled neurophysiologists. Quantification, mapping, and statistical comparison with normative data serve to improve the visibility of information contained within scalp-recorded electrophysiologic data and enhance its sensitivity and utility in clinical diagnosis.

REFERENCES

1. Arezzo, J. A., Pickoff, A., and Vaughan, H. G. J. (1975): The sources and intracerebral distribution of auditory evoked potentials in the alert rhesus monkey. *Brain Res.*, 90:57–73.
2. Bear, D. M. (1979): Temporal lobe epilepsy—a syndrome of sensory-limbic hyperconnection. *Cortex*, 15:357–384.
3. Bear, D. M., and Fedio, P. (1977): Quantitative analysis of interictal behavior in temporal lobe epilepsy. *Arch. Neurol.*, 34:454–467.
4. Bickford, R. G. (1968): Properties of the microreflex system—human and animal studies. *Proc. Int. Union Physiol. Sci.*, VII.
5. Bickford, R. G., Cody, D. T., Jacobsen, J. L., and Lambert, E. H. (1964): Fast motor systems in man: Physiopathology of the sonomotor response. *Trans. Am. Neurol. Assoc.*, 89:56–58.
6. Bickford, R. G., Jacobson, J. L., and Cody, D. T. (1964): Nature of average evoked potentials to sound and other stimuli in man. *Ann. NY Acad. Sci.*, 112:204–223.
7. Buchsbaum, M. (1979): Neurophysiological aspects of the schizophrenic syndrome. In: *Disorders of the Schizophrenic Syndrome*, edited by L. Belak. Basic Books, New York.
8. Buchsbaum, M. S., Ingvar, D. H., Kessler, R., et al. (1982): Cerebral glucography with positron tomography. Use in normal subjects and in patients with schizophrenia. *Arch. Gen. Psychiatry*, 39:251–259.
9. Callaway, E. (1969): Diagnostic uses of the averaged evoked potential. In: *Average Evoked Potentials*, edited by E. Donchin. NASA, Washington, DC.
10. Chiappa, K. H. (1983): *Evoked Potentials in Clinical Medicine.* Raven Press, New York.
11. Cody, D. T., Jacobson, J. L., Walker, J. C., and Bickford, R. G. (1964): Averaged evoked myogenic and cortical potentials to sound in man. *Ann. Otol.*, 73:763–777.
12. Cooley, W. W., and Lohnes, P. R. (1971): *Multivariate Data Analysis*, John Wiley, New York.
13. Cracco, R. Q., and Bodis-Wollner, I. (1986): *Frontiers of Clinical Neuroscience III: Evoked Potentials.* Alan R. Liss, New York.
14. Davis, H. (1965): Slow cortical responses evoked by acoustic stimuli. *Acta Otolaryngol. (Stockh.)*, 59:179–185.
15. Dawson, G. D. (1950): Cerebral responses to nerve stimulation in man. *Br. Med. Bull.*, 6:326–329.
16. Donchin, E. (1979): Event-related brain potentials: A tool in the study of human information processing. In: *Evoked Brain Potentials and Behavior*, edited by H. Begleiter. Plenum Press, New York.
17. Donchin, E., and Cohen, L. (1967): Average evoked potentials and intramodality selective attention. *Electroencephalogr. Clin. Neurophysiol.*, 22:537–546.
18. Donchin, E., Ritter, W., and McCallum, W. C. (1978): Cognitive psychophysiology: The endogenous components of the ERP. In: *Event-Related Brain Potentials in Man*, edited by E. Callaway. Academic Press, New York.
19. Duffy, F. H. (1982): Topographic display of evoked potentials: Clinical applications of brain electrical activity mapping (BEAM). *Ann. NY Acad. Sci.*, 388:183–196.
20. Duffy, F. H., Bartels, P. H., and Burchfiel, J. L. (1981): Significance probability mapping: An aid in the topographic analysis of brain electrical activity. *Electroencephalogr. Clin. Neurophysiol.*, 51:455–462.

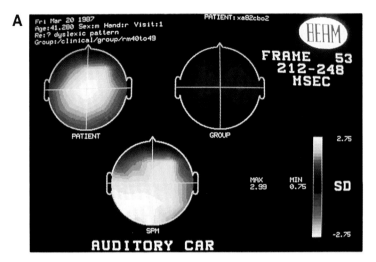

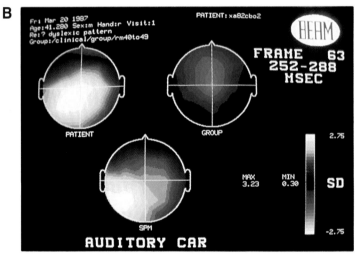

FIG. 8. Abnormal left temporal AER topography in an adult dyslexic. Two sets of three BEAM images are shown as for Fig. 6. Note the augmented left posterior-temporal/parietal AER positive activity for 212 to 248 msec (**A**) and 252 to 288 msec (**B**). The patient is a 41-year-old former dyslexic. Such AER abnormalities are characteristics of adult dyslexia (see text).

21. Duffy, F. H., Burchfiel, J. L, and Lombroso, C. T. (1979). Brain electrical activity mapping (BEAM): A method for extending the clinical utility of EEG and evoked potential data. *Ann. Neurol.*, 5:309–321.
22. Duffy, F. H., Denckla, M. B., Bartels, P., and Sandini, G. (1980): Dyslexia: Regional differences in brain electrical activity by topographic mapping. *Ann. Neurol.*, 7:412–420.
23. Duncan-Johnson, C. C., and Donchin, E. (1977): On quantifying surprise: The variation in event-related potentials with subjective probability. *Psychophysiology*, 14:456–467.
24. Farkas, T., Reivich, M., and Alavi, A. E. A. (1980): The application of F-deoxy-2-fluoro-D-glucose and positron emission tomography in the study of psychiatric conditions. In: *Cerebral Metabolism and Neural Function*, edited by J. V. Passonneau. Williams and Wilkins, Baltimore.
25. Fenton, G. W., Fenwick, P. B. C., and Dollimore, J. E. A. (1980): EEG spectral analysis in schizophrenia. *Br. J. Psychiatry*, 136:445–455.
26. Flor-Henry, P. (1976): Lateralized temporal-limbic dysfunction and psychopathology. *Ann. NY Acad. Sci.*, 280:777–797.
27. Franzen, G., and Ingvar, D. H. (1975): Absence of activation in frontal structures during psychological testing of chronic schizophrenics. *J. Neurol. Neurosurg. Psychiatry*, 38:1027–1032.
28. Garfield, E. (1982): Autism: Few answers for a baffling disease. *Current Contents*, 7:5–15.
29. Giannitrapini, D., and Kayton, L. (1974): Schizophrenic and EEG spectral analysis. *Electroencephalogr. Clin. Neurophysiol.*, 36:377–386.
30. Goodin, D. S., Squires, K. S., Henderson, B. H., and Starr, A. (1978): Age-related variations in evoked potentials to auditory stimuli in normal human subjects. *Electroencephalogr. Clin. Neurophysiol.*, 44:447–458.
31. Halgren, E., Squires, N. K., Wilson, C. L., Rohrbaugh, J., Babb, T, and Crandall, P. (1980): Endogenous potentials generated in the human hippocampal formation and amygdala by infrequent events. *Science*, 210:803–805.
32. Halliday. A. M. (1987): Fourth Dawson Memorial Lecture. *Clin. Evoked Potentials*, 5:2–10.
33. Ingvar, D. H. (1980): Abnormal distribution of cerebral activity in chronic schizophrenia: A neurophysiological interpretation. In: *Perspectives in Schizophrenia Research*, edited by C. Baxter and T. Melnechuk. Raven Press, New York.
34. Ingvar, D. H., and Franzen, G. (1974): Abnormalities of cerebral blood flow distribution in patients with chronic schizophrenia. *Acta Psychiatr. Scand.*, 50:425–462.
35. Ingvar, D. H., and Franzen, G. (1974): Distribution of cerebral activity in chronic schizophrenia. *Lancet*, ii:1484–1486.
36. Itil, T. H. (1977): Qualitative and quantitative EEG findings in schizophrenia. *Schizophr. Bull.*, 3:61–79.
37. Jacobson, J. L., Cody, D. T., Lambert, E. H., and Bickford, R. G. (1964): Physiological properties of the post-auricular response (sonomotor) in man. *Physiologist*, 7:167.
38. Jasper, H. H. (1958): The ten-twenty system of the International Federation. *Electroencephalogr. Clin. Neurophysiol.*, 10:371–375.
39. Jeffreys, D. A., and Axford, J. G. (1972): Source locations of pattern-specific components of human visual evoked potentials. *Exp. Brain Res.*, 16:1–40.
40. Jewett, D. L., and Williston, J. S. (1971): Auditory-evoked far fields averaged from the scalp of humans. *Brain*, 94:681–696.
41. Kaufman, L., and Williamson, S. J. (1982): Magnetic location of cortical activity. *Ann. NY Acad. Sci.*, 388:197–213.
42. Larsen, B., Skinhoj, E., and Lassen, N. A. (1978): Variations in regional cortical blood flow in the right and left hemispheres during automatic speech. *Brain*, 101:193–210.
43. Lassen, N. A., Ingvar, D. H., and Skinhoj, E. (1978): Brain function and blood flow. *Sci. Am.*, 239:62–71.
44. Mesulum, M. M., and Geschwind, N. (1978): On the possible role of neocortex and its limbic connections in the process of attention and schizophrenia: Clinical cases of inattention in man and experimental anatomy in monkey. *J. Psychiatr. Res.*, 14:249–259.
45. Morihisa, J. M., Duffy, F. H., and Wyatt, R. J. (1983): Brain electrical activity mapping (BEAM). In: *Investigation of Schizophrenia in Brain Imaging, in Psychiatry, and Neurology: PETT and Other Specific Techniques*, edited by M. Buchsbaum, E. Usdin, W. Bunney, and D. Ingvar. Boxwood/Synapse, Pacific Grove, CA.
46. Morstyn, R., Duffy, F. H., and McCarley, R. W. (1983): Altered P300 topography in schizophrenia. *Arch. Gen. Psychiatry*, 40:729–734.
47. Morstyn, R., Duffy, F. H., and McCarley, R. W. (1983): Altered topography of EEG spectral content in schizophrenia. *Electroencephalogr. Clin. Neurophysiol.*, 65:263–271.
48. Newlin, D. B., Carpenter, B., and Golden, C. J. (1981): Hemisphere asymmetries in schizophrenia. *Biol. Psychiatry*, 16:561–582.
49. Posner, M. I. (1975). Psychobiology of attention. In: *Handbook of Psychobiology*, edited by M. S. Gazzaniga. Academic Press, New York.

50. Roth, W. T. (1977): Late event related potentials and psychopathology. *Schizophr. Bull.*, 3:105–120.
51. Scherg, M., and Von Cramon, D. (1985): Two bilateral sources of the late AEP as identified by a spatio-temporal dipole model. *Electroencephalogr. Clin. Neurophysiol.*, 62:32–44.
52. Shagass, C., Roemer, R. A., and Straumanis, J. (1979): Temporal variability of somatosensory, visual, and auditory evoked potentials in schizophrenia. *Arch. Gen. Psychiatry*, 36:1341–1351.
53. Sherwin, I., Peron-Magnan, P., and Bancaud, J. (1982): Prevalence of psychoses in epilepsy as a function of the laterality of the epileptogenic lesion. *Arch. Neurol.*, 39:621–625.
54. Stevens, J. R. (1973): An anatomy of schizophrenia? *Arch. Gen. Psychiatry*, 29:177–189.
55. Sutton, S., Tueting, P., and Hammer, M. (1978): Evoked potentials and feedback. In: *Multidisciplinary Perspectives in Event-Related Brain Potential Research*, edited by D. A. Otto. Environmental Protection Agency, Washington, DC.
56. Tueting, P. (1978): Event-related potentials, cognitive events, and information processing: A summary of issues and discussion. In: *Multidisciplinary Perspectives in Event-Related Brain Potential Research*, edited by D. A. Otto. Environmental Protection Agency, Washington, DC.
57. Weinberger, D. R., and Wyatt, R. J. (1980): Structural brain abnormalities in chronic schizophrenia: Computer tomography findings. In: *Perspectives in Schizophrenia Research*, edited by C. F. Baxter and T. Melnechuk. Raven Press, New York.
58. Widen, L., Bergstrom, M., and Blomquist, C. (1981): Glucose metabolism in patients with schizophrenia: Emission computed tomography measurements with C-glucose. International Congress of Biological Psychiatry, Stockholm, Sweden.
59. Wood, C. C., Allison, T., and Goff, W. R. E. A. (1980): On the neural origin of P300 in man. *Prog. Brain Res.*, 54:51–56.

Subject Index

A

Acetylcholine, as efferent cochlear neurotransmitter, 394–396

Acetylcholinesterase, efferent nerve terminal location, 395

Acoustical stimuli coding. *See* Sound stimuli coding

Acoustic input, definition, 37

Acoustic meatus, external. *See* Ear canal, external

Acoustic spatial information, neural coding, 415–418
  azimuth/interaural disparity magnitude and, 415–416
  cerebral hemispheres and, 417–418
  free-field studies, 416,417,418
  lateral superior olivary nucleus and, 417
  pinna and, 415–416

Actin
  filamentous, 53,189
  hair cell content, 187,463,464,465
  spiral ligament content, 195

α-Actinin, spiral ligament content, 195

Adaptation, to sound stimuli, 365–367
  by cochlear nerve, 365–367
  in sound stimuli coding development, 440,444
  in temporal coding, 440,444

Adenosine, as hair cell neurotransmitter, 399

Adenosine triphosphate, as hair cell neurotransmitter, 399

Admittance, in cochlear impedance, 111–112,113,115–116,117,121

Adrenergic nerve plexus, of inner ear, 214–215

Aesculapius, 1,8

Afferent neurons
  of cochlea, 201–210
    adaptation, 365–367
    axoplasm structure, 205
    electrophysiology, 359–384
    innervation density, 201,202–203
    number, 201
    peripheral distribution, 202–205
    type I neurons, 201,202,203,205,206, 207–208,209,210
    type II neurons, 201–202,203,205, 206–207,208,210

of cochlear nerve, 359–384
  axons, 359
  broadband click stimuli response, 368
  combination tones response, 370–371
  discharge rate changes, 365
  intensity coding, 365
  nerve fiber responses, 360–371
  noise masking, 370
  noise stimuli response, 368–370
  in pathological cochleas, 363,376–380
  phase locking, 367–368,369–370,376
  pure tone response, 360–364
  resting activity, 360,361
  speech sounds response, 371–376
  temporal coding, 367–368
  tonotopic arrangement, 359
  two-tone suppression, 370,371
of vestibular system, 215–216, 466–467

Afferent synaptic transmission, cochlear
  hair cell glutamate hypothesis, 387–394
  neurotransmitters, 385–394

Alcmaeon, 2

Alexandria, anatomists of, 4–5

Alpha antagonists, cochlear blood flow effects, 332

Aminoadipate, hair cell neurotransmission and, 390–391,392–393

Aminoglycoside antibiotics, hair cell and, 492–493

Amniotes, auditory nerve regeneration in, 479–481

Anastomosis
  arteriovenous, 328
  of Oort, 176,210,211

Angiotensin II, cochlear blood flow effects, 329–330,332

Annular ligament, 226,227

Anteroventral cochlear nuclei, 407,408–410,412
  bushy cells, 410
  frequency selectivity, 435
  stellate cells, 410

Antidromic conduction test, of facial nerve, 135

Antihypertensive therapy, cochlear blood flow and, 334–335

Aristotle, 3–4,5,10,15

Arnold's nerve, 44

Reactance, 110
Receptor potentials, 279–286
    alternating current, 279,280,282,284,285,
        286
    cochlear microphonic, 279,280,281,282,
        283,287
    direct current, 279,280,282,284,285,286
    neurotransmitter release and, 360
    resting, 278–279
    stimulus, 279–298
Reissner, Ernst, 19
Reissner's membrane
    anatomy, 159,162,167
    discovery, 19
    embryonic development, 233
    ultrastructure, 196–197,341
    vasculature, 299,306,308,311,313
Resistance, 110,113
Resonance theory, of hearing, 22,23
Resonant frequency, 116–117,118
Response latency, 440,441–444,449
Resting potentials, 278–279
Reticular lamina, 19,22
Retzius, Magnus Gustaf, 19–20,21,159
Reverse correlation technique, 368–370
Rosenthal, Friedrich Christof, 17
Rosenthal's canal, 175,176
Rotational test, for vestibular function, 25
Rufus of Ephesus, 5

S
Saccule
    anatomy, 175
    embryonic development, 227,230
    functional morphology, 457,458,459,461
Salicylates, outer ear developmental
        effects, 223
Saline, cochlear blood flow effects, 335
Saliva, secretion, 132
Scala media
    anatomy, 174,175
    embryonic development, 233
    endolymph, 278–279
    perilymph, 345–346
    receptor potential, 279,280,282
    structure, 341,342
    vasculature, 297,300–301,312
Scala tympani
    anatomy, 175
    embryonic development, 233
    perilymph, 344–345
        flow, 351–352
    structure, 341,342
    vasculature, 237,297,301–303,304,313
Scala vestibuli
    anatomy, 174,175

blood flow measurement, 328
embryonic development, 233
perilymph, 344,350–352
structure, 341,342
vasculature, 297,298–300,304,312,350–
    351
Scarpa, Antonio, 15,16–17,19,24
Scarpa's fluid, 16
Schelhammer, Gunther Christoph, 12–13
Schirmer test, for lacrimation, 133
Schizophrenia, brain electrical activity
    mapping, 512–514,519,520
Schwann cell, 229,478
Sclerotic cell system, chronic ear disease
    and, 92
Sebaceous glands, of external ear canal,
    46,48
Secretory component, in otitis media with
    effusion, 68,69,70,71
Senile dementia, 400
Serratia marcescens, cerumen and, 48
Short wave theory, of cochlear signal
    processing, 253
Signal processing. See Sound stimuli
    coding
Skein bone, embryonic, 149,150
Smith, Catherine, 24
Sniffing, 91,93–94,95
    autophonia and, 93–94,95,96
    control, 97
    hyperacusis and, 94,96
Sniff test, 93,98
Sodium
    plasma membrane distribution, 271,272
    tectorial membrane content, 467
Sodium channels, in hair cells, 492
Sonometry, 99
Sound intensity, psychophysical dynamic
    range, 365
Sound pressure transformation, 31–38
    acoustic input definition, 37
    binaural, directional hearing, 31–33
    concha effects, 34,35
    ear canal effects, 33,34,35,36
    earphone calibration couplers and, 37–
        38
    in enclosed ears, 37
    head effects, 31–33
    middle ear impedance and, 107
    pinna effects, 33,35
    torso effects, 31
    tympanic membrane impedance and, 36
Sound stimuli coding, by cochlea, 243–270
    afferent cochlear neuronal response,
        359–384
        axons, 359
        broadband click stimuli response, 368